SCHOOL NURSING

A framework for practice

SCHOOL NURSING

A framework for practice

SUSAN J. WOLD, R.N., M.P.H.

Assistant Professor, University of Minnesota
School of Nursing, Minneapolis, Minnesota

with 55 illustrations

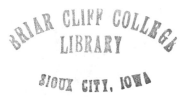

The C. V. Mosby Company

ST. LOUIS • TORONTO • LONDON   1981

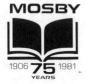
LB
3407
.W63

The C. V. Mosby Company
11830 Westline Industrial Drive, St. Louis, Missouri 63141

Library of Congress Cataloging in Publication Data

Wold, Susan J   1946-
   School nursing.

   Bibliography: p.
   Includes index.
   1. School nursing. I. Title. [DNLM: 1. School
nursing. WY 113 W852s]
LB3407.W63   371.7′12   80-27711
ISBN 0-8016-5611-7

AC/M/M 9 8 7 6 5 4 3 2   01/D/086

Contributors

MARY LOU CHRISTENSEN, P.N.A., M.P.H.

Associate Director, Ramsey County Public Health Nursing Service, St. Paul, Minnesota

NANCY V. DAGG, R.N., M.P.H., P.N.A.

Director of Public Health Nursing, Anoka County Community Health and Social Services Department, Anoka, Minnesota

JOANNE GINGRICH-CRASS, R.N., M.S.N.

Assistant Professor, New Program Development, Metropolitan State University, St. Paul, Minnesota

JUDITH B. IGOE, R.N., M.S.

Associate Professor and Project Director, School Nurse Practitioner Program, University of Colorado Health Sciences Center, Denver, Colorado

JEAN O'LEARY, B.S.N., M.S.

Formerly Diabetes Instruction Coordinator, Hopkins Independent School District No. 274, Hopkins, Minnesota

ELLEN D. SCHULTZ, R.N., M.S.

Assistant Professor, College of Nursing, Clemson University, Clemson, South Carolina

To

Delphie J. Fredlund

teacher, mentor, colleague, and friend

and

Florence M. Reuter

my late grandmother

with thanks for their abiding faith, unconditional love
and support, and endless encouragement

Preface

In the United States, school nursing emerged as a public health nursing specialty following the experimental placement of a public health nurse in a New York City public school in 1902. The success of that first school nurse, Lina Rogers Struthers, in reducing absenteeism due to communicable diseases led to the employment of other nurses in New York City and elsewhere. The role of these early school nurses quickly expanded to include an emphasis on wellness and disease prevention, health education, and a broadly defined client population including children, their families, school personnel, and the community.

Despite wide acceptance and praise for the contributions of school nurses during the first half of the twentieth century, the number of nurses employed in schools has steadily declined in recent years, due in part to escalating costs and consequent budgetary cutbacks in school districts across the country. As a result, today's school nurses too often have unrealistic and unwieldy student-nurse ratios and are typically expected to serve more than one school. Because school nurses must serve larger numbers of students, demands on their time are increasing. In addition to coping with budgetary cutbacks, elimination of school nursing positions, and the resulting increase in student-nurse ratios, school nurses must also contend with conflicting expectations of their role. Although school nurses may envision their role as focused on health education and counseling, others—including principals, teachers, other school personnel, parents, and students—may view the school nurse's role as that of a Band-Aid supplier and record keeper. Too often, the unhappy results of these problems are underuse of school nurses' skills and expertise and a corresponding overemphasis on immediate results and visible functions, such as first aid and record keeping, at the expense of less tangible, more long-range outcomes, such as development of healthy and health-educated young adults.

Although school nurses' problems of role confusion and underuse are partially the result of others' misperceptions and inappropriate expectations, school nurses must accept partial responsibility for these problems themselves. Indeed, school nurses have too long *allowed* others to define their role and direct their practice. Even among school nurses themselves, there has been no consensus regarding such basic issues as appropriate roles and functions or educational preparation and employment experience needed for school nursing. In short, school nursing has consistently lacked direction as a discipline. This lack of leadership and direction is no doubt reflected in the sparse, largely non-research-based school nursing literature, in which the last major textbook on school nursing was published in 1963.

The continuing decline in numbers of nurses employed in schools is particularly ironic during a period in which wellness, health promotion, and child health in particular are receiving increased attention and commitment both nationally and internationally. On the one hand, we hear that promotion of health and prevention of disease are worthy goals of our health care system, while at the same time, funding for school health and many other preventive health programs is rapidly evaporating. Obviously, if school health, school nursing, and similar health promotional programs are to succeed and become more than empty rhetoric, changes in philosophy and action are needed.

This book represents an attempt to spur such changes in action by suggesting a philosophy and roles and goals for school nursing practice and a compatible conceptual framework to guide their implementation. The concepts included in this book (public health, adaptation, helping relationships, tools, and systematic process) constitute the scope and focus of school nursing as I view it. This conceptual framework is presented as *a* sound approach to school nursing practice; it is not, nor does it pretend to be, *the* only sound school nursing approach. The concepts presented in this book are intended to *guide* school nursing practice. This is *not* a "cookbook" or a how-to-do-it approach.

This book is directed toward several audiences. First, currently employed school nurses should find it a useful reference and textbook. Within baccalaureate nursing curricula, this book can be used as a textbook in introductory courses on school nursing or as a resource for students completing supervised field experience. Within master's level nursing curricula, including school nurse practitioner (SNP) programs, this book can also be used, with an emphasis on the identified problems confronting school nursing, such as lack of leadership, research, and documentation of practice outcomes, and attention to creative and effective solutions. In fact, believing in the importance of school nurses with master's degree preparation, I view graduate students as an important audience for this book. Finally, through its clarification of the role of the school nurse, this book should help reduce the existing communication barriers among school nurses; between school nurses and other nursing specialties; between school nurses and school administrators and other school personnel such as teachers, psychologists, and social workers; and between school nurses and others in the community, including physicians and other health personnel. I hope that many of these "significant others" will read and discuss this book.

Regarding the format, this text is divided into seven parts. The first part, Dimensions of School Nursing, includes a historical overview of the school nurse role, a discussion of the philosophy behind this book and the corresponding roles and goals suggested for school nursing practice, and a description of the conceptual framework on which the remainder of the book is based. Parts II to VI are each devoted to concepts relating to the five strands of the framework, beginning with public health (Part II) and progressing through adaptation (Part III), helping relationships (Part IV), tools (Part V), and systematic process (Part VI). Part VII, Future Perspectives on School Nursing, explores the role of the school nurse practitioner and concludes with a discussion of the major problems confronting school nurses, suggesting goals for those problems and proposing strategies for achieving them. Part VII is followed by an appendix of primarily reprinted articles concerning children with special needs. Topics included are chronic illnesses and their effects on school-age children, adolescents, and their families; children with chronic respiratory diseases, diabetes, or cancer; abused children and their families; and, in addition to the previously mentioned article about chronically ill adolescents, a discussion of the unique nutritional needs of adolescents.

With regard to the style in which the book is written, the reader will notice that the school nurse is consistently referred to as "she" throughout the text; this has been done to avoid the cumbersome use of "he/she" or similar designations. Although I recognize and welcome the entrance of increasing numbers of men into nursing, most nurses today are women, so the feminine pronoun has been used. Similarly, to avoid confusion and awkward grammatical forms, the student or client is referred to as "he." Finally, although I also recognize (from my former stature as a Latin scholar) that the word *data* is a plural noun, the current collegiate dictionary indicates that data is a collective noun and can be used with *either* a singular or plural verb; my own preference has been to use a singular verb with "data," a choice that I hope will not distress most readers.

Obviously, completion of a book this size requires the support and involvement of many persons, whose contributions must be acknowledged. First, the conceptual framework on which this book is based grew out of the conceptual framework taught in the baccalaureate nursing curriculum in the School of Nursing at the University of Minnesota; that framework (including the strands of adaptation, systematic process, helping relationships, and tools) was developed by the faculty teaching in that program. Although the framework presented in this book is in many ways different from theirs, I am indebted to the faculty teaching in that curriculum, since their thinking has directly influenced mine.

I am also most grateful to all the contributing authors, whose chapters have added breadth and depth to this text. I am particularly indebted to Nancy Dagg, with whom I collaborated from the very beginning, and to Joanne Gingrich-Crass, for her comprehensive and innovative chapters on adaptation, for reviewing portions of the manuscript and providing honest feedback, and for her support and encouragement throughout the development of this book. I must also publicly acknowledge the contributions of Delphie Fredlund, whose enthusiastic support for this project from its earliest beginnings and whose unflagging support throughout helped sustain my motivation to see it through. But perhaps more than anyone else, I am indebted to Nancy Evans, who believed in me and in the merits of this project, who provided thoughtful and incisive editing and commentary, and who displayed infinite patience and support as the manuscript took shape; without her contributions, this book would not exist.

I am also grateful to all the publishers, authors, and others who so generously gave permission to reprint their materials; their generosity enabled me to include illustrations and ideas that enhance the quality of this book. Furthermore, I would like to thank Susan G. Hartman for her careful typing of the manuscript and her unruffled nature in the face of impossible deadlines.

Finally, while it seems woefully inadequate to do so, I would like to thank my friends and family, especially my husband Lauren E. Wold, for their tolerance in the face of my reclusive life-style and evasion of social involvements during the past months. I appreciate your patience, and I hope that when you finally see this in print, you'll think it was all somehow worth it.

Throughout the writing of this book, I have remained staunchly committed to the role of school nursing as a critically important public health nursing specialty that can contribute positively and significantly to the health, health attitudes, and health behaviors of today's children and, consequently, tomorrow's adults. However, I also recognize that if school nurses hope to achieve that goal, they must begin now by critically appraising current practices and standards and revising and upgrading them as needed. I hope that this book can stimulate school nurses to begin and persist in their efforts to restore school nursing to its original stature as a profession of unquestioned value in the school setting. The health of tomorrow's adults may well depend on the outcomes of their efforts.

Susan J. Wold

Contents

PART I

Dimensions of school nursing

CHAPTER 1

School nursing: a passing experiment?

SUSAN J. WOLD and NANCY V. DAGG

An in-depth look at school nursing would be incomplete without some attention to its history. As nursing historian Minnie Goodnow (Fig. 1-1) observed:

. . . History repeats itself. This is discouraging, because it reveals to us the difficulties which may lie ahead. It is also encouraging, because it teaches us that progress may sometimes be quick and at the same time secure. It shows that what was thought to be a dream was in reality a vision of what was to come (Goodnow, 1943:1).

The vision identified by early school nursing leaders has not yet been realized. Our search through nursing archives produced a wealth of ideas and role concepts that remain underdeveloped and are not yet part of contemporary school nursing practice.

The purpose of this chapter is to share the excitement, frustration, and challenge experienced as as we turned the dusty pages of old history books. The excitement came from our discovery that the role of the early school nurse was public health and wellness-oriented. In addition, the school nurse's client system included not only the child, but also his family, other school personnel, and the community. Her impact was observable in such areas as reduction of communicable disease, decreased absenteeism in schools, and involvement of the school nurse in daily classroom health education. At that time, the value of the school nurse role was unquestioned. Indeed, Gardner (1926:320) stated that ". . . wherever [the school] nurse has made her entry her value has been recognized." Unfortunately, Gardner was unable to foresee that the value of the school nurse's contributions would not be sustained through the next 50 years.

Hawkins (1971:751) concludes that withdrawing nurses from school systems

". . . would entail no immediate apparent loss for either themselves or the schools." The present status of school nursing supports Hawkins' conclusion. Over the past 50 years, the role of the school nurse has diminished in scope and value. It has emphasized episodic care and record keeping at the expense of preventive care, health education, and community involvement.

We are further frustrated by our recognition that the educational background of many school nurses is inadequate. First-level educational programs in nursing generally do not adequately prepare their graduates to assume the responsibilities of the school nurse role. In addition, continuing education opportunities for school nurses vary from state to state. Consequently, numerous inequities exist in the educational backgrounds of school nurses throughout the country. Still another frustration is the realization that standards of care for school nursing practice have only recently (1974) been developed (American School Health Association, 1974) and are not widely known or applied. Finally, there is disparity among the states regarding the need and criteria used for certification of school nurses. In fact, one state has only two requirements for certification of its school nurses: a registered nurse (RN) license and proof (by college transcript or test score) of knowledge of the state and federal constitutions (Castile and Jerrick, 1976).

Despite these frustrations, we are optimistic about the future of school nursing. The challenge is to regain the public health focus lost in the last 50 years and to expand the contribution of the school nurse so that dreams from the past do become realities in the future. To provide insight into the historical perspectives of this unmet challenge, in the remainder of this chapter we will discuss the following: (1) general nursing history, including concurrent forces and

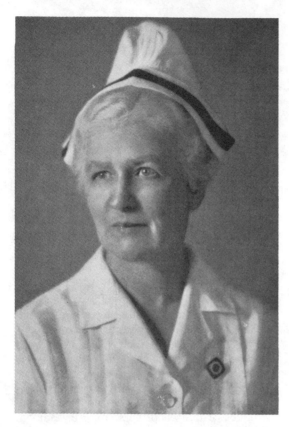

Fig. 1-1. Minnie Goodnow. (From Dolan, J. A.: 1978. Nursing in society: a historical perspective, 14th ed., W. B. Saunders Co., Philadelphia.)

world events that influenced the history; (2) public health and particularly school nursing history; and (3) implications for the future.

NURSING HISTORY IN BRIEF

The art of nursing has existed for centuries because illness, disability, and the need for maternity services have existed throughout civilization. However, little is known about the details of early nursing practice because nursing care was part of everyday life, and no one thought it important enough to write down until the cities had grown so large that care of the sick became a public problem (Goodnow, 1943). Women have traditionally been the primary providers because nursing was thought to be an extension of the "mothering" role.

The development of nursing has been heavily influenced by religion and wars. Although many of the early hospitals were run by religious orders, the influence of religion on the care of the sick declined during the Reformation when control of the hospital fell into the hands of politicians. Not only did the quality of care suffer, but also the quality of the caregiver declined. Nursing became an undesirable occupation, and the average nurse was lacking in both skills and morals. For example, Charles Dickens' character, Sairey Gamp (Fig. 1-2). depicted a woman given to habitual drunkenness, indifference to her patients' needs, and actual enjoyment of deathbed scenes (Goodnow, 1943).

Little improvement was seen until the arrival of Florence Nightingale, who provided long-needed leadership. As Goodnow noted:

The general dissatisfaction with the nursing of that day, the not-always-successful attempts of doctors and others to train a better kind of nurse, and the good work of the deaconess orders, all paved the way for the coming of a woman whose ability was equal to the task before her, that of putting nursing into the high place where it belongs.

She cannot be considered as a product of her time, since she was ahead of and beyond it; but the season was ripe for her genius to do its work, and for her to become *the founder of modern nursing* (Goodnow, 1943:62-63).

Although Florence Nightingale's accomplishments were many, one of the most important was the establishment in London of the first fully endowed and therefore independent school of nursing in 1860. Physicians voiced a great deal of opposition to the school for several reasons. First, nurses in particular and women in general had very little status in society and were clearly dominated by men. Thus a move toward expanding their educational opportunities was potentially threatening to physicians. Another likely reason for their opposition was that in this new school, for the first time, nurses would be educated by nurses and not by physicians. Some physicians no doubt recognized that this independence of nursing education would ultimately result in nursing being an autonomous profession, recognized as such by the patient, with the possible loss of economic and social status by the physicians. Specific objections voiced by physicians surveyed at the time would cause any modern-day feminist to cringe:

A nurse is a confidential servant, but still only a servant. . . . She should be middle-aged when she begins nursing; and if somewhat tamed by marriage and the troubles of a family, so much the better (Goodnow, 1943:74).

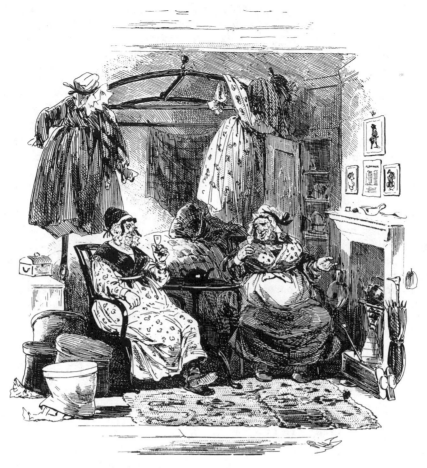

Fig. 1-2. Sairey Gamp proposes a toast. (From Dickens, C. A.: Martin Chuzzlewit, Oxford Illustrated Dickens edition, 1951, Oxford University Press, Oxford, England.)

Another important contribution of Florence Nightingale, which influenced the origins of school nursing, was her emphasis on asepsis. Although the germ theory was established during her lifetime but not accepted by her, Miss Nightingale did recognize the relationship between dirt and disease. She was instrumental in reforming hospital conditions and later published extensively on the subject. She also devoted 40 years to the development of a health program for India, a project that no women and few men had previously undertaken. Although the project was widely hailed as a masterpiece of public health planning (Goodnow, 1943), the published report gave no credit to Miss Nightingale. The omission of her name was further evidence of the continuing low status and lack of political power held by women and nurses. Miss Nightingale stated:

I am convinced that political power is the greatest it is possible to wield for human happiness, and until women have their part in it in an open, direct manner, the evils of the world can never be satisfactorily dealt with (Goodnow, 1943:77).

Florence Nightingale's achievements in the area of improved hospital conditions, the development of the Indian Health Plan, and her outspoken insistence on increased political power and independence for women paved the way for the evolution of public health nursing.

THE EUROPEAN ORIGINS OF SCHOOL NURSING

Organized public health nursing had its origin in Liverpool in 1858 when the first "district" nurses were employed to provide home care for the sick poor (Goodnow, 1943). The extension of public health services into the schools began in France in 1837 with the passage of a royal ordinance mandating health supervision of schoolchildren and enforcement of sanitary conditions by school authorities. Although further development in France was slow in coming, Brussels, Belgium, in 1874 became the first city to employ regular school physicians and to establish a city-wide system of school inspections (Gardner, 1926).

The first employment of a nurse in the schools was in London in 1892 when Amy Hughes was hired for the purpose of investigating the nutrition of schoolchildren. Within 6 years, her efforts had resulted in the establishment of the London School Nurses' Society. The London School Board was reluctant to finance the school nursing service but grudgingly agreed to provide a salary for one nurse. It was not until 1904 that the London County Council took matters into its own hands and financed the appointment of a staff of school nurses who worked under a superintendent (Gardner, 1926). Even today, financial support for school nursing services continues to be a problem and a political issue.

THE DEVELOPMENT OF SCHOOL NURSING IN THE UNITED STATES

Early public health and school nursing work in England contributed to the development of school health services in the United States. Transatlantic exchange visits by the secretary of the London School Nursing Society and by Lillian Wald (Fig. 1-3) of New York City inspired both countries to expand and define the role of school nurses (Gardner, 1916).

In fact, Miss Wald was instrumental in directing the focus of both public health nursing and school nursing practice in this country. In 1893, Lillian Wald and a friend, Mary Brewster, developed the first nurses' settlement in the United States. The purpose of the Henry Street Settlement, located in New York's worst slum, was to influence by example as well as by teaching. This represented innovation in "public health nursing," a term which Miss Wald coined. As she explained:

We called our enterprise "public health nursing." Our basic idea was that the nurse's peculiar introduction to the patient and her organic relationship with the neighborhood should constitute the starting point for a universal service to the region. Our purpose was in no sense to establish an isolated undertaking. We planned to utilize, as well as to be implemented by, all agencies and groups of whatever creed which were working for social betterment, private as well as municipal. Our scheme was to be motivated by a vital sense of the interrelation of all these forces. For this reason we considered ourselves best described by the term "public health nurses" (Wales, 1941:xi).

The first school health services in the United States were medical inspections begun in the Boston schools in 1894. These inspections were designed to identify for exclusion from school those students with serious communicable disease, such as scarlet fever, diphtheria, pertussis, chickenpox, and mumps. A short time later these inspections were broadened to include screening for parasitic diseases such as scabies, impetigo, and ringworm (Gardner, 1936). The problem with medical inspections was that no follow-up was done on those children who were excluded from school because of communicable diseases. The finding by Henry Street Settlement workers of a 12-year-old boy who never attended school because of a tiny sore on his head led to an investigation that proved he was only one of many such truant children. Agitated by these findings, Miss Wald challenged New York City officials and the Board of Educuation to allow her to place a public health nurse in selected schools on an experimental basis to increase school attendance by educating school officials, parents, and children regarding disease control procedures and by home visit follow-up of known cases. This first public health school nurse was Lina Rogers Struthers (Fig. 1-4).

In November, 1902, Miss Wald placed Lina Rogers as the first school nurse in the four New York City schools with the greatest number of exclusions. It was hoped that through her health education efforts and follow-up of individual cases, she could not only decrease the length of exclusion, but that she could reduce the number of exclusions as well. The results were so convincing that the Board of Education hired twenty-five more nurses shortly thereafter. A statistical comparison of the number of students excluded for communicable diseases in the New York City schools before and after the hiring of school nurses reveals a startling difference: in September, 1902, 10,567 students were sent home, whereas in September, 1903, only 1101 students were excluded (Gardner, 1926). Thus the impact of school nursing was clearly dem-

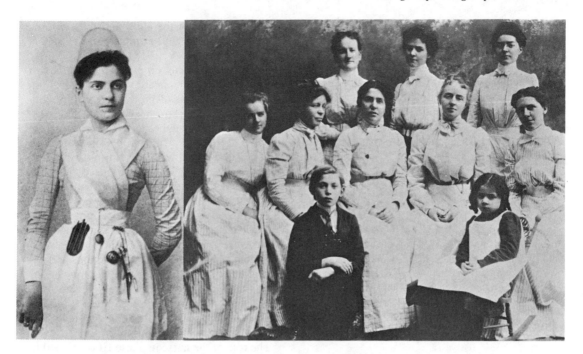

Fig. 1-3. Lillian Wald in her student uniform (left) and with her staff at Visiting Nurse Service of New York (right); Miss Wald is seated in the middle of the second row. (From Dolan, J. A.: 1978. Nursing in society: a historical perspective, 14th ed., W. B. Saunders Co., Philadelphia; courtesy Visiting Nurse Service, New York.)

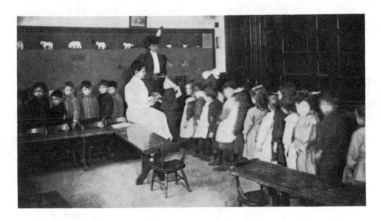

Fig. 1-4. Miss Lina Rogers, the first school nurse, inspects schoolchildren. (From Dolan, J. A.: 1978. Nursing in society: a historical perspective, 14th ed., W. B. Saunders Co., Philadelphia.)

onstrated (Gardner, 1926; Cromwell, 1963; Brand, 1972).

It was not long until medical inspection, defined as "the search for communicable disease," was replaced by "medical examination," which included "the search for physical defects, many of which furnish the soil for contagion" (Gardner, 1936:355). It was soon re-

cognized that such a focus on case finding and disability limitation was shortsighted because it totally ignored primary preventive aspects of health. This realization resulted in the incorporation of health education into the school curriculum.

The development of the role of the school nurse paralleled this expansion of school health services. Three phases can be identified in the early development of the schools nurse's role (Table 1-1). In phase I, the thrust of the school health program was *medical inspection,* the goal of which was to prevent the spread of contagious diseases by continuing attention to the physical health of the children. Kelly and Bradshaw provide the following colorful description of the routine inspection performed by the school nurse:

Nurses should make routine inspection of all children in their schools once in two months, or oftener if possible. . . . The eyelids, throat, skin, and hair of each pupil are examined, and the general condition as regards cleanliness, nutrition, etc., noted. In making this inspection the nurse need not touch the child, who should be instructed to open the mouth, pull down the eyelids, and show hands and wrists. In examining the hair the nurse should use two toothpicks, or, if she is economically inclined, one toothpick broken in two, lifting and separating the hair so as to expose the scalp (Kelly and Bradshaw, 1918:35-36).

The nurses at the Henry Street Settlement recognized that medical inspection without follow-up resulted in the loss of valuable school time by those children who could least afford it. Aware of the importance of such follow-up, these early school nurses made home visits as needed to advise the parents regarding home

care procedures for the child and thus ensured his early recovery and prompt return to school (Kelly and Bradshaw, 1918).

The phase II focus on *medical examination* grew out of the realization that medical inspection as a means of protecting healthy children from those who had communicable diseases was inadequate because it overlooked the total health of the child. In their search for physical defects, physicians and nurses carried out periodic medical examinations of all children within the school. The role of the school nurse was similar to that in phase I. She assisted the physician with the actual examination and conducted home visits to ensure that the defects found were corrected.

Recognizing that medical inspections and examinations offered little long-range prevention, in phase III school health workers began to incorporate health education into the school curriculum. Their goal was that students learn and practice responsible health behaviors.

The role of the nurse in phase III continued to include assisting the physician with inspections and examinations and making home visits to follow-up known cases. The involvement of the nurse in the newly added health education program proceeded through three stages. In the first stage, the nurse developed and implemented her own program without regard for the

Table 1-1. The developing role of the school nurse during the 1920s and 1930s

Phase	School health program activity	Goal	School nurse's role
I	Medical inspection	Control of contagion	Assist school physician with inspection *or* independently inspect children in classroom Visit homes for follow-up
II	Medical examination	Identification of physical defects	Assist school physician with examination
		Disability limitation through correction of defects	Visit homes for follow-up
III	Medical inspection Medical examination	Same as for phase II	Same as for phase II
	Health education	Student attainment of responsible health behavior	Stage one: develop and implement own health education program Stage two: incorporate health education program into teacher's program
		Student and parental attainment of responsible health behavior	Stage three: mutual planning of health education program by teacher and nurse

rest of the curriculum. Originally, the topics of the nurse's 3- to 5-minute talks included cleanliness, food, teeth, and proper rest and sleep for the growing child. These talks often preceded or followed inspections for cleanliness. Chayer (1931) reports that although the teacher usually remained in the classroom during the nurse's talk, she did not participate. The goals of the nurse and the teacher were not coordinated. In addition, there was not necessarily any logical connection between one health talk and the next, nor was there necessarily any adjustment of the content or delivery of the talk to reflect the comprehension abilities of students in the different grade levels.

Thus, from its early focus on medical inspection and examination in phases I and II, the role of the school nurse was expanded in phase III to include implementation of an integrated health education program.

At about the same time (1920s), school nursing became a real force in rural America as well, after comparative studies revealed that rural children had more physical defects and aftereffects from childhood diseases than did urban children (American National Red Cross, 1931). Through their work in the schools, rural American Red Cross nurses realized the importance of health education in improving the health status of rural children, and therefore expanded their activities to include health teaching.

The role and services of the school nurse continued to expand in the 1930s. By that time school nurses were so overextended in their efforts to meet all the needs of the school children, they were doing nothing well. Educators and nurses were shocked when the 1934 survey of public health nursing conducted by the National Organization for Public Health Nursing (NOPHN) showed that the poorest quality of any phase of public health nursing was that being done in the schools (Gardner, 1936; Wales, 1941). Troop (1963) speculates that the poor quality of school nursing stemmed from the inadequate hospital-based education received by nurses.

In 1923 the Committee for the Study of Nursing Education, whose work was financed by the Rockefeller Foundation and directed by C. E. A. Winslow and Josephine Goldmark, published the results of their survey in a book entitled *Nursing and Nursing Education in the United States.* This report recognized the need for specialized postgraduate preparation for the

practice of public health nursing, and went on to recommend that nurses working full-time in the school setting strengthen their public health background. However, many school nurses believed that they were more closely allied with educators than nurses and did not even consider themselves public health nurses. This role confusion gave rise in the 1920s to the use of such labels as "school nurse teacher" and "teacher-nurse" (Troop, 1963). After the Winslow-Goldmark report was published, state boards of education set up certification requirements for nurses, which helped to improve the quality of school nurses. However, certification requirements were and unfortunately often still are unrelated to the education and practice of school nursing.

During the 1930s, while the school nurse grappled with problems of overextension and role confusion resulting from allegiances to public health and education, the renewed interest of the American Medical Association (AMA) in school health propelled the school physician into a position of leadership within the school health program (Randall, 1971). Physicians expanded their services to include examinations for physical education, screening for athletes in competitive sports, special examination for food handlers and faculty members, and preemployment examinations for other school staff members (Randall, 1971).

With the advent of World War II school health and school nursing services faced reevaluation and possible curtailment. The war required that citizens submerge their personal needs and wants and focus instead on safeguarding the national interest. With so many persons and goods being diverted to the war effort, many domestic services had to be revised and cut back. Paradoxically, the health of schoolchildren received increased emphasis during this time from educators and civilians for two reasons: (1) because this was a mechanized war, large numbers of healthy young men were needed for the draft and (2) Selective Service data regarding prospective draftees revealed that approximately one fourth of the registrants were rejected because of physical defects (Palmer, 1944). Thus the discovery that a large number of supposedly healthy young males had physical defects became a potential threat to the national security and resulted in renewed interest in preventive aspects of school health.

Randle (1943:482) of the NOPHN identified

the following four school nursing services that needed to be maintained during the war:

1. Advisory service to school administrators regarding the school health program and the expanded use of community resources to supplement it
2. Guidance and in-service education for teachers regarding health services they were now expected to perform
3. Interpretation of student health examination data to parents, teachers, and children with referral to community resources for needed follow-up
4. Home visiting to interpret children's health needs to their parents, to discover the family's health needs for interpretation to other school personnel, and to assist the family and school to meet these needs

To guarantee that the nurse would be able to carry out these essential services, those tasks which frequently were carried out by the nurse, but did not actually require nursing skills were delegated to others, including volunteers, aides, and teachers (Palmer, 1944). Dilworth (1944) acknowledged the merits of delegating nonnursing duties to others and urged that this be seriously considered not only as an emergency wartime measure, but also as a long-range approach to improvement of school nursing services. Dilworth recommended that older students be recruited as volunteers to help with some of these tasks. Among the tasks that she believed could be appropriately delegated to trained volunteers or interested teachers were vision and hearing screening, periodic weighing and measuring of the children, and the daily health inspection of students.

Perhaps as an outgrowth of this wartime need to delegate some of the nurse's tasks, involvement of the classroom teacher in the health service aspects of the school health program was increased. Emphasis began to be placed on the value of the teacher's day-to-day observations of her students as a means of detecting significant changes in appearance, behavior, and health (Wilson, 1945). During this time the teacher also began to become directly involved in another aspect of health services: first aid for sick and injured children in the school. Again, because the teacher had continuing contact with the children and because she was always present in the school, she was the logical person to take responsibility for emergency care. Thus the role of the school nurse regarding first aid and emergency care became that of in-service

educator for the teacher, regarding first aid techniques, necessary emergency equipment, and appropriate community resources for emergency medical care, such as ambulance services, physicians, and clinics (Grant, 1942).

According to an NOPHN editorial (NOPHN, 1944), approximately half of all the public health nurses in the United States were engaged in the practice of school nursing at that time. Of that group, one half were working full time in the school, and the other half were working within more generalized public health nursing programs and were therefore providing part-time service in the school. Between 1944 and 1948 the United States Public Health Service reported a significant increase in the numbers of nurses employed for school nursing. In 1944 boards of education had employed 3722 nurses; in 1948, that figure was increased to 5091. In 1944 local official health agencies that provided school nursing as part of their generalized programs reported that they employed a total of 10,343 nurses; by 1948 that number was 11,171 (Dilworth, 1949). This trend toward increased employment of nurses for school health no doubt reflects the prevalent belief that even during wartime, school nursing services were essential.

The trend toward delegation of health service tasks to the teacher freed the school nurse to redirect her time and energies to other priorities. As a result, during the 1940s school nursing became more identified as a kind of public health nursing. As previously noted, at least half of the available public health nurses were practicing in the school, which most likely enhanced the public health orientation that became prominent in school nursing. This increased public health emphasis was reflected in the school nurse's renewed concern with family-centered care. It became obvious that many of the defects found when children entered school could have been prevented or minimized with earlier recognition and intervention. Thus the school nurse expanded her focus during the home visits she made to the families of school children and addressed herself to the needs of all the family members, including infants and preschoolers (Wales, 1941). This renewed conviction that school health services are essential to the promotion of community health and the fact that school nurses were now extending their practice into the family in the community indicated the need for coordination of community nursing services. Nurses were encouraged (Axelson, 1944; Dilworth, 1944) to avoid duplication of services with careful and thoughtful planning by those public health nurses employed by health departments, visiting nurse associations, and schools.

Communicable disease control continued to be an important part of the school health program during the 1940s because the means of infection, immunization, and prevention of certain diseases such as scarlet fever and polio were still not fully understood (Grant, 1942). School health programs during this decade also included such innovations as special classes for handicapped children, such as those crippled by polio, sight-saving classes for children whose corrected vision was 20/70 or worse, and classes for hard-of-hearing children, in which they learned to read lips and improve their speech (Ayling and Johnson, 1949). The importance of dental health as part of the school health program also gained prominence during this period. Although the services provided were largely educational in nature, some periodic dental inspection was included, with children referred to private dentists or clinics for reparative work (Ayling and Johnson, 1949).

Periodic medical examinations also continued to be a part of the school health program during the 1940s, although in many instances these examinations were little more than cursory inspections (Hubbard et al., 1949). However, the purpose of the medical examinations was modified gradually until school medical examinations were touted as "desirable educational process[es]" (Grant, 1942:201). This was an important shift in emphasis and had far-reaching effects; in place of the previous emphasis on the numbers of students examined and referred for follow-up, there was now an emphasis on the outcome of those referrals. The term "health or medical examination" was replaced with "health counseling or guidance," which by definition included both the health examination and follow-up procedures (Wilson, 1945). In accordance with the prevailing public health philosophy, this approach to health counseling had as its goal helping students to solve their own health problems and to assume responsibility for protecting, maintaining, or improving their health. This belief that individuals should be responsible for their own health included not only the children but also their families:

The school health service should be of such educational value that children learn how to protect their health, to secure medical care when it is needed, and

to accept reasonable responsibility for their own health and that of others. Moreover, the parents should be taught how to give their children the care necessary to promote health and maintain efficiency and happiness (Grant, 1942:194-195).

Freeman (1945) identified four major changes in emphasis in the school health program, which she believed had implications for the role of the school nurse. The first of these changes was the increasing emphasis on the importance of the classroom teacher's involvement in teaching health. A closely related change was the increased attention to health as a school subject area; this interest carried over into the development and expansion of physical fitness programs and instruction about the home care of ill persons. A third change was the increased acceptance of the need to correlate health instruction and health practice with school and home behavior. The final change that Freeman discussed concerned the increased participation and collaboration by students, teachers, parents, administrators, special health personnel, and community representatives in planning and implementing health programs. Thus, during this era, the responsibility for the school health program shifted from the school nurse and school physician being solely responsible to sharing of responsibility by teachers, students, and health personnel, and a coordinated and integrated health education curriculum was proposed (Dilworth, 1944).

These developments, according to Freeman (1945), would leave the nurse with some new responsibilities. Instead of focusing on routine inspection and vision and hearing testing, she could now take on an expanded role in guidance and consultation. The nurse would then need to be familiar with the subject matter to be taught as "health" and would need some understanding of classroom teaching to help the teacher integrate the health content into the curriculum. This expanded role would necessitate the following additional educational preparation by the school nurse (Freeman, 1945):

1. Increased technical expertise based on accurate and current scientific data
2. Better preparation for leadership, including courses on research methods, decision making, and methods of influencing the behavior of others
3. Expanded background in educational methods and family health guidance
4. Interdisciplinary course work with other school personnel, such as teachers, physi-

cians, and administrators, to accustom these professionals to group or team problem-solving methods in the school

In fact, by the late 1940s efforts were being made to upgrade school nursing by specifying the preparation needed for nurses wishing to practice in the school setting. By 1949, sixteen state departments of education required certification of the nurse for work in the school, and four other states required a certificate for the nurse if she taught any classes (Dilworth, 1949).

The 1950s were largely devoted to expansion and development of programs and priorities established during the 1940s, with an overall emphasis on stabilization of the positive changes that had occurred during the previous decade. Many school nurses were still kept busy with such tasks as exclusion and readmission of sick children, since school administrators, wishing to be relieved entirely of that responsibility, emphasized this as the most important function for the nurse (Sellery, 1950).

By the 1950s, it was generally accepted that "health is the first objective of education" and that the goal of the school health program should be to develop "optimum health" for every schoolchild, healthful school surroundings, and to "imbue him with this kind of climate [so] that he will want to have the same for his family and eventually, his community" (Brown, 1952:220). Optimum health was now recognized to be more than physical fitness and the absence of defects; health included mental, spiritual, and emotional elements as well (Brown, 1952).

Although the school nurse during the 1950s was still expected to prepare children for the school physician's examinations and to assist the physician with the examination, the idea developed during the 1940s that the physical examination should be a learning experience was expanded during this decade. School health personnel finally realized that discovery of defects was unimportant in the long run unless the child could be motivated to correct them. Hence, the emphasis was not so much on what the physician found as a result of medical examination, but on how the child responded and on what he learned as a result of the examination (Sellery, 1950). This change in emphasis was closely correlated with the prevalent belief that the quality of a school health program was more appropriately evaluated based on changed behavior rather than on statistics alone (Sellery, 1950).

Another important trend that surfaced during this period was the shift toward completion of periodic medical examinations of students by private physicians rather than by a physician provided in the school. This required more responsibility on the part of students and their parents and created a coordination problem between the school and the family physician. To obtain needed information from the private physician after his examination of the child, the school had to develop some kind of reporting form to be filled out by the physician and returned to the school. This in turn raised some ethical questions regarding the appropriateness of sharing information. The complexities of following up the known health problems of the children resulted in the adoption of a cumulative health record form for each child in the school. However, this too had its drawbacks; the question now raised was who should keep the records, make them out, and file them (Cromwell, 1952)? The issue of record keeping continues to be a problem today.

With the change in overall emphasis from defect finding to health education, the school nurse's most important role was that of health educator (Dierkes, 1951; Brown, 1952). The school nurse fulfilled her role as health educator through a variety of activities. She was able to provide both formal and informal health teaching in one-to-one conferences with students and parents. Some school nurses met with groups of parents in addition to their individual conferences to educate the parents regarding their children's health needs. The school nurse was also called on to provide in-service education for classroom teachers to enhance their ability to assess the health and growth and development of children in their classes. The nurse was also requested to provide brief talks in the classroom for students and to recommend health education materials and visual aids for teachers in planning their health classes. Finally, the school nurse was often looked to for leadership in developing the family life education program, an emphasis that was just beginning to take hold in the school (Sellery, 1950).

In addition to the beginning interest in family life education in the school, two other areas of the school health program were expanded. The first of these was nutrition for the school-age child. The relationship between sound nutrition and normal growth and development had long been recognized. This new emphasis on health education provided a vehicle for stressing sound nutritional habits. To improve nutrition, the school lunch program was born, with the hope that through provision of balanced and nutritionally complete meals, students would learn proper eating habits and would therefore grow and develop at normal rates. The second area of expansion within the school health program was the increased emphasis on positive mental health for the students. The emotional stresses that accompany school entrance and adolescence were known to require considerable adjustment by the students. Thus the importance of providing a supportive learning environment and promoting positive self-concepts was emphasized. This focus on mental health required extra effort from all school personnel, including the teacher and school nurse (Wallace, 1959).

As part of the emphasis on stabilization of changes in the school health program that had begun during the 1940s, the "teamwork" philosophy was expanded. Cromwell (1952) stressed the importance of collaboration by the teacher and nurse in planning and implementing routine screening procedures and in initiating other case-finding activities. Again, the prevailing philosophy was that the teacher is best qualified to assess changes in the children in her classes because of her ongoing contact with them, which greatly facilitates observation.

A direct consequence of the expanded interest in teamwork in the school health program was the development of the "school health council" concept, which grew out of the new philosophy that the school health program is a responsibility to be shared by the teacher, administrator, and nurse (Brown, 1952). Wallace (1959) recommended that the council include representation from involved community agencies and from the lay consumer group. According to Wallace, the council provided a means of coordinating the services of the agencies involved with the school population and had major responsibility for formulation of policies and development of programs and services for school-age children in the community. The council also had a role in evaluating the outcome and effectiveness of the school health program.

In addition to comments regarding the role and activities of the school nurse, some writers of the 1950s attempted to provide insights into the personal qualities and attributes needed by the school nurse. According to Sellery (1951: 123):

The school nurse of today must be strong in her understanding of other people's needs. She must be able to counsel people without protruding personal feelings of superiority, and without inciting feelings of inadequacy and guilt on the part of those being counseled. She avoids giving advice in such a way that the implied criticism causes the parent's [sic] to become defensive in their reactions. On the contrary she must have the skill to develop relationships with parents and children which are so warm and friendly that they voluntarily seek her professional advice and counsel. All this requires that the school nurse shall be a very mature comfortable person.

Hilliard (1951:138) went on to describe the physical appearance of the school nurse in a series of comments that are particularly shocking in view of today's emphasis on feminism:

All administrators want to hire a combination of Lana Turner, Betty Grable, Florence Nightengale [sic] and Albert Einstein—all in one package with a degree in Public Health and in Education. She must be between the ages of 21 and 25 and have 5 years experience. You and I know that school teachers and public health nurses are not known for their beauty. If they were, they would be married and have their own children to cope with.

The early 1960s brought an end to the political and fiscal conservatism that characterized the 1950s in this country. The 1960s provided a decided contrast to the previous decade with the liberalization of government, which resulted in the "New Frontier" and the "Great Society." Our national involvement in the unpopular Viet Nam War had a divisive effect on society, with many of our youth feeling alienated and hostile. The antiwar sentiment produced a peace movement of sorts, organized and manned primarily by disillusioned college students and other disgruntled youth. Thus the 1960s became an era of rapid and often precipitous social change, characterized by the proliferation of health and welfare programs, many of which were poorly planned and short lived.

This expanded concern for the health and welfare of American citizens carried over into the school health program. The goal of the school health program according to Tipple (1964) was twofold: maintenance of optimal health by the schoolchild so that he might benefit maximally from his educational opportunities and development of positive health attitudes and practices for the child to ensure a "lifetime of healthful productivity" (Tipple, 1964:99). Within these goals and in keeping with the national interest in social programs, the school health program, like the educational system as a whole, found itself addressing the issues of "equality of educational opportunity" and special needs of the "culturally deprived child" (Cromwell, 1964:44). Because he was believed to be both culturally and educationally deprived, the handicapped child began to receive special attention within the school health program. This emphasis on the needs of the handicapped child within the regular school program was continued and further expanded in the 1970s and had a definite impact on the role of the school nurse.

From 1952 to 1962, the number of nurses engaged in school health work more than doubled. The greatest increase was in the number of school nurses employed by boards of education; in 1952 the number of nurses reported as employees by boards of education was 6456. In 1962 that figure had risen to 12,119, an increase of 87.7% (Bryant and Hudson, 1962:105; Coakley and Parker, 1965). Thus there was now a definite trend toward the employment of school nurses by boards of education rather than health departments or other voluntary agencies.

School nurses faced increasing problems in defining their role and position within the school health program during this era. That there was a general lack of agreement as to the appropriate role and goals for the school nurse is evidenced by this definition of school nursing (Gair, 1966:401):

School Nursing is a varying combination of what an administrator wants, teachers expect, students need, parents demand, the community is accustomed to, the situation requires and what the nurse, herself, believes.

The nurse's problems in role definition were partly attributable to her inadequacy in clarifying and communicating her proper role. McAleer (1965) speculated that this was partially due to the age-old stereotypical view of the nurse as "a person who took orders but was not supposed to think, question or make any suggestions or decisions" (McAleer, 1965:50). The need for the school nurse to educate coworkers in the school regarding her role and to exercise more leadership in carrying out her responsibilities was emphasized.

As a consequence of her inability to define her role, the school nurse often found herself carrying out highly inappropriate functions such as arranging school bus schedules and delivering faculty paychecks (McAleer, 1965). Although the school nurse's lack of assertiveness

in defining her role within the school created problems due to conflicting expectations, research studies during this decade revealed that a significant number of school nurses themselves had less than ideal beliefs about the goals and roles for school nursing. In her study of school nursing practice in Illinois, Fricke (1967) surveyed 614 school nurses, asking them to rank a list of twenty-three school nurse functions according to the importance attached to each function in a model (or ideal) program. The following represents the ratings of 75% of the nurses regarding functions that were deemed "very important" to the daily program (Fricke, 1967: 27):

Function	Reporting (%)
Elementary	
1. Assumes responsibility for screening procedures (vision, hearing)	89.1
2. Maintains student health records	86.0
3. Provides emergency care for seriously ill and injured	84.5
4. Uncovers health problems through observations, interviews, and analyses of records	75.0
Secondary	
1. Gives emergency care for seriously ill and injured	89.8
2. Maintains student health records	87.9
3. Gives first aid in accordance with established policies	85.1
4. Assumes responsibility for screening procedures	79.5

Fricke and other school nursing proponents were understandably disappointed to learn that school nurses themselves attached more importance to such activities as record keeping and first aid than to activities within the realm of guidance, counseling, advising, and consulting. Fricke's finding that first aid was considered a relatively important school nursing function was supported by Forbes' study (1967) in which teachers' perceptions of the nurse's role reinforced the emphasis on first aid activities. Indeed, the role of the nurse was increasingly perceived as task oriented with the typical list of duties (O'Brien, 1969:346) for the school nurse in a school health program consisting of the following:

1. Prepares the session for the doctor
2. Issues all medical forms
3. Does vision and hearing screening and height and weight measurements

4. Escorts children to their homes
5. Makes home visits to check on attendance
6. Total first aid program
7. Sends out appointments for doctor sessions
8. Multiple clerical duties
9. Inventory and requisitioning supplies

Thus despite the emphasis in the literature on prevention activities (Tipple, 1964) and on the importance of the relationships between the nurse, child, family, school health team, curriculum, and community (Fredlund, 1967), school nursing became increasingly focused on more visible functions such as record keeping and first aid.

One of the conclusions reached by Fricke (1967) in her study was that the preparation level of the school nurse influenced her perception of her role. Of the nurses included in her study, more than 90% of those prepared at the baccalaureate level or above rated the need for leadership in identifying students with health needs that interfere with learning as a very important function; only 78% of the diploma nurses identified leadership as an important function for the nurse in a model program.

The discovery that school nurses were engaging in nonessential activities, such as record keeping, first aid, and attendance monitoring, led to a renewed interest in the use of auxiliary personnel in the school health program, a concept that had been widely proposed during World War II. In addition, the concept of the school health team was being broadened to include other disciplines, such as psychologists, counselors, health teachers, and social workers; the school health team was now becoming known as "pupil personnel services" (Dukelow, 1960; Cromwell, 1964). Perhaps because her perception of her role was so limited, the school nurse's position within the school was actually threatened by the addition of these new professionals to the school staff. Especially with regard to the social worker, problems with duplication of functions surfaced. The area of greatest overlap and ambiguity of function between the social worker and the school nurse was probably home visiting. With increased focus on tasks like first aid and record keeping, the school nurse had less time to devote to follow-up activities and made fewer home visits. Thus when the social worker became a part of the school health team, she "took over" in this area, which had traditionally been the stronghold of the public health–oriented school nurse.

In addition to the inclusion of other professionals in the school, there was an increasing trend toward the use of nonprofessional assistants to relieve the nurse of many of the nonessential tasks that had occupied so much of her time. Although this was in principle a sound and cost-effective means for freeing the nurse for more important activities that required her knowledge and skills, there were some very real problems as Tipple (1964:100) explained:

. . . In reality, one of two undesirable practices occurs. The auxiliary personnel may be assigned to perform a segment of the professional responsibilities of the qualified school nurse. Or, the activity may be carried out as an isolated technical process completely losing its educational significance. In actual practice, I have found, auxiliary personnel in most situations are not serving as assistants. They are serving in place of professional nurses.

Solving the problems that now confronted and even haunted school nurses was recognized as a complex challenge. Educational preparation of the school nurse now received closer scrutiny, and there was a renewed campaign to encourage the school nurse to seek at least a baccalaureate degree, preferably including public health nursing so that her educational credentials would more closely approximate those of her fellow faculty members. It was also hoped that through upgrading her preparation, the nurse would get back to an emphasis on the preventive aspects of school health. Some authorities went a step further (Fredlund, 1967; Stobo, 1969) and advocated preparation at the graduate level for the school nurse, recommending that such preparation include maternal and child health, mental health, public health nursing, administration and supervision, and interdisciplinary courses to be taken with other disciplines who are part of pupil personnel services.

By the late 1960s school districts across the nation were faced with fiscal problems that resulted in the widespread need to trim the school budget. Because the benefits of the school health program were generally long-range and less obvious and tangible than were the outcomes of other school programs, such as intramural athletics, many districts began to regard the school health program as a luxury (Fredlund, 1967). This resulted in reduction and sometimes elimination of services that had once been highly valued and indispensable features of the school's program. Administrators and school boards became primarily concerned with the cost of school health services, and budget decisions were made on that basis alone, a practice that Tipple (1964:101) deplored:

How can we reconcile the cost of school health programs? Let us recognize that the costs for education and health represent much more than payment for service rendered. They represent an investment in the future and the dividends cannot be measured only in terms of dollars and cents. The production of healthier, happier, better human beings is much more than a commodity to be purchased.

By the 1970s the school nurse found herself in a position that could be described as being "between a rock and a hard place." On one hand, there was talk about expanding roles, improved educational preparation, and increased community health involvement for the school nurse. On the other hand, the budgetary cutbacks that had begun to challenge the nurse's once secure position in the school were increasing, and the school nurse faced loss of job security, role confusion, and role reduction.

At the same time, the health needs and concerns of the school-age child were changing, which necessitated some changing of priorities by the school nurse. Chemical and drug use and abuse had increased among young people during the social upheaval of the 1960s. By the 1970s chemical dependency had become a critical health problem, and the school health program began to focus some of its educational efforts toward reduction of this problem. The family as an institution had lost some of its influence over the behavior of its members, and sexual permissiveness and divorce were increasing. Experimentation with sex, alcohol, and other chemicals resulted in an increase in problems related to chemical abuse, including delinquency, venereal disease, and adolescent pregnancy. The trend in continuing education for pregnant minors was to keep them in their home schools, rather than isolate them in special institutions. Thus some nurses found that they were providing health supervision and guidance for pregnant girls as part of the school health program.

The national emphasis on equal opportunities for all, which grew out of the civil rights legislation of the 1960s, worked to the advantage of handicapped children. Whereas the philosophy for many years had been to provide "separate but equal" educational opportunities for handicapped youngsters, during the 1970s main-

streaming those children into regular classes with nonimpaired children became the accepted practice. This too had implications for the role of the school nurse, since she now became an advocate for these children and focused her energies on facilitating their positive adaptation within the school.

Some authorities (Fredlund, 1970) continued to emphasize the importance of home visiting as a means of providing primary prevention for preschool siblings of the school-age child, with the goal of eliminating health problems before they become "entrenched." Along with this renewed commitment to family-centered care and home visiting came a broadened emphasis on the role of the school nurse in the promotion of positive mental health for schoolchildren. Her activities for promoting mental health included emotional support, crisis intervention, and counseling (Crosby and Connolly, 1970; Brand, 1972; Fricke, 1972).

Despite renewed commitment to family-centered care and mental health, the school nurse of the 1970s continued to suffer from role confusion. Hawkins (1971:745) explains the problem as follows:

In summary, school nurses perform tasks outside the context of healer and patient, with no clear professional guidelines, under nonmedical norms, and with goals and means for achieving them largely divorced from the basic model of nursing.

Hawkins goes on to say (1971:746) that the school nurse is ". . . expected to provide guidance in poorly defined areas, to coordinate activities of which she is only vaguely a part, and to cooperate in health education on terms dictated largely by others."

As previously noted, the nurse's inability to define her role clearly contributed to her difficulties in being a member of the pupil personnel services team within the school. Thomas' study (1976) of the school nurse as a member of the school health team, revealed that teamwork was a major problem area for the nurse. Specific problems regarding teamwork included relationship problems between the nurse and teachers, counselors, school administrators, and parents; breakdown of staff-team communication; and lack of acceptance of the nurse by school staff.

To upgrade the quality of school nursing, increased attention was paid to the issue of certification of the nurse to work in the school. By 1976 twenty-three of the fifty states had mandatory school nursing certification requirements, and ten states had permissive requirements (Castile and Jerrick, 1976).

Improved educational preparation of the nurse as a means of upgrading the quality of practice was also a recurrent theme. In accord with the recommendation of the American Nurses' Association that minimum preparation for the practice of professional nursing be a baccalaureate degree from an accredited nursing program, the American School Health Association (ASHA) adopted the baccalaureate degree as the accepted minimum preparation for school nursing as well. ASHA (1974:10) further recommended that the baccalaureate graduate should have acquired the "professional competency necessary for beginning practice in school nursing under supervision." ASHA acknowledged that there were significant numbers of capable nurses currently employed in the schools who did not yet have baccalaureate degrees and recommended that schools of nursing begin to plan programs and courses of study to enable these nurses to obtain their degrees. Other authors recognized the value of master's level preparation (Marriner, 1971; Brand, 1972) for the school nurse to enhance her ability to be a leader within the school health program and to be a responsible participant in comprehensive health planning in the community.

During the early 1970s another educational and practice-related trend developed in school nursing: the evolution of the school nurse practitioner (SNP) role. Developed in Denver in 1970 (Igoe, 1975), the SNP concept required a minimum 4-month postbaccalaureate training program to expand the nurse's skills in such areas as history taking, physical appraisal, and developmental assessment. With her expanded skills and the support of administrators in the school, it was hoped that the school nurse could participate more effectively and responsibly within the school health program. The SNP could also be expected to have a clear definition of her role, which should help improve her relationship with other members of the pupil personnel services team.

Despite these attempts to clarify and expand the school nurse's role during the 1970s, the national trend toward cutbacks in school health and elimination of school nursing positions continued for a number of reasons. First, the costs of education continued to escalate during the 1970s; as a result, all school personnel and services "not directly and demonstratively bene-

ficial to the learner" (Coleman and Hawkins, 1970:121) were subject to close scrutiny and possible elimination. Because the outcomes of school nursing services were long-range and at times intangible, school nurses were often among the first personnel to be cut from the school's budget. Second, the trend begun in the 1960s toward employment of nonprofessional assistants in the school health program continued. As Tipple (1964) had predicted, some districts trimmed their budgets by replacing their nurses with health clerks and school health aides. The result was that no one coordinated the program for meeting the child's total health needs, and school health services became fragmented. As Lum (1973:357) reports:

. . . School health services became primarily a tool for resolving immediate health problems and for minimally fulfilling state mandates; secondly, a means for identifying selected health problems; and only incidentally, a service aimed at improving the health status of children so that they may attain the greatest benefit from their educational experiences.

However, perhaps the most truthful explanation for continued reduction in the number of school nursing positions in school districts around the country was that offered by Ford (1970). Her frank opinion was that nursing had failed to demonstrate to the public that its services were *worth* the cost. School nurses had not taken the initiative to "sell" the merits of their services to school boards, administrators, or even consumers. By the time the need to do so was recognized it was virtually too late; the reductions were well underway.

The future of school nursing may depend on how well school nurses heed Dickinson's (1971) advice. He proposed that school nurses, like all other threatened services, demonstrate their accountability and contributions to the educational program through the use of behavioral objectives to describe how the student is different as an outcome of nursing intervention. By writing and evaluating objectives in terms of changed consumer (student) behaviors rather than in terms of the process and intervention used by the nurse, outcomes of school nursing service can be more readily evaluated. This would enable the nurse to "sell" herself as an indispensable part of the school health program.

Ultimately, the continued failure of school nurses to demonstrate clearly their contribution within the school will result in the complete elimination of school nursing and would support Hawkins' (1971:751) contention that:

For nurses to withdraw completely from school systems would entail no immediately apparent loss for either themselves or the schools. The profession could accommodate them elsewhere, and only minor vested interests would seem to be involved.

It is our belief that school nursing has a vital role to play in promoting and safeguarding the health of school populations. Therefore this book will attempt to clarify the contributions to the school health program made by the nurse and present a framework for practice that will allow the nurse to become accountable in the educational setting, proving that she is not after all a "passing experiment."

REFERENCES

American National Red Cross: 1931. Rural school nursing: an outline for Red Cross public health nurses, The American Red Cross, Washington, D.C.

American School Health Association: 1974. Guidelines for the school nurse in the school health program, American School Health Association, Kent, Ohio.

Axelson, A. J.: 1944. School nursing: what is its future? Public Health Nurs. **36**(9):441-442.

Ayling, W. E., and Johnson, E. F.: 1949. The nurse-teacher in a school health program, Public Health Nurs. **41**(4):179-186.

Brand, M. L.: 1972. The potential of school nursing in the '70s, ANA Clin. Sess., pp. 3-9.

Brown, E. S.: 1952. The role of the nurse in the school health program, J. School Health **22**(8):219-224.

Bryant, Z., and Hudson, H. H.: 1962. The census of nurses in public health, Am. J. Nurs. **62**(12):104-107.

Castile, A. S., and Jerrick, S. J.: 1976. School health in America, American School Health Association, Kent, Ohio.

Chayer, M. E.: 1947. Nursing in modern society, G. P. Putnam's Sons, New York.

Coakley, J. M., and Parker, J. M.: 1965. Education of nurses for school nursing, Am. J. Nurs. **65**(11):84-87.

Coleman, J., and Hawkins, W.: 1970. The changing role of the nurse: an alternative to elimination, J. School Health **40**(3):121-122.

Committee for the Study of Nursing Education: 1923. Nursing and nursing education in the United States, The Macmillan Publishing Co., Inc., New York.

Cromwell, G. E.: 1952. Teammates—teachers and school nurses, J. School Health **22**(6):165-171.

Cromwell, G. E.: 1963. The nurse in the school health program, W. B. Saunders Co., Philadelphia.

Cromwell, G. E.; 1964. The future of school nursing, J. School Health **34**(1):43-46.

Crosby, M. H., and Connolly, M. G.: 1970. The study of mental health and the school nurse, J. School Health **40**(7):373-377.

Dickinson, D. J.: 1971. School nursing becomes accountable in education through behavioral objectives, J. School Health **41**(10):533-537.

Dierkes, K.: 1951. The nurse in a generalized program, J. School Health **21**(4):131-135.

Dilworth, L. P.: 1944. Essential school nursing in wartime, Public Health Nurs. **36**(9):443-447.

Dilworth, L. P.: 1949. The nurse in the school health program, Public Health Nurs. **41**(8):438-441.

Dukelow, D. A.: 1960. 1960 White House conference recommendations on school health, J. School Health **30**(9):334-341.

Forbes, O.: 1967. The role and functions of the school nurse as perceived by 115 public school teachers from three selected counties, J. School Health **37**(2):101-106.

Ford, L. C.: 1970. The school nurse role—a changing concept in preparation and practice, J. School Health **40**(1):21-23.

Fredlund, D. J.: 1967. The route to effective school nursing, Nurs. Outlook **15**(8):24-28.

Fredlund, D. J.: 1970. Juvenile delinquency and school nursing, Nurs. Outlook **18**(5):57-59.

Freeman, R.: 1945. Developments in education of public health nurses for school health work, Public Health Nurs. **37**(9):454-455.

Fricke, I. B.: 1967. The Illinois study of school nursing practice, J. School Health **37**:24-28.

Fricke, I. B.: 1972. School nursing for the '70s, J. School Health **42**(4):203-206.

Gair, C.: 1966. What is School Nursing? J. School Health **36**(9):401-402.

Gardner, M. S.: 1916. Public health nursing, The Macmillan Publishing Co., Inc., New York.

Gardner, M. S.: 1926. Public health nursing, 2nd ed., The Macmillan Publishing Co., Inc., New York.

Gardner, M. S.: 1936. Public health nursing, 3rd ed., The Macmillan Publishing Co., Inc., New York.

Goodnow, M.: 1943. Nursing history in brief, 2nd ed., W. B. Saunders Co., Philadelphia.

Grant, A. H.: 1942. Nursing: a community health service, W. B. Saunders Co., Philadelphia.

Hawkins, N. G.: 1971. Is there a school nurse role? Am. J. Nurs. **71**(4):744-751.

Hilliard, P.: 1951. Nurse in a jointly administered program, J. School Health **21**(4):136-139.

Hubbard, J. P., Bain, K., and Pennell, M. Y.: 1949. School health services, J. School Health **19**(6):143-148.

Igoe, J. B.: 1975. The school nurse practitioner, Nurs. Outlook **23**:381-384.

Kelly, H. W., and Bradshaw, M. C.: 1918. A handbook for school nurses, The Macmillan Publishing Co., Inc., New York.

Lum, M. C.: 1973. Current concepts in the use of nonprofessional assistants in school health services—a selected review, J. School Health **43**:357-361.

Marriner, A.: 1971. Opinions of school nurses about the preparation and practice of school nurses, J. School Health **41**(8):417-420.

McAleer, H. S.: 1965. What's new in school nursing, J. School Health **35**(2):49-52.

NOPHN: 1944. School nurse and community, Public Health Nurs. **36**(9):442.

O'Brien, M. J.: 1969. A nurse in school—why? Nurs. Clin. North Am. **4**(2):343-349.

Palmer, M. F.: 1944. Essentiality of school nursing, Public Health Nurs. **36**(5):221-222.

Randall, H. B.: 1971. School health in the seventies, J. School Health **41**(3):125-129.

Randle, B. B.: 1943. Wartime essentials in school nursing, Public Health Nurs. **35**(9):482-483.

Sellery, C. M.: 1950. Where are we going in school health education? J. School Health **20**(6):151-159.

Sellery, C. M.: 1951. The nurse in the school health program—the administrator's point of view, J. School Health **21**(4):119-124.

Stobo, E. C.: 1969. Trends in the preparation and qualifications of the school nurse, Am. J. Public Health **59**(4): 669-672.

Struthers, L. R.: 1917. The school nurse, G. P. Putnam's Sons, New York.

Thomas, B.: 1976. The school nurse as a member of the school health team: fact or fiction? J. School Health **46**(8):466-470.

Tipple, D. C.: 1964. Misuse of assistants in school health, Am. J. Nurs. **64**(9):99-101.

Troop, E. H.: 1963. Sixty years of school nurse preparation, Nurs. Outlook **11**(5):364-366.

Wales, M.: 1941. The public health nurse in action, The Macmillan Publishing Co., Inc., New York.

Wallace, H. M.: 1959. School health services, J. School Health **29**(8):283-295.

Wilson, C. W.: 1945. Health counseling in schools, Public Health Nurs. **37**:436-438.

SUGGESTED READINGS

Cary, H. A.: 1951. Development of a school health program, J. School Health **21**(9):283-286.

Macdonough, G. P.: 1972. Comparison of nursing roles, J. School Health **42**(8):481-482.

CHAPTER 2

Philosophy, roles, and goals of school nursing

SUSAN J. WOLD and NANCY V. DAGG

The practice of nursing is influenced by an individual's *philosophy* about the nature of nursing, its roles and goals, and the qualifications needed by its practitioners. Consequently, that philosophy or set of guiding beliefs influences the professional roles an individual plays and the goals toward which practice is directed.

The purpose of this chapter is to present a philosophy of school health and school nursing and to explore the roles and goals that we believe are appropriate for the practice of school nursing based on this philosophy. The philosophy presented in this chapter is the basis for the remainder of the book.

PHILOSOPHY OF SCHOOL NURSING PRACTICE

We subscribe to the following beliefs about school health and school nursing as written and endorsed by the ASHA and the American Nurses' Association (ANA) (ASHA, 1974:3):

- Every child is entitled to educational opportunities which will allow each to reach full capacity as an individual and to prepare him or her for responsibility as a citizen.
- Every child is entitled to a level of health which permits maximum utilization of educational opportunities.
- Every school has a legal and moral obligation to provide a school health program which will promote and protect the health of its children and youth.
- The school health program should be consistent with the philosophy and objectives of the school program.
- The school health program, through the components of health service, health education and concern for the environment, provides knowledge and understanding on which to base decisions for the promotion and protection of individual, family and community health.

- A dual preparation in health and education best qualifies professional personnel for participation in the intraprofessional and interdisciplinary approach to school health.
- Activities of the school health program play a primary role in establishing a viable working relationship with home and community.
- Parents have the basic responsibility for the health of their children; the school health program activities exist to assist parents in carrying out their responsibilities.
- The community has the responsibility of providing comprehensive health and related services; the school health program will assist parents and youth to utilize such community services effectively.
- School health program activities should include participation in regional, state, and local comprehensive health planning to identify and interpret health needs, and to coordinate health services for children and youth, and their families.

In addition to the foregoing statements, we also believe the following:

- The school nurse is an important member of the school health team; she contributes to the success of the school health program through her participation in the planning, implementation, and evaluation phases.
- The school nurse should have academic credentials comparable to those of other faculty members in the school. She should have at least a bachelor's degree in nursing and should meet requirements for certification as a public health nurse and as a school nurse. Her academic background should include courses in public health nursing and school nursing and a supervised clinical experience in both areas. She should have courses in child growth and development, educational theories and methods, school health administration, psychology, sociology, and health assessment.
- The appropriate roles of the school nurse in the school health program include manager of health care; deliverer of health services; advocate for the health rights of children; counselor for health con-

cerns of children, families, and staff; and educator for school/community health concerns.

These thirteen statements make up our philosophy of school nursing. Our philosophy permeates the rest of the book because it is our "perceptual filter" in discussing school nursing.

The major portion of this chapter discusses the roles and goals of the school nurse in the school health program. Before we proceed to a discussion of the roles and goals of the nurse within the school health program we will clarify (1) the role of the school in providing for the health of its population and (2) the nature and thrust of the school health program.

The school is a community institution with an age-specific population; it is a heterogeneous group actually mandated by state law. Since parents cannot totally protect the health of their children in this heterogeneous community, they must delegate some of this responsibility to the school. Therefore, the school has an obligation, moral if not legal, to protect and promote the health of its students and staff through the development and implementation of the school health program.

COMPONENTS OF THE SCHOOL HEALTH PROGRAM

The school health program is generally described as having three basic functions: (1) provision of a safe and healthful school environment, (2) implementation of an ongoing and effective health education curriculum, and (3) delivery of health services to students and staff. In our discussion of the school health program, we have deviated somewhat from the "three-pronged" focus and have instead identified six areas of responsibility that we believe should be part of the school health program. These six areas are incorporated within the three functions just identified and merely provide a more specific breakdown of the components of the school health program. The order in which they are discussed does not indicate priority.

The first of the six basic responsibilities of the school health program is to identify and exclude from school those students and staff with communicable diseases and initiate appropriate follow-up to ensure their prompt readmission. This responsibility has always been a part of school health programs. In fact, school health programs came into existence (Chapter 1) because of the excessively high absenteeism in schools due to communicable diseases. It is ob-

vious that a child who is frequently ill and unable to attend school will not benefit as fully from the learning opportunities available in the school program as he could if he were healthy. Although the family and child are ultimately responsible for the child's health, the school is responsible for minimizing health threats in the school environment that might cause illness and interfere with the child's learning.

The second obligation of the school health program is to prevent the outbreak and spread of communicable diseases through consistent enforcement of existing laws and school policies regarding immunizations for students and school personnel. With the advent of immunizations against childhood diseases that were once considered inevitable, such as measles (rubeola), rubella, and mumps, the control of communicable diseases has become an easier task. However, as a result of the recent national trend toward complacency and laxity in seeking immunizations for children, communicable diseases within school populations are not as well controlled as they should be. Hence, the need for the school health program to focus on communicable disease control persists. This includes referral to community resources to obtain needed immunizations or arranging an in-school immunization clinic.

The third function of the school in protecting the health of its students is to limit disability through early diagnosis and prompt treatment for such potentially chronic problems as hearing loss, impaired vision, and scoliosis. At one time the school health program was responsible not only for screening school populations, but also for treating students for defects or impairments (Chapter 1). Because it is now generally believed that students and families are responsible for their own health, the treatment aspect is no longer part of the school health program. However, the school continues to provide periodic screening for vision and hearing and, in recent years, for scoliosis as well, since these kinds of correctable defects can interfere with a student's ability to learn. This function is carried out, then, by means of periodic screening of age-specific groups and/or those groups known to be at risk. Once defects are discovered, referrals are made to the appropriate community resource for treatment, and follow-up is initiated if needed to ensure that the defects are corrected.

The fourth responsibility of the school regarding the health of its students and staff is to maintain a safe and healthful school environment so that conditions that might interfere with the teaching-learning climate are minimized. This includes elimination of safety hazards, provision of sanitary food and water supplies, and installation and maintenance of adequate lighting, heating, and ventilation systems in accordance with existing laws and policies, and adequate supervision of the students' play and recreation areas.

The fifth task to be completed within the school health program is to develop a practical and appropriate system for providing first aid and emergency care for students and staff who become injured or ill at school. When the responsibility for maintaining a safe and healthful school environment is adequately addressed, the need for first aid and emergency services should be decreased. However, some accidents and illnesses are not preventable, and the school must provide first aid and emergency care episodically. The school should have clearly written guidelines and procedures established for such services. It is also important that a number of faculty, staff persons, or volunteers in the school be trained in first aid techniques and that at least one of these persons be available in the school during all school functions. Despite the tendency toward using the school nurse for routine first aid and emergency care, this is *not* advisable and is not the most effective use of her skills.

The sixth specific health responsibility delegated to the school is perhaps the most important and certainly the most difficult. It is the development, implementation, and evaluation of a comprehensive health education curriculum to prepare students to assume responsibility for their own health. It has long been recognized that a child who is not healthy cannot benefit from the educational opportunities available to him; therefore the school must educate the child and his family to understand the nature of the health-disease continuum and to incorporate into daily life those practices and routines which prevent disease and promote health.

Responsibility for planning, implementing, and evaluating the outcome of the school health program is generally delegated to the school health *team,* which includes administrators, principals, school nurses, teachers, social workers, psychologists, school health aides, volunteers, and parents. Although the superintendent of the school system or the administrator (principal) of a particular school may be ultimately *responsible* and *accountable* for the health program, the collaboration of *all* team members during all phases of the program is critically important to its success. However, since the focus of this book is on school nursing, the remainder of this chapter will deal with the specific contribution of the school nurse to the success of the school health program.

ROLES AND GOALS OF THE SCHOOL NURSE

Based on our philosophy of school nursing and on our modifications of portions of the ASHA guidelines (1974), we have identified five basic roles for the nurse in the school health program and a corollary goal for each (Table 2-1). Although the roles and goals will be discussed sequentially, the school nurse may find herself playing multiple roles. She will also find that some tasks and goals overlap and are included in more than one role-goal dyad.

Table 2-1. Roles and goals of the nurse in the school health program

Roles	Goals
Manager of health care within school health program	To participate in planning, implementation, and evaluation of school health program
Deliverer of health services	To deliver needed health services to client system using systematic processes to assess needs, plan interventions, and evaluate outcomes so that high-level wellness can be achieved
Advocate for health rights of children	To act as advocate for health rights of children and their families both within school setting and between school and community at large
Counselor for health concerns of children, families, and staff	To provide health counseling and guidance for client system on individual basis or within group setting
Educator for school/community health concerns	To participate in health education program activities for children, youth, school personnel, and community

The school nurse as manager of health care within the school health program

GOAL: *To participate in planning, implementation, and evaluation of a school health program.*

Customarily, the objectives of the school health program are determined at the school district level. Thus the superintendent or other designated school district administrator is ultimately responsible for the development of guidelines and goals for school health. The administrator in the individual school, that is, the principal, is then charged with the responsibility for interpreting the guidelines and goals, arranging for their implementation, and participating in the evaluation of their outcomes.

Clearly, then, it is *not* the responsibility of the school nurse to independently plan and implement the school health program. Rather, as a nurse who recognizes that management* is essential for the successful practice of nursing within the school setting, the school nurse takes on the role of manager as she participates in planning, implementation, and evaluation of the school health program (Fig. 2-1).

During the planning phase, the school nurse can provide useful data regarding the health needs of children in the school so that appropriate objectives and activities can be designed.

---

*Scanlan (1974:12) defines management as ". . . the coordination and integration of all resources (both human and technical) to accomplish specific results."

Because of her frequent contacts with students, school personnel, family members, and other interested community members, the nurse is uniquely and amply qualified to provide this information. Using her knowledge of health and education, the school nurse collaboratively formulates specific objectives and policies for the school's health program, maintaining consistency with the school district's philosophy and overall goals for school health.

The school nurse further participates in planning the school health program by making recommendations regarding the budget. If she believes that the needs of schoolchildren indicate that a particular objective of the overall health program should be given heavy emphasis and high priority, she suggests appropriate budgetary increases and/or spending shifts to ensure that this phase or goal of the school health program is accomplished.

The school nurse's role as manager carries over into the implementation phase of the school health program as well. This involves organization and completion of activities to meet objectives formulated during the planning phase. Again, during this phase, the school nurse works collaboratively with the school health team and is careful to plan activities that conform with existing pertinent school district policies. Specifically, the nurse has seven tasks to achieve in this phase (Fig. 2-1).

First, the nurse must establish open and di-

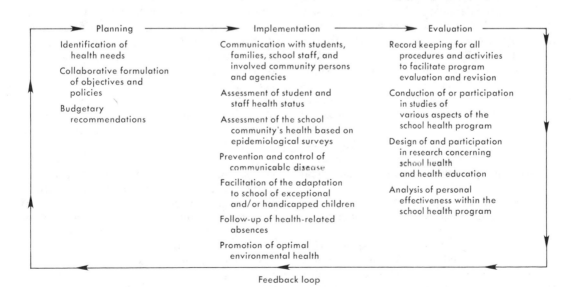

Planning	Implementation	Evaluation
Identification of health needs	Communication with students, families, school staff, and involved community persons and agencies	Record keeping for all procedures and activities to facilitate program evaluation and revision
Collaborative formulation of objectives and policies	Assessment of student and staff health status	Conduction of or participation in studies of various aspects of the school health program
Budgetary recommendations	Assessment of the school community's health based on epidemiological surveys	Design of and participation in research concerning school health and health education
	Prevention and control of communicable disease	Analysis of personal effectiveness within the school health program
	Facilitation of the adaptation to school of exceptional and/or handicapped children	
	Follow-up of health-related absences	
	Promotion of optimal environmental health	

Feedback loop

Fig. 2-1. School nurse as manager of health care within the school health program.

rect communication with students, families, school staff, and involved community persons and agencies with whom she works. Maintaining good communication patterns is essential throughout all three stages (planning, implementation, and evaluation) and requires that the nurse know and practice effective helping relationship skills (Chapter 10). It is especially important, however, to maintain open communication with the client, whether child, parent, teacher, or any other person or group, during the implementation phase, because the nurse's ability to implement her plan of activities depends on her ability to gain acceptance, cooperation, and trust.

The school nurse's second implementation task is providing for assessment of the health status of individual students and staff members as needed. Most school districts have policies and guidelines indicating at what intervals or grade levels physical assessments (including dental checkups) are to be done. The nurse is responsible for procedural aspects, such as carrying out the physical appraisals and/or completing health histories, referring students and staff to other school and community resources for these services, or arranging an in-school screening program for vision, hearing, scoliosis, and/or other health appraisals.

In addition to concern for individual and periodic health appraisals, a third concern of the nurse is assessment of the school community's health. This can be accomplished through the use of epidemiological process (Chapter 16), such as an epidemiological survey. Such surveys can help the nurse more clearly identify the health needs of the school population as a whole and can be invaluable as tools in setting priorities for implementation activities. These surveys further reveal trends in the health status of the population, for example, shifting rates of communicable disease such as an increase in venereal disease. Once these trends are identified, the school health program can be revised accordingly. This helps maintain consistency between the planned program and the "real world."

Closely related to the task of school community health assessment is the fourth implementation task of the school nurse, which is to prevent and control communicable diseases. This includes writing and implementing procedures for identifying and excluding those children and school staff members who have communicable diseases and who are endangering the health of others by their presence in the school. Such procedures must be consistent with the school district's policies and local and state laws concerning communicable disease and need to include specific recommendations regarding readmission to school once the period of communicability has ended. In addition, the nurse makes recommendations regarding environmental disinfection when needed and may arrange for health screening/appraisal of the at-risk population if warranted.

However, to be successful, the long-term approach to prevention and control of communicable disease requires ongoing health education of students, families, and staff. This can be handled on an episodic basis by reinforcing principles of prevention and control in the existing school health education curriculum. The nurse, as a resource person and consultant, ensures incorporation of this content into the health curriculum through participation in the planning and implementation phases.

A fifth implementation task for the school nurse-manager is to facilitate adaptation of exceptional and/or handicapped students within the school setting. This task also involves writing and implementing procedures to enact the school district's policies for incorporation of these children within regular and special school programs and modification of the physical plant to meet their needs. With her knowledge of health, education, pediatrics, and growth and development, the school nurse is well-qualified to assess the particular needs of these children and to help arrange for their identified needs to be met within the school. Her interventions with and on behalf of these special children will require that she carry out the roles of "manager of health care," "deliverer of health services," and "advocate" as she coordinates the school experiences for these children. For example, she will wear all three "hats" as she initiates and/or participates in team conferences for a particular child to work out the details of daily classroom experiences, needed rest periods, counseling sessions, physical health care procedures, and so forth. School nurses are becoming increasingly concerned with the needs of handicapped children because of the trend toward mainstreaming these children into regular schools (Chapter 6).

A sixth task for the school nurse in implementing the role of manager is to follow up on illness-related absences. This does *not* mean that the school nurse should be considered the school's truant officer with the responsibility of calling the homes of all absent students to determine the cause. It does mean that those children who are known to be absent for health-related reasons for long periods of time or on a "patterned" basis should be followed up to determine if they are receiving the care they need to facilitate their recovery and prompt return to school. Those students who have no resource for care for their illnesses will need referral to community agencies. For those cases where absences are due to other stresses within the individual or family, the nurse may make a home visit and/or refer the student and family to other school health team members, such as the social worker or psychologist or to a community resource.

The seventh and last specific task for the nurse-manager during the implementation of the school health program is to promote optimal environmental health. In addition to planning environmental modifications to aid handicapped children and recommending environmental sanitation measures to prevent and control the spread of communicable disease, the school nurse has a fundamental interest in promoting optimal environmental health for all students and staff. Thus she may consult with school engineers and maintenance staff to ensure compliance with the district's policies on ventilation, heating, and lighting.

The final stage of the school nurse-manager's involvement in the school health program is evaluation. Evaluation may be done formatively, that is, on an ongoing basis while the program is being implemented, or summatively, at the conclusion of the program. In some instances both formative and summative evaluations may be used to allow for ongoing revisions as well as evaluation of the total program's effectiveness. The specific evaluative measures and tools used will depend on the variable being evaluated and on the purpose of that evaluation.

For the school nurse, an important source of data for both formative and summative evaluation is the student health record. The resolution of health problems can be readily evaluated when the school nurse correctly and consistently uses a problem-oriented health record (POHR) format (Chapter 12). However, beyond the evaluation of her one-to-one student contacts via the POHR format, the nurse must collect and record all pertinent data to help her realistically evaluate and revise all the programs

and activities she is charged with implementing. The importance of such data collection and analysis cannot be overstated because the evaluation process provides an important "feedback loop" (Fig. 2-1) to the planning stage, so that the school health program continues to be relevant to the needs of the school population.

Other evaluative measures that are appropriate for the school nurse to use include studies relating to various aspects of the school health program, such as nurse-pupil ratio, staffing patterns, and time use. The nurse may conduct such studies on her own initiative or may be a participant only.

Although studies of specific aspects of the school health program, for example, nurse-pupil ratio, are important sources of data for program planning, priority-setting, and program evaluation, other kinds of research also need to be done. As part of her role in evaluating the school health program, the school nurse may design and/or participate in research concerning school health and health education. Specifically, there is a need for school nurses to complete studies documenting their roles and the outcomes of school nursing intervention strategies. With the current budgetary crises faced by school districts across the country, there is an increasing need for all departments and personnel in the schools to clearly document their contributions and the importance of their services if they expect school districts to continue to provide funds for their programs. The notion that research belongs in the laboratory or ivory tower and is solely the province of the elite and those with advanced education is neither accurate nor realistic. Nurses in all practice settings and at all levels need to conduct research to improve their practice and to evaluate their effectiveness. However, the need is especially acute right now in school nursing; unless school nurses can provide data to justify their continued employment within the school, they can reasonably expect that in the future they will be replaced by lay personnel.

The final evaluative responsibility of the school nurse is to develop and consistently use appropriate means to analyze her personal effectiveness within the school health program. Although the nurse's employer, whether it be a public health agency, board of education, or board of health, generally evaluates her performance annually, in many cases the criteria used are not specific or particularly meaningful.

Thus the nurse is not provided with a means for ongoing evaluation of her practice.

It is the nurse's responsibility as a health professional to determine some means for providing meaningful performance feedback for herself. This problem can be approached in several ways. First, school nurses working in a given school district or geographic region might collaboratively develop a performance tool including behaviors common to all of their school settings. Second, nurses might negotiate individually with the school nursing supervisor or the designated administrator for a "performance contract" for a particular school year. This contract would be based on the district's expectations of the nurse and on any additional objectives the nurse might have for her professional growth. A third approach might be for school nurses to develop a system of peer review in which criteria agreed to by all school nurses in the district would be used to provide periodic feedback to one another after direct observation of performance, review of records and statistics, and/or conferences with the nurse, other school personnel, and clients (children, families, staff, and community residents). Most important to successful implementation of any of these methods is the development of behavioral objectives or goals for the nurse's performance. These goals should be broken down into specific measurable behaviors that can be used as evaluative outcome criteria (EOCs), allowing for objective comparison of the nurse's performance with the criteria to determine if a particular goal was achieved.

The school nurse as deliverer of health services

GOAL: *To deliver needed health services to the client system using systematic processes to assess needs, plan interventions, and evaluate outcomes so that high-level wellness can be achieved.*

In the role of deliverer of health services, the school nurse is directly concerned with the health of the client system and with those measures needed to correct health problems. Her specific activities as deliverer of health services should flow from and be consistent with the school health program's goals, policies, and procedures, which the nurse helped formulate in her role as manager of health care. There is an obviously close relationship between the role as manager during the implementation phase and the role as deliverer of health services (Fig. 2-1). Many activities that are part of implementing the school health program are also activities involving delivery of service, such as assessment of student and staff health status.

Since one of the primary goals of this book is to provide school nurses with a framework on which to base delivery of services and because we wish to avoid overlapping and repetitive discussion, the remainder of this discussion will not provide a detailed description of how services can be delivered by the school nurse but will instead identify only the basic activities that are part of the nurse's role in delivering health services.

As previously mentioned, the specific services "delivered" by the school nurse will depend on the goals and objectives established for the health program in a particular school in a given school district. The kinds of services delivered by the nurse are also influenced by her own philosophy as to what is an appropriate service to offer and by her knowledge and skills.

Despite the influence of such individual differences among nurses and variations in program objectives from one school or district to another, some activities are common to most school nurses in carrying out the role of deliverer of health services. First, the role of the nurse as deliverer of health services depends on the nurse's ability to identify the health status and health needs of schoolchildren through the following means:

1. Periodic and episodic physical health appraisal using appropriate examination techniques such as inspection, palpation, auscultation, and percussion
2. Collection of a health history
3. Assessment of growth and development and psychosocial health
4. Periodic screening of at-risk populations to detect visual problems, hearing loss, scoliosis, or other conditions
5. Periodic conferences with teachers, other school staff, the child and his family, and other relevant persons for early detection of health problems or learning and perceptual disabilities
6. Observation of students in the classroom and during play or recreation periods as a means of casefinding

The second area of focus for the school nurse as deliverer of health services is planning and carrying out appropriate interventions once health needs are known. This may include referring a student to his physician or to another community resource for follow-up and treatment. It may also involve setting up a school health team conference to plan and intervene on behalf of the child. It may be limited to health education or to other personal counseling to enable the child and his family to correct the problem.

To maximize the nurse's contribution to the school health program and minimize unnecessary funneling of time into tasks that lay personnel can be taught to do, the school nurse as deliverer of health services should not routinely be involved in first aid procedures. Rather, she can assist the school in setting up guidelines and procedures for first aid and emergency care and can help instruct teachers or volunteers to provide these services. In the event of a serious accident or other emergency at the school the nurse can certainly participate in handling the crisis if she is in the building or nearby; however, the school should not plan for her to routinely handle all first aid, since this is not good use of her time and skill and interferes with her ability to achieve other goals of the school health program.

The third focus of the nurse in delivering health services in the school is to follow up on those children and school personnel with known illnesses or health problems to ensure their full recovery and prompt return to school. This may involve a variety of means, including telephone calls and home visits to check progress toward heath. It may also involve establishing lines of communication with specific community agencies to facilitate both referral for treatment and evaluation of referral outcomes.

The school nurse as an advocate for the health rights of children

GOAL: *To act as an advocate for the health rights of children and their families both within the school setting and between the school and community at large.*

In working toward this goal, the school nurse is asked to assume the role of advocate for the health rights of children. Webster's New Collegiate Dictionary defines an advocate as "one that pleads the cause of another" or someone who gives "support." It is extremely important that this role be clearly defined—what the role *is* and *is not*. The nurse is asked to speak for the health rights of individual children and groups of children. As needs are identified, she makes them known to families and to health care resources in the community. The nurse does *not* assume a surrogate parent role and take on responsibilities that belong to the family. The nurse is a facilitator who sees that a child's health care needs are met by seeking out resources and giving support to the family as they make the actual arrangements for the needed service. Specifically, it is not the role of the nurse to make medical and dental appointments for children; by so doing, the nurse is denying the family the opportunity to recognize or develop their own skills. These skills are increasingly needed as the health care delivery system becomes more complex.

The role of advocate for children's health rights is delegated to the school nurse because of her unique position in the school community as a professional confronted daily with the needs of individual children. Because of her public health orientation, she gathers information that includes not only the acute care needs of the child but also information about the health of the child's family. She gathers this data from school personnel and families. Her reputation as a "helping" professional is recognized by students and families, and she is often sought by students, families, and staff to discuss health concerns. The school nurse confers with school personnel to interpret the identified health concerns of students. Based on these conferences, adaptations are made in the school class schedule, the school's physical plant, physical education activities, and class lesson plans. Following are specific examples of each:

1. The school class schedule—a youth with school phobia may have his favorite class scheduled first.
2. The school physical plant—ramps may be installed for students confined to wheelchairs; special bathroom facilities may be required in older school buildings.
3. Physical education activities—a child with hemophilia will be restricted from playing contact sports; a child recovering from brain surgery will be required to wear a plastic helmet.
4. Class lesson plans—science projects requiring animals will be altered if students in the class have allergies.

The school nurse also confers with other health professionals and community groups to increase their awareness of locally identified needs.

Through these discussions, the school nurse can stimulate development of community resources.

In addition to conferring with the school and community, the school nurse as an advocate needs to be aware of and lobby for legislative programs that may have an impact on school health services and health education. This may be accomplished through membership in professional organizations such as the ANA, National Association of School Nurses (NASN), American Public Health Association (APHA), and ASHA.

The school nurse as health counselor for individuals and groups

GOAL: *To provide health counseling and guidance for the client system on an individual basis or within a group setting.*

By maintaining relationships with health professionals in the community, the school nurse will develop an awareness of existing health care resources. By investing some additional time, the school nurse can explore new resources and keep up with changes in existing resources. This is a wise investment of time, since an important part of the health counseling done in a school is informing youth, parents, and school personnel about professional health care services for the identified health problem or concern.

The responsibility of the school nurse may end when the client system is referred to a health care provider. However, if the health concern is chronic rather than acute, the nurse may be asked to help the parent, child, and school personnel to understand and adjust to the changes and limitations stemming from the health problem. This may be accomplished through discussions, information giving, and problem solving.

The school nurse will make a nursing assessment and counsel parents, youth, and school staff when illness creates absenteeism. In addition, the school nurse may arrange for homebound education or for gradually increasing school attendance hours based on the child's energy level.

As health problems are identified in the school setting, the school nurse works with families and groups of students to identify how their information, attitudes, and values affect their health behavior and level of wellness. The nurse must be sensitive to and knowledgeable about socioeconomic and cultural influences if she is to effectively counsel in this area.

Whenever possible the school nurse works with groups rather than individuals because peer group influence is important to the child or youth. For example, a diabetic child may be resistant to eating a snack at a particular time of the day. By having a group of diabetic children discuss their nutritional needs and the timing of snacks, the child refusing snacks may change his attitude.

An additional benefit of group work is that more students can be reached at one time. Therefore it is more cost-effective than one-to-one counseling. When school districts and health departments are trying to contain costs, it is imperative that groups be used for health counseling whenever feasible.

The school nurse as health educator in the school health program

GOAL: *To participate in health education program activities for children, youth, school personnel, and the community.*

The school nurse is one of many people who participate in the health education program in the school. She may be the coordinator of the health education program or that role may be assigned to an educator. Either way, the school nurse makes significant contributions through several activities.

The school nurse correlates her direct service activities, such as health appraisal and screening procedures, with the health education curriculum. Prior to implementing screening procedures, which may be viewed as routine by school personnel, the nurse alerts teachers and provides them with sufficient information or a prepared lesson plan so they can incorporate this content into their health classes. Another example is a health talk about a communicable disease outbreak such as streptococcal infections. After the nurse assesses that there is an outbreak in the school, she may prepare a health talk in an attempt to prevent the spread of streptococcal infections to other children.

A second activity in health education is collaborating with teachers in areas for which the school population is at high risk, including topics such as drug use and abuse, venereal disease, family living, personal hygiene, and suicide. Depending on the community, these topics may be sensitive issues, and it is very appropriate for the nurse to invest time in developing the skills needed to work effectively in these areas. The school nurse may also provide in-service education on health topics for school personnel based on needs of the school population.

A broad background in health and knowledge of resource materials enable the school nurse to provide consultation regarding appropriate health education materials. She can also be part of the team responsible for evaluation of the health curriculum for kindergarten to twelfth grade. Ideally, the nurse also participates in community planning, implementation, and evaluation of the adult health education programs. Programs for the adult population may be on topics that have a direct relationship to the school population, for example, parenting and child care classes, first aid, and nutrition.

Last, but of equal importance to all of these activities, is the direct one-to-one health education that occurs when the child, youth, or parent consults the nurse about a health problem. At this point, because the health problem or concern has been identified, the nurse is in a good position to help the student or parent get into the health care system to receive treatment. If treatment has already been obtained, the nurse may explain the treatment and help the student sort out his feelings about the problem or treatment. The nurse wears the ''hats'' of counselor and educator in this situation.

Participation in the school health education program gives the school nurse an opportunity to emphasize health and wellness rather than disease and illness. The result sought by both the educator and the school nurse is a health-educated young adult who is capable of making responsible decisions regarding health.

CONCLUSION

In this chapter we have presented our philosophy of and beliefs about school nursing. We have discussed the importance of the school health program as part of the overall school program and have proposed a list of roles and goals to guide the school nurse as she participates in planning, implementation, and evaluation of the school health program.

In the next chapter, we will discuss a conceptual framework that the school nurse can use to guide her day-to-day practice as she implements the roles and goals we have presented.

REFERENCES

American School Health Association: 1974. Guidelines for the school nurse in the school health program, American School Health Association, Kent, Ohio.

Scanlan, B. K.: 1974. Management 18: a short course for managers, John Wiley & Sons, Inc., New York.

CHAPTER 3

A framework for practice

SUSAN J. WOLD and NANCY V. DAGG

As a consequence of the broad client system to be served and the duality of the school nurse's expected allegiances (to nursing and to education), school nursing today is a complex clinical practice specialty. The population served by the school nurse includes children of all ages, from preschool through late adolescence. The needs of these children change rapidly as they grow and develop; therefore successful nursing intervention demands that the school nurse have a strong background in growth and development theories, child and adolescent psychology, and pediatrics. The school nurse also addresses herself to the needs of the families of schoolchildren, which may involve some outreach activities such as home visiting. In addition, the school nurse concerns herself with promoting and maintaining the health of school personnel and individuals or groups in the surrounding community through activities such as health education programs, screening clinics, and immunization clinics. Serving a broad client group requires her to have sufficient flexibility to adapt her approach for a variety of clients.

The practice of school nursing is further complicated by the duality of allegiances inherent in the term ''school nursing.'' The fact that she practices in the *school* requires that the school nurse be committed to the goals and philosophy of the educational program offered. This in turn requires that she have an adequate background in educational theories and instructional philosophies and methodologies so she can contribute effectively to the achievement of the school's educational mission. However, she is constantly reminded that she is first and foremost a *nurse* and that she must therefore retain a strong allegiance to the nursing camp. Unfortunately, this division of her loyalties is often compounded by the conflicting expectations imposed on her by nursing and education. Each profession, it seems, believes she should be *more* concerned with their particular mission and *less* concerned with that of the other group. This conflict becomes more overt when the school nurse finds herself accountable to both camps. An example of this is the school nurse who reports not only to the principal in the school building, whose primary concern is the *education* of the children in that school, but also reports to the district's school nursing supervisor, whose primary concern is the *health* of the children being educated in that school. This ''dual boss'' situation is a clear violation of the ''unity of command'' principle of management, which provides that an employee be accountable to only one superior. All too often the result of this territorial battle is that the school nurse is unable to effectively meet the expectations of *either* group.

As if the complexities of a broad client system and conflicting dual professional allegiances are not sufficiently challenging for the school nurse, the proposed roles and goals for the practice of school nursing are so comprehensive that they are at times overwhelming. Implementation of the roles and goals presented in Chapter 2 requires not only a tremendously broad knowledge and experiential base, but it also requires some way of effectively *applying* knowledge and skills to actual practice.

The purpose of this chapter is to present a conceptual framework that we believe provides an effective means for the school nurse to organize her knowledge and skills so as to more readily apply them within her daily practice. By using a conceptual framework to structure her practice, the school nurse can more adequately implement her roles and goals. The conceptual framework that we propose grew out of our philosophy of school nursing. Although there have been other conceptual frameworks developed for the practice of nursing, we have found this particular framework to be most compatible with our beliefs, and we think it provides a viable structure for the practice of school nursing.

In the remainder of this chapter we will:
1. Define ''conceptual framework'' and ''concepts''
2. Discuss the five strands of our framework, including a definition of each, our rationale for incorporating that strand into our framework, and example(s) illustrating the application of the concepts to school nursing practice

CONCEPTUAL FRAMEWORK AND CONCEPTS

By definition, a conceptual framework is a cluster of concepts that relate to a particular phenomenon or discipline. This cluster or grouping of ideas provides a frame of reference to help clarify one's thinking and to focus one's behaviors or actions. A conceptual framework is made up of individual strands or *concepts,* which Aldous (1972:4) defines as useful ideas that ''. . . enable man to learn from experience, to identify current events, to behave appropriately, and to study systematically such phenomena . . .'' as school nursing. The number of concepts in a given framework can be few or many, at the discretion of those who devise it. The particular concepts selected for inclusion in a conceptual framework represent the philosophy and value system of the individuals who have developed it; thus there is no one ''right''

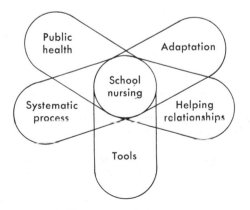

Fig. 3-1. Conceptual framework model for school nursing. Area where the five concepts or strands overlap constitutes the scope and focus of school nursing.

framework in an absolute sense of the word.

Based on our philosophy of school nursing (Chapter 2), we have chosen these five strands as the basis for our school nursing framework: public health, adaptation, helping relationships, tools, and systematic process (Fig. 3-1). In this chapter, we will demonstrate the relevance of these concepts to the practice of school nursing and provide examples illustrating their application.

SCHOOL NURSING CONCEPTUAL FRAMEWORK
Public health

In the first two chapters we noted that the origins of school nursing are directly related to public health. For that reason, we believe strongly that school nurses should consider themselves public health nurses and should practice accordingly. Specifically, this means that school nurses need a working knowledge of public health theory.

In its broadest sense, public health may be thought of as ''. . . a continuum of activities to protect the health of the community'' (Rapoport, 1965:129). Leavell and Clark (1965:20) have organized these activities into the following three levels:
1. *Primary prevention,* which includes health promotion and specific protection (Chapter 4)
2. *Secondary prevention,* which includes early diagnosis, prompt treatment, and disability limitation (Chapter 5)
3. *Tertiary prevention,* which focuses primarily on rehabilitation (Chapter 6)

When public health practice and nursing practice are synthesized, the result is *community health nursing* (ANA, 1973), or *public health nursing.* Public health nursing as a specialty area is further characterized by its community focus. The community as a whole is considered to be the nurse's client system, whether the actual unit of service is the community at large, subgroups of the community, families, or individuals. The public health nurse does not restrict her services to clients of particular age groups or diagnostic categories. Rather, she is concerned with all aspects of the community's health and offers comprehensive services that emphasize distributive or preventive care rather than episodic illness-related care. The public health nurse further demonstrates her commitment to promoting and preserving the health of the community by becoming involved in comprehensive health planning and in the legislative process on issues that affect the community's health and well-being.

The school population is a subgroup or subsystem of the total community. In health-related areas, this relationship of the school subsystem to the community system means that a change in health status of either one (the school or total community) will affect the other. For example, an outbreak of measles or rubella within the school population threatens the health status of the entire community and requires the full cooperation of the citizens. Because of this interdependent relationship between the school population and the overall community, the school nurse must retain her identity as a public health nurse or community health nurse. In other words, in all her actions on behalf of the consumer, whether the consumer is an individual, a family, school personnel, or others, the school nurse must consider the level of prevention needed and must also be certain that all relevant persons and groups are included in her planned interventions.

The following examples demonstrate the applicability of public health concepts to the practice of school nursing. At the primary prevention level, an immunization program illustrates both health promotion and specific protection activities. Successful implementation of any immunization program for schoolchildren requires active coordination of the efforts of all involved personnel by the school nurse in planning, implementation, and follow-up (including delegation of appropriate tasks) (Table 3-1).

At the secondary prevention level, the school nurse conducts various screening programs such as vision, hearing, and scoliosis. In each program the nurse is involved with planning, implementation, and follow-up activities. Although the primary recipient in these screening programs is the child, the family and community are also involved. The nurse initiates contact with the family when deviations are noted and facilitates their referral to existing community resources for necessary follow-up. In the event that no resource is readily available for such follow-up (a fact that should be known before the screening program is initiated), the public health–oriented school nurse will intervene at the community level to stimulate appropriate agencies or groups to develop a resource.

At the tertiary prevention level, the school nurse facilitates the positive adaptation of a handicapped child in the school setting. She coordinates the care of the child with input from school personnel, the family, and other health care providers such as the child's primary physician. She provides for special class schedule changes, rest, nutrition, medication, and treatment needs during the school day. She counsels the child, his peers, and school personnel to enhance his acceptance within the school environment. She also advises school personnel regarding necessary modifications of the physical plant such as the addition of ramps, handrails, and rest rooms. To ensure continuity of care between the school and home, she makes home visits as needed for assessment, counseling, and emotional support.

Adaptation

Adaptation is a concept that has been used and defined by many authors. For our purposes,

Table 3-1. The school-based immunization program: activities for the school nurse as health team coordinator

Planning	Implementation	Follow-up
Consults with local health department officials, school administrators, and community representatives in setting goals, objectives, and means Promotes successful achievement of goals and objectives through health education with children, families, school personnel, and community	Works with school administrators and families to identify specific immunization needs for school children Orders or delegates ordering of supplies Coordinates clinic: recruits and orients volunteers, sets up clinic routing patterns Screens community recipients regarding immunization needs and contraindications Manages emergency situations	Records immunizations Reads and records results of tuberculin testing Monitors reactions Refers clients to other community resources for completion of immunization schedule Participates in evaluation of program's goals and objectives

the most useful definition is that advanced by Byrne and Thompson (1972:22), which states that *adaptation* is ". . . the positive, constructive end results . . . that occur when adjustments are made to either an internal or external environmental change." Since adaptation focuses on the positive, constructive results of one's interaction with his environment, it is a useful concept for the public health–oriented school nurse.

Byrne and Thompson (1972:40) suggest that the nurse focus on the orderliness, consistency, and coherency of clients' behaviors as a means of assessing adaptation. Specifically, they suggest that the following questions be addressed:

1. What are the limitations with which the client must cope?
2. To what degree is he utilizing the potential of which he is capable?
3. How does the client view or evaluate his situation?
4. What are the environmental resources available to him and how can they be utilized more effectively?

In applying this concept to school nursing practice, an appropriate example to consider is that of the diabetic child leaving an elementary school and entering a junior high school. Because of hourly classroom changes, the child will face expanded peer group influences and varied teacher expectations. In addition to these external environmental changes, the child must cope daily with internal changes resulting from the developmental tasks that confront him as an adolescent. The child's need for a structured diabetic management regimen is threatened by these new needs. By using Byrne and Thompson's four questions, the child's past behavior and new needs can be reordered into a new regimen compatible with his physical requirements, social needs, and new school environment.

In this example, it is the responsibility of the school nurse to anticipate and plan for these necessary changes by consulting and communicating with the child, his family, involved school personnel (including the school nurse from his former school), and physician as needed.

Helping relationships

Like other helping professions, such as medicine, social work, and guidance counseling, nursing is concerned with "people problems." This requires nursing practitioners to focus on ". . . helping people achieve more effective relationships between themselves and others or the world in which they live" (Combs et al., 1971:3). Such a focus is consistent with the adaptation frame of reference just discussed (and in Chapters 7 to 9) and with our belief that the goal of nursing is the promotion of health for the client system.

Successful intervention by the nurse in promoting the client's health depends on the establishment of an effective *helping relationship,* which may be defined as ". . . the effective use of the helper's self in bringing about fulfillment of his own and society's purposes" (Combs et al., 1971:6). According to this definition, the effectiveness of the relationship depends on the nurse's ability to use her "self" as an instrument or tool. How she does this will depend on her beliefs about herself as a person and as a "helper," her beliefs about the client, her beliefs about nursing as a profession, and her beliefs about the nature and purposes of humans and society. Although there are many "techniques" that can be learned to assist an individual in becoming a "helping person," such as interviewing and listening techniques, establishing a truly "helping" relationship requires an attitude of the helper, which Rogers (1969) describes as genuineness or "realness." This means simply that the helper is "being himself" in his encounters with the client and is avoiding any facade which could jeopardize the relationship.

The ability to establish and maintain helping relationships is of obvious importance for the school nurse. The school nurse is generally viewed as a helping person who, unlike the teachers and administrative personnel in the school, has no direct authority or control over the students' lives; therefore the school nurse can be a trusted adult to assist students with their problems. However, her effectiveness depends on her ability to assess needs, plan interventions, and evaluate the outcome based on the establishment of a helping relationship.

A real challenge to the school nurse's helping relationship skills might be posed by the pregnant adolescent who confides her fears and uncertainties about pregnancy to the nurse. Development of a helping relationship in this instance requires first of all that the nurse be in touch with her own feelings and beliefs regarding unwed pregnancy so that she can be nonjudgmental, or "real." Having worked through her feelings about the student's pregnancy, the school nurse should be able to develop rapport and trust so that a realistic contract can be negotiated. This contract might reasonably include the psychological support of the student in telling her family about the pregnancy, referral of the student to appropriate community resources for pregnancy testing and follow-up, facilitation of the student's problem solving by helping her identify and sort out her alternatives, and communication of the outcome of this planning to the appropriate school personnel.

Tools

The fourth concept in this framework's cluster is *tools.* According to Webster's a tool is ". . . an instrument or apparatus . . . necessary in the practice of a vocation or profession." Nurses use tools to assess clients' needs, adaptation, and level of wellness. Their tools include history taking, systematic assessment of functional areas, and nursing diagnosis (Murray and Zentner, 1975) as well as apparatus such as audiometers, sphygmomanometers, and otoscopes. The format used for collecting and recording a health history or determining a nursing diagnosis will vary according to the educational preparation, professional work experience, and nursing philosophy of the individual practitioner. Systematic assessment of the functional areas may be accomplished using empirically tested tools or tools developed by the nurse herself within her practice setting.

An example of the school nurse's use of tools is reflected in her role functions at a preschool screening clinic. She might use a locally developed health inventory, an empirically tested tool such as the Denver Developmental Screening Test, as well as apparatus for testing visual and auditory acuity. If health problems are identified as a result of using these tools, she may use a structured or nonstructured interview format to gather data for a health history. The child's completed physical examination form and the nursing history provide the data base for determining a nursing diagnosis. The diagnosis in turn generates a plan for follow-up to facilitate the child's adaptation to kindergarten.

Systematic process

The last concept or strand included in this framework is *systematic process,* which Webster's defines as a methodical series of actions or operations employed for the achievement of specific results. Use of such a process ensures a holistic and comprehensive approach for identifying and meeting the nursing needs of clients. Many systematic processes are directly ap-

plicable to the practice of nursing, including the following:

1. Nursing process
2. Contract-setting process
3. Health education process
4. Research process
5. Epidemiological process
6. Administrative/management process
7. Planned change process
8. Legislative process

These processes may be used singly, consecutively, or concurrently, depending on the situation. An example of the multiple use of these processes might be an outbreak of rubeola (red measles) in an elementary school population. Initially, the school nurse would be confronted by a small number of children with vague symptoms such as fever, rhinitis, and malaise. Her use of the nursing process would begin with physical examination skills (tools) and interviewing techniques (helping relationships) to obtain a nursing *assessment.* The assessment would become the basis for her *intervention,* which would involve exclusion from school of the ill children and health teaching for parents about symptomatic treatment and the importance of medical follow-up. When her subsequent *evaluation* reveals an increased incidence of rubeola, she will need to employ epidemiological investigative techniques to identify the reservoir of the infection. Once identified, those students who constitute the reservoir would also be excluded from school. The nurse would need to use the health education process with school personnel, children, and families to explain the etiology and control of the disease and to encourage specific protection such as immunization for the susceptible population within the school, family, and community. If the number of susceptible individuals is sufficiently large, it may be advisable to plan and conduct an immunization clinic, which would require use of the administrative/management process.

CONCLUSION

Today's school nurse faces a crisis that her predecessors could not have envisioned. A review of nursing history reveals that for about 50 years the school nurse played an important role in maintaining optimum health within the school population. Her contributions to the success of the school health program were universally recognized and highly valued. The biggest problem facing many of these early school nurses was finding ways to increase their ranks sufficiently so that the nurse-pupil ratio could be improved, thus enabling them to continue and expand their services within the school. As we explained in Chapter 1, the school nurse's position within the school has been increasingly challenged in recent years. The result is that the major problem confronting today's school nurse is *survival*.

Therefore today's school nurse must be prepared to explain and defend her practice and skills and to document her unique contributions to the school health program and the school community. The consistent, conscientious application of the conceptual framework presented in this chapter provides the school nurse with the basis for effectively articulating, documenting, and communicating her interventions and their outcomes, so that she can survive the budgetary cutbacks that threaten the continued existence of school nursing.

REFERENCES

Aldous, J.: 1972. The developmental approach to family analysis. Vol. 1: The conceptual framework, University of Minnesota, Minneapolis.

American Nurses' Association: 1973. Standards: community health nursing practice, ANA, Kansas City, Mo.

Byrne, M. L., and Thompson, L. F.: 1972. Key concepts for the study and practice of nursing, The C. V. Mosby Co., St. Louis.

Combs, A. W., Avila, D. L., and Purkey, W. W.: 1971. Helping relationships: basic concepts for the helping professions, Allyn & Bacon, Inc., Boston.

Leavell, H. R., and Clark, E. G.: 1965. Preventive medicine for the doctor in his community, McGraw-Hill Book Co., New York.

Murray, R., and Zentner, J.: 1975. Nursing concepts for health promotion, Prentice-Hall, Inc., Englewood Cliffs, N.J.

Rapoport, L.: 1965. Working with families in crisis: an exploration in preventive intervention. In Parad, H. J., editor: Crisis intervention: selected readings, Family Service Association of America, New York.

Rogers, C. R.: 1969. Freedom to learn, Charles E. Merrill Publishing Co., Columbus, Ohio.

PART II

Public health concepts in school nursing practice

CHAPTER 4

Primary prevention: health promotion and specific protection

NANCY V. DAGG

The public health strand of the conceptual framework (Chapter 3) gives the school nurse two general concepts that provide the foundation for her public health nursing practice: *prevention of disease or injury* and *promotion of health*. It is important to understand what is meant by each of these concepts before examining the three levels of prevention in Chapters 4 to 6.

DEFINITION OF CONCEPTS

According to Leavell and Clark (1965:19), prevention at any level of application, primary, secondary, or tertiary, is related to the natural history of the disorder, disease, or injury. This fits with Webster's definition of prevention: "the act of coming before, anticipating, or forestalling." Therefore "levels of prevention" refer to specific interventions at various points or times in the natural history of a disease or injury (Fig. 4-1).

Levels of prevention

Prevention may be accomplished in the period before a person is diseased by interventions designed to promote optimum health, by specific protection measures against the disease agent, or the establishment of a disease agent barrier in the environment. Prevention by either of these methods, health promotion or specific protection, is *primary prevention*.

When the disease process is established in humans, either in the subclinical state or the clinical state, *secondary prevention* may be accomplished through early diagnosis and by prompt, adequate treatment. Through early intervention and treatment, the disease process may be halted, or the negative consequences of the disease or accident may be lessened. Secondary prevention is more closely associated with episodic care and is what many people associate with medical or health care.

Tertiary prevention deals with disease or accident outcomes. If a person is left with a defect or disability, rehabilitation is needed. Rehabilitation is more than stopping a disease process; it is the prevention of complete disability after the anatomical and physiological changes are stabilized. The goal of tertiary prevention is to return the affected person to a useful place in society, with maximum use of remaining capabilities or abilities (Leavell and Clark, 1965).

Fig. 4-2 summarizes the relationship of the levels of prevention to the disease process in humans. There are actually five phases in the continuum of prevention. These phases are not static or isolated; they correspond to and can be compared to the natural history of the disease.

Primary prevention: specific protection and health promotion

Prevention at any level of application is based on the premise that any disorder, disease, or accident may have multiple causes related to host, agent, and environmental factors. Health is a dynamic process—the host, agent, and environment are constantly interacting. Whether prevention does or does not occur depends on whether the causes can be intercepted or counteracted. Specific protection measures, such as immunizations or attention to personal hygiene, intercept or counteract the disease agent before the disease process is established in humans. Environmental barriers can also block the disease process. In general, prevention strategies at all three levels are directed toward persons under some specific stress or risk.

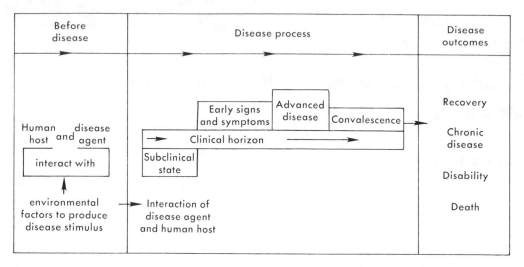

Fig. 4-1. Disease process in man. (Modified from Leavell, H. R., and Clark, E. G.: 1965. Preventive medicine for the doctor in his community: an epidemiological approach, 3rd ed., McGraw-Hill, Inc., New York.)

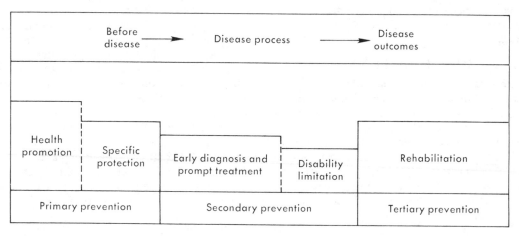

Fig. 4-2. Relationship of levels of prevention to natural history of disease. (Modified from Leavell, H. R., and Clark, E. G.: 1965. Preventive medicine for the doctor in his community: an epidemiological approach, 3rd ed., McGraw-Hill, Inc., New York.)

In contrast to specific protection measures, health promotion strategies are not directed at specific diseases, disorders, or accidents. Rather, health promotion strategies are directed toward the general population and situations of normal growth and development (McPheeters, 1976). This is a basic difference between disease prevention and health promotion. Disease prevention focuses on ill or soon to be ill people, whereas health promotion focuses on well people.

Promotion of health is further defined using the continuum of health illustrated in Fig. 4-3. The illness portion of the continuum of health represents the natural history of disease discussed earlier. On this continuum, health is referred to as the "absence of disease signs and symptoms," which is how health is generally viewed in our culture. The concept "health" is often described in philosophical terms that are difficult to grasp or measure. The Preamble to the Constitution of the World Health Organiza-

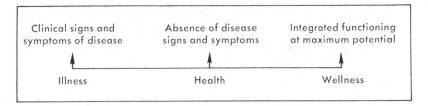

Fig. 4-3. Continuum of health.

tion defined health as a "state of complete physical, mental, and social well-being, and not merely the absence of disease or infirmity" (Dunn, 1961:1). Although this definition emphasizes a positive direction for health, it needs expansion if it is to be used as a guide or measurement of health promotion. Dubos (1959) presents a more practical and useful "health" definition when he states that health is the manner in which humans adapt.

The concept "promotion of health" implies that there are levels or degrees of health or adaptation. Dunn (1961) coined the term *high-level wellness* to represent the optimal level of integrated functioning. Dunn's definition is also abstract and philosophical. How can "optimal level of integrated functioning" be measured or assessed? One way to approach an assessment of optimal functioning is through an examination of the developmental stage and age-specific developmental tasks for each child or adult. This is a practical way to measure optimal integrated functioning or wellness. In this chapter, the terms promotion of health and promotion of wellness are used interchangeably.

The preceding distinctions between prevention of disease and promotion of health provide the principles on which prevention strategies and health promotion programs are built. The school nurse selects target populations for specific prevention interventions and selects different strategies to promote health in the general school population. The remainder of this chapter will apply and expand these concepts in the school setting. Second, this chapter will relate primary prevention strategies to developmental stages and tasks of school-age children; the school nurse can use this information to begin assessing the "level of wellness" in individual children. Finally, the primary prevention challenges for the school nurse and school health team, whose work in primary prevention has just barely begun, will be discussed.

THE SCOPE OF PRIMARY PREVENTION IN THE SCHOOL

The school community is composed of students, teachers, administrators, other professional staff, and support staff such as secretaries, cooks, janitors, bus drivers, and volunteers. Indirectly, students' families might also be included as part of the school community. When all of these are included, no other community setting even approximates the magnitude of the school setting in providing a captive audience in which health can be given educational emphasis during the impressionable childhood years. The school has both the opportunity and the social mandate to produce "health-educated young adults." It also has a professional commitment: the NEA recently reaffirmed health as the primary objective of education (Jerrick, 1978).

Unfortunately, there is no strong constituency demanding primary prevention in the school setting. Adults usually react to health concerns when they are ill or confronted with illness. In general, the majority of the school-age population is healthy, that is, without signs or symptoms of illness. Therefore adults in the schools do not routinely focus on the future health consequences of their students. Presently, schools are being asked to respond to and provide solutions for complex social problems. Primary prevention strategies, including both specific protection and health promotion, can and should be part of the approach used to find solutions or alternatives to personal and community health problems.

Specific protection in the school

Specific health protection measures are applicable to both diseases and injuries. These measures are designed to intercept causes of the disease or accident before they affect humans. In the school setting, immunization programs are the most obvious example of specific health

---

AMERICAN ACADEMY OF PEDIATRICS
RECOMMENDED SCHEDULE FOR ACTIVE IMMUNIZATION
OF NORMAL INFANTS AND CHILDREN

2 months	DTP*	TOPV†
4 months	DTP	TOPV
6 months	DTP	TOPV‡
1 year		Tuberculin test§
15 months	Measles,‖ rubella‖	Mumps‖
1½ years	DTP	TOPV
4 to 6 years	DTP	TOPV
14 to 16 years	Td¶ —repeat every 10 years	

*DTP—diphtheria and tetanus toxoids combined with pertussis vaccine.

†TOPV—trivalent oral poliovirus vaccine. This recommendation is suitable for breast-fed as well as bottle-fed infants.

‡A third dose of TOPV is optional but may be given in areas of high endemicity of poliomyelitis.

§Frequency of repeated tuberculin tests depends on risk of exposure of the child and on the prevalence of tuberculosis in the population group. For the pediatrician's office or outpatient clinic, an annual or biennial tuberculin test, unless local circumstances clearly indicate otherwise, is appropriate. The initial test should be done at the time of, or preceding, the measles immunization.

‖May be given at 15 months as measles-rubella or measles-mumps-rubella combined vaccines.

¶Td—combined tetanus and diphtheria toxoids (adult type) for those more than 6 years of age, in contrast to diphtheria and tetanus (DT) toxoids which contain a larger amount of diphtheria antigen. *Tetanus toxoid at time of injury:* For clean, minor wounds, no booster dose is needed by a fully immunized child unless more than 10 years have elapsed since the last dose. For contaminated wounds, a booster dose should be given if more than 5 years have elapsed since the last dose.

□ Copyright American Academy of Pediatrics 1977. American Academy of Pediatrics: 1977. Report of the committee on infectious diseases, American Academy of Pediatrics, Evanston, Ill.

---

protection against disease. Mumps, measles, rubella, polio, diphtheria, pertussis, and tetanus are all preventable by administration of a series of immunizations that can be given according to the American Academy of Pediatrics schedule (1977) (see above).

In states requiring these immunizations for school entry, the school nurse may supervise a health record audit of new students and may exclude unprotected students until they begin their immunization series. In states without mandatory immunization laws, immunizations can be encouraged by making them available at preschool roundup sessions. Some school districts have obtained standing orders that authorize the school nurse to give required immunizations on written authorization by the parent. What works in one community may not meet the needs of another community; each school health team needs to be familiar with state health laws and design an immunization program to meet the assessed need.

Other examples of specific protection strat-

egies are given in Table 4-1. History has shown that the most effective strategies are those which require the least personal cost and effort—usually strategies directed toward the environment (McPheeters, 1976). A fluoridated city water supply can help to significantly reduce dental caries without individual effort or cost. Although a public health–sponsored school-wide fluoride mouth rinse program in rural areas without fluoridated water supplies can accomplish the same outcome, more effort and cost are involved in the mouth rinse program. A successful mouth rinse program requires that a public health dentist or dental hygienist convince the school administration that the improved oral health of their student population will occur with minimal time spent by teachers in the classroom. Next, parents have to be informed and give their consent. Third, the hygienist needs to demonstrate mouth rinsing and then to monitor the program throughout the year.

Another example of controlling the environ-

Table 4-1. Specific protection prevention strategies

Strategy	Health problems	Target population
Dietary restrictions	Disease or metabolic disorders	Diabetics; children with malabsorption problems
Removal of environmental health hazards	Carcinogens	Smokers; schools with asbestos ceilings
Seasonal play restrictions	Asthmatic attacks or seasonal allergies	Children with asthma or respiratory allergies
Fluoride mouth rinse programs	Dental caries	Children whose homes do not have a fluoridated water supply
Safety programs	Accidents and injuries	Children who walk to school; all children who ride bikes; teenagers learning to drive automobiles, mopeds, and motorcycles
Referral for medical care	Chronic disease such as rheumatic fever or nephritis	Children with possible streptococcal infections
Venereal disease education and treatment programs	Spread of venereal disease; sterility and infertility	Sexually active teenagers
Poison prevention programs	Accidental ingestion	All elementary schoolchildren
Exclusion from school	Communicable diseases	Children exhibiting signs and symptoms of communicable diseases

ment is the school playground. It is far easier to control the environment on the school playground by selecting safe play equipment than by teaching children how to use or not to use certain equipment. It is also easier to control the physical school environment to minimize noise and distractions than it is to work with disruptive behavior problems. Some of the following questions should be asked about each school building:

1. Are class sizes appropriate for the space provided?
2. Does the school provide quiet individual activity as well as group activity?
3. Can the temperature of each room be controlled for comfort?

These physical school environment variables are much easier to address than behavior or discipline problems.

However, most of the examples addressed in Table 4-1 do not deal with environmental interventions because in contemporary school settings, environmental factors are carefully considered. Rather, the school health team is confronted by those variables which do require personal effort on the part of school personnel, parents, and students. As problems or groups at risk are identified, the school health team needs to identify and implement appropriate prevention strategies. The team will need to be creative and innovative as they design programs to meet their specific needs.

Health promotion in the school

Specific protection health strategies are only part of the focus of primary prevention in the school setting. Health promotion strategies are equally important. Health promotion strategies are directed toward well people in routine growth and development situations. The goal of these strategies is to strengthen the adult or student so he can reach a higher level of wellness. Examples of health promotion strategies include health education, food and nutrition programs, income supplementation, programs to strengthen group and family supports, and health supervision such as anticipatory guidance, genetic counseling, and recreation. Health promotion strategies such as those listed are aimed toward sociocultural and behavioral factors that affect health or wellness.

The major thrust of health promotion in the school is health education. The setting may be a formal structured class or it may be the "teachable moment" when a student comes in for first aid or because he's ill. No other community setting comes close to providing the health educational input that grades kindergarten to twelve can provide *if* health is a priority concern in the school curriculum.

Health education is not simply providing health information or a one-time talk on a health education problem such as hygiene, sex, drugs, or alcohol. A National Task Force on Consumer Health Education (Somers, 1976:75) adopted a health education definition that includes the following six activities:

1. Inform people about health, illness, disablity, and ways in which they can improve and protect their own health, including more efficient use of the delivery system
2. Motivate people to want to change to more healthful practices
3. Help them learn the necessary skills to adopt and maintain healthful practices and life-styles
4. Foster teaching and communication skills in all those engaged in educating consumers about health
5. Advocate changes in the environment that will facilitate healthful conditions and healthful behavior
6. Add to knowledge through research and evaluation concerning the most effective ways of achieving these objectives

Stated succinctly, health education is a process linking health information with positive "healthful" behavior changes. Life-styles or health habits are difficult to change and maintain.

Our society is aware of linkages between health behaviors or habits and specific diseases. Table 4-2 demonstrates these behavior-disease linkages. However, although awareness often exists, it is difficult to get children and teenagers who are living in and for the present to change health habits that *may* affect them at some time in the future. Comprehensive health education curricula need to be designed and implemented in all grades to promote positive health habits in nutrition, physical exercise, accident prevention, smoking control, alcohol and drug usage, sex education, dental health, stress reduction, crisis intervention, and the appropriate choice and use of health resources.

Health education should emphasize positive behaviors rather than identify negative behaviors or relationships. Studies from the Human Population Laboratory indicate a strong relationship between daily habits and health and mortality. As outlined by Breslow (1977:247), the following habits are hypothesized to influence health:

1. Eating breakfast
2. Eating regularly (no snacking between meals)
3. Eating moderately (normal weight for height)
4. Not smoking cigarettes
5. Drinking moderately (if at all)
6. Sleeping 7 to 8 hours a night regularly
7. Exercising moderately

These seven habits should be emphasized in school health education programs because they are relevant for all ages and because the earlier these habits are begun and reinforced, the more likely they are to continue as a life-style. Activities that promote normal development or age-specific developmental tasks are worthwhile targets for health promotion strategies. The next section discusses how health promotion strategies can promote optimal functioning or wellness in the preschool, school-age, and adolescent stages by facilitating successful completion of age-specific developmental tasks.

PRIMARY PREVENTION APPLIED TO DEVELOPMENTAL STAGES

According to Erikson (1963), the human life cycle consists of developmental stages that proceed in an ordered sequence. Each stage of psychosocial development proceeds by critical steps or turning points. These critical steps are systematically related to all preceding and later turning points. A delay or acceleration in one stage will influence all subsequent stages. Because development proceeds in an ordered sequence, it is important to know the client's developmental stage as well as chronological age when primary prevention strategies are planned, implemented, and evaluated. The specific strategy and implementation approach should vary according to the developmental stage in the life cycle.

Table 4-2. Linkages between health behaviors and specific diseases

Health behavior	Specific diseases
Cigarette smoking	Lung cancer; emphysema
Overeating and obesity	Heart disease
Iron-deficient diet	Anemia
Overuse of alcohol	Cirrhosis of the liver
Nonuse of seat belts	Automobile accident injuries
Promiscuous sexual behavior	Venereal disease
Early multiple sexual contacts	Cervical cancer
Drug taking	Drug addiction
Use of refined sugar	Dental caries

Table 4-3 reviews the developmental stages of the preschool child, school-age child, and adolescent. Each stage has specific developmental tasks; successful achievement of all the tasks for a given stage results in a positive resolution of the developmental crisis. However, failure to complete developmental tasks at any stage will result in unhappiness, disapproval by society, and difficulty with later tasks (Duvall, 1971). To attain high-level wellness or optimal integrated functioning, an individual must successfully complete developmental tasks along with physical growth. School health education curricula should be structured to augment or complement normal everyday activities so that all children reach their optimal potential.

The preschool child

A brief look at the developmental tasks of preschool children will increase understanding of the expected accomplishments or abilities of children entering school. According to Duvall (1971:260-262), the developmental tasks of the preschool stage are as follows:

1. Settle into a healthful daily routine of rest, activity, and elimination
2. Master good eating habits
3. Develop large- and small-muscle coordination and movement skills
4. Become a participating member of the family
5. Begin to master impulses and conform to parental expectations
6. Develop healthy emotional responses for a wide variety of experiences
7. Communicate effectively with others
8. Develop ability to respond correctly to potentially hazardous situations
9. Use initiative tempered by his own conscience
10. Lay the foundation to understand the meaning of life, the physical world, and the spiritual world

The preschool child begins to reach beyond the family's sphere of influence and establish relationships with others. His curiosity to explore, together with an immature understanding of danger and illness, make him very susceptible to accidental injuries. Specific health protection measures to prevent accidents are very important during this stage of development. In addition, entry into kindergarten greatly increases the preschool child's exposure to communicable diseases; therefore the preschool child needs booster immunizations to ensure protection against diphtheria, pertussis, tetanus, and polio. To promote the health of the preschool child, activities should enhance or encourage the development of social skills, motor skills, internal values, emotional control, and curiosity.

Success with the preschool developmental tasks results in continued initiative or trying new and old tasks to develop competency. "I can't, I can't," sets the stage for decreased exploration. Failure results in guilt and the possible beginnings of a poor self-concept.

The school-age child

At 5 or 6 years of age, the preschool child reaches a developmental milestone: beginning school. Although elementary schoolchildren vary greatly within the range of "normal" physical, mental, and social development, they all face the same developmental crisis: industry versus inferiority (Erikson, 1963). School-age children risk a sense of inferiority if they experience repeated failure. As children experience success, they develop their capacity to enjoy work and play.

The developmental tasks of this stage include reinforcing and reworking the preschool tasks

Table 4-3. Developmental stage and crisis by age

Stage	Chronological age	Developmental crisis*
Preschool	2 to 5 years	Initiative versus guilt
Schoolchild		
Juvenile	6 to 9 or 10 years	Industry versus inferiority
Preadolescent	9 or 10 years to ?	
Adolescence	12 years to ? years	Identity versus role confusion
Adulthood	Not clearly defined, usually high school or college graduation	Intimacy versus isolation

*Modified from Erikson, E. H.: 1963. Childhood and society, W. W. Norton & Co., Inc., New York.

plus accomplishing specific new tasks. The school-age developmental tasks (Duvall, 1971: 289-291) are as follows:

1. Mastering basic fundamental skills and a rational approach for problem solving
2. Developing concepts and reasoning abilities for everyday adult living
3. Mastering age-appropriate physical and self-care skills
4. Developing a socially accepted understanding of money: how to get it, how to spend it, and how to save it
5. Assuming an active, responsible, cooperative role within the family
6. Relating effectively to peers and other adults outside the family, that is, making and keeping friends
7. Handling feelings, emotions, and impulses appropriately
8. Learning age-appropriate sex behaviors and adjusting to prepubertal body changes
9. Developing self-respect for one's own behavior and individuality
10. Developing loyalties to religion, culture, moral values, and social institutions
11. Accepting the eternal realities of birth, death, and infinity

Success with these tasks depends on the opportunities the child has in the family, school, and community and also requires that adults recognize developmental readiness and then encourage the child's attempts to master these tasks. It is crucial that opportunities are provided which are within the child's capability.

Specific protection activities for school-age children include those already mentioned in the preschool section. Because of increasing skills and risk taking to test those skills, safety programs need to be geared toward emerging physical abilities. Survival skills such as swimming, traffic safety, and wearing seat belts are an important part of learning to take care of oneself. Children with chronic or communicable illnesses need individualized nursing assessments and interventions to meet their identified health needs.

Health promotion activities include providing adequate exercise, rest, and nutrition. However, the main emphasis is not merely on physical skills. Social skills, cognitive abilities, and self-concept development should also have an equal emphasis. The school health team needs to structure the health education curriculum so that social skills development and self-concept

development are given equal consideration or time when compared with physical skills and cognitive development.

In addition, the health education class should not be limited to a survey of information about health and disease; rather, it should help elementary schoolchildren identify their own health needs and make decisions about their own health. What many children have learned about health in the past has been abstract and difficult to apply to their lives. The desired outcome is for children to take action to maintain their health and prevent illness (self-care). If they are ill, children should know what to do or from whom to seek help both at home and at school.

Health values, health habits, and behavior patterns established during this stage form the basis for adult life-styles. If positive health behaviors are absent, modeling by teachers and reinforcement by peers can help to shape positive health habits in schoolchildren. Promoting optimal growth and shaping positive health behaviors will contribute to successful resolution of the industry versus inferiority developmental crisis.

The adolescent

With the establishment of an initial relationship to the world of skills and tools (industry) and with the onset of puberty, childhood ends and adolescence, or the teenage stage, begins. Rapid body changes and new sexual maturity cause a questioning of self, accepted beliefs, and ways of doing things. Developmental tasks completed earlier are reworked and reevaluated. The developmental crisis of the adolescent stage is identity versus role confusion (Erikson, 1963). The reintegration of self or successful resolution of the crisis results in identity formation. Erikson (1963:261) states that identity is the "confidence that the inner sameness and continuity prepared in the past are matched by sameness and continuity of one's meaning for others. . . ." In contrast, failure results in role confusion. Continued uncertainty about one's lifework or frequent changes in occupations and jobs during the adult stage are indicators that role confusion persists during adulthood.

To resolve the identity formation versus role confusion developmental crisis, the following tasks need to be accomplished (Duvall, 1971: 325-327):

1. Accepting one's changing body and learning to use it effectively
2. Achieving a satisfying and socially accepted masculine or feminine role
3. Finding oneself as a member of one's own generation and establishing mature relations with peers
4. Achieving emotional independence of parents and other adults
5. Selecting and preparing for an occupation and economic independence
6. Preparing for marriage and family life
7. Developing intellectual skills and social sensitivities necessary for civic competence
8. Developing a workable philosophy of life that makes sense in today's world

It should be noted that Table 4-3 does not list a chronological age for the end of the adolescent stage. Some adolescents remain in this stage for an extended period, especially if they continue to be financially supported by their parents through college and graduate school. Regardless of how long this stage lasts, there are important achievements during this time. Family, friends, school, and other social institutions provide feedback regarding the adolescent's physical, social, and psychological changes. If an adolescent establishes economic independence and gets married, society expects him to behave as an adult. Whether the remainder of the developmental tasks have or have not been accomplished, the adolescent is thrust into a new place in society.

Prevention strategies can be applied to numerous adolescent health problems: motor vehicle accidents, drowning, football and sport injuries, obesity, acne, pregnancy, venereal disease, drug abuse, and suicide (Murray and Zentner, 1975). Specific protection strategies such as driver education can be implemented to prevent accidents. Venereal diseases can be treated. Contraceptives can provide an alternative to an unplanned pregnancy and possible abortion. Sex education and responsible sexual behavior can prevent these problems related to sexual activity. Dietary regimens may be prescribed for acne and obesity problems. It is hoped that primary prevention health promotion activities at earlier stages can prevent or reduce the number or severity of these health problems.

Health promotion activities for this stage should continue to emphasize positive health values, health habits, and life-styles. Health education classes should introduce teenagers to alternative sources of "highs," such as yoga, meditation, and exercises, rather than pointing out the pitfalls of chemical highs. The school health education curriculum should continue to emphasize the development of personal health decisions and self-care. Adolescents should be allowed to structure minihealth courses to meet their perceived health needs. Increased responsibility for determining health needs is imperative if students are to become self-sufficient health-educated young adults.

THE SCHOOL HEALTH TEAM'S CHALLENGE

The school health team faces challenges in all three areas of prevention. Primary prevention simultaneously presents unique problems and unique opportunities. The scope of problems is broad, and there is no specific protocol or specific cookbook approach that will meet the needs of every school. Health team members must identify health needs, know their community resources, know their state laws and school regulations, and develop primary prevention activities and strategies to meet their needs. In addition, the school health team needs to evaluate the school health curriculum. Each school should have a comprehensive integrated health education plan for grades kindergarten to twelve.

The goals of the school health team should be to establish healthful behavior practices in all students. This will require informing the students, motivating them to change or adopt healthy behaviors, and then reinforcing or modeling healthy behaviors. The result will be "health-educated young adults" who can identify their health needs and who know the community resources so they can get help for their health problems.

The school health team has the added responsibility of being an advocate for environmental changes in the school and community. Environmental changes in the school, such as class sizes, noise level, and temperature, can have an impact on the physical and emotional health of the students.

Last, it is important for the school health team to document their successes and failures and to evaluate their health programs so schools can learn from each other, and existing primary prevention programs can be strengthened. The challenges are present in all schools—they have not yet been met.

REFERENCES

American Academy of Pediatrics: 1977. Report of the committee on infectious diseases, American Academy of Pediatrics, Evanston, Ill.

Breslow, L.: 1977. A policy assessment of preventive health practice, Prev. Med. 6(2):242-251.

Dubos, R.: 1959. Mirage of health, Anchor Books, Garden City, New York.

Dunn, H. L.: 1961. High level wellness, R. W. Beatty Co., Arlington, Va.

Duvall, E. M.: 1971. Family development, J. B. Lippincott Co., Philadelphia.

Erikson, E. H.: 1963. Childhood and society, W. W. Norton & Co., Inc., New York.

Jerrick, S. J.: 1978. Mental health in schools, J. School Health 48(9):559-563.

Leavell, H. R., and Clark, E. G.: 1965. Preventive medicine for the doctor in his community: an epidemiological approach, 3rd ed., McGraw-Hill Book Co., New York.

McPheeters, H. L.: 1976. Primary prevention and health promotion in mental health, Prev. Med. 5(1):187-198.

Murray, R., and Zentner, J.: 1975. Nursing assessment and health promotion through the life span, Prentice-Hall, Inc., Englewood Cliffs, N.J.

Somers, A. R., editor: 1976. Promoting health: consumer education and national policy, Aspen Systems Corp., Germantown, Md.

SUGGESTED READINGS

Bruhn, J. G., and Cordova, F. D.; 1977. A developmental approach to learning wellness behavior. Part I: Infancy to early adolescence, Health Values: Achieving High-Level Wellness 1(6):246-254.

Bruhn, J. G., and Cordova, F. D.: 1978. A developmental approach to learning wellness behavior. Part II: Adolescence to maturity, Health Values: Achieving High-Level Wellness 2(1):16-21.

Bruhn, J. G., Cordova, F. D., Williams, J. A., and Fuentes, R. G., Jr.: 1977. The wellness process, J. Community Health 2(3):209-221.

Gellman, D. D., Lachaine, R., and Law, M. M.: 1977. The Canadian approach to health policies and programs, Prev. Med. 6(2):265-275.

Haggerty, R. J.: 1977. Changing lifestyles to improve health, Prev. Med. 6(2):276-289.

James, G.: 1972. Preventive medicine: management of the disease process, Prev. Med. 1(1):6-9.

Kiefer, N.: 1973. Accidents—the foremost problem in preventive medicine, Prev. Med. 2(1):106-122.

Kristein, M. M.: 1977. Economic issues in prevention, Prev. Med. 6(2):252-264.

Lee, P. R., and Franks, P. E.: 1977. Primary prevention and the executive branch of the federal goverment, Prev. Med. 6(2):209-226.

Lindsay, G. M.: 1978. Implications of Piagetian theory for health education, Health Values: Achieving High-Level Wellness 2(2):68-73.

Nader, P. R., editor: 1979. School-related health care, Report of the Ninth Ross Roundtable on Critical Approaches to Common Pediatric Problems, Columbus, Ohio.

Taintor, Z. C.: 1976. What the schools can do to promote mental health, J. School Health 46(2):86-90.

Wallace, H. M., and Oglesby, A. C.: 1972. Preventive aspects of maternal and child health, Prev. Med. 1(4): 554-558.

CHAPTER 5

Secondary prevention: theoretical and ethical issues

SUSAN J. WOLD

As discussed in Chapter 4, primary prevention is the preferred intervention level for school nurses and other health professionals. However, primary prevention efforts do not always succeed and in some situations effective primary prevention strategies may not exist. Therefore secondary or perhaps tertiary prevention measures may need to be initiated. In the remainder of this chapter, secondary prevention will be discussed with particular attention focused on screening and the role of the school nurse.* Tertiary prevention is discussed in Chapter 6.

SECONDARY PREVENTION: A DEFINITION

According to Leavell and Clark (1965), secondary prevention activities are divided into two categories: (1) early diagnosis and prompt treatment and (2) disability limitation. The goal of early detection and prompt treatment is to detect the disease process early in pathogenesis and apply prompt and effective treatment to cure or arrest the disease process so that sequelae can be avoided or at least minimized. If the disease in question is communicable, such as syphilis, secondary prevention is important not only as a means of preventing complications for the identified patient but also as a means of preventing the spread of the disease to others.

If detection of disease is delayed until the

disease process is more clinically advanced, then secondary prevention activities initiated are necessarily focused on *disability limitation.* Prevention efforts at this level are primarily therapeutic and directed toward the host to prevent further disability or sequelae. The need for intervention at this stage clearly indicates failure of prevention efforts earlier in the natural history of the disease.

Obviously, the success of a secondary prevention program depends on early detection of disease so that treatment can be initiated before the disease has progressed beyond the earliest detectable stage. As defined by Wilson and Jungner (1968), *early disease detection* refers to *all* forms of early detection, including screening and physical examination.

SCREENING AND RELATED TERMS

One of the most widely used methods of early detection, especially in school populations, is *screening.* As defined by the Commission on Chronic Illness (1957:45), screening is "the presumptive identification of unrecognized illness or defect by the application of tests, examinations, or other procedures which can be applied rapidly." According to this definition, the primary purpose of screening for disease is to sort out apparently well persons who probably have a disease from those who probably do not. However, it is important to remember that a screening test is not intended to be diagnostic; persons with positive or "suspicious" findings should be referred to a physician for a diagnostic workup and for treatment if indicated (Commission on Chronic Illness, 1957; Thorner and Remein, 1961; Whitby, 1974; Wilson and Jungner, 1968). In discussing their definition of screening, Wilson and Jungner note that it includes identification of *un-*

---

*Systematic assessment, including history taking and physical appraisal can also be a secondary prevention strategy. Although the discussion in this chapter will arbitrarily focus on screening, systematic assessment will be discussed at length in Chapter 12. The terminology and examples presented in this chapter focus primarily on screening for disease. Obviously, developmental screening is also an important secondary prevention measure for the school nurse; discussion of developmental screening will be included in Chapter 13.

recognized symptomatic as well as *presymptomatic* disease. They also point out that physical examination can be considered a means of screening as long as it is "rapid." Wilson and Jungner also note that tests which are usually considered "diagnostic" may be used as part of screening, although the intent of the screening itself is not to diagnose. Finally, in clarifying the meaning of this definition's reference to "other procedures," they suggest that the methods of screening may also include the use of questionnaires or other tools.

Depending on the population to be screened and the purpose of that screening, different labels are applied. To clarify the terminology associated with screening, these labels will be briefly discussed.

A term that is often used interchangeably with the word screening is *surveillance*. According to Webster's dictionary surveillance is the "close watch kept over someone or something." This implies a continuous, long-term observation of the health of a population group as opposed to the short-term testing of an at-risk population within a screening program. For that reason, in the remainder of this book, Wilson and Jungner's definition of surveillance (1968: 12) as "a long-term process where screening examinations are repeated at intervals" will be used.

Another label associated with screening is *case finding*. According to Wilson and Jungner (1968:12), case finding is "that form of screening of which the main object is to detect disease and bring patients to treatment." Thus case finding can be contrasted with *population or epidemiological surveys,* which are intended to provide data concerning the prevalence, incidence, and natural history of particular variables, conditions, or diseases. Case finding may be an outcome of such surveys but is not the purpose of population or epidemiological surveys (Wilson and Jungner, 1968).

The last group of screening terms clarified by Wilson and Jungner (1968) includes labels describing the population to be screened or the extent of the screening. The first of these is *mass screening,* which refers to the large-scale screening of entire populations. This term is commonly used to refer to screening in which no selection of population groups is made. In contrast, the term *selective screening* denotes screening of selected high-risk groups within the population; selective screening may be done on a large-scale basis and can be considered a

form of population screening. In recent years *multiple, or multiphasic, screening* has gained in popularity. Defined by the Commission on Chronic Illness (1957:45) as "the application of two or more screening tests in combination to large groups of people," multiphasic screening has been widely accepted because it is more economical to offer two tests at one time than to offer them separately.

During the past decade, screening has begun to rival the periodic physical examination as a popular means of early disease detection. School nurses have been involved in implementing screening programs for some time and will no doubt continue to be involved. For these reasons, in the remainder of this chapter screening and the role of the school nurse will be discussed.

SCREENING: A TOOL FOR EARLY DIAGNOSIS AND PROMPT TREATMENT

Bergman (1977) reminds health professionals that, contrary to public opinion, uncovering health problems by means of screening is not always a good thing, nor is it always justifiable. The decision to screen or not to screen should be based on a careful review of the relevant principles of screening and an honest evaluation of situational factors.

Because schoolchildren are to some degree a captive population, it is especially important that their availability does not result in their exploitation by individuals or groups under the guise of screening. Therefore, to assist the school nurse in planning and implementing responsible screening programs, in the remainder of this chapter the following will be discussed:

1. Goals and benefits of screening
2. Evaluation of screening results
3. Principles of screening for early disease detection
4. Selecting the appropriate screening level
5. The role of the school nurse in the screening program

Goals and benefits of screening

As discussed previously, one of the primary purposes of screening is the early detection of disease in apparently well individuals. The goal is to detect the disease process in the presymptomatic or unrecognized symptomatic stages so that prompt treatment can be initiated. Through such prompt treatment measures, the development of permanent or severe sequelae can be decreased or prevented altogether; in this way the extent of the person's disability can be limited.

Within a school population, a second and related goal of a screening program might be the identification of children within the population screened who may have special needs requiring some kind of anticipatory planning or special program development. An example could include children who are found to have some kind of vision or hearing impairment. Such children might have special classroom seating requirements and may need adaptive equipment such as glasses or hearing aids; special classes may also be indicated.

A third goal of a screening program might be to promote the importance of primary and secondary prevention efforts. Again, within a school setting the routine and periodic screening of children for vision and hearing problems or scoliosis could be included within the health education curriculum. Children could be taught about normal vision and hearing and body alignment and could then better understand explanations of conditions for which they will be screened, how the testing will be done, and what can be done to remedy any defects noted. The complexity of the information shared with the students can be geared to their developmental and cognitive stages. In this way, the students can begin to develop positive health attitudes and behaviors through combined health education (primary prevention) and screening (secondary prevention) efforts. Children will also be more likely to cooperate during the screening procedure if they have some understanding of the purpose and likely outcome.

Another potential goal of a screening program would be evaluation of existing primary prevention efforts through data collection and analysis. For example, in a school with an established dental health education curriculum emphasizing preventive efforts such as brushing, flossing, and dietary modifications, periodic dental screening can provide some index of the effectiveness of that curriculum in improving the overall dental health of the student population. To provide some additional comparisons, such an evaluation could be set up as a research design with both experimental and control groups.

In addition to the achievement of the stated goals, there are some other benefits of a screening program in the schools, including several benefits for the individual screened. One of the primary individual benefits is that screening provides the individual with data concerning his health status, which he can then use to make some responsible decisions about his health and life-style. A child who, on repeated dental screenings, is found to have poor oral hygiene and resultant dental caries can be helped to learn the relationship between his behavior and the consequences. Then with appropriate reinforcement from his family and involved health professionals he can learn to behave more responsibly in the care of his teeth. Another benefit for the individual screened is that early diagnosis and treatment are frequently less costly than diagnosis and treatment which occur later in the disease process. An example of a condition for which early diagnosis and treatment are usually less costly is scoliosis. If the condition can be treated before permanent deformity occurs, the complexity and duration of treatment can be reduced, thus minimizing expense. Another benefit of screening is that early treatment reduces the psychological trauma for the individual and facilitates his adaptation to the condition. Scoliosis can again be cited as an example. If scoliosis can be diagnosed when the child is preadolescent, permanent deformity can be avoided, treatment costs reduced, and emotional trauma to the child minimized. Adolescents are very body conscious and tend to worry about many seemingly minor afflictions such as acne. If an adolescent is found to have a potentially serious and disabling condition such as scoliosis, his ability to cope psychologically may be hampered by other doubts and traumas he faces simply because he is an adolescent.

Other benefits of a school screening program accrue not only to the individuals screened but to the population and the administrators of the school as a whole. The first of these is that data yielded from a school screening program can be useful for the incorporation of special education opportunities within the school. If screening reveals a significant number of vision or hearing impaired children, for example, perhaps a special class or teacher will be needed to facilitate their learning. If the screening is part of a research design, data analysis can indicate changes in the population screened. These changes may have implications for general planning or modifications of the school health program, including the health education curriculum.

Table 5-1. The efficiency of a screening test*

Screening result	True disease classification of apparently well population	
	Diseased persons	Persons without disease
Positive	With disease and with positive test (true positives)	Without disease but with positive test (false positives)
Negative	With disease but with negative test (false negatives)	Without disease and with negative test (true negatives)
Total	Total unknown cases of disease	Total persons without disease

$$\text{Sensitivity\dagger} = \frac{\text{Diseased persons with positive test}}{\text{All persons in population with disease}} \qquad \text{Specificity\dagger} = \frac{\text{Nondiseased persons with negative test}}{\text{All persons in population without disease}}$$

*From Wilson, J. M. G., and Jungner, G.: 1968. Principles and practice of screening for disease, Public Health Papers no. 34, World Health Organization, Geneva, Switzerland.
†These values are often expressed as percentages.

Evaluation of screening results

According to the Commission on Chronic Illness (1957), the following six parameters are to be considered when evaluating the results of screening procedures:

1. Validity
2. Reliability
3. Yield
4. Cost
5. Acceptance
6. Follow-up services

This discussion will focus on the first three; the rest will be considered on pp. 54 to 57.

As defined by the Commission on Chronic Illness (1957), the *validity* of a screening test is the ability of the test to separate those individuals who have the condition or variable sought from those who do not; that is, the validity measures the frequency with which the test result can be confirmed by an acceptable diagnostic procedure. When a given population, such as a group of schoolchildren, is screened using a particular test or procedure, the results obtained fall into four categories (Table 5-1).

Individuals whose test result is positive make up two groups: *true positives,* those with a positive result who actually have the disease, and *false positives,* those with a positive test result who do not have the disease. Individuals with a negative test result also make up two groups: *true negatives,* those with a negative result who do not have the disease, and *false negatives,* those whose test result is negative but who actually do have the disease.

The ability of a test to give a positive result when the person tested actually has the disease in question is called its *sensitivity;* in other words, the sensitivity is a measure of the false-negative rate (Thorner and Remein, 1961; Wilson and Jungner, 1968). As illustrated on p. 53, sensitivity is calculated by dividing the true positives by the sum of the true positives and false negatives and multiplying by 100.

The ability of a test to give a negative result when the individual tested is actually free of the disease or condition is its *specificity;* that is, the specificity measures the false-positive rate (Thorner and Remein, 1961; Wilson and Jungner, 1968). Specificity is calculated by dividing the true negatives by the sum of the true negatives and false positives and multiplying by 100.

Another factor to consider in determining the validity of a test is the *predictive value of a positive test result,* which is defined as the "percentage of positive results that are true positives when the test is applied to a population containing both healthy and diseased subjects" (Galen and Gambino, 1975:12). Three variables are used in determining the predictive value of a test: sensitivity, specificity, and prevalence or incidence. The predictive value of a positive result is calculated by dividing the true positives by the sum of the true and false positives and multiplying by 100 (p. 53).

Prevalence is probably one of the most important, yet least understood, factors influencing the usefulness of a test result. Since some confusion persists among health professionals about the definitions of prevalence and inci-

---

CALCULATION OF TEST VALIDITY*

$$\text{Sensitivity} = \frac{TP}{TP + FN} \times 100$$

$$\text{Specificity} = \frac{TN}{TN + FP} \times 100$$

$$\text{Predictive value of a positive result} = \frac{TP}{TP + FP} \times 100$$

*TP, True positives; FP, false positives; TN, true negatives; FN, false negatives. (From Galen, R. S., and Gambino, S. R.: 1975. Beyond normality: the predictive value and efficiency of medical diagnoses, John Wiley & Sons, Inc., New York.)

---

dence, it is appropriate to clarify those terms here. As distinguished by Galen and Gambino (1975), the *prevalence* rate of a disease equals the number of persons who have the disease *at the time of the testing* per 100,000 population. In contrast, the *incidence* is always associated with a stated time period and equals the *number of persons who develop the disease in a given year* per 100,000 population. Thus the incidence of a chronic disease can be low (few new cases per year) even though the prevalence (total number of persons who have the disease) may be high, because the duration of the disease may be lifelong. On the other hand, the incidence of an acute disease may be high, whereas its prevalence is very low. Such might be the case with an outbreak of influenza; a large number of new cases may occur in a given year, but if the disease has a short duration, the prevalence will be low. To avoid distortion and confusion, Galen and Gambino suggest that in determining the prevalence of a disease, the incidence should be multiplied by the duration. Prevalence will be further discussed later in this chapter, since it directly affects the yield of a screening program.

The second parameter to consider in evaluating screening results is *reliability,* or *efficiency.* This is the consistency with which a given test measures what it is designed to measure. In other words, efficiency represents the percent of all the test results that are true results, both positive and negative (Galen and Gambino, 1975:33):

Efficiency =

$$\frac{\text{True positives} + \text{True negatives}}{\text{Grand total}} \times 100.$$

As Wilson and Jungner point out (1968), assuming that the screening test selected is a good indicator of the disease it is meant to detect, the reliability, or efficiency, of the test will depend on two factors: the variation of the method or procedure itself and the variation of the observer (also referred to as interrater reliability).

The third parameter to be assessed is *yield.* According to Wilson and Jungner (1968:23-24), the yield from screening "may be regarded as the measure of previously unrecognized disease (whether overt or latent), diagnosed as the result of screening and brought to treatment." They further note that another form of yield is provided by individuals with known disease who have allowed treatment efforts to lapse. Obviously, the yield from any screening program will be related to the prevalence of the disease or condition within the population being studied and to the availability and use of health care facilities. Thus the highest yields will result from screening for highly prevalent diseases or conditions in a population with minimal availability and underuse of health care resources. In areas where health care delivery is good, less new disease will be discovered by screening, even though the disease may be quite common (Wilson and Jungner, 1968). In addition, as noted in the discussion of reliability of screening results, the efficiency of a test is another factor that directly affects the yield.

Obviously, an ideal test is one that will always give positive results in anyone with the disease and negative results in anyone who does not have the disease. Unfortunately, there are no ideal tests. Therefore in planning a screening program, one must decide whether to use the test with the highest sensitivity, highest specificity, highest predictive value for a positive result, or highest efficiency. This decision should be made by considering the prevalence and severity of the disease, cost of the test, and advantages and probability of early treatment (Galen and Gambino, 1975). According to Galen and Gambino (1975:50-51):

The highest sensitivity (preferably 100%) is desired in the following situations:
The disease is serious and should not be missed.
and
The disease is treatable.
and
False-positive results do not lead to serious psychologic or economic trauma to the patient.
EXAMPLES: phenylketonuria, venereal diseases, and other treatable infectious diseases

The highest specificity (preferably 100%) is desired in the following situations:
The disease is serious but is *not* treatable or curable.
and
The knowledge that the disease is absent has psychologic or public health value.
and
False-positive results can lead to serious psychologic or economic trauma to the patient.
EXAMPLES: multiple sclerosis, most occult cancers, and other serious and untreatable diseases

A high predictive value for a positive result is essential in the following situation:
Treatment of a false positive might have serious consequences.
EXAMPLE: occult cancer of the lung (for which the only available treatment is surgery or radiation; performance of such radical treatment on a patient without cancer could have dire consequences)

The highest efficiency is desired in the following situation:
The disease is serious but treatable.
and
False-positive results and false-negative results are essentially equally serious or damaging.
EXAMPLE: diabetes mellitus, myocardial infarction, lupus erythematosus, and some forms of leukemia and lymphoma

Thus selection of a screening test requires some decisions that are made on the basis of value judgments.

Principles of screening for early disease detection

In their world-renowned book *Principles and Practice of Screening for Disease,* commissioned by the World Health Organization, Wil-

son and Jungner (1968) identify ten principles of early disease detection, which, according to Bergman (1977), should be "required reading for all who dabble in screening" (1977:601-602). The principles of early disease detection follow (Wilson and Jungner, 1968:26-27):

1. The condition sought should be an important health problem.
2. There should be an accepted treatment for patients with recognized disease.
3. Facilities for diagnosis and treatment should be available.
4. There should be a recognizable latent or early symptomatic stage.
5. There should be a suitable test or examination.
6. The test should be acceptable to the population.
7. The natural history of the condition, including development from latent to declared disease, should be adequately understood.
8. There should be an agreed policy on whom to treat as patients.
9. The cost of case finding (including diagnosis and treatment of patients diagnosed) should be economically balanced in relation to possible expenditure on medical care as a whole.
10. Case finding should be a continuing process and not a "once and for all" project.

Importance of the disease as a health problem

As Wilson and Jungner explain, for a disease or condition to be considered an important health problem it need not be highly prevalent. Some diseases, such as the common cold and other viral respiratory tract infections, are highly prevalent but are characterized by relatively mild symptoms, varying durations, and often a low response to treatment. Although these diseases are inconvenient and uncomfortable, their overall importance as health problems is not sufficient to warrant screening programs to detect them. In contrast, a disease of relatively rare occurrence, such as phenylketonuria (PKU), can have severe and lasting consequences if not discovered and treated early in life. In this instance screening is warranted despite the low prevalence of the condition.

Obviously, the importance of a disease as a health problem needs to be assessed from the perspective of both the individual and the community. Thus diseases that have serious and lasting outcomes for the patient and his family may justify a relatively uneconomical screening program. On the other hand, screening may also be justified for conditions that produce only mild illness in patients but which have potentially serious effects on the community if not discovered and treated early; obesity has been cited as an example of the latter (Wilson and Jungner, 1968).

Existence of an accepted treatment

Wilson and Jungner believe that the ability to adequately treat the diagnosed disease or condition is probably the most important of their ten principles. They point out that the provision of an accepted treatment, whether or not it has scientifically proven merit, is an ethical obligation. However, earlier detection of disease poses two questions (Wilson and Jungner, 1968:28):

1. Does treatment at the presymptomatic borderline stage of a disease affect its course and prognosis?
2. Does treatment of the developed clinical condition at an earlier stage than normal affect its course and prognosis?

In answer to the first question, they emphasize the importance of research efforts to determine effects of early treatment of borderline stages on the overall course and prognosis of the disease. Until there is data to indicate that such early treatment has a beneficial result, Wilson and Jungner believe that persons who are in the borderline range should be told that they are not diseased. The second question falls within the realm of what is accepted clinical practice. Using diabetes mellitus as an example, despite the fact that there is lack of agreement among researchers concerning the long-range impact of early treatment, it is generally accepted that early treatment prevents some complications; therefore screening to detect persons with signs of clinical diabetes is defensible. However, for some conditions early diagnosis and treatment do not improve the prognosis for most patients. In such cases as lung cancer it is probably better to screen only selected high-risk groups like cigarette smokers and to concentrate

greater efforts on health education of the public. In summary, then, early detection should be undertaken *only* when the chances of treating the disease or condition are at least reasonable.

Availability of diagnostic and treatment facilities

Not only is it essential that the condition for which screening is done have an accepted treatment available, it is also critically important that there be available and accessible facilities to diagnose those referred after the screening and to treat any identified patients. Again, this seems so obvious that to state it insults one's intelligence. However, in far too many instances, mass screening is undertaken without any plans being made for responsible follow-up! Bergman (1977) cites the federal Early Periodic Screening Diagnosis and Treatment (EPSDT) program as an example of what he calls "naive shortsightedness"; in that program, which provides screening for millions of children, no money was appropriated for continuing medical care for uncovered illnesses and defects! Unless there are available and accessible (geographically, psychologically, and financially) facilities for the diagnosis and treatment of individuals who are suspected of having the disease or condition, it is morally and ethically irresponsible to screen for that condition!

Recognizable latent or early symptomatic stage

For a disease to be detected and treated early in its pathogenesis, there needs to be a clinically recognizable stage at which symptoms are either not present or not blatant. Many chronic diseases and some acute communicable diseases have a latent stage; however, other diseases such as multiple sclerosis and rheumatoid arthritis do not meet this criterion (Wilson and Jungner, 1968).

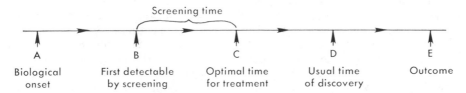

Fig. 5-1. Screening time related to course of disease. (From Frankenburg, W. K.: Selection of diseases and tests in pediatric screening, Pediatrics **54**(5):613, Nov., 1974. Copyright American Academy of Pediatrics 1974.)

Frankenburg (1974) has identified another relevant criterion: the optimal (defined as "most effective and economical") time for treatment should precede the usual time of diagnosis and treatment (Fig. 5-1). If, as he explains, point *C* (the optimal time of treatment) occurs *after* point *D* (the usual time of discovery), screening to provide early diagnosis is of little value. He also points out that the "screening time" (the interval between points *B* and *C*) must be adequate. Some diseases such as tuberculosis have long screening times; others like PKU have relatively limited screening times.

Availability of a suitable test or examination

In deciding whether a test is suitable, a number of factors must be considered. Obviously, as previously discussed, one of those factors is the validity of the test, as measured by the number of false positives and false negatives it yields. Another factor is the ease of application or simplicity of the test; some tests are considered suitable on that basis, although they may not be very good indicators of the disease or condition being sought. Still another factor affecting the suitability of a test is the extent to which it is a direct indicator of the disease. Generally, the more direct the index provided by the test, the less the chance of diagnostic error. The use of blood glucose levels in diabetes is an indirect index of the disease and is therefore subject to errors of both observation or measurement and interpretation; in contrast, measurement of hemoglobin level to determine anemia is considered a direct and highly precise indicator (Wilson and Jungner, 1968).

Acceptability of the test to the population

If a screening program is to be successful, it must secure the cooperation of the population to be screened; the cooperation of the population will definitely depend on the acceptability of the test(s) or procedure(s) to be used. Generally, tests that are simple, rapid, convenient, and physically and psychologically comfortable are acceptable to those being screened, whether they are adults or children (Frankenburg, 1974; Wilson and Jungner, 1968). Indeed, the importance of acceptability cannot be overstated; despite the diagnostic validity and reliability of tests like the Pap smear and proctosigmoidoscopy, these tests are considered unpleasant by many individuals and have definite limita-

tions in mass screening programs for that reason.

Adequate understanding of the natural history of the disease

Since the goal of screening is case finding so that early treatment can be sought, it is necessary in planning the screening program to decide who will be advised to seek treatment and who will not; thus a decision must be made about what signs and symptoms constitute disease. Wilson and Jungner (1968:32) identify the following three questions that need to be answered in understanding the natural history of the disease:

1. What changes should be regarded as pathological and what should be considered physiological variations?
2. Are early pathological changes progressive?
3. Is there an effective treatment that can be shown either to halt or to reverse the early pathological changes?

Accepted policy on whom to treat

As noted earlier in the discussion of existence of accepted treatment, the problem of individuals in the borderline range needs to be addressed. If only those patients with clinically established disease are to be treated, then some plan for follow-up of borderline cases is in order. If an individual is screened by his personal physician with whom he has an ongoing relationship, follow-up for borderline results can be done more readily and without alarming the patient. When the individual is screened within a community agency, such as a school or health department, the problem of following up becomes more complex. Also, as Frankenburg (1974) points out, when individuals screened are to be referred to health facilities and professionals who did not participate in the planning or implementation of the screening program, it is essential to secure the cooperation of those practitioners. If the health facilities to which the individual is referred do not agree with the criteria used to refer clients for diagnosis, adequate follow-up may not be received. In addition, the client may lose faith in the screening program and may refuse to participate in future screenings. The client may also feel that the money spent on follow-up was wasted. This is especially of concern to parents of schoolchildren who may be referred for eye examinations only to be told by the examiner that "nothing" is wrong.

Economic balance between case finding and medical care

The cost of case finding by screening depends in part on the test or procedure used. If the test is simple, rapidly administered, and can be given by auxiliary health workers, technicians, or volunteers, then the cost is less than administering a complex test that requires the skills of a physician. It is sometimes tempting to overstate the economy of screening by pointing out the per capita cost of the screening procedure and contrasting that with the cost of medical care for the condition. This is misleading, however, because the total cost of screening actually includes the costs of diagnosis and treatment. The true cost balance between case finding and medical care is best determined, according to Wilson and Jungner (1968), through prospective surveys to determine the reduction in morbidity and improvement in productivity of the screened population as compared with a nonscreened population.

Case finding as a continuing process

Frequently, screening programs are one-time-only efforts as part of a "health fair" or a particular disease "drive" or a national "week" to call attention to a given disease. As Wilson and Jungner (1968) point out, these one-shot screenings are of only limited value because (1) often only a small proportion of the population is screened—usually those who are least at risk and (2) the screening only identifies those persons in the population who happen to have the disease at that time; it cannot provide data concerning future incidence. Therefore continuing periodic screenings are more beneficial; as noted earlier in this chapter, this ongoing attention to the health of a population by repeated screening is called surveillance. Plans for surveillance of a population through repetitive screening can reduce the problem of follow-up for individuals in the borderline range, since they can be monitored through rescreening.

Selecting the appropriate screening level

Before any screening program is undertaken, the ten principles advanced by Wilson and Jungner must be employed; the omission of any one of them may result in the planning and implementation of an irresponsible, ineffective, and inefficient program. Assuming, then, that the planners of a screening program have followed those guidelines in deciding what conditions are to be sought, the next problem is determining the *appropriate screening level,* which is the value or score at which the test is considered positive. Selection of the level at which the test is considered positive is an important decision, since a change in the screening level that *increases* sensitivity (the number of false negatives) will *decrease* specificity (the number of false positives). In other words, the planners must decide how true and false negatives and positives will affect both the individuals screened and the community at large. Thorner and Remein (1961:4-6), reporting on work done in 1957 by Blumberg, discuss six questions to be considered in determining the screening level:

1. *What is the outlook for a person with the disease?* A true positive is more valuable if the patient's chances for a cure or a shorter convalescence are improved through early detection. If case finding provides no health benefits, then screening is not advisable.

2. *What facilities exist for treating cases found?* If treatment facilities are inadequate, the value of a true positive is decreased; it is not profitable to find more cases than can be treated (unless the long-range effect is to provide more adequate treatment facilities).

3. *What mental status accompanies knowledge or suspicion of the disease?* If suspicion of disease creates potentially debilitating anxiety, then a true negative could provide reassurance and health benefits. If fear from being labeled falsely positive also creates undue anxiety, this can be harmful too and can be minimized by careful wording of the directive to the client asking him to seek diagnostic study.

4. *Who is going to do the diagnostic follow-up?* False positives can be a burden to diagnostic facilities, although they are less harmful if the facilities are adequate and the diagnostic workup relatively inexpensive. As previously noted, false positives can discredit the screening procedures and screeners in the eyes of both those screened and the health professionals to whom they are referred for follow-up.

5. *What is the likelihood of repeat screening within the community?* If it is unlikely that screening will be repeated soon, then false negatives could be harmful. If

screening will be repeated soon and if the disease is not communicable or rapidly progressive, then false negatives are less harmful, since the disease may be discovered the next time.

6. *Are healthy individuals being sought?* If so (as in the case of selection of candidates for armed services or specific employment) false negatives may be very costly, whereas false positives may not be.

THE ROLE OF THE SCHOOL NURSE IN THE SCREENING PROGRAM

Involvement of the nurse in development, implementation, and evaluation of a screening program depends primarily on her success in her role as manager of health care (Chapter 2). In planning a screening program there are a number of important decisions to be made, and the participation of the school nurse in the decision-making process is essential. Decisions can be made for an entire school district or for individual schools.

Among the first decisions to be made are those concerning who is to be screened and for what disease or condition. As discussed in Chapter 2, in both the planning and implementation phases of her role as manager, the school nurse is concerned with the unique health needs of the school population. The nurse may use such methods as epidemiological surveys to identify health needs and to determine which individuals are high risk and therefore need to be the target group for a selective screening program. The school nurse's expertise as a health professional will be essential in then deciding for which disease or condition the population selected is to be screened. As discussed previously, these criteria must be met: the condition sought should be an important health problem, accepted treatment should be available for identified patients, facilities for diagnosis and treatment should be available and accessible, the disease should have a recognizable latent or early symptomatic stage, the natural history of the disease should be understood, and the cost of case finding should be economically balanced with the cost of medical care.

Once the purpose of the screening has been established, the procedure or test to be used must be selected. The school nurse's expertise is again needed for this aspect of planning. Not only must she be sure that the funds budgeted for the screening program will be adequate to meet the costs, but she must also ensure that the mechanics of the screening procedure are completed. She may elect to carry out some of these functions personally or she may delegate them to others. Specifically, some of these mechanics include ordering supplies, securing parental consent for screening, recruiting and orienting volunteers to help with the procedure, determining the screening flow patterns (facilities to be used, room arrangement, number of students to be screened per hour, who will do the actual screening, etc.), recording findings, arranging for rescreening of borderline or questionable cases, and planning follow-up mechanisms. Her input into the actual choice of the test to be used in the program should be based on whether sensitivity, specificity, predictive value of a positive result, or efficiency is most important, and on the availability of a test that is suitable and acceptable. The last decision to be made concerning the screening test is determination of the screening level. This is done by reviewing the six questions posed by Blumberg (1957) (p. 57).

The successful outcome of a school screening program also requires collaboration of the school health team, particularly the school nurse, with area health professionals and resources. As previously noted, such collaboration in determining and communicating the criteria to be used in deciding which persons screened to refer for diagosis and possible treatment is critically important in securing the cooperation of these professionals. Collaboration should also be used to determine who will do the actual follow-up, including confidential handling of data, interpretation of screening results to students and their parents, home visits or telephone calls to assess the outcome of the referral or treatment, education of the patient and family regarding the disease and its treatment, communication of results of the screening to appropriate school personnel such as the teachers of students found to have the disease, and participation in anticipatory planning for children who will need special facilities or learning opportunities because of the disease or condition. The school nurse may personally follow up many or all of these areas or may continue to collaborate with community health resource persons. The final, but by no means the least important, area requiring collaboration between the school nurse and the rest of the health team with area resources, is in deciding who will be treated as patients. Because this is often a gray area, the decision will be based on both theoretical and ethical issues. However, the importance of agreement by those involved concerning which individuals to treat cannot be overstated; failure to reach agreement can result in sabotage of the screening program.

The planning of the screening program is incomplete if attention is not paid to long-range plans for continued case finding. Because there are limitations to the effectiveness of one-shot screening efforts, plans for periodic rescreening or other forms of early detection should be made. As a leader within the school health team, it is the nurse's responsibility to direct attention to this need.

Another area in which the school nurse can contribute effectively to the success of the screening program is by encouraging the incorporation of content concerning the disease being sought through screening, the outcome and treatment for those with the disease or condition, and the screening procedure itself into the health education curriculum. The nurse may accomplish this by acting as resource person to the classroom teacher or by direct participation in the classroom. In this way, the students can better understand the purposes and benefits of screening as a preventive health practice.

The role of the school nurse in a screening program should include, when feasible, the design and implementation of research studies to evaluate the outcomes of the screening program. Especially in these times of economic cutbacks in school health, research can provide

Table 5-2. Usefulness of screening tests*

	Importance	Prevalence	Diagnostic criteria	Effective treatment	Early treatment more effective	Adequate screening time	Adequate treatment resources	Effective screening test	Acceptable direct costs	Acceptable cost of false positives	Acceptable cost of false negatives
Phenylketonuria	+	±	+	+	+	+	+	+	+	+	+
Galactosemia	+	±	+	+	+	+	+	+	±	+	+
Other inborn errors of metabolism	+	±	+	±	±	+	+	+	±	?	+
Anemia	+	+	+	+	+	+	+	+	+	+	+
Sickle cell diseases	+	−	−	±	+(1)	+	?	+	+	+	+
Hemoglobin S and C traits	?	+	+	?	+(2)	+	?	+	−	+	+
Bacteriuria	?	+	+	+	?	+	+	+	+	+	+
Impaired hearing	+	+	±	+	+	+	+	±	+	?	+
Impaired vision	+	+	±	+	?	+	+	±	+	?	+
Middle ear effusion	?	+	±	?	?	±	±	+	+	?	?
Heart murmurs	?	+	+	+	±	+	+	+	+	0	?
Deviant physical growth	+	+	?	±	±	+	+	+	+	?	+
Deviant psychomotor development	+	+	?	±	±	+	?	+	?	?	?
Glucosuria	+	0	+	+	0	0	+	+	+	?	?
Albuminuria	?	+	?	?	0	?	?	+	+	0	+
Cystic fibrosis	+	±	+	+	?	+	+	?	?	?	?
High blood pressure	?	?	0	?	?	+	?	±	+	0	+
Hypercholesterolemia	?	?	?	?	?	+	?	+	?	?	+
Deviant behavior	+	+	?	?	?	+	0	?	?	?	?
Intestinal parasites	?	+	+	+	?	+	+	?	0	?	?
Dental diseases	+	+	+	+	+	+	±	±	0	+	0
Lead absorption	?	?	±	±	+	±	±	±	±	?	?
Tuberculosis	+	0	+	+	+	+	+	+	+	0	+
Occult stool blood	?	+	?	?	?	+	+	+	+	0	?

*+, Problem or test appears to meet this criterion; ±, problem or test appears to partially meet this criterion; 0, problem or test appears to fail this criterion; ?, evidence appears insufficient for judgment; (1), only when discovered in first 6 months of life; (2), only for persons pregnant or planning pregnancy. (From North, A. F.: 1974. Screening in child health care: where are we now and where are we going?'' Pediatrics **54**(5):634, Nov. Copyright American Academy of Pediatrics 1974. Updated by North, 1978.)

persuasive data documenting the cost-effectiveness of school health services. Research studies can be effectively used to evaluate the adequacy of the screening procedures, prevalence and severity of the condition in the population studied, and long-range effects of the school health program on the prevalence and severity of the disease.

Finally, perhaps as an additional benefit of research concerning the screening program and its outcome, the school nurse may be aware of the need to develop or expand certain community health resources. As a manager of health care and as a responsible health professional the school nurse is obligated to facilitate development of needed community resources for diagnosis and treatment. This can be done through involvement in the legislative process, directly or indirectly, or by other kinds of community participation.

SUMMARY

Because of the popularity of screening as a means of early detection of health problems and because schoolchildren comprise an essentially captive population, school nurses and other members of the school health team must be especially vigilant to prevent abuses of this population through what are generally well-intentioned screening efforts. The decision to have a screening program must be carefully and responsibly determined, based on sound theoretical and ethical principles. What may be a very appropriate screening program in one school or school district may be inappropriate in another, due to differences in the populations and in the values held by the officials responsible for the planning and administration of the programs. Table 5-2 provides a suggested evaluation of the merits of screening children for specific conditions.

Although such tables can be used as a guide for decision making, it is important to remember that such areas as importance of the condition as a health problem and adequacy of treatment resources depend on the value system of the decision maker. Thus in planning, implementing, and evaluating screening programs, the school nurse must be sure that her decision making is based on sound evaluation of the theoretical and ethical issues involved.

REFERENCES

Bergman, A. B.: 1977. The menace of mass screening, Am. J. Public Health **67**(7):601-602.

Blumberg, M. S.: 1957. Evaluating health screening procedures, Operations Res. **5**:351-360.

Commission on Chronic Illness: 1957. Chronic illness in the United States. Vol. I. Prevention of chronic disease, Harvard University Press, Cambridge, Mass.

Frankenburg, W. K.: 1974. Selection of diseases and tests in pediatric screening, Pediatrics **54**(5):612-616.

Galen, R. S., and Gambino, S. R.: 1975. Beyond normality: the predictive value and efficiency of medical diagnoses, John Wiley & Sons, Inc., New York.

Leavell, H. R., and Clark, E. G.: 1965. Preventive medicine for the doctor in his community: an epidemiologic approach, 3rd ed., McGraw-Hill, Inc., New York.

Thorner, R. M., and Remein, Q. R.: 1961. Principles and procedures in the evaluation of screening for disease, U.S. Department of Health, Education, and Welfare, U.S. Public Health Service Monograph no. 67, Washington, D.C.

Whitby, L. G.: 1974. Screening for disease: definitions and criteria, Lancet **2**(7884):819-821.

Wilson, J. M. G., and Jungner, G.: 1968. Principles and practice of screening for disease, Public Health Papers no. 34, World Health Organization, Geneva, Switzerland.

SUGGESTED READING

North, A. F.: 1974. Screening in child health care: where are we now and where are we going? Pediatrics **54**(5):631-640.

CHAPTER 6

Tertiary prevention: mainstreaming handicapped children

SUSAN J. WOLD

As discussed in Chapters 3 to 5, there are three levels of disease and disability prevention: (1) primary prevention, which includes health promotion and specific protection; (2) secondary prevention, which includes early detection and prompt treatment and disability limitation; and (3) tertiary prevention, which encompasses rehabilitation efforts. Although primary and secondary prevention programs are the preferred methods for delivering health care, tertiary prevention also has its role. To clarify the role and purpose of tertiary prevention programs as they affect the health and well-being of school-age children and youth, this chapter will discuss the following:

1. The scope and thrust of tertiary prevention
2. Mainstreaming handicapped children: legal mandates
3. Mainstreaming handicapped children: the role of the school

THE SCOPE AND THRUST OF TERTIARY PREVENTION
Relevant definitions

Tertiary prevention may be considered the last resort for halting progression of a disease or disability; it occurs *after* both primary and secondary prevention methods have, for whatever reason, failed to either completely prevent development or adequately limit progression and complications of a particular disease state, disabling injury, or other condition. Once defect and disability become fixed or stabilized, *tertiary prevention* is accomplished by means of rehabilitation (Leavell and Clark, 1965). More specifically, as conceptualized by Leavell and Clark, tertiary prevention includes such activities as (1) provision of rehabilitative facilities

and programs for those in need, (2) education of the general public and industry executives regarding the employability of handicapped persons, (3) establishment of sheltered workshops and similar facilities to enable profoundly retarded or disabled persons to be employed, (4) efforts to ensure full employment for all handicapped persons within the limitations imposed by their disability, and (5) provision of housing units adapted to the needs and limitations of the handicapped, to enable them to live as independently as possible.

As implied by this list of tertiary prevention activities, *rehabilitation* involves more than merely halting disease progression; it includes "prevention of complete disability after anatomic and physiologic changes are more or less stabilized" (Leavell and Clark, 1965:26). That is, rehabilitation is a *restorative* process (Boroch, 1976), the goal of which is to "return the individual to a useful place in society and make maximum use of his remaining capacities" (Leavell and Clark, 1965:26). As just defined, rehabilitation incorporates physical, mental/emotional, and social aspects (1965:26). Rehabilitation must view the client holistically, considering not only his physical or mental impairments but also environmental constraints.

The need for tertiary prevention among children and youth
Prevalence of chronic and/or handicapping conditions

According to Webster's dictionary, a *handicap* is "a disadvantage that makes achievement unusually difficult." Although physical disability is cited as perhaps the most obvious kind of handicap, a handicap can be physical, mental, emotional, or social in nature—or some com-

61

bination thereof. It should also be noted that Webster's nonspecific definition lends itself to liberal interpretation; therefore a handicap might also be construed as being any condition or problem that the affected individual perceives as being a "disadvantage" making it "unusually difficult" for him to achieve his goals and interfering with his sense of well-being. Thus handicaps may range from severe physical disabilities like cerebral palsy or muscular dystrophy to sensory impairments involving loss of vision or hearing to chronic and/or debilitating physical conditions/diseases such as diabetes, epilepsy, and severe allergies. Other less tangible problems are in the psychosocial areas of emotional or mental illness, learning disabilities and behavior problems, delinquency, low self-esteem, or, based on the student's perception of his problem, such seemingly minor problems as shyness, being overweight, or having severe and persistent acne. Although not all of these conditions or problems (shyness and acne, for example) would probably be viewed as handicaps by many health professionals or teachers, to the affected child or youth they may seem as devastating and debilitating as blindness or cerebral palsy. Therefore the school nurse and others engaged in counseling, educating, or providing other services to students need to elicit students' perceptions of their health and well-being and consider those perceptions when planning nursing interventions on behalf of students.

For statistical and programmatic purposes, schoolchildren's handicaps are more conventionally defined in terms of obvious physical, mental, intellectual, emotional, sensory, or social impairments. Thus according to P.L. 94-142, a *handicapped* child is one with mental retardation, hearing impairment (including deafness) or speech impairment, visual handicap, serious emotional disturbance, orthopedic or other health impairment, or specific learning disabilities, who needs special education and related services in order to learn (Jones, 1979; Nader, 1979).

The prevalence of handicapping conditions among children and youth is difficult to precisely ascertain due in part to differences in diagnostic criteria and labeling among professionals; thus although one professional might label a particular child as mentally retarded, another might diagnose the same child as "slow" or "dull normal." Efforts to accurately estimate the prevalence of handicapping conditions among children and youth are further hampered by the fact that too often these conditions are undetected. A child whose seizures are infrequent and/or mild and unobtrusive may not be identified as epileptic until he is well into his academic career. Thus for these and other reasons, statistical estimates of the prevalence of handicapping conditions (as defined in P.L. 94-142) are probably *conservative,* underestimating the scope of the problem to an undetermined extent.

Although these figures are probably low, Table 6-1 estimates the number of American children with handicaps as ranging between 6 to 9 million. In an effort to make such statistics more "real," Mayshark et al. (1977:235) report that out of every 1000 students, sixty will have physical handicaps, another forty will have mental ability that "deviates considerably" from the average; of the forty students in the latter category, twenty will be mentally re-

Table 6-1. Prevalence of handicapped children in the United States

	Percent of population	Number of children ages 5 to 18*
Visually impaired (includes blind)	0.1	55,000
Hearing impaired (includes deaf)	0.6 to 0.8	330,000 to 440,000
Speech handicapped	3.5 to 5.0	1,925,000 to 2,750,000
Crippled and other health impaired	0.5	275,000
Emotionally disturbed	2.0 to 3.0	1,100,000 to 1,650,000
Mentally retarded (both educable and trainable)	2.5 to 3.0	1,375,000 to 1,650,000
Learning disabilities	2.0 to 4.0	1,100,000 to 2,200,000
	11.2 to 16.4	6,160,000 to 9,020,000

*Number of children based on 1978 population estimates. (From Gearheart, B. R., and Weishahn, M. W.: 1976. The handicapped child in the regular classroom, The C. V. Mosby Co., St. Louis.)

tarded, and the other twenty will include "gifted" students. Thus it seems clear that regardless of the statistical procedures used and the presumed underestimation they provide, the prevalence of handicapping conditions in school-age populations is more than just a few isolated cases—there are significant numbers of schoolchildren in need of special education and/or support services.

Unfortunately, as shown in Table 6-2, many handicapped children who are in need of such services do not receive them. Those handicapped students whose needs seem to be most overlooked or neglected are "crippled and other health impaired" and "emotionally disturbed," 80% and 85% of whom (respectively) fail to receive needed services (Gearheart and Weishahn, 1976). Again, without belaboring the point or digressing to discuss it in detail, the reasons for lack of services to these large numbers of students include lack of suitable services and personnel and difficulty in identifying those students with handicapping conditions who need additional services.

Primary and secondary prevention failures

Having established that there are significant numbers of school-age children with chronic and/or handicapping conditions, many of whom are not even receiving needed

and legally mandated supportive and special education services, it is appropriate to briefly discuss why so many children progress to the tertiary prevention level before effective intervention occurs.

Regarding the primary prevention level, one basic failure is the failure to educate the public (including children and youth) about the *importance* of primary prevention as an approach to health care. As a result, the emphasis in our health care delivery system is on episodic, illness-oriented care, with very little attention to prevention. In addition, other health promotion strategies (besides health education), such as genetic counseling and nutritional guidance, tend to be underused. Persons with hereditary diseases in their families may not be aware of the existence of or need for genetic counseling as a means of preventing (or at least calculating the risks of) future births of affected children. Similarly, despite active and ongoing research in the realm of food science and nutrition, many Americans continue to have inadequate nutrition, due both to lack of information as well as lack of compliance with recommended dietary principles.

Another reason for failure at the primary prevention level concerns specific protection measures such as immunizations. Part of the problem is that for many conditions or diseases, in-

Table 6-2. Handicapped children receiving service and those in need but not receiving service*

	Total number of children†	Percent receiving service	Number receiving service	Percent remaining in need of service	Number remaining in need of service
Visually impaired	55,000	35	19,250	65	35,750
Hearing impaired	330,000	25	82,500	75	247,500
Speech handicapped	1,925,000	55	1,058,750	45	866,250
Crippled and other health impaired	275,000	20	55,000	80	220,000
Emotionally disturbed	1,100,000	15	165,000	85	935,000
Mentally retarded	1,375,000	55	756,250	45	618,750
Learning disabled	1,100,000	‡	330,000	‡	770,000
	6,160,000		2,466,750		3,693,250

*We have elected to use the more conservative prevalence data from Table 6-1 and to round off recent estimates of those receiving services to the nearest 5%, rounding upward (increasing the percent presumed to be receiving services) to reflect a slow increase in the percent of children served owing to mandatory legislation. This will tend to result in a conservative estimate of children remaining in need of services.

†Number of children based on 1978 population estimates (Table 6-1).

‡Services to children with learning disabilities have been increasing rapidly and any estimate of number and percent of children served may quickly become inaccurate. In addition, much of the reported data in state studies reflects a definition of learning disabilities that includes more moderate and mild learning problems than those indicated by the 2% (1,100,000 children) figures used to reflect the total number of children who should receive service. However, information from a variety of sources leads us to estimate that 30% of the 1,100,000 children were receiving some service as of 1976. (From Gearheart, B. R., and Weishahn, M. W.: 1976. The handicapped child in the regular classroom, The C. V. Mosby Co., St. Louis.)

cluding cancer, there are *no* available specific protection measures. In addition, many of the specific protection measures that *are* available, such as immunizations for measles, rubella, and mumps, too often are not used; thus in recent years there have been numerous outbreaks of preventable diseases like measles, largely due to parental complacency regarding the need for immunizations.

At the secondary prevention level, in which the goal is early diagnosis and prompt treatment, screening is the predominant activity (Chapters 5 and 13). However, some problems and consequent prevention failures are associated with screening and follow-up activities as well. One obvious problem associated with screening is the lack of valid and reliable screening procedures for some diseases and conditions. For certain kinds of diseases and conditions (Chapter 5), there may be no specific protection (primary prevention) measures nor early detection (secondary prevention) methods; as a result, individuals who develop these diseases/conditions are more likely to progress through to the tertiary prevention level before the disease process can be halted and/or reversed.

Another problem associated with the secondary prevention level is the failure to screen the appropriate at-risk population. If, for example, a school's scoliosis screening program focused primarily on first-grade boys, the yield (Chapter 5) would be small, since 80% to 90% of cases of idiopathic scoliosis occur in *girls* and are most readily detected in the *early adolescent* age group (Chapter 13). In this instance, the girls at risk of having the condition would not be detected, since they are not included in the population screened, which would increase the chance that those girls with scoliosis would not be diagnosed and treated in time to prevent progression of the curve.

Another problem associated with secondary prevention screening efforts is the occurrence of false-negative and false-positive test results (Chapter 5). Occurrence of false negatives leads to failure to identify those persons needing additional follow-up (diagnostic work and/or treatment). Since early detection and prompt treatment therefore become less likely, the person's illness or other condition may progress to the tertiary level. False positives, on the other hand, not only increase health costs for unnecessary follow-up of healthy persons, but also may undermine people's confidence in screening procedures altogether; if that happens, people may be even more inclined to neglect their health until diseases or other health problems progress to the tertiary level.

Finally, it should be noted that a certain degree of blame for primary and secondary prevention failures can be attributed to the economics of health care delivery. It is no secret that third-party reimbursement (payments by insurance companies and programs like Medicaid on behalf of clients who have received health-related services) is *most* readily available for treatment of disease and *least* available for preventive services. As long as this reality persists, health care costs will continue to escalate while countless persons will continue to needlessly experience progression of disease and disability to the tertiary level. Furthermore, the traditional and continuing use of the medical model (pathophysiology orientation) in the educational curricula of physicians and other health care professionals (including nurses) perpetuates the episodic, disease-treatment approach to health care delivery, thereby minimizing opportunities for and commitment to primary (and sometimes secondary) prevention. Because costs of disease diagnosis and treatment are greater than the costs of disease and disability prevention, health professionals' continuing focus (beginning with their basic educational curricula) on *curing* rather than *preventing* fuels the escalation of health care delivery costs and may also force many people to delay necessary treatment in an effort to avoid to health care costs, resulting in further disease progression and ultimately greater costs (financial and emotional).

Thus, for a number of reasons, primary and secondary prevention efforts often may not succeed and in some cases may not even be attempted. Consequently, significant numbers of persons—including school-age children and youth—experience tertiary level illness and disability and are therefore in need of rehabilitative and supportive educational and health services. In the following discussion, the legal mandates for provision of such services to school-age children and youth will be detailed.

MAINSTREAMING HANDICAPPED CHILDREN: LEGAL MANDATES
Mainstreaming: origins and intent

As Gearheart and Weishahn (1976:15) point out in their carefully documented historical overview of trends in the education of the handicapped, "in the past, the handicapped have been eliminated [through infanticide or later execution], ignored, made to work as indentured servants, and institutionalized, in that approximate order." Although the precise nature and extent of such reactions varied around the world, these societal responses to the handicapped predominated until about 1900.

Shortly after the beginning of the twentieth century, special classes for handicapped children within the public school were common and quite popular. Although such classes were a positive step away from earlier suspicious and punitive approaches to the handicapped and toward provision of educational opportunities for affected children, these classes were eventually misused, overused, and badly in need of reform (1976).

This reform began in earnest during the 1960s—during the social reform campaigns of the Great Society—with the full support of certain major political figures such as John Kennedy and Hubert Humphrey, whose personal interest was sparked by the presence of handicapped persons within their own families (1976). In addition, at about the same time, the political savvy and lobbying expertise of special interest groups like the National Association for Retarded Children (NARC) was increasing. For these and perhaps other reasons, the federal government and the judicial system (through a series of court tests) aided this reform movement.

As a result of these and other forces, the most recent and hopeful trend in the education of handicapped children has been away from segregation—even in special classes—and toward a concept called *mainstreaming*. Although this concept is subject to a variety of definitions and interpretations, *mainstreaming* of handicapped children generally refers to efforts to provide them with "maximum integration in the regular class, combined with concrete assistance for the nonspecial education teacher" (Gearheart and Weishahn, 1976:2). Thus the intent of mainstreaming is to incorporate handicapped children into regular classes along with their nonhandicapped peers to the fullest possible extent.

At the same time, as defined in the preceding paragraph, mainstreaming also includes provision of "concrete assistance" for the classroom teacher who is not prepared in special education; such assistance might include (1) attendants to assist handicapped students with personal care; (2) teacher aides, special education teachers, health care professionals, and other personnel to act as resource persons and consultants; and (3) special and/or adaptive equipment and instructional aids to enhance the comfort and learning of handicapped students. The emphasis is on both integrating these special children *and* providing supportive assistance to teachers to ensure the success of this integration.

P.L. 94-142: The Education for All Handicapped Children Act

The culmination of the social reform of the 1960s was the eventual realization that, like all other children, handicapped children deserve equal opportunities to fully develop whatever abilities and talents they possess (Gearheart and Weishahn, 1976). Furthermore, it was recognized that such opportunities should be available to *all* handicapped children, regardless of their parents' ability to pay. To ensure the availability and fiscal accessibility of these opportunities, in 1975 the Ninety-fourth Congress enacted P.L. 94-142: the Education for All Handicapped Children Act.

Needless to say, passage of P.L. 94-142 was a widely heralded milestone in the education of the handicapped. This act, which has been supplemented by additional legislation in a number of states, includes certain key provisions and requirements that affect not only handicapped children but also the teachers, administrators, and other school personnel (including school nurses) charged and entrusted with the responsibility of providing the specified services and programs. These key provisions and requirements of P.L. 94-142 are discussed at length by Best (1978), Jones (1979), and Rose (1980) and will be summarized in the succeeding paragraphs.

Essentially, P.L. 94-142 (1975) requires that *all* handicapped children between the ages of 3 and 21 years, regardless of the severity and extent of their handicap, must be provided a "free appropriate education"; exceptions to this requirement may be made for children between ages 3 and 5 and/or 18 and 21 when this requirement conflicts with state laws or policies or with any court order (P.L. 94-142: Section 162). The act is permanent (nonexpiring) legislation that provides federal financial assistance to states and local school districts based on the number of handicapped children served. In addition, the stipulation that the education must be "free" is strictly interpreted to mean that parents are not expected to pay directly for services, although third party payments are permissible (Jones, 1979).

In addition to the required "free appropriate education" for all handicapped children between the ages of 3 and 21, following are seven other important components of P.L. 94-142:

1. *An individualized education program (IEP)*, which is to be a written plan for meeting the educational needs of a particular handicapped child, collaboratively developed and annually updated by appropriate school personnel, the parents, the child (if appropriate), and any other persons invited by the parents or school, based on assessment of the child's needs and abilities. The IEP must include (1) a statement of the child's present educational performance levels; (2) a statement of annual goals, including short-term instructional objectives; (3) an explicit statement of the specific educational services the child will receive and the projected extent to which the child will be able to participate in regular educational programs; and (4) the projected dates for beginning and terminating these services, and the evaluation criteria, schedules, and procedures to be applied in evaluating achievement of the instructional objectives (P.L. 94-142: Section 4).
2. *Nondiscriminatory testing and placement*, which means that procedures used to identify handicapped children and determine their most appropriate educational placement or setting must avoid racial or cultural discrimination. Assessment procedures and tests must be selected and administered in a manner that avoids racial or cultural discrimination; for example, tests must be administered in the child's native language, and a child may not be classified as handicapped solely on the basis of one test or procedure (Rose, 1980).
3. *Least restrictive environment*, which simply means that to the "maximum extent appropriate," handicapped children should be educated with nonhandicapped children; removal of handicapped children from the "regular educational environment" for separate classes and/or separate schooling should occur *only* "when the nature or severity of the handicap is such that education in regular classes with the use of supplementary aids and services cannot be achieved satisfactorily" (P.L. 94-142: Section 612). This includes the expectation that each school district will provide a "continuum of alternative placements" (Jones, 1979:149) such as that suggested by Gearheart and Weishahn (1976); this continuum will probably include alternatives like regular classes, resource rooms, itinerant instruction, special schools, homebound instruction, and instruction provided in hospitals and other institutions.
4. *Parental involvement*, which encourages parents to participate in the educational planning for their children; this provision includes parents' rights to (1) be consulted prior to any proposed change in their child's educational placement, (2) participate on advisory boards, and (3) have "unrestricted access" to their child's school records (Rose, 1980:30).
5. *Data confidentiality*, which requires that parental consent be obtained before releasing any "personally identifiable" information to anyone; among its other specific provisions, this data confidentiality clause requires the school to notify parents when this personally identifiable information is no longer needed for providing educational services to the child; at that point, the parents may request that it be destroyed (Jones, 1979).
6. *Due process*, which means that if parents do not believe that their child is receiving a "free appropriate education" or if they wish to challenge the identification/labeling of the child as "handicapped" or his evaluation and educational placement, they may request a due process hearing. This hearing must be conducted by someone not employed by or affiliated with the school or other agency responsible for education and/or care of the child (Jones, 1979).
7. *Personnel development*, which must be incorporated into the annual program plans of both the school district and the state education agency, including plans for provision of in-service training for teachers based on needs assessment; in-service education plans must also identify incentives such as release time, tuition reimbursement, and salary step credits to ensure teachers' participation (Jones, 1979).

Although the preceding seven components do not provide a detailed and comprehensive discussion of the letter and intent of P.L. 94-142, they embody the essential elements of the law and illustrate the tremendous responsibility placed on local educational systems to meet the needs of handicapped children and youth. With this brief overview of P.L. 94-142 as a common frame of reference, the remainder of the chapter will more fully explore the role of the school in mainstreaming handicapped children.

MAINSTREAMING HANDICAPPED CHILDREN: THE ROLE OF THE SCHOOL

The recent and continuing trend toward mainstreaming handicapped children into regular classrooms or the least restrictive environment has required some adaptation by students, school systems, and school personnel. Since the passage of P.L. 94-142, there is no longer much debate as to whether or not the school has a role in working with handicapped children; rather, the primary focus is now on deciding more precisely *what* the school's role should be and how it can be most effectively and efficiently carried out. To simplify discussion of the school's role in mainstreaming handicapped children, this discussion will be subdivided into two general topics: educational issues and concerns and health needs and the role of the school nurse.

Educational issues and concerns

Although the mutual learning benefits of mainstreaming for both handicapped and non-handicapped children are generally widely recognized, the actual achievement of these benefits depends on the school's efforts to ensure the success of mainstreaming. That is, if all children are to maximally benefit from the opportunity to be educated with children who may be physically, mentally, and/or emotionally different from themselves, then mainstreaming *programs* must be carefully designed, implemented, and evaluated, which may necessitate some potentially major and costly changes in the school's physical plant, curriculum, class size, teacher qualifications and job description, and faculty/staff composition and preparation. The remainder of this discussion will identify and discuss five specific school needs to ensure successful mainstreaming. For more detailed discussion of these areas the reader is referred to the Suggested Readings at the end of the chapter.

One of the most obvious changes often needed to ensure success in mainstreaming handicapped children is to expand the accessibility of the school's physical plant so that children in wheelchairs or with other mobility problems can move about to their classes and restrooms as independently and unimpeded as possible. Regulations concerning accessibility standards and policies/procedures for removing or otherwise modifying architectural barriers have been developed at the federal, state, and local levels of government. Schools built since the enactment of P.L. 94-142 should already be barrier-free. However, older schools may need a variety of modifications, such as widening of hallways and/or doors, installation of ramps for wheelchairs, handrailings in hallways, widening of toilet stalls to accommodate wheelchairs, raised toilets, and installation of elevators. Such modifications not only improve handicapped students' mobility and integration into the school, but they also promote safety and minimize the risk of further injury and disability, which might require removal of the affected child to a more restrictive educational setting.

Another important action needed to ensure the success of mainstreaming efforts is development and implementation of a carefully planned and thoughtfully executed program for incorporating handicapped students into the school population. The term *program* is used in contrast with the too common practice of providing a proliferation of *services,* which are often poorly coordinated, resulting in gaps and overlap in services (Chapter 13). Development of a *program* for mainstreaming handicapped children is advocated in recognition of the fact that although all children have certain basic needs in common, including the need to be educated to the extent of their abilities and aspirations (Best, 1978), the needs of handicapped children may be exaggerated. Indeed, handicapped children may not only have increased difficulties *learning* (depending on the nature and extent of their handicap), but may also have problems in the areas of social/emotional adjustment and mental health (American Academy of Pediatrics, 1977). To ensure careful assessment of *each* (handicapped) child's educational and health needs and appropriate planning to meet those needs, a program—complete with goals, objectives, and evaluation methods—must be developed and implemented.

A third area of need to be addressed to ensure success in mainstreaming is the need for adequate numbers of qualified teachers. As indicated in the earlier discussion of P.L. 94-142, schools are required to provide in-service education opportunities for teachers and other school staff to better prepare them to work with handicapped students. Although the intent is *not* to expect all teachers to become proficient in special education, there *is* a need for all teachers working with handicapped students to understand the nature of the students' handicaps, the likely effects of those handicaps on students' learning needs and abilities, predictable and unpredictable complications of their handicaps and/or therapies (including possible drug reactions and side effects), special personal needs resulting from the handicaps or therapies (such as need for extra restroom visits or preferential classroom seating), and emergency and first aid procedures should the need arise.

In addition to this need for adequately prepared faculty, there is a need for sufficient numbers of teachers to maintain manageable student-teacher ratios. Because handicapped children need (and are required by P.L. 94-142 to have) IEPs, the presence of these children in regular classrooms obviously demands that some of the teacher's attention be diverted away from the nonhandicapped students. Therefore teachers who may be accustomed to having twenty-eight students in their classes will probably *not* be able to effectively maintain that ratio if some of those students are handicapped; in that event, the school will need to reduce the student-teacher ratio and/or provide supplementary resources (equipment and personnel) for the teacher.

A fourth area of concern in schools where mainstreaming is occurring is the need for supportive or special services to meet the needs of handicapped children. As just noted, teachers may need additional staff such as teacher aides to assist them in classroom management; these teacher aides would then serve to some extent as "teacher extenders," thereby reducing the student-teacher ratio without hiring additional teachers. However, handicapped children may also need the services of a physical therapist, occupational therapist, speech therapist, psychologist, social worker, nurse, special education consultant, or other specialist in order to maintain or improve their health while benefiting maximally from their learning opportunities at school. Schools may have these specialists employed full time within their buildings or may contract for their services as needed. No matter which procedure is followed for securing such needed services, it is the school's moral and legal obligation to ensure that handicapped students' needs are met to enable them to continue their education within the letter and spirit of P.L. 94-142.

Another area of need to be addressed concerns curriculum and instructional modifications to meet the needs of handicapped children. Although the nature of these modifications depends in part on the specific handicap encountered, it is important for each school or school district planning a mainstreaming program to consider the curriculum and the usual instructional methods employed in implementing it to determine what if any changes are warranted. For example, McNab (1978) emphasizes the importance of adequate sex education for all students, including the handicapped, and points out that handicapped students may need a sexuality curriculum that considers their unique learning *and* sexual needs. McNab (1978) discusses sex education for the handicapped, focusing on four specific groups (hearing- and vision-impaired, paralyzed students, and the mentally retarded) to illustrate the need to modify the instructional approach used (as with hearing- and vision-impaired students) and the content and instructional goals (as with mentally retarded students).

Sex education has been cited as an example of the kinds of curricular modifications that may be needed when handicapped students are mainstreamed, but other aspects of the overall curriculum must also be reviewed for possible modification. For example, a school or particular teacher may wish to begin using more self-instructional teaching-learning strategies to allow children (handicapped and nonhandicapped) to progress at their own pace or to use equipment and methods individualized to their learning needs and preferred learning styles (Safford, 1978b).

The preceding five basic educational issues and concerns must be addressed to some extent by nearly all schools involved in mainstreaming efforts. Obviously, depending on the nature of a given mainstreaming effort, the relative priority of these areas may vary, and new areas of concern may arise. The point to be made here, however, is that to successfully meet the unique educational needs of mainstreamed handicapped children, schools must philosophically commit themselves to the concept of mainstreaming and must modify their structure and programs accordingly.

Health needs and the role of the school nurse

In addition to the resulting educational issues and concerns, mainstreaming handicapped children also poses a challenge to the school health program and to the school nurse in particular. The purpose of this discussion, then, is to focus on the role of the school nurse in relation to meeting the health needs of handicapped children. For clarity and consistency, the school nurse's involvement will be approached using the five basic school nurse roles discussed in Chapter 2; suggested tertiary prevention actions will be presented for each of the five school nurse roles (Table 6-3).

The first basic school nurse role is manager of health care within the school health program; among the sample suggested actions for carrying out this role is to lead and/or participate in interdisciplinary team conferences for the pur-

Table 6-3. School nurse roles and tertiary prevention actions

School nurse role	Sample tertiary prevention actions
Manager of health care within school health program	Lead and/or participate in interdisciplinary conferences to plan child's IEP and to monitor his progress toward achievement of stated educational goals Apply principles of staffing and delegation to effectively and efficiently meet handicapped students' health needs while at school
Deliverer of health services	Develop and implement appropriate nursing care plans for handicapped students based on careful assessment of their health status and needs Provide for safe and effective administration of indicated treatments, medications, and other therapies for handicapped students at school
Advocate for children's health rights	Serve as advocate for particular handicapped students to ensure school's responsiveness to their educational and health needs Become politically active and involved at local and state levels to pass legislation providing legal and financial support for equal and adequate educational opportunities for handicapped students
Counselor for health concerns of children, families, and staff	Provide supportive counseling to families of handicapped students to assist them in coping with "crisis" of having disabled child Provide one-to-one and/or small group counseling for handicapped students to help them cope with their limitations Provide individual and/or small group counseling for handicapped students' nonhandicapped peers, teachers, and other school personnel to help them deal with their feelings about handicapped students and to help them more fully integrate handicapped students into school population
Educator for school/community health concerns	Provide (through in-service training or individual consultation) health information and anticipatory guidance for teachers and other school staff regarding particular students or groups of students with similar handicaps to enable them to more effectively and appropriately plan learning activities consistent with handicapped students' needs and limitations Provide health education for handicapped students in such areas as nature and extent of their handicap, self-care activities, coping strategies, and sexuality Provide health education for families of handicapped children regarding such topics as self-care, family dynamics and coping, nature and extent of handicap(s), rationale for prescribed therapies, and availability of community resources

pose of planning a child's IEP and monitoring his progress toward meeting the stated learning goals. Because the school nurse is a health expert and is therefore knowledgeable about the child's handicap and health management, she is a key person to assist in planning an appropriate IEP for him that takes into account his unique needs and problems.

At the same time, in her role as manager of health care, the school nurse must use principles of staffing and delegation (Chapter 18) to ensure that the child's health needs are effectively and efficiently met. Thus the school nurse will need to delegate all aspects of a child's care not requiring her own education and expertise; specially trained volunteers (including fellow students) or other personnel (teacher aides, LPNs, and so on) may be recruited to assist in

the day-to-day delivery of needed health services to affected students.

With regard to her role as deliverer of health services, the school nurse should develop and implement an appropriate nursing care plan for each handicapped child under her jurisdiction; each care plan should be based on careful assessment of the student's health status and needs. In addition, the school nurse's role includes providing for safe, effective administration of ordered treatments, medications, and other therapies for handicapped children at school. It is important to note that this action does *not* necessarily entail administration of the particular drug or treatment *by the nurse herself;* although she is responsible for planning for compliance with specific treatment needs, she may (and in many instances *should*) delegate responsibility for completion of a given treatment or task to someone else.

In her role as advocate for children's health rights, the school nurse may find herself serving as advocate for particular handicapped students to ensure the responsiveness of school officials to their unique educational and health needs. Thus if the nurse believes that certain needs of students are being overlooked and underserved, she can lobby and otherwise pressure administrators to provide the necessary resources to correct the problem. In a broader sense, the role of the school nurse as advocate includes the need to become politically active and involved (Chapter 19) at the local and state levels to pass legislation that provides legal and financial support for efforts to ensure equal and adequate educational opportunities for handicapped students.

As counselor for health concerns of children, families, and staff, the school nurse may take several actions. One action might be to provide supportive counseling to the families of handicapped children (especially those newly diagnosed or disabled) to assist them in coping with the "crisis" of having a disabled child (Barnard and Erickson, 1976). As with any kind of loss, families may be expected to grieve the diagnosis or prognosis of their handicapped children and may need help to adapt positively to this crisis. Because handicapped children may have secondary emotional, mental, and social problems/needs (Barnard and Erickson, 1976; Buscaglia, 1975; Mattsson, 1979; Safford, 1978a), the school nurse may also provide one-to-one and/or small group counseling for handicapped students and/or their families to help the students cope with their limitations while developing and maintaining positive self-concepts. Finally, but of equal importance, the school nurse may provide individual and/or group counseling for the nonhandicapped peers of handicapped students, and for their teachers and other school personnel, to help them deal with *their* feelings about and reactions toward the handicapped students and to help them integrate these handicapped young people into the mainstream of school life. At the same time, the nurse must avoid overemphasizing the handicapped child's differences and disabilities, since that can further hamper efforts to more fully incorporate him into all aspects of school life.

Finally, in her role as educator for school/community health concerns, the school nurse is concerned with providing health information and anticipatory guidance to teachers and other school staff regarding particular students or groups of students with similar handicaps to enable them to more effectively and appropriately plan learning activities that are consistent with the needs and limitations of handicapped students. This action may be taken either through in-service classes provided to faculty and staff groups or through one-to-one consultation with teachers as needed. In addition to thus providing such health information and consultation to teachers and other staff, the school nurse in her role as educator may also provide health education *directly* to handicapped students; areas she might include would be self-care activities, information on the diagnosis and treatment of the child's handicap, availability of social and recreational resources in the community, and sex education, to name a few. Similarly, and perhaps in conjunction with her counseling role, the school nurse may also provide direct health education to the families of handicapped children, incorporating some of the same areas just mentioned, including self-care, the nature of the handicap and rationale for specific treatment or therapy methods, and availability of pertinent community resources.

Through careful attention to her five roles as modified to meet the tertiary prevention needs of handicapped children in the school, the school nurse contributes significantly to the education and integration of these children into the mainstream of school life and activity, thus helping prepare them for productive, self-sufficient lives as adults.

REFERENCES

American Academy of Pediatrics: 1977. School health: a guide for health professionals, American Academy of Pediatrics, Evanston, Ill.

Barnard, K. E., and Erickson, M. L.: 1976. Teaching children with developmental problems, 2nd ed., The C. V. Mosby Co., St. Louis.

Best, G. A.: 1978. Individuals with physical disabilities: an introduction for educators, The C. V. Mosby Co., St. Louis.

Boroch, R. M.: 1976. Elements of rehabilitation in nursing: an introduction, The C. V. Mosby Co., St. Louis.

Buscaglia, L.: 1975. The disabled and their parents: a counseling challenge, Charles B. Slack, Inc., Thorofare, N.J.

Gearheart, B. R., and Weishahn, M. W.: 1976. The handicapped child in the regular classroom, The C. V. Mosby Co., St. Louis.

Jones, E. H.: 1979. P.L. 94-142 and the role of school nurses in caring for handicapped children, J. School Health **49**(3):147-156.

Leavell, H. R., and Clark, E. G.: 1965. Preventive medicine for the doctor in his community: an epidemiologic approach, 3rd ed., McGraw-Hill, Inc., New York.

Mattsson, A.: 1979. Long-term physical illness in childhood: a challenge to psychosocial adaptation. In Garfield, C. A., editor: Stress and survival: the emotional realities of life-threatening illness, The C. V. Mosby Co., St. Louis.

Mayshark, C., Shaw, D. D., and Best, W. H.: 1977. Administration of school health programs: its theory and practice, 2nd ed., The C. V. Mosby Co., St. Louis.

McNab, W. L.: 1978. The sexual needs of the handicapped, J. School Health 48(5):301-306.

Nader, P. R.: 1979. Opening remarks—the handicapped child in school, The Seventh Annual Schering Symposium, Oct. 13, 1978, Dearborn, Mich., J. School Health 49(3):139.

P.L. 94-142: 1975. Education for All Handicapped Children Act of 1975. U.S. Government Printing Office.

Rose, T. L.: 1980. The Education of All Handicapped Children Act [P.L. 94-142]: new responsiblities and opportunities for the school nurse, J. School Health 50(1): 30-31.

Safford, P. L.: 1978a. Mental health counseling dimensions of special education programs, J. School Health 48:541-547.

Safford, P. L.: 1978b. Teaching young children with special needs, The C. V. Mosby Co., St. Louis.

SUGGESTED READINGS

Amundson, M. J.: 1975. Nurses as group leaders of behavior management classes for parents, Nurs. Clin. North Am. 10(2):319-327.

Anderson, C. L., and Creswell, W. H.: 1980. School health practice, 7th ed., The C. V. Mosby Co., St. Louis.

Anfenson, M.: 1980. The school-age child with cystic fibrosis, J. School Health 50(1):26-28.

Bean, M. R., and Bell, B. J.: 1975. Nursing intervention in the care of the physically handicapped, severely retarded child, Nurs. Clin. North Am. 10(2):353-359.

Bleck, E. E.: 1979. Integrating the physically handicapped child, J. School Health 49(3):141-146.

Brewer, G. D., and Kakalik, J. S.: 1974. Improving services to handicapped children: summary and recommendations, Rand McNally & Co., Skokie, Ill.

Bryan, E.: 1979. Administrative concerns and schools' relationship with private practicing physicians, J. School Health 49(3):157-163.

Bryan, E., Warden, M. G., Berg, B., and Hauck, G. R.: 1978. Medical considerations for multiple-handicapped children in the public schools, J. School Health 48(2):84-89.

Bumbalo, J. A., and Seidel, M. A.: 1975. Identifying and serving a multiply handicapped population: deaf-blind children and their families, Nurs. Clin. North Am. 10(2):341-352.

Clapp, M. J.: 1976. Psychosocial reactions of children with cancer, Nurs. Clin. North Am. 11(1):73-82.

Connolly, B. H., and Anderson, R. M.: 1978. Severely handicapped children in the public schools: a new frontier for the physical therapist, Physical Therapy 58(4):433-438.

Daniel, W. A.: 1977. Adolescents in health and disease, The C. V. Mosby Co., St. Louis.

DelCampo, E. J., and Josephson, D. B.: 1978. Accommodating the severely retarded child in our schools, MCN 3(1):34-37.

Fergusson, J. H.: 1975. Late psychologic effects of a serious illness in childhood, Nurs. Clin. North Am. 11(1): 83-93.

Haslam, R. H. A., and Valletutti, P. J., editors: 1975. Medical problems in the classroom: the teacher's role in diagnosis and management, University Park Press, Baltimore, Md.

Hussey, C. G.: 1979. Surviving a handicap in everyday life: how to help, MCN 4(1):46-50.

Jenne, F. H., and Greene, W. H.: 1976. Turner's school health and health education, 7th ed., The C. V. Mosby Co., St. Louis.

MacDonough, G. P.: 1978. Nursing is the name of the game, J. School Health 48(1):618.

Motz, P. A.: 1978. The school-aged child, the law, and the school nurse, J. School Health 48(9):568.

Norris, G. J.: 1975. National concerns for children with handicaps, Nurs. Clin. North Am. 10(2):309-318.

Pattullo, A. W.: 1975. The socio-sexual development of the handicapped child: a preventive care approach, Nurs. Clin. North Am. 10(2):361-372.

Roberts, F. B.: 1979. The child with heart disease. In Garfield, C. A., editor: Stress and survival: the emotional realities of life-threatening illness, The C. V. Mosby Co., St. Louis.

Rose, M. H.: 1975. Coping behavior of physically handicapped children, Nurs. Clin. North Am. 10(2):329-339.

Rusk, H. A.: 1977. Rehabilitation medicine, 4th ed., The C. V. Mosby Co., St. Louis.

Steele, S., editor: 1977. Nursing care of the child with long-term illness, 2nd ed., Appleton-Century-Crofts, New York.

Swisher, J. D.: 1978. Developmental restaging: meeting the mental health needs of handicapped students in the schools, J. School Health 48(9):548-550.

VanPutte, A. W.: 1979. Relationship of school setting to self-concept in physically disabled children, J. School Health 49(10):576-578.

PART III

Adaptation concepts in school nursing practice

CHAPTER 7

Assessing and promoting adaptation in school populations

SUSAN J. WOLD

In Chapter 3, the conceptual framework for school nursing, which has been the focus of this book, was introduced, and its five strands (public health, adaptation, helping relationships, tools, and systematic process) briefly described. In Chapters 4, 5, and 6 the public health strand was further explored and discussed, with an emphasis on levels of prevention and promotion of wellness.

Chapter 7 is the first of three chapters designed to explore and develop the concept of adaptation as applied to school populations and will be followed by discussion of structural variables affecting adaptation (Chapter 8) and concepts of stress and crisis (Chapter 9). To provide a basis for understanding and assimilating the ideas to be presented in Chapters 8 and 9, Chapter 7 will focus on the following three major areas of discussion:

1. Defining adaptation
2. Understanding and assessing adaptation of children, youth, and their families
3. Promoting adaptation: the role of the school nurse

DEFINING ADAPTATION

Attempting to define as ethereal a concept as adaptation is a risky and even foolhardy undertaking. Indeed, as Dubos (1965:257-258) points out:

. . . the word adaptation is treacherous because it can mean so many different things to different persons. The layman, the biologist, the physician, and the sociologist use the word, each in his own way, to denote a multiplicity of genetic, physiologic, psychic, and social phenomena, completely unrelated in their fundamental mechanisms. These phenomena set in motion a great variety of totally different processes, the effects of which may be initially favorable to the individual organism or social group involved, and yet have ultimate consequences that are dangerous in the long run. Furthermore, an adaptive process may be successful biologically while undesirable socially.

However, despite the inherent dangers of attempting to define and apply concepts of adaptation, it is important and necessary to do so because ". . . states of health or disease are the expressions of the success or failure experienced by the organism [person, group, or community] in its efforts to respond adaptively to environmental challenges" (Dubos, 1965:xvii). Thus adaptation is an important area for study, since it promotes understanding of people's attempts to cope with their life situations. For nurses and other health care professionals, an adaptation frame of reference provides a means of viewing clients holistically in assessing their needs and planning and delivering pertinent nursing care, thus avoiding the too frequent tendency to regard clients as fragmented parcels of biological, psychological, spiritual, and social needs (Levine, 1966, 1971; Martin and Prange, 1962).

Definitions and/or models of adaptation have been proposed by a number of authors (Boland et al., 1975; Byrne and Thompson, 1978; Hames, 1978; Jones, 1978; Martin and Prange, 1962; Roy, 1980). Although it may be heretical to say so, some of these definitions and models seem to be too vague and abstract to be generally useful and applicable for nurses and others involved in giving direct nursing care to clients. For that reason, only three definitions—arbitrarily selected for intelligibility and ease of application—will be highlighted in this discussion.

In a definition that is process oriented (as opposed to outcome oriented), Boland et al. (1975:158) define adaptation as a process through which "... man, either individually or in groups, constructively copes with conditions imposed internally or externally in order to meet his needs." Boland et al. further believe that these "conditions" may be stimuli, forces, stressors, or pathological processes (diseases), which are either totally beyond people's control or are the consequences of freely chosen alternatives. These authors further assert that in their view "adaptation" and "life" are synonymous because both terms involve the whole person or organism.

Byrne and Thompson also begin their discussion of adaptation with an emphasis on the process of adapting. Their preliminary definition describes adaptation as "the process or utilization of coping behaviors by an individual when faced with new, different, or threatening stimuli." They note that "behavioral adaptation occurs at each of the behavioral levels: cellular, organ, organ system, organismic, primary group, or community" (1978:28).

However, to enhance the precision and accuracy of client/patient assessment, Byrne and Thompson (1978:28) believe that a distinction must be made between constructive and nonconstructive adaptation. Thus they propose the following outcome-oriented definitions:

Adaptation is . . . the positive, constructive end results, for the person as an ongoing functioning unit, that occur when adjustments are made to either an internal or an external environmental change. Maladaptation then refers to the nonconstructive or destructive consequences for Man as an integrated behavioral unit.

It should be noted, however, that the distinction between an adaptive and maladaptive behavior is not always clear. Thus an individual attempting to preserve the integrity of one body part or system may find that his behavior is actually maladaptive rather than adaptive. For example, a person with arthritis may avoid moving and exercising a swollen, painful joint to reduce discomfort and trauma; however, the long-range outcome of "favoring" the joint may be atrophy and contractures, which may be irreversible (Byrne and Thompson, 1978).

As Byrne and Thompson further point out, a behavior, such as crying, that was originally adaptive may, if continued, actually be maladaptive. When a child or adult cries because he is physically or psychologically "hurt," crying relieves some tension and may also gain the attention and support of other people. However,

if he continues to cry, whine, and complain, the behavior is then maladaptive, resulting in loss of attention and support and increased isolation and tension. Thus, as these examples point out, the distinction between adaptive and maladaptive behavior is not always clear.

The last definition of adaptation to be presented in this chapter is that offered by Martin and Prange who define *adaptation* as "all conscious and unconscious forms of adjustment to actual or supposed environmental conditions—past, present, and future—which confront man." Their definition also regards *environment* as "both that which is exterior and interior to man" (1962:235). This definition is fairly broad, including unconscious as well as conscious efforts to cope with internal or external stimuli or stressors (environmental conditions).

Regardless of which of the preceding definitions is adopted for use, following are some basic assumptions common to all of these definitions:

1. Man is an integrated biopsychosocial being (Byrne and Thompson, 1978; Roy, 1980).
2. Man is constantly interacting with a changing and challenging environment (Roy, 1980).
3. To cope with his changing environment, man uses both innate and acquired biological, psychological, and social means (Roy, 1980).
4. "Health and disease are patterns of adaptive change" (Levine, 1966:2452) and are an "inevitable dimension of life" (Roy, 1980:181).
5. To respond positively (and not merely react) to his changing environment, man must adapt (Roy, 1980).
6. "The person's adaptation level is determined by the combined effect of three classes of stimuli: (1) focal stimuli, or stimuli immediately confronting the person; (2) contextual stimuli, or all other stimuli present; and (3) residual stimuli, such as beliefs, attitudes, or traits which have an indeterminate effect on the present situation" (Roy, 1980:181).
7. "Nursing intervention must be founded not only on scientific knowledge, but specifically on recognition of the individual's behavioral responses which *indicate the nature of the adaptation taking place*" (Levine, 1966:2452).

However, since adaptation appears to be a

vogue concept in nursing and other professions, many different models have been proposed (Byrne and Thompson, 1978; Jones, 1978; Riehl and Roy, 1980), each with its own set of assumptions. Therefore this list is intended to include only those assumptions which appear to be widely accepted and espoused in the literature and are (presumably) the basic tenets of adaptation theory on which Chapters 7 to 9 can be built.

Attributes of adaptation

In the baccalaureate curriculum in the University of Minnesota School of Nursing, one of the strands of the nursing conceptual framework is adaptation. In developing and refining the adaptation strand, the faculty has identified three attributes of man that are believed to significantly influence adaptive behavior; they are *energy, perception,* and *integration.* The importance of these fundamental characteristics or field properties is described by Ryden (1977: 72):

The adaptive process by which the individual copes with changing life events is thus seen as a function of the interrelationships among these attributes. To the extent that one of these attributes is enhanced or diminished, the adaptive process is affected.

Energy

According to the definition adopted by the University of Minnesota School of Nursing faculty, *energy* is "a field force sustaining a living system's capacity to act and to maintain the functions integral to the adaptive process" (University of Minnesota, 1979:32). In a description of man as "a manifestation of energy," Dunn (1961:18-21) discusses five basic types of energy found in the human body: (1) energy bound into matter, (2) energy bound into form, (3) communication energy, (4) stored energy, and (5) expendable energy.

As Dunn explains, *energy bound into matter* includes energy "bound" into the substances that make up the human body, such as water, salts, and other chemicals. The second type of energy he describes, *energy bound into form,* is the force that binds together the cells, tissues, and organs of living organisms. The third type of energy is *communication energy,* which is the type of energy needed to maintain the organism's integrity and to "keep the cells and the various systems in relationship with one another" (1961:19); that is, communication en-

ergy helps coordinate the organism's total activities. As Dunn points out, communication energy is probably equivalent to what Selye (1976) calls *adaptation energy.* Selye believes that each person inherits a finite, genetically determined amount of adaptation energy, which must be budgeted throughout his life span. He can choose to spend it rapidly in pursuit of a colorful, exciting life, or he can spend it thriftily, living what Selye describes as a "long but monotonously uneventful existence" (1976: 82). In either case, however, the quantity of adaptation energy is limited, and individuals therefore need to set their priorities accordingly. The fourth type of energy described by Dunn is *stored energy,* including fat and glycogen, which are stored in the body as reserves until they are needed. The fifth and last kind of energy Dunn describes is *expendable energy,* which is available for use on a continuing basis, such as the energy from daily dietary caloric intake. Expendable energy is needed in large quantities and is directly related to health and wellness, since "the more well we are, the more expendable energy we seem to have in our bodies, available for our purposes" (Dunn, 1961:20). Sleep is no doubt the body's way of recharging its expendable energy "battery," so that energy is available when needed for various activities.

In addition to the five kinds of energy described by Dunn, the University of Minnesota School of Nursing faculty identifies two other types of energy: stimulus energy and psychic energy (University of Minnesota, 1979). *Stimulus energy* or information is used in the process of perception, for which it is transformed into chemical and electrical energy. Stimulus or information energy is stored by the brain as short-term or long-term memory. Although it is less well understood than the various forms of physiological energy, *psychic energy* is thought to be a form of internal stimulus energy; thus *drives* (human needs that motivate individuals) act as "energizers."

Obviously, one's energy requirements depend on a number of factors, including age, body size or surface area, rate and amount of current growth, climate, body temperature, and activity level. How and to what extent any of these factors influence an individual's energy needs and usage will depend in part on individual differences. Despite such individual differences, all organisms (persons) must achieve a balance between energy input and energy expenditure if their adaptation is to be healthy and successful. In other words, "successful adaptation—health—is dependent upon having sufficient energy, transforming it properly, and expending it wisely" (University of Minnesota, 1979:34). Thus all individuals must carefully conserve their energy by setting priorities for its use, since the more energy that is used for basic maintenance functions and survival activities, the less energy will be available for mobility and growth (University of Minnesota, 1979).

In other words, energy is required for achieving individuals' adaptive goals. Because nurses are concerned about their clients' adaptation, they need to carefully assess clients' energy by considering the following questions (University of Minnesota, 1979:35):

1. How adequate are the client's basic physiological energy sources, such as nutrients, oxygen, water, and rest?
2. Are there any indications of problems in energy transformation, such as problems with digestion, respiration, circulation, and fluid balance?
3. What basic needs or goals are acting as energizers for the individual?
4. What are the main areas of energy expenditure? That is, for what primary activities is the individual expending his available energy?
5. Is the individual's current energy intake adequate for meeting his expenditures?
6. Has the individual experienced changes in his life situation requiring and resulting in reallocation of his energy expenditure?
7. What are the factors (such as age, body size, activity level) presently influencing the individual's energy requirements?

Perception

The second attribute of man that significantly influences adaptation is *perception*. As used in this chapter, *perception* may be defined as "the process of receiving and interpreting incoming sensory data from the internal and external environment" (University of Minnesota, 1979:22). As an attribute affecting adaptation, three aspects of perception are generally included: physiology, psychology, and self-concept. Although each of these three aspects will be briefly described, the reader is encouraged to consult reliable texts and other literature in the fields of physiology, general psychology, and perceptual psychology for more comprehensive discussion.

Probably the most obvious forms of physiological perception are the sensory processes such as vision, hearing, taste, smell, and touch. These senses depend on the functioning of receptor cells within sensory organs such as the eyes, ears, tongue, nose, and skin. Sensory perceptions such as vision and hearing also depend on transformation of the energy (in the form of light or sound waves) received from the environment into a transmissible form or code, which can then be sent to the central nervous system for interpretation and determination of an appropriate adaptive response (University of Minnesota, 1979). Similarly, receptors sensitive to changes in body posture and positioning, as in the semicircular canals of the inner ear, help man maintain equilibrium. Thus physiological perception involves: (1) a peripheral nervous system (including receptors and their structures, collectively referred to as peripheral neural activity), (2) central nervous system activity (central neural events), and (3) central neural storage, which includes the neural events and changes that occur in response to past stimulation. These three elements combine to produce the "phenomenal events of perception" (University of Minnesota, 1979:22).

The psychological aspects of perception generally include two elements: *selection* and *organization* (University of Minnesota, 1979). *Selection* includes attention or readiness to select sensory data or stimuli from the environment; that is, selection is the means by which stimuli capture one's attention or are "received." This selection process is influenced by the intensity, size, repetition, and change in a given stimulus. Thus a teenager's parents may "select" the sound of loud "acid rock" music, played over and over on the family stereo and may react by demanding that it be turned down (or preferably off!), and yet their teenager may not perceive that same music at the chosen volume as being more than mere background sound for doing homework or studying.

The second psychological element of perception is *organization,* which is the process by which a selected stimulus (that is, one which has caught the person's attention) is organized and becomes meaningful. This organization process is influenced by past experience, knowledge, and attitudes and beliefs. Again, using the example of rock music, if the teenager's parents have always disliked rock music, believe that it can damage one's hearing, and associate loud rock music with "negative social elements," such as "free love" and drug abuse, they are likely to try to limit its influence on their teenage children and to restrict the frequency and volume at which it is played at home. However, if their teenagers love rock music, believe that it has to be loud to be experienced fully, and associate rock music with the joy of living, including parties and other good times, then the stage is set for a potentially full-scale war between parents and their teenagers concerning musical taste and volume.

In addition to the physiological and general psychological aspects of perception is a third very important perceptual aspect: self-concept. According to Combs et al. (1978:17), *self-concept* includes "all those aspects of the perceptual field to which we refer when we say 'I' or 'me.' It is the organization of perceptions about self that seems to the individual to be who he or she is." Furthermore, the self-concept is a composite of many perceptions of varying "clarity, precision, and importance in the person's peculiar economy." In other words, one's self-concept is the frame of reference for viewing and experiencing the world, a "personal reality, the vantage point from which all else is observed and comprehended" (Combs et al., 1978:19). Thus objects are perceived as being closer or farther away or to the right or left of oneself. In addition, one's self is likewise the "yardstick" for making various judgments; others are viewed as taller, smarter, older, happier, or more self-assured than oneself. Because the self is the center or basis for these judgments, this perceptual yardstick changes as the self inevitably changes due to aging and other life changes. One's judgments and beliefs change over time, so that perceptions of what is "old" and what is politically "conservative" may be quite different at age 21 as compared with age 65.

The following basic characteristics of self-concept that affect adaptation (Combs et al., 1978:17-26) provide further clarification and a common frame of reference for this chapter:

1. Self-concept is an integration of both the physical and psychological self; thus, it includes both bodily characteristics (such as height, weight, hair and eye color) and one's values and attitudes about those characteristics and other traits.

2. One's self-concept acts as a screen or perceptual filter for viewing and experiencing the world; as such, it acts as a selectively permeable barrier between the person and his environment.

3. Experiences and perceptions that are congruent with one's existing self-concept tend to be readily accepted, whereas those which are incongruent may be discomforting and anxiety-producing. Thus, a once obese teenage girl who has succeeded in losing her excess weight may nonetheless continue to view herself as "fat" and unattractive, even though she may now be a svelte size 5. In extreme cases, such an adolescent girl might persist in her dieting and weight loss efforts even to the point of developing an eating disorder, which may involve overeating or food binges followed by self-induced vomiting to avoid weight gain. On the other hand, a teenager growing up in a family in which everyone is significantly overweight may have a positive body image and self-concept, viewing herself as comparatively "average" or "normal."

4. The self-concept is self-corroborating; that is, the self-concept tends to support existing beliefs about the self, thus maintaining and reinforcing its existence. In other words, the self-concept is circular, perpetuating the idea that "I am because I think I am." This circular property can be either positive or negative for the individual; a person who feels and projects an aura of self-confidence, will probably be more successful in winning others' confidence than will a person of equal ability who feels and acts uncertain.

5. Because of this self-perpetuating and self-corroborating property, the self-concept has a high degree of stability and is therefore difficult to change once it has been solidly established. As Combs et al. (1978:22) note, this often results in persons becoming "victims" of their own limited self-perceptions who remain on the "treadmill of self-corroboration," thereby contributing to such pervasive social problems as poverty and unemployment. For health professionals (including school nurses), this self-perpetuating property of self-concept can be a two-edged sword; to a client who has always been "able to eat anything," the restrictions of a diabetic diet may be intolerable and may therefore be ignored. In contrast, a client whose health has always been of

tantamount importance may readily incorporate seemingly radical life-style changes without protest or difficulty and may even get "carried away" with his health and treatment regimens, embracing them with an almost religious fervor.

6. One's self-concept is *learned,* based on one's experiences and interactions with the physical environment and with other people, especially those persons viewed as "significant others." From these experiences and interactions emerges a sense of identity or "personness," which guides the individual's behavior for the rest of his life. Therefore children who "learn" early in life that they are unlovable, unattractive, and/or "bad," may be haunted by those perceptions for the rest of their lives, which is one reason why school health programs should include components intended to help children develop positive and healthy self-concepts early in life.

Because one's perception of the world determines how one adapts to his physical and psychological environment, nurses must focus their assessments on the client's perception of himself, his health, and his life situation. Nurses must also remember that clients will respond or react to stimuli *as they perceive them,* regardless of the situation's reality (University of Minnesota, 1979). Furthermore, a person's behavior represents his perception of the most appropriate behavior at that time and must be judged accordingly. Even when a client's behavior seems bizarre or inappropriate to the nurse or others, that behavior "makes sense" to the client at that moment. Therefore to fully understand clients' behavior and to assist them to adapt positively to their life situations, nurses must use their helping relationship skills to gain clients' perceptions and should assess those perceptions based on the following questions (University of Minnesota, 1979):

1. How adequate is the client's perceptual apparatus? That is, can he hear, see, touch, smell, and taste? Is his nervous system functioning properly? Does he have any psychological or mental health problems?
2. What stimuli does the client select to perceive? That is, which stimuli capture his attention?
3. How does he view his situation?
4. How accurate are his views (perceptions)?
5. What information or data is available concerning the client's self-concept?
6. How does the client view others?
7. Concerning the amount of stimulation the client receives, is he experiencing stimulus overload? Does he lack adequate stimulation?
8. How do his past experiences affect his current perceptions?

Integration

The third attribute of man believed (in addition to energy and perception) to significantly influence adaptive behavior is *integration,* which is defined as "the process by which the contributing parts and functions of a system are organized, regulated and coordinated to achieve the integrity and well-being of the whole" (University of Minnesota, 1979:28). Integration allows the person or organism to function holistically by unifying his adaptive behavior. When an individual's body systems work together in harmony and unity, he can interact more effectively with his environment and can better achieve a balance between internal and external environmental demands and expectations. This holistic, integrated view of man is reflected in Byrne and Thompson's belief that "man as a whole is different from and more than the sum of his component parts" (1978:4).

As an attribute of individuals and groups, integration is necessary for effective functioning (University of Minnesota, 1979). According to Levine (1971), integration or integrity can be thought of as occurring on three dimensions: structural, personal, and social. *Structural integrity* refers to maintenance of bodily structure (physical and physiological) or "wholeness"; examples of bodily efforts to promote structural integrity are blood clot formation and the inflammatory reaction that occur following cuts or other breaks in the skin. Structural integrity thus includes all physiological processes and phenomena that preserve the body's structure and enhance its functioning. *Personal integrity* concerns an individual's *perceptions* of himself as a "whole" person; that is, his identity and feelings of self-worth. Thus although a person may be *structurally* (physically and physiologically) integrated, unless he *perceives* himself as "whole" and as a person of worth, he may lack *personal* integration. An individual's integration depends on *both* structural (physical) *and* personal (psychological/perceptual) integrity. The third dimension of integrity described by Levine is *social integrity*, which includes both an individual's socialization into groups such as the family, as well as the group process or communication dynamics of the group as a whole (which is actually an "integration" of individuals). Indeed, the group dynamics within a family or other important social group can directly affect the structural and personal integrity and overall health of the individual. For that reason, nurses must carefully assess all three dimensions of their clients' integration.

Although integration may seem to be a hazy concept to understand and apply, perhaps the following example can help clarify its usefulness. After delivering her first baby, the postpartum woman is abruptly propelled into a period of rapid physiological and psychological change. Because labor and delivery greatly deplete her energy stores and because she has lost blood volume during those processes, her structural integrity is threatened; she needs adequate nutrition and rest, plus surveillance of her vital signs, lochia, and fundal firmness to ensure structural integration. In addition, after the arrival of the infant, the woman must now begin perceiving herself in the new role of mother and as an adequate mother if she is to maintain her personal integrity. Finally, with the arrival of the infant, the family's roles and social patterns become more complex; effective socialization or incorporation of the baby into the family will require parental time, energy, and communication if the family is to maintain its social integrity as a group. Thus such a common occurrence as the birth of an infant can affect structural, personal, and social integration.

As Levine (1971) points out, the goal of nursing care is to conserve or maintain clients' structural, personal, and social integrity—that is, to "promote wholeness." However, if nurses are to support clients' integrative processes and efforts, they must first assess present levels of integration so that an appropriate plan of care can be established. Although they are not intended to be exhaustive, the following lists are suggested as guides for assessing clients' integration. In assessing structural integration, these areas/factors should be considered (University of Minnesota, 1979):

1. Functional adequacy of regulators of physiological homeostasis, such as fluid and electrolyte balance, respiration, circulation, and gastrointestinal function
2. Structural and functional integrity of the nervous system

3. Adequacy of endocrine function
4. Adequacy of metabolic processes
5. Adequacy of neuromuscular integration, as determined by assessment of coordination, locomotion, speech, and vision

Assessment of personal integrity, which depends on the client's perceptions, is accordingly more difficult and less precise than assessment of structural integrity. Following are areas/factors to be considered:

1. Cognitive integration; that is, ability to "learn, understand, see relationships, problem solve, analyze, synthesize" (University of Minnesota, 1979:29).
2. Personality integration: a sense of identity or "unity of self"—"having it together" (University of Minnesota, 1979:29).
3. Possession of a sense of purpose to one's life and a sense of life's meaning to begin answering the question "What's it all about?" Development of life philosophy, values, and goals.
4. Ability to meet basic human needs and to achieve balance among the spheres of one's life; avoid putting "all one's eggs in one basket."
5. Integration of new developmental tasks and new roles appropriate for age; ability to cope with developmental and situational change and stress and to assimilate changes into one's self-concept (University of Minnesota, 1979:29).

In contrast with structural and personal integration, which focus on the individual, assessment of social integration considers the individual's interactions and involvement with others and may also include assessment of a *group's* integration, such as a family or a work group. In assessing an individual's social integration into groups, the following questions may be helpful (University of Minnesota, 1979):

1. What (if any) evidence is there of the individual's sense of "belonging" or identification with groups such as family, ethnic/cultural group, community, nation, and the world?
2. Is there evidence of alienation from any of these groups?
3. Does the individual's present adaptation include becoming a member of a new social group? Does it demand reintegration into a group to which he formerly belonged (such as a former client of a mental hospital being discharged into the community, or a child with a chronic illness

returning to school after a long absence)? In assessing the social integration of a group as a whole, it is suggested (University of Minnesota, 1979) that the following questions be addressed:

1. Is the group cohesive? If so, to what extent?
2. Does communication within the group facilitate or interfere with integration?
3. Are the group's activities guided by a clear sense of purpose?
4. How does the group organize itself to achieve its goals?
5. Are the activities of group members coordinated?

Levels of adaptive behavior

Adaptive behavior may be viewed as occurring on three levels: compensation, mobility, and growth (University of Minnesota, 1979). Indeed, these levels may be thought of as a hierarchy, beginning at the bottom with compensation and culminating at the top with growth (Ryden, 1977). Since assessment of an individual's adaptive behavior requires attention to the level of that behavior, each of these three behavioral categories or levels will be briefly discussed.

Compensation

As defined by the faculty at the University of Minnesota School of Nursing, *compensation* involves "the maintenance and restoration of biophysical and psychosocial equilibrium" by means of "protective, defensive, regulatory, and homeostatic behaviors" (University of Minnesota, 1979:5); the primary focus of compensation behaviors is *internal*. Examples of compensatory level behaviors include two basic categories:

1. *All* physiological responses, such as eating, sleeping, fainting, and vital signs such as temperature, pulse, respiration, and blood pressure (University of Minnesota, 1979)
2. Internally focused psychological defense mechanisms intended to maintain or restore psychological equilibrium, such as denial, withdrawal, or repression (University of Minnesota, 1979; Ryden, 1977)

School phobia, as evidenced by the child who becomes physically "sick" before or during school or who withdraws physically or psychologically from his classmates, may be viewed as compensatory level behavior, because the goal of the behavior, whether conscious or unconscious, is to restore *internal* physical and psychological equilibrium by avoiding a perceived stressful situation (school).

Mobility

The second level of adaptive behavior is *mobility*, which involves active coping with the *external* environment; that is, mobility includes attempts to "explore, deal with and master the environment" (University of Minnesota, 1979:5) and has an *external* focus. Examples of mobility level behaviors include work, social interactions, sports and hobbies, problem solving, and "aggressive response to threat" (University of Minnesota, 1979:5; Ryden, 1977:74). School-age children who are actively involved in their studies, participate in athletics, and are active members of clubs, church groups, and the like are engaging in mobility behaviors (and, if new behaviors and learning are involved, are also demonstrating *growth*).

Growth

The third and highest level of adaptive behavior is *growth*, including psychosocial, biological, and cognitive growth. Growth entails development of "new behaviors, new skills, new insight" (University of Minnesota, 1979:6). Examples of growth level behaviors include physical growth (increased height and weight), pregnancy (conception and development of new life), mastery of new skills (learning to read or write), and "learning evidenced by changed behavior" (University of Minnesota, 1979:6), such as the preschool child who learns to verbally ask for food and toys, rather than merely pointing at the desired object.

The individual's adaptive level depends in part on his available energy. If his energy is limited, he may remain internally focused and may therefore operate at a compensatory level. If he has more energy than that needed for compensation, he may be motivated to expand his focus to the *external* environment, achieving mobility and/or growth. Although growth is the highest behavioral level, individuals demonstrating growth behaviors also demonstrate compensatory (life-sustaining) and mobility (external coping) behaviors. Because growth is built on compensatory and mobility levels, an individual demonstrating growth is by definition also demonstrating some compensation and mobility. Therefore assessment of individuals' adaptive behaviors may reveal evidence of all three levels.

Up to this point, adaptation has been defined,

its attributes (energy, perception, and integration) identified and discussed, and levels of adaptive behavior described. With this content as background and a common frame of reference, application of adaptation theory in understanding and assessing the adaptation of children, youth, and their families will be discussed.

UNDERSTANDING AND ASSESSING ADAPTATION OF CHILDREN, YOUTH, AND THEIR FAMILIES

Because the primary population with whom the school nurse works includes children (preschool and school age), youth (adolescents), and their families, it is important for her to be able to understand and assess their adaptation if her interventions are to be appropriate and effective. However, because this population is so large and diverse and because of the large volume of literature available that addresses adaptation of children, youth, and families, it is impossible for this chapter (or *any* one chapter) to adequately and thoroughly discuss their adaptive needs and ways of assessing their adaptation. For that reason, this discussion will be somewhat generalized. The following arbitrarily selected areas will be included:

1. Understanding and assessing expected growth and development of children and youth
2. Nutritional needs of children and youth
3. Life events and their effect on the adaptation of children and youth
4. Family development and assessment

Understanding and assessing expected growth and development of children and youth

To discuss expected growth and development, a review of several basic ideas introduced in Chapter 4 is in order. As noted in that chapter, human growth and development generally proceed in an ordered sequence based on discernible developmental stages. Although the precise labeling of those stages depends on the theorist and developmental area (psychosocial, cognitive, moral) studied, growth and development are regarded as epigenetic processes; that is, each new stage is built on the preceding stages and thus depends on successful resolution of critical developmental tasks at each stage. For example, an infant learns to crawl or creep before he walks, since walking is "built" on the muscular development and coordination used for crawling and creeping. Similarly, an infant must resolve his "trust versus mistrust" crisis before he can feel secure enough to work on the "autonomy versus shame and doubt" conflict of the next developmental stage (Erikson, 1963). Thus according to Duvall (1971: 139), although successful achievement of developmental tasks results in happiness and success with later tasks, failure results in "unhappiness in the individual, disapproval by society, and difficulty with later tasks." In other words, individuals' early development affects their later development, which reinforces the importance of primary prevention and health promotion.

While achievement of one's stage- and age-appropriate developmental tasks is critically important, interpretation of individuals' developmental progression must be cautiously done to allow for individual differences. Although most developmental theorists such as Erikson (1963; 1968), Duvall (1971), and Piaget (Ginsburg and Opper, 1969) identify approximate ages that correspond with specific developmental stages and tasks, it is important to remember that these are *only* approximations. *Every child is unique and develops at his/her own pace.* Indeed, as the AAP (1977) points out, there is a wide range of "normal" development; walking into any classroom and observing the vast differences in height, weight, and body build among children of the same age and sex is partial proof of that fact. Although developmental screening tests and other assessment tools can help determine the extent of a child's development *at that point in time* compared with other children of the same age, allowances for children's individual differences must be made in interpreting results. A child's *overall pattern* of growth and development and his overall progression toward maturity *are of greater consequence than the precise age at which he achieves a given developmental task.* Failure to remember this too often results in the harmful mislabeling of some children as "slow" or "retarded"—a label that can handicap them for the rest of their lives.

With the preceding review of basic concepts of growth and development as a common frame of reference, the remainder of this discussion will be devoted to specific areas of individual growth and development, including physical growth and cognitive, psychosocial, and moral development. Physical growth, cognitive development, and psychosocial development are summarized in Table 7-1; moral development is summarized in Table 7-3. However, readers are

Table 7-1. Expected growth and development of children and youth by age group

	Age group			References
	Preschool (ages 3 to 5)	School age (ages 6 to 12)	Adolescence (ages 13 to 20)	
Physical				
Growth rate	Height, 2 to 2½ inches (5 to 6.3 cm); weight gain of 5 pounds (2.3 kg) per year	Height, 2 inches (5 cm) per year; weight gain is 10% of total body weight per year; head growth nearing completion by age 6; by age 12, brain reaches adult size	Ages 12 to 13, girls begin puberty, completed by age 15 to 16; boys' puberty begins at age 13 to 14, completed by 17 to 19	AAP (1977) Brower and Nash (1979) Frankenburg et al. (1975)
Body build	Tall and thin	Wiry, slender, long legged (ages 6 to 9); lean bodies, narrow shoulders and hips (ages 9 to 12)	Ages 12 to 14, appear to be "all arms and legs," but most growth actually occurs in trunk; ages 15 to 18, most growth occurs in arms and legs; range of builds is from short and stocky to tall and thin	Murray et al. (1979c)
Motor skills	Age 3 years: throws ball overhand; walks up and down stairs, alternating feet; builds tower of four to eight blocks; copies circle; rides tricycle Age 4 years: balances on one foot for 5 to 10 seconds, hops on one foot; uses scissors; heel-toe walks; copies cross Age 5 years: catches bounced ball; heel-toe walks forward and backward; runs and skips with agility and speed; copies square; draws man with three to six distinct parts	Physically active ("energetic"); balance and coordination improving; manual skill and eye-hand coordination improving	Activity level varies: may become involved in organized competitive athletics	
Cognitive	*Preoperational thought period: preconceptual phase (ages 2 to 4)* Egocentric, limited perceptions, and "centering" of thoughts within self Associates objects as representative of other objects Uses symbolic and imaginary play; for example, thinks his tricycle is a police car and his toy gun is real	*Preoperational thought period: intuitive phase (ages 4 to 7)* Thinking becomes more complex and elaborate Egocentrism gives way to social interaction and social signs More flexible language use, including use of "because," indicating beginning awareness of cause-effect relationships	*Period of formal operations (ages 11 to 15)* Uses wider range of symbolic processes and logic than during previous stage No longer focuses only on "real," but is now able to consider and operate with "possible" Systematically solves hypothetical, mental, and verbal problems and uses scientific reasoning; no longer uses trial and error	Ginsburg and Opper (1969) Kaluger and Kaluger (1979) Maier (1969) McClinton and Meier (1978) Murray et al. (1979c) Piaget (1952)

Continued.

			References
Play occupies waking hours; with its focus on "how" and "why" becomes the child's primary adaptive tool—child "plays his way through life"	Begins to use language for communicating thoughts to others	Capable of imaginative, creative thought, and may theorize, test hypotheses, and critically evaluate his own logic	AAP (1977)
Magical thinking and animism	Centering persists		Duvall (1971)
Lacks concept of reversibility	Believes that things are as they appear		Erikson (1963, 1968)
Inability to state cause-effect relationships; belief that proximal events are related	Animism persists		Kaluger and Kaluger (1979)
Egocentric language: talks aloud to self or to objects; may talk in "monologues" even when others are present (collective monologues); *assumes* others understand him	May be able to count and may know right hand from left, but does not yet understand *concepts* of numbers and right and left		Murray and Zentner (1979a)
	Period of concrete operations (ages 7 to 11)		Murray et al. (1979c)
	Uses perceptions of concrete reality to form mental images		O'Neil et al. (1977)
	Thinking becomes decentered, dynamic, and reversible		Siemon (1978)
	Operations characteristic of this stage: conservation, reversibility, classification, seriation, nesting, and multiplication		Smart and Smart (1972)
	Can imagine object or situation from another person's perspective, and can see others' viewpoints		

Psychosocial

Developmental crisis		
Initiative versus guilt	Industry versus inferiority	Identity versus identity confusion
Developmental tasks		
Formation of gender or sex-role identity	Successful school entrance and achievement: *competence*, especially in academic arena	Establishing "sense of self," including sexual identity
Development of healthy self-concept and body image	Expanding one's social network: *belonging* to gang	Choosing occupation/vocation and planning for eventual economic independence
Increased peer associations	Development of close relationship with one same-age and same-sex peer	Adopting stable life-style, based on socially responsible attitudes and behaviors, which provides opportunities for commitment and close relationships with significant others
Solitary, then parallel play, evolving into cooperative play		Emancipation of one's self from family, while maintaining loving relationship with them

Table 7-1. Expected growth and development of children and youth by age group—cont'd

	Age group		References
Preschool (ages 3 to 5)	School age (ages 6 to 12)	Adolescence (ages 13 to 20)	
Developmental tasks—cont'd		Becoming responsible, contributing citizen guided by socially acceptable set of values and moral principles	
Adaptive mechanisms Introjection, primary and secondary identification, fantasy, and repression	Ritualistic behavior, reaction formation, undoing, isolation, fantasy, identification, regression, malingering, rationalization, projection, and sublimation	Compensation, sublimation, and identification	
Language Vocabulary develops from 900 words (age 3) to 1500 words (age 4) to 2100 words (age 5); by age 5 can count to 10 and name four colors	Six-year-old has oral vocabulary of approximately 2500 words; uses sentences about five words long; uses all parts of speech; can recognize some printed letters of alphabet and few words; language use more socialized; comprehends some abstract uses, such as jokes, puns, and figures of speech; develops written communication skills: first printing, then longhand; learns to read at age 6	Peer group dialect commonly used; continued growth in use of language skills and expansion of vocabulary, depending on educational and social opportunities and norms	

cautioned to use these tables only as guides in assessing individual children and youth; this information is *not* intended to be used as a bible or screening tool.

Physical growth

Childhood is obviously a period of rapid physical growth, as children progress toward adult stature and somatotype. Their growth is generally evaluated by recording periodic measurements of height, weight, and (especially for infants) head circumference and by plotting those measurements by age and sex on a growth grid (Chapter 12). Use of such grids allows comparison of children's growth with other children of the same age and sex, while at the same time providing a record of each child's growth over time. Again, it is important to use growth charts and grids discriminately, bearing in mind that a child's overall growth progression is more significant than his actual percentile rank on a growth chart or grid. Thus a child whose height and weight are consistently at the 40th percentile *may* nonetheless be growing ''normally'' and consistently with his heredity. School nurses and other health professionals may occasionally need to reassure parents and children themselves that a particular child's comparatively ''small'' or ''large'' size is normal for that child (assuming, of course, that growth defects, delays, or other related health defects are not present). Table 7-1 describes the average or usual rate of growth for preschool and school-age children and adolescents and their corresponding body build changes.

Cognitive development

The second area of growth and development is *cognitive development* (Table 7-1), which may be defined as the development of ''a logical method of looking at the world, utilizing one's perceptual and conceptual powers'' (Kaluger and Kaluger, 1979:493).

The late Jean Piaget is considered one of the foremost researchers and theorists in the area of cognitive and intellectual development. Based on his descriptive and experimental studies of children (using his own children as his first subjects), Piaget theorized that human cognitive development involves the following four basic ''periods,'' one of which includes two distinct phases (Piaget, 1952):

    I. Sensorimotor period (ages 0 to 2)
    II. Preoperational thought period (overall, ages 2 to 7): preconceptual phase (ages 2 to 4), intuitive phase (ages 4 to 7)
    III. Period of concrete operations (ages 7 to 11)
    IV. Period of formal operations (ages 11 to 15)

Because this book does not include infants as part of its direct focus, the sensorimotor period will not be discussed and is not included in Table 7-1. However, in the remainder of this discussion of cognitive development, periods II, III, and IV will be highlighted.

Preoperational thought period: preconceptual phase. During the preconceptual phase, which begins at about age 2 and concludes at about age 4, the child's thinking is characteristically *egocentric;* that is, he is unable to take another's point of view. In addition, the child's thoughts are *centered,* or focused, on only a single aspect of an object or situation. Therefore when asked to sort a group of red and yellow shapes (such as spheres, squares, and triangles), a child in this phase would be able to sort only by shape *or* color, not by shape *and* color, because his thought is ''centered'' on only one attribute (shape or color).

During this phase, the child also begins to acquire use of symbols, and enjoys symbolic and fantasy play. Thus he may think of his tricycle as a police car and his toy gun as ''real.'' Play becomes his predominant activity during waking hours and is his ''primary adaptive tool,'' since it teaches him ''how'' and ''why''; indeed, the child seems to ''play his way through life'' (Maier, 1969:119). Also during this period, the child uses magical thinking and *animism,* which is the belief that inanimate objects are actually alive (McClinton and Meier, 1978). Thus when he trips over a chair, the child may scold the ''bad'' chair for ''kicking'' him.

In addition, the child in the preconceptual phase is characterized by his use of *irreversible thought,* which is the inability to ''undo mentally that which has been done in reality'' (McClinton and Meier, 1978:194). For example, if the child walks with an adult or other person through an unfamiliar neighborhood to visit at someone's home, he will not be able to reverse or retrace his steps back to his starting point. In this phase, the child is further hampered by his inability to state cause-effect relationships; instead, he is likely to believe that two events that occur close together (in time) are related. An example might be the child who is singing happily in the bathtub when the lights suddenly go out; he may erroneously conclude that his singing caused the power failure and may therefore be afraid to sing during his bath again.

A final characteristic of the preconceptual phase is the child's use of language, which tends to be egocentric, in that he talks aloud to himself or to inanimate objects in a kind of "monologue." Even in the presence of others, the child may talk aloud to no one in particular. When two or more children in the preconceptual phase are observed, these monologues become "collective," with each child talking aloud without expecting others to listen or respond. As further evidence of his egocentric language, when the child does "communicate" with others, as in the telling of a story, he makes no effort to explain or elaborate as he talks and may as a result omit crucial details of the story or event he is narrating (McClinton and Meier, 1978).

Preoperational thought period: intuitive phase. By about age 4, the intuitive phase begins, during which the child's thinking becomes more complex and elaborate and his egocentrism gives way to "social interaction and social signs" (Kaluger and Kaluger, 1979:186). Although animism and centered thought may persist during this time, the child is beginning to use language for communicating his thoughts to others and is less likely to talk aloud to himself. Language use becomes more flexible as well; the child's increasing use of the word "because" indicates his beginning awareness of cause-effect relationships. However, his thought processes are still immature and intuitive, because when asked "to give a reason for a certain happening, he will give some coincidentally occurring characteristic such as 'The sun sets because people want to go to bed' " (Kaluger and Kaluger, 1979:186).

Also, during this phase the child judges experiences and events on the basis of their outward appearance and results; he believes that things are as they appear. Thus, if the child's environment is altered or rearranged, such as by moving his bed to a new room, the bed becomes "new" or foreign to him. It is also significant that despite his ability to count and to distinguish his right hand from his left, the child in the intuitive phase does not yet *understand* concepts such as numbers or right and left (Kaluger and Kaluger, 1979; Maier, 1969).

Period of concrete operations. The period of concrete operations begins at about age 7 and continues until about age 11. As defined by Murray et al. (1979c:172), this stage involves "systematic reasoning about tangible [concrete] or familiar situations." The child's thought is now *operational* in that the child has "the mental capacity to order and relate experience to an organized whole" (Maier, 1969:136). Piaget divides operational thought into two stages: concrete operations and formal operations. This division is based on Piaget's observations that children's initial performance of mental operations (ages 7 to 11) relies on their perceptions of "concrete reality," whereas older children (ages 11 to 15) can use symbolism and abstractions, which characterize the period of formal operations.

The child in the period of concrete operations uses perceptions of concrete reality to form mental images. In addition, his thinking becomes decentered, dynamic, and reversible. The child's thinking is *decentered* in the sense that he can consider more than one aspect or characteristic of an object or situation; thus he can now sort wooden blocks by color and shape. During this stage the child's thought processes have also moved from static to *dynamic;* that is, the child is able to "attend to transformations between end states and gain usable information" (McClinton and Meier, 1978:196). For example, in testing a child's ability to *conserve,* that is, to see "that mass or quantity remains the same even if it changes shape or position" (Murray et al., 1979c:173), using different sized glasses and a fixed quantity of water or any liquid, the child in the preoperational phase whose thinking is static, will invariably, after watching the tester pour the water from one container to another of a different shape without spilling a drop, say that the quantity of water has increased or decreased simply because it "looks" different. The child is unable to "use" his observations of the water being poured from one glass to another without spilling to accurately conclude that the water volume has not changed. The child in the concrete operational phase, in contrast, whose thinking is now dynamic, *is* able to use his observations and thus is able to conserve as well. Finally, the child's thinking is also *reversible,* which means that he can mentally "undo" what he has observed (McClinton and Meier, 1978) and can "follow a line of reasoning back to its starting point" (Murray et al., 1979c:173). The child can see, for example, that to return home from his friend's house requires that he "reverse" the series of right turns he made on the way there to left turns.

In addition to the operations of *conservation* and *reversibility,* in the concrete operational phase, the child can perform the following operations: *classification, seriation, nesting,* and *multiplication.* According to the definitions of Murray et al. (1979:173), *classification* entails "sorting objects in groups according to attributes" such as shape or color. *Seriation* refers to "ordering objects according to increasing or decreasing measure" such as height or weight. *Nesting* involves being able to understand "how a single concept fits into a larger concept"; for example, the child could identify that cups and saucers (single concept) are dishes (larger concept) or that dogs (single concept) are also animals (larger concept). The final operation associated with this period is *multiplication,* which refers to "simultaneously classifying and seriating, or using two attributes together"; an example of multiplication is the child who can sort his blocks according to both color and shape.

The final characteristic of the concrete operational phase is the child's ability to imagine or envision an object or situation from another angle or perspective; thus, for example, the child can rearrange a group of dolls to show how they would appear to someone sitting on the opposite side of the table. In addition, the child is now able to see another's point of view, rather than focusing egocentrically on his own views, and, as a result, his communication with others is enhanced (McClinton and Meier, 1978).

Period of formal operations. The period of formal operations roughly corresponds with adolescence, beginning at about age 11 and continuing until approximately age 15 (Kaluger and Kaluger, 1979; Maier, 1969; Murray et al., 1979c). A principal distinction between this stage and concrete operations is that the youth uses a wider range of symbolic processes and logic than during the previous stage (Murray et al., 1979c).

In addition, he no longer focuses only on the "real," but is now able to consider and operate with the "possible" (Kaluger and Kaluger, 1979); he can now anticipate the consequences of his own and others' actions. The adolescent is also able to systematically (rather than randomly or by trial and error) solve problems, whether they are hypothetical, mental, or verbal, and can use scientific reasoning (Murray et al., 1979c). As a result, the adolescent is capable of imaginative, creative thought, which may lead to theorizing, hypothesis testing, and critical evaluation of his own logic (Kaluger and Kaluger, 1979; Murray et al., 1979c). However, as McClinton and Meier (1978:197) point out, the hazard of this period of formal operations is that the adolescent's self-absorption and preoccupation with his own thoughts and logic may lead him to believe that he can "change the world." Thus although this period is a maturation of cognition, it also represents a limited return to egocentrism.

Children's understanding and perceptions of death as reflections of their cognitive development. Although discussion of children's perceptions of death may at first seem out of place in a book about school nursing, it is included because nearly all children have some encounter with death during their early childhood, such as the death of a pet, family member, schoolmate, or friend.

According to Kastenbaum (1967:93), there is a close relationship between a child's development of notions regarding death and his general cognitive development: ". . . the child's concept of death is dependent upon the total pattern of mental processes and resources available to him at a particular stage in his development." Thus a brief discussion of children's developing perceptions of death may serve as an illustration of the cognitive developmental stages previously described.

Although children's perceptions of death develop in conjunction with the cognitive developmental stages identified by Piaget, the age groupings used by Piaget and by researchers and theorists studying children's understanding of death are slightly different. For that reason, the age groupings included in this discussion and in Table 7-2 will be less specific than in the foregoing discussion of cognitive development; the ages included are preschool (ages 3 to 5), school age (ages 5 to 12), and adolescence (ages 12 or 13 to maturity at about age 21).

As indicated in Table 7-2, during the preschool age, which approximates Piaget's period of preoperational thought, children view death as a temporary, reversible state. Because preschoolers also view death as a separation or departure, which is often the most significant aspect of the death to them, they are likely to ask questions such as: "Where did he go? When will he come back? What is he doing?"

Table 7-2. Cognitive development of children's understanding and perceptions of death by age group

Preschool	School age	Adolescence	References
Death viewed as separation or departure	Personification of death as person (boogeyman) or spirit	Ability to think about one's own death	Barnes (1978) Fredlund (1977)
Main characteristic of death is immobility; death seen as reversible	Begin working (at age 5) toward acceptance (ages 9 to 12) of death as final, inevitable, universal, and personal	Use of denial to control anxiety resulting from realization of their mortality	Grollman (1967; 1976) Hostler (1978) Kastenbaum (1967)
Cause of death is seen as accident or act of violence	By ages 10 to 12 realization that death can happen to to anyone at any age	Engage in risk-taking behaviors to "test" vulnerability to death	Nagy (1948) Sahler (1978) Shuler (1978)

(Fredlund, 1977:534). Death is recognized by the apparent immobility of the "victim," as in the case of a dead dog found motionless by the side of the road. At this age, death is viewed as something that happens to other people, especially the elderly, and not to oneself (Grollman, 1967; Kastenbaum, 1967). In addition, young children believe that death generally results from accidents or violence (muggings, murder, assault). Young children do *not* view death as inevitable, but rather see it as *avoidable;* that is, "people may live forever if they are fortunate and careful" (Grollman, 1976:29).

School-age children tend to personify death, as reflected in their preoccupation at times with notions of "the boogeyman" or ghosts and other spooky phenomena and stories. Children ages 5 and older gradually (by age 10 or 12) come to view death as "final, inevitable, universal, and personal" (Kastenbaum, 1967:101-104). No longer do they voice the expectation that the dead person or animal will return, since they now realize that "dead is dead" (Grollman, 1976:29). As Fredlund (1977:534) further notes, by ages 10 to 12, children realize that "death can happen to anybody at any age." School-age children thus begin to deal with death as an event that will someday happen to them.

Adolescents, who are entering Piaget's period of formal operations, have the cognitive tools to begin dealing with abstractions and possibilities as well as actualities; for that reason, they may begin to think about their own deaths and may have a renewed curiosity about death during this stage. Contemplating one's own death can of course be anxiety producing; adolescents may therefore use denial to cope with the anxiety generated by thoughts of their even-

tual deaths and by realization of their mortality (Hostler, 1978). It should also be noted that adolescents may "test" the "personal" and "inevitable" properties of death by "daring it to happen." Thus adolescents may engage in risk-taking behaviors such as playing "chicken," hitchhiking, reckless driving, and drug use (Fredlund, 1977).

Obviously, one's perceptions of death and one's vulnerability to it change and develop even after adolescence is safely over. Personal experiences and life events will help shape those perceptions and ideally will also help ready an individual to accept and meet his own death. Although this discussion of developing one's concept of death has been necessarily brief, this is an important area for school nurses and other school staff to study and in which to develop some counseling proficiency, so that children's reactions to death can be understood, accepted, and their healthy adaptation to death and dying facilitated and promoted.

Psychosocial development

The term *psychosocial development* tends to be so very loosely and generally applied by many authors that it often refers to all kinds of growth and development except physical growth. For the purposes of this chapter, however, the term psychosocial development will include personality development, language, and social-interactional development. Discussion of moral development will follow.

Unquestionably, one of the most widely known and respected human development theorists is Erik Erikson, whose major texts *Childhood and Society* (1963) and *Identity: Youth and Crisis* (1968) are generally regarded as classics. Erikson's theory of human development is built on and adapted from Freud's psychoanalytical theory and views development as an epigenetic process in which one stage is built on another. It is important to note that Erikson regards personality development as a lifelong process: "an individual never *has* a personality, he is always redeveloping his personality" (Maier, 1969:29).

Erikson's theory of human development includes the following eight stages, which he refers to as the "Eight Ages of Man" (1963; 1968):

1. Trust versus mistrust
2. Autonomy versus shame and doubt
3. Initiative versus guilt
4. Industry versus inferiority
5. Identity versus identity confusion
6. Intimacy versus isolation
7. Generativity versus stagnation
8. Integrity versus despair

However, only the three stages pertaining to preschool and school-age children and adolescents will be discussed in this chapter.

Psychosocial development of the preschool child. For the preschool child, the *developmental crisis,* which is the central problem or dilemma to be faced and "mastered" during a particular developmental stage (Maier, 1969) is "initiative versus guilt" (Erikson, 1963). That is, the child must achieve a sense of *initiative* or "enjoyment of energy displayed in action, assertiveness, learning, increasing dependability, and ability to plan," while avoiding *guilt,* which is the "sense of defeatism, anger, feeling responsible for things which he is not really responsible for, feeling easily frightened from what he wants to do, feeling he is bad, shameful, and deserving of punishment" (Murray et al., 1979c:151). This sense of guilt can result from sibling rivalry and from restrictions on the child's fantasy and activities, such as when parents "do things for" the child when he could do them himself. On the other hand, development of a sense of initiative is enhanced by encouraging the child to use his imagination and to explore his environment within the limits of safety and socially acceptable behavior. The child's imagination and activity should not be stifled as long as they pose no threat to the safety and well-being of the child or others (Murray et al., 1979c).

In addition to resolving the developmental crisis of initiative versus guilt, the preschooler has other developmental tasks to master, including those identified by Duvall (1971) and

highlighted in Chapter 4. Among the important developmental tasks for preschoolers identified by Murray et al. (1979c) is gender or sex-role *identification,* which comes about through imitation of the same-sex parent's behavior as well as through internalization or adoption of sexual, moral, social, and occupational attitudes, values, and roles. If the child does not identify with the same-sex parent or a same-sex caretaker, he may be confused and may have difficulty forming his sense of identity and sexuality during adolescence and adulthood. Closely related to gender and sex-role identification is the child's self-concept and body image. The preschooler's "sense of self" and his "body boundaries" become more definite during this stage (Murray et al., 1979c) and are influenced in part by others' reactions to his body and behavior. If the child receives messages that he is "not OK," for example, if he cannot run and climb as well as other children, or if, due to overly protective parents, he is not allowed to explore his environment or test his skills, then his self-concept will probably not be positive and healthy. The child may become fearful, anxious, passive, withdrawn, and inhibited. In short, he may lack a sense of initiative, having instead an overwhelming sense of guilt.

In the area of play, which is an important developmental and learning activity for the child, the preschooler is making great strides away from solitary (by himself) play, toward parallel play (playing alongside another child without cooperation or sharing), and ultimately toward cooperative play (Kaluger and Kaluger, 1979). The child's development of cooperative play is facilitated by his increasing opportunities for peer associations within his neighborhood and at church, day care centers (or babysitters), or nursery (preschool) school. This is the beginning of his gradual shift of orientation from family to peer group (Murray et al., 1979c), which seems to peak during adolescence.

Murray et al. (1979a:71) have identified "adaptive mechanisms" used at each stage of development throughout the life span. According to their definition, *adaptive mechanisms* are "learned behavioral responses that aid adjustment and emotional development." For the preschool child, the important adaptive mechanisms are introjection, primary and secondary identification, fantasy, and repression (Murray et al., 1979c). *Introjection* refers to "taking attitudes, information, and actions into the self through empathy and learning" (1979:152); this internalizing of facts, attitudes, and values assists the child in developing a sense of himself or a self-concept. This development of a sense of self is further enhanced by *primary identification* or imitation of others' (family and peers) attitudes and behavior, which in turn allows *secondary identification,* the internalizing of "standards, moral codes, attitudes, and role behavior, including gender, as his own and in his own unique way" (1979:152), to occur. *Fantasy* or imagination is another adaptive mechanism used by the preschool child and provides tension release and a means of testing reality and learning to master the environment; the child's delight in fairy tales and magic illustrates use of fantasy. The final adaptive mechanism associated with the preschool child is *repression,* which is the unconscious removal from awareness of "the thoughts, impulses, fantasies, and memories of behavior which are unacceptable to the self" (Grohar et al., 1979: 105). Although some repression must necessarily occur as the child's parents and his culture require his compliance with rules and his orientation to reality, excessive repression, which may be due to guilt feelings, severe punishment, and/or the child's perception that others strongly disapprove of him or his behavior, may ultimately result in "constricted creativity and restricted behavior" as well as unhappy memories of his preschool years (Murray et al., 1979c:153). Thus repression, like fantasy, may be either a helpful, adaptive mechanism or an unhealthy, maladaptive coping mechanism.

The final area of psychosocial development to be included in this discussion is language. Although language development is a lengthy, complex, and continuous process throughout childhood and adolescence, for the purposes of this chapter the language achievement of the preschool child will be briefly summed up by noting that the child's vocabulary increases from approximately 900 words at age 3 to 1500 words at age 4 and to 2100 words at age 5—a net gain of 600 words per year—and by age 5 the child can count to ten and name four colors (Murray et al., 1979c). For more detailed discussion of language development refer to the Suggested Readings at the end of the chapter.

Psychosocial development of the school-age child. The developmental crisis to be resolved by the school-age child is "industry versus inferiority" (Erikson, 1963). As defined by Leonard et al. (1979:186-188), *industry* is "an interest in doing the work of the world, the child's feeling that he can learn and solve problems, the formation of responsible work habits and attitudes, and the mastery of age-appropriate tasks." The child takes great pride in doing things well both at school and at home and applies himself with great concentration to that end. Although different personality traits emerge and subside year by year between ages 6 and 12, the period of industry is generally characterized by independence, self-control, loyalty, and an overriding sense of justice and fairness. According to Erikson (1963), if the school-age child does not achieve a sense of industry during this period, he is likely to be left with a sense of *inferiority,* or "feeling inadequate, defeated, unable to learn or do tasks, lazy, unable to compete, compromise, or cooperate, regardless of his actual competence" (Leonard et al., 1979:188).

In addition to resolving the developmental crisis of industry versus inferiority, the school-age child has other developmental tasks to accomplish, including those identified by Duvall (1971) and listed in Chapter 4. Obviously, one of the most important developmental tasks confronting the school-age child is successful school entrance and academic achievement. When the child enters school, he is officially "launched" from the bosom of his family into the outside world; as a result, he must now conform to the expectations of adults (such as teachers) other than his parents and to the demands and expectations of his widening peer group (classmates).

This task is complicated by the fact that others not only expect him to relate and communicate effectively with his new associates, but at the same time expect him to succeed academically. The child is expected to meet age-appropriate achievement standards in reading, writing, arithmetic, and other academic areas. The child needs to develop a sense of *competence:* the feeling that he can master his environment and exercise some control over it. Development of this sense of competence is facilitated by giving the child tasks that he is capable of mastering and then recognizing and rewarding his efforts. However, the child also needs to work on developing his sense of initiative, and he should therefore have the opportunity to take risks and experiment, with standby problem-solving assistance available if (and only if) he needs it (Siemon, 1978).

In addition to his academic pursuits, the

school-age child is busily expanding his social network. Besides identifying himself as a member of a family, neighborhood, and school, the child is now aware of his membership in a nationality, an ethnicity, and a social class (Siemon, 1978). By middle childhood (approximately 8 years old), the child may be involved with a loose-knit group, such as a celebrity fan club, although such clubs tend to be short-lived. The child's involvement with a loose-knit group gradually is replaced with membership in a *gang,* a social group in which "membership is earned on the basis of skilled performance of some activity, frequently physical in nature" (Leonard et al., 1979:183); the gang's stability and identity are often expressed through such formal symbols as secret passwords or uniforms. Such gangs contribute to children's development by providing them with an opportunity to "discharge hostility and aggression against peers rather than adults and [to] begin to work out their own social patterns without adult interference."

By age 9 or 10, the "chum" stage usually occurs, during which the child transfers his affection from his group or gang to a *chum,* "a special friend of the same age and sex." Development of a close relationship with a same-age and same-sex peer is an important developmental task for the school-age child, since it helps him to know himself (his similarities to and differences from his chum and others) and to accept himself. Leonard et al. (1979) believe that the chum relationship provides the basis for intimate heterosexual relationships in adulthood as well as preparing the child to later develop close friendships with both men and women. According to their view, there may be dire consequences for a child who does not have a chum relationship, because "he has little capacity for adolescent heterosexuality or adult intimacy. Fixation at this level results in *homosexuality,* an inability to focus love upon a member of the opposite sex" (Leonard et al., 1979:183).

As Siemon (1978) notes, if the school-age child is to develop a healthy self-concept, he must develop both a sense of competence and a sense of belonging. Formation of peer group, gang, and chum relationships contributes to the child's sense of belonging. However, the child's family patterns also play an important role in his feelings of belonging. A child whose family moves frequently, due to military or corporate transfers or the itinerant nature of his parents' employment (as in the case of migrant

workers who harvest various crops around the country), may have difficulty developing gang and chum relationships and feeling that he is part of his school or neighborhood because he may not be in one place long enough to be accepted and to make friends. In addition, if the child's family is internally unstable, due to parental alcoholism, unemployment, or other factors, he may not view home as an emotionally "safe" and secure place; as a result, the child may be unable to relax at home and work on assimilating his new knowledge, skills, and expanding peer relationships and may therefore have difficulty achieving the sense of competence and belonging essential for development of a mentally healthy self-concept.

Thus the school-age child continues to develop his positive self-concept (begun in earnest during the preschool years) by focusing on achievement of a sense of competence and a sense of belonging. As Siemon (1978:215) points out, the opinions of others—especially adults—are very important to the school-age child because a "child comes to accept himself as a person of worth to the extent that he experiences the love and understanding of significant adults." Siemon goes on to list three "primary antecedents" for promoting self-esteem that adults should keep in mind: (1) a high degree of acceptance of the child by parents and others, (2) provision of clear and consistent limits for the child's behavior, and (3) allowing enough flexibility within those behavioral limits to permit individual actions and choices. Although these factors seem to be obvious and basic expectations for parents and others who work with children, Siemon (1978) notes that potential emotional development problems often relate to the first two factors; that is, such problems may result from lack of recognition and acceptance for the child, as well as from lack of limits for his behavior. Therefore however basic these ideas may be, they merit repetition.

There are a number of adaptive mechanisms used by the school-age child. One that is commonly observed is *ritualistic behavior* or "consistently repeating an act in a situation" as a means of evading imagined harm and increasing one's sense of being in control (Leonard et al., 1979:192); an example of such behavior is the child who carefully avoids stepping on cracks in the sidewalk, believing that if you "step on a crack, you'll break your mother's back."

Reaction formation, "replacing his original

idea and behavior with the opposite behavior characteristics'' (Grohar et al., 1979:105), may be used by the child to deal with his hostile feelings, which he finds unacceptable. Thus a child who resents his parents for making him babysit with his younger siblings may suddenly become a responsible, cheerful babysitter who even volunteers to sit before he is asked; in this way, the child finds a socially acceptable way to deal with his feelings of anger, resentment, and hate.

Another adaptive mechanism used by the school-age child is *undoing*, or ''unconsciously removing an idea, feeling, or act by performing certain ritualistic behavior'' (Leonard et al., 1979:192). Thus the child who accidentally steps on a crack in the sidewalk may ward off the supposed danger to his mother (that is, breaking her back) by carrying out a chant or some other action to reverse the expected dire consequences. A related adaptive mechanism is *isolation*, which is a means of ''unconsciously separating emotion from an idea because the emotion would be unacceptable to the self'' (Leonard et al., 1979:192). The adaptive mechanism of isolation keeps the idea (for example, the death of a child's kitten) in the conscious awareness, while the feelings associated with the idea or event (such as grief for the death) remain in the unconscious. Thus a child using isolation to deal with the death of his kitten might be expected to talk very matter-of-factly about the kitten and its death, displaying little emotion.

School-age children also use *fantasy* or imagination as an adaptive mechanism in compensating for such feelings as inadequacy, inferiority (''I'm not OK''), or failure (Leonard et al., 1979). The child who is shy and has difficulty making friends may have imaginary playmates, or the child who is not athletically inclined may imagine himself to be a major league baseball player. Fantasy is generally recognized as being closely related to creativity and should therefore not be discouraged unless the child's preoccupation with his fantasies interferes with his reality orientation to and participation in the real world.

Another adaptive mechanism used by many children is *identification*, defined by Webster's as the ''psychological orientation of the self in regard to . . . a person or group . . . with a resulting feeling of close emotional association.'' For school-age children, such identification generally takes the form of hero worship

of a teacher, older relative, such as an aunt, uncle, or older brother or sister, or anyone else whom the child respects and admires (Leonard et al., 1979).

Among the less socially accepted adaptive mechanisms used by the school-age child are regression, malingering, and rationalization (Leonard et al., 1979:194). *Regression* entails ''returning to a less sophisticated pattern of behavior'' and is a defense that helps protect the child from anxiety and pain. An example of this is the child who expresses his jealousy toward his new baby brother by regressing to use of babytalk or temper tantrums. *Malingering*, in contrast, involves ''feigning illness in order to avoid unpleasant tasks''; an example is the child who reportedly feels too sick to go to school on the day of a big test or the child who deals with his ''math anxiety'' by becoming ill each morning during arithmetic but feels fine after that class period. *Rationalization*, or giving excuses for failing to complete tasks or achieve expected standards, is often used by children regarding their school performance; thus a child who fails a test may dismiss the test grade as ''unimportant'' or insist that the test was ''too hard'' or ''unfair.''

Other adaptive mechanisms used by school-age children include projection and sublimation. *Projection* is attributing one's own feelings or behaviors to someone else (Grohar et al., 1979). The child who is angry with his mother for punishing him may loudly insist ''You hate me!'' which is actually his own feeling at that moment. *Sublimation*, in contrast, is ''channeling impulses into socially acceptable behavior rather than expressing the original impulse'' (Grohar et al., 1979:106). The child may funnel his aggressive impulses into organized athletics such as a Little League baseball team. Sublimation is an important mechanism during the school-age period and is the basis for developing a sense of industry, which is, of course, the overriding developmental task for the school-age child (Leonard et al., 1979).

The school-age child also continues to grow in the area of language skills. By age 6, the child has an oral vocabulary of approximately 2500 words. In addition, he can use sentences that are generally five words long and uses all parts of speech, such as nouns, verbs, adjectives, adverbs, and conjunctions. He is also likely to know some of the alphabet and to recognize some letters in their printed form; he may also be able to recognize some simple words in their printed form, as in his storybooks (Kaluger and Kaluger, 1979).

During the school-age period, the child's use of language moves away from the egocentric patterns of the preschool years toward more socialized use of language; that is, he uses language consciously as a means of communicating his thoughts, desires, and feelings to others. As he continues to refine and expand his language skills, the child also is increasingly able to understand more abstract language forms and uses, such as jokes, puns, and figures of speech. During this period the child is also beginning to develop skills in written communication, beginning with simple printing at age 6 and expanding to use of legible longhand at a comfortable pace by about age 10. Finally, it also important to note that during this period the child is learning to read, beginning with simple words and stories in the first grade, and gradually progressing to more complicated and lengthy books. His involvement with reading is an important means for increasing his vocabulary and improving his grammar, as well as providing him with a new source of intellectual stimulation and knowledge.

However, as Leonard et al. (1979) point out, the child's use of language and ability and motivation to develop skills in both self-expression and reading are jeopardized by an uncensored overdose of television. Because television is a passive, one-way communication medium, children who spend many unsupervised hours watching cartoons, slickly produced commercials, and programs that often depict violence and sexism, may grow up not only with a distorted sense of values, but may also have limited abilities to use correct grammar and enunciation and diminished motivation and ability to read and interpret what they read.

Psychosocial development of the adolescent. Although adolescence is generally regarded as the chronological period between ages 12 or 13 and age 21 (the age of legal majority), designation of an age range to characterize such a complicated, confusing, trying, and little understood developmental stage is totally inadequate. It must also be noted, that while adolescence is generally thought to take place during the 8- or 9-year period just described, in actuality adolescence may begin earlier than age 12 and may continue beyond age 21. Indeed, some people seem to never grow up and may remain adolescents despite attainment of chronological and physiological adulthood.

Among the many and diverse definitions of adolescence and adolescents in the literature are several that will be mentioned here to further clarify the meaning of these terms. The simplest and most basic definitions are those in Webster's dictionary: *adolescence* is "the state or process of growing up" or "the period of life from puberty to maturity terminating legally at the age of majority," whereas an *adolescent* is therefore "one that is in the state of adolescence." These definitions allude to the approximate time period described in the foregoing paragraph, while at the same time pointing out that adolescence begins with the onset of *puberty,* the "period of physiological change when male and female sexual organs mature" (Nolan et al., 1979:206). For girls, puberty usually begins at about age 10 or 11 and continues to age 14; during this 3-year span *menarche* or onset of menses (menstruation) usually occurs. For boys, attainment of physiological maturity requires 4 or more years to complete, beginning at about age 12 and continuing until age 16 (Nolan et al., 1979).

While there is general agreement that puberty marks the onset of adolescence, there is obviously more to adolescence than mere physiological maturing. Adolescence is variously referred to as a transitional period between childhood and adulthood (Powell, 1963), an "in-between" stage, or a time of physical, social, and emotional "metamorphosis" (Kaluger and Kaluger, 1979). A more tongue-in-cheek view of adolescence is that offered by Wallinga (1973:91), who characterizes adolescence as ". . . the last of the common childhood diseases, from which most individuals recover spontaneously but occasionally it evolves into a chronic illness from which recovery is slow."

For the purposes of this chapter, the most useful definition is that advanced by Nolan et al. (1979:206), which describes *adolescence* as "the period in life which begins with puberty and extends for 8 or 10 years, or longer, until the person is physically and psychologically mature, ready to assume adult responsibilities and be self-sufficient because of changes in intellect, attitudes, and interests." As these authors point out, however, there are individual variations in the rate and extent of maturity and psychological growth. Thus some persons will be adolescents longer than others, while a few individuals may *never* achieve psychological maturity. Thus, definitions such as the foregoing must be applied with caution to individuals, and sweeping generalizations should be avoided. Nolan et al. (1979) further divide adolescence into the following four subperiods:

1. *Preadolescence,* or prepuberty, which generally begins at age 9 or 10 and continues until age 12. This period is characterized by increased hormonal production and a "new capacity to love, when the satisfaction and security of another person of the same sex is as important to the child as his own satisfaction and security" (Leonard et al., 1979:159).

2. *Early adolescence,* the period beginning with puberty during which physical growth is occurring. Approximate ages included are 12 to 14 for girls and 14 to 16 for boys. During this phase, involvement and close relationships with same-sex peers decrease, interest in the opposite sex increases, rebellion against parental and other adult authority increases, and peers' standards and values become more important.

3. *Middle adolescence,* beginning when physical growth is complete. Inclusive age groups are 15 to 18 for females and 16 to 20 for males. The focus during this period is on establishing one's identity, forming relationships with members of the opposite sex, developing an interest in the future, and beginning to plan for future choices of occupation, education, and life partner/spouse.

4. *Late adolescence,* which may occur between ages 20 and 25. Although the late adolescent may have already established a stable identity and sense of values, he may not have chosen a life-style (such as marriage) or an occupation, although he might be a student or an apprentice; in other words, he "still questions his relationship to existing social, vocational, and emotional roles and life-styles" (1979: 207).

While school nurses employed in collegiate settings are primarily concerned with middle and late adolescents (as well as adults, of course), the discussion of adolescents/adolescence in this chapter will focus primarily on the first three subperiods, excluding late adolescence.

The developmental crisis to be resolved during adolescence is "identity versus identity confusion" (Erikson, 1968; 1963). The adolescent must know who he is and where he is going in life and must find a purpose for his exis-

tence—a sense of how he fits into the world. Formation of an identity, then, "implies an internal stability, sameness, or continuity, which resists extreme change and preserves itself from oblivion in the face of stress or contradictions" (Nolan et al., 1979:224). If the adolescent fails to achieve a sense of identity for himself due to a variety of reasons such as lack of adequate role models and support from parents and other adults with stable identities and values, identity confusion will result (Erikson, 1963, 1968; Nolan et al., 1979). The adolescent experiencing identity confusion (also referred to as "identity diffusion" and "role confusion") may feel insecure, powerless, confused, alienated, doubtful, self-conscious, overwhelmed, and lost. He has difficulty making decisions, is unable to defer gratification of his needs, often appearing "brazen or arrogant." He has difficulty in his interpersonal relationships at work, with his friends, and in intimate or sexual relationships. An everpresent risk is that he may take on antisocial behavior in his pursuit of an identity, apparently believing that "it's better to be bad than nobody at all" (Nolan et al., 1979:225).

In addition to achieving a sense of identity, there are other developmental tasks to be addressed by the adolescent; many of these specific tasks have been identified by Duvall (1971) (Chapter 4). Five of the most important adolescent developmental tasks, as adapted from Duvall (1971) and O'Neil et al. (1977), will be briefly discussed here. As already noted, the primary task for the adolescent is to establish an identity or "sense of self," including a sexual identity. This process depends on the adolescent's ability to synthesize biopsychosocial traits from a variety of sources, including his own earlier gender/sex-role identity, family, peers, and from membership in cultural, ethnic, religious, and/or occupational groups (Nolan et al., 1979). With so many sources of input and feedback, which may often conflict, this obviously becomes a herculean task.

A second major task confronting the adolescent is the need to choose an occupation/vocation and to plan for eventual economic independence. This requires the youth to adopt a future orientation, with attention to needed education or training to carry out his chosen career. For adolescents who are not yet past middle adolescence, this task is difficult, since they do not usually have many work and life experiences to guide their choice and must therefore rely on others' opinions, experiences, and recommendations. A wrong choice can be disastrous or at least highly inconvenient because of economic losses while the adolescent changes his focus in employment and/or education and because of inevitable delays in advancing up the career ladder resulting from his decision to start over in a new occupation.

A third important developmental task for the adolescent is the need to adopt a stable lifestyle, based on socially responsible attitudes and behaviors, which provide opportunities for commitment and close relationships with significant others. Thus by the time he completes adolescence and becomes an adult, the individual is expected to have settled down into a socially approved life-style, which may or may not include marriage. His life-style should reflect an ability to solve problems and make reasonable decisions and plans, anticipating possible consequences of his various alternatives. The young person who drifts from job to job or who parties until all hours, uses drugs, or enters a succession of purely sexual relationships in which he has no commitment to or real interest in his partner is obviously not meeting this task and is therefore still an adolescent.

A fourth important developmental task for the adolescent is to emancipate himself from his family, while maintaining a loving relationship with them. This, too, is no easy task. Some adolescents lack the necessary self-confidence to move out of their parents' home and to establish a separate residence. Adolescents who go on to college or pursue other education may ease this transition away from their parents' home if they attend a school out of town, which necessitates at least a part-time change of residence. If such students can live in a dormitory or other group housing facility where some of the comforts of home are provided, their adaptation to this change in their life-style will be smoother.

However, simply moving out of the parental home is only one part of the task confronting the adolescent. Perhaps the more difficult aspect of this developmental task is trying to maintain close, loving ties with family without forfeiting independence. It is difficult for both the adolescent and his parents to "let go," and time and effort are therefore necessary to help both parties renegotiate their relationship away from a parent-child focus, toward an adult-adult focus. Too, if the adolescent's quest for freedom and independence has been overly aggressive and rebellious, and/or if it has been met with strong parental resistance, it may be particularly difficult for him and his parents to

sustain a loving, emotionally supporting relationship, although the importance of doing so cannot be overstated.

The fifth developmental task for the adolescent is the expectation that he will become a responsible, contributing citizen guided by a socially acceptable set of values and moral principles. This includes the societal (and parental!) expectation that he will become self-supporting, maintaining consistent and reliable employment. Beyond this expectation that he will be economically independent by seeking and maintaining employment are other expectations of fiscal responsibility, including prompt payment of bills, avoidance of unnecessary debts or those he cannot afford, and reasonable, appropriate spending of his income and other fiscal resources. In addition, this developmental task implies the societal expectation that the adolescent will obey laws, be a good neighbor, and demonstrate interest in supporting the common good in his community by voting responsibly in all elections and becoming involved in appropriate ways in the political process. His behavior is expected to meet socially accepted standards of morality, as defined by law and custom, which require that he develop and follow a philosophy of life and social responsibility.

Because of the obvious complexity and importance of achieving the foregoing developmental tasks, it is no wonder that adolescence is a difficult, traumatic, and anxiety-producing stage of life for many young people. To cope with this myriad of seemingly conflicting and overwhelming expectations, the adolescent uses a variety of adaptive mechanisms, including any or all of those discussed and defined earlier in this chapter. However, three mechanisms in particular are generally used: compensation, sublimation, and identification. *Compensation* is defined as a "form of compromise" (Nolan et al., 1979:229) and can be used by the adolescent as a means of arriving at reasonable expectations of himself in light of his personal or environmental limitations. Thus the student who lacks athletic abilities may compensate for his inability to make the team by becoming its manager. According to Nolan et al., compensation, sublimation, and identification (the latter two of which were defined in the discussion on the school-aged child) are particularly helpful for the adolescent because they can help him improve interpersonal relationships and achieve goals that are appropriate to his abilities and resources. In addition, insofar as they help him develop an appropriate sense of self and form an identity that is consistent with his abilities and limitations, these mechanisms help shape his personality and character.

Before concluding this discussion of adolescent psychosocial development, it is necessary to briefly discuss language development, which is interwoven with both cognitive and social development. As Nolan et al. (1979) point out, use of slang or jargon is typical of adolescents and serves as a *peer group dialect* or "a highly informal language which consists of coined terminology and of new or extended interpretations attached to traditional terms." Such "in" language helps peer group cohesion and identification, while at the same time prevents adults from intruding and invading their privacy; in fact, teen jargon can be effectively used to unleash hostility and aggression on unsuspecting and bewildered adults, reminiscent of the way children exclude, taunt, and exercise control of younger children through use of "pig latin" or secret passwords. Adolescence is also a time of continued growth in the use of language skills (speaking, writing, creative expression, heightened awareness of correct grammatical forms) and expansion of vocabulary, although growth in these areas depends on educational and social opportunities and expectations (norms).

Moral development

Although moral development is discussed in the literature by a variety of authors, probably the foremost author and researcher in the area of moral development is Lawrence Kohlberg.

Kohlberg views moral development as being closely related to cognitive development, believing that increasing cognitive development enables the child to mature in his moral judgments (Sutterley and Donnelly, 1973). Although cognitive maturity is essential for eventual maturity of moral judgment, it is not in itself sufficient for developing a morally mature adult; an adult or adolescent may have readily achieved the cognitive stage of formal operations, but there is no guarantee that he will use his critical and abstract thinking processes in moral and socially responsible ways.

According to Kohlberg (1964; 1968), moral development proceeds in an invariant sequence along three levels: preconventional or premoral, conventional, and postconventional or principled (Table 7-3). The *preconventional* level, which generally includes children ages 4 to 10, is the first level of moral thinking. Although the child at this level is usually well behaved, his

ideas of what is right and wrong or good and bad depend on the physical consequences (punishment, reward, or exchange of favors) of actions and on the physical power of those who make the rules and affix the labels of "right" and "wrong" (Kohlberg, 1968). At the *conventional* level, which is generally associated with preadolescence, obeying the rules and meeting the expectations of one's family, group, or nation is seen as valuable in and of itself. The emphasis at this level is on both *conformity* with the social order and *maintenance,* support, and justification of it. The third, or *postconventional,* level, which corresponds with middle and late adolescence and with adulthood (if this third level is ever achieved), is characterized by "a major thrust toward autonomous moral principles which have validity and application apart from authority of the groups or persons who hold them and apart from the individual's identification with those persons or groups" (Kohlberg, 1968:26). According to some authorities (Kaluger and Kaluger, 1979), most adults operate at the conventional level, although very few—5% to 10% of the population—ever reach stage six within the postconventional level (Table 7-3). As indicated in Table 7-3, within each of these three levels are two distinct identifiable stages, for a total of six stages. Stages 1 and 2 occur at the preconventional level, stages 3 and 4 during the conventional level, and stages 5 and 6 during the postconventional level.

Again, it should be emphasized that the age groupings given are only approximations, since the actual stage of an individual's moral development depends not only on his level of cognitive development, but also on his values and philosophy (Kaluger and Kaluger, 1979). In addition, the individual's development of a philosophy and set of values depends, in turn, on his problem-solving experience, reasoning/thinking ability, and on the amount and kind of information he has available to guide his thinking; therefore the person who receives little or no information may be left with "moral and religious uncertainty," since he is forced to work out answers to many questions by himself without guidance, resulting in a "kindergarten theology" that is useless for problem solving in the "adult world of reality" (Kaluger and Kaluger, 1979:357).

As a postscript to this discussion, it should be noted that although the right and/or obligation of schools to teach and stimulate development

Table 7-3. Summary of Lawrence Kohlberg's levels and stages in moral development

Level I—preconventional Moral value resides in external, quasiphysical happenings, in bad acts, or in quasiphysical needs rather than in persons and standards		Level II—conventional Moral value resides in performing good or right rules in maintaining the conventional order and expectancies of others		Level III—postconventional Moral value resides in conformity by the self to shared or shareable standards, rights, or duties	
Ages 4 to 10 years in American middle class		**Preadolescence**		**Adolescence**	
Stage 1	Stage 2	Stage 3	Stage 4	Stage 5 (A and B)	Stage 6
Punishment and obedience orientation and nonquestioning deference to superior power. The physical consequences of action regardless of their human meaning or value determine his goodness or badness. He obeys rules to avoid punishment.	Instrumental relativism. Instrumental hedonism and concrete reciprocity. Right action consists of that which instrumentally satisfies one's own needs of others. Elements of fairness, reciprocity, and equal sharing are present but are always interpreted in a physical, pragmatic way, not a matter of loyalty, gratitude, or justice.	Orientation to interpersonal relations of mutuality; orientation to approval, affection, and helpfulness. Good-boy, good-girl; seeks approval by being "nice," much conformity to stereotype of what is majority or natural behavior. Behavior is often judged by intention—"he means well" and is often overused.	Orientation to maintaining a social order, of rules and rights. Right behavior consists of doing one's duty, showing respect for authority, conforming to the fixed rules, and maintaining the given social order for its own sake. The maintenance of the expectations of the individual's family, group, or nation is perceived as valuable in its own right.	A. Social contract legalism A social-contract orientation generally with legalistic and utilitarian overtones. Right action in terms of general rights and in terms of standards which have been critically examined and agreed upon by society as a whole. Right or wrong is a matter of personal opinion. Awareness of this relativism necessitates an emphasis upon procedural rules for reaching consensus. This is the legal point of view but with an emphasis upon the possibility of changing law in terms of rational considerations of social utility (official morality of American government). Outside of legal realm, free agreement and contract are binding elements of obligation. B. Orientation to internal decisions of conscience but without clear rational or universal principles—a higher law and conscience orientation.	Orientation to universal moral principles. An orientation toward ethical principles appealing to logic, comprehensiveness, universality, and consistency. Most principles are abstract and ethical (the Golden Rule, the categorical imperative). They are not concrete moral rules like the Ten Commandments. They are the universal principles of justice, of the reciprocity and equality of human rights, out of respect for the dignity of human beings as individual persons.

Below is an example of how a moral issue would be judged according to each of the stages of moral development.

Issue: "Value of Human Life"

Confused with the value of physical objects and is based on social status or physical attributes of the possessor.	Seen as instrumental to the satisfaction of the needs of its possessor or other persons.	Value of human life based on the empathy and affection of family members and others toward its possessors.	Life is seen as sacred in terms of its place in a categorical moral or religious order of rights and duties.	Life is valued both in terms of its relation to community and in terms of being a universal right.	Belief in the sacredness of human life as representing a universal value of respect for the individual regardless of status or property.

*From Sutterley, D., and Donnelly, G.: 1973. Perspectives in human development, J. B. Lippincott Co., Philadelphia, p. 226.

of morality has come under fire in recent years, researchers and theorists like Kohlberg believe that the school and, particularly, the teacher "has increasing responsibility for stimulating conceptions of success which involve some moral dimensions" (1964:427). In addition, Kohlberg notes that whether or not character building is seen as an explicit goal in the classroom, there is a significant amount of moralizing inherent in day-to-day classroom teaching, and the teacher, in addition to the parent, can therefore strongly influence children's moral standards. For that reason, it is important for schools to begin to recognize the role they have in shaping the moral standards of tomorrow's adults and to begin efforts to consciously stimulate moral development—with particular attention to those children whose moral development seems to be delayed or severely lacking.

Nutritional needs of children and youth

According to Webster's dictionary, *nutrition* is the "act or process of nourishing or being nourished," although the term more specifically refers to all processes by which an individual takes in and uses food substances. Because the way in which an individual takes in and uses his food directly affects his growth and development, nutritional adequacy is a relevant and important area for the school nurse to assess in her work with school community populations. However, due to limitations of space, content, and primary focus (school nursing), this discussion of the nutritional needs of children and youth will be limited. For more in-depth discussion of nutritional needs, patterns, recommended dietary (food) sources of specific nutrients, and assessment of nutritional status and adequacy, refer to the Suggested Readings at the end of the chapter.

The importance of nutritional adequacy in promoting normal growth and development of children and youth has been well documented in the literature (Getchell and Howard, 1975; Pearson, 1977; Pipes, 1981). As these sources point out, both physical growth and psychosocial development are affected by nutrition, which may explain the derivation of the phrase "You are what you eat." Children whose nutrition is inadequate in some respect may be shorter in stature than peers of the same sex and age and may be either underweight or overweight (including obesity, which, although due to intake of more calories than the body can burn off, may be accompanied by deficiencies in specific nutrients). In addition, if nutrition is

inadequate during so-called critical periods of growth, growth of specific body organs may be permanently adversely affected. For example, the critical period for brain growth is believed to extend from midgestation (during pregnancy) into the child's second year of life; interference with brain growth during this critical time, whether due to malnutrition or other causes, will result not in *delayed* brain development, but will likely result in *lessened* brain growth, which may forever limit the child's intellectual capability (Pipes, 1981).

While the effects of nutrition on physical growth may seem rather obvious, the impact of nutritional adequacy on psychosocial development may not be so readily apparent. Of course, children whose physical size (height and/or weight) is significantly different from their peers may experience emotional stress due to teasing, poor body image, and the misery of knowing they are "different" and are consequently not fully accepted by their peers. In this sense, then, the psychosocial effects of malnutrition may be overt. However, less obvious but equally hazardous is the possibility that inadequate nutrition during childhood and/or adolescence may result in an unhealthy relationship with food. For example, children who for one reason or another may have difficulty relating with their peers or families, may seek solace in food, leading to overeating and possible obesity. On the other hand, adolescents (especially girls) who are very conscious of their body image, may become preoccupied with the pursuit of thinness, resulting in skipped meals, omission of essential nutrients, and in some extreme cases, development of anorexia nervosa.

While there are undoubtedly other examples available to document the interrelationship among nutritional adequacy, physical growth, and psychosocial development, the point is that nutritional behaviors, patterns, and attitudes developed during childhood and adolescence may have a profound and lasting effect on the individual's adult body size (height, weight, and physique) and lifelong relationship with food. Thus, adequate and appropriate nutrition during childhood and adolescence is essential for the development of physically, mentally, and socially healthy adults.

Ensuring nutritional adequacy: recommended dietary allowances and suggested food sources

To assist individuals or groups in planning meals and eating patterns and in evaluating intake adequacy, the Food and Nutrition Board of the National Research Council of the National Academy of Sciences compiles and periodically updates a table of *recommended dietary allowances (RDAs)*. This table of RDAs recommends levels for daily intake of calories (energy), protein, fat, and water-soluble vitamins (with specific levels identified for each nutrient), and minerals (Table 7-4).

The RDAs include built-in margins of safety to allow for individual variations among healthy people in the U.S. Thus due to individual variations in nutritional needs, the RDAs may exceed the actual needs of some individuals. On the other hand, the RDAs do *not* allow for the additional nutritional needs of individuals experiencing illness, trauma (physical or emotional), or "prolonged inadequate nutritional intake or utilization." (Getchell and Howard, 1975:185). RDAs, then, are *suggested* intake levels to promote and maintain optimal nutrition and health for *most healthy* American people. However, the table must be cautiously and judiciously applied in assessing the nutritional status of particular individuals, and one should *never* conclude that "individual food intakes short of recommendations constitute inadequacies" (Getchell and Howard, 1975:185). Finally, for those readers who may find the multitude of acronyms commonly used by health professionals to be more than a little confusing, it is important to note that recommended dietary allowance (RDA) is different from the term *minimum daily requirement (MDR)*, which denotes the *least amount* of a particular nutrient "that will promote an optimum state of health" (Getchell and Howard, 1975:185).

Although it would have been relatively easy to edit the RDAs for infants and adults out of Table 7-4, obviously that has not been done. The rationale for including the RDAs for infants and adults is that although the school nurse works most directly and consistently with school-age children and adolescents, she also maintains a family and community focus. Therefore the school nurse must be aware of nutritional and other health-related needs as they change throughout the life span, since the school community population invariably includes persons of all ages. Table 7-4 also includes RDAs for pregnant and lactating females; while those RDAs may at first seem applicable only to women elsewhere in the community, the rising pregnancy rate among adolescents and the importance of the school nurse serving as a health counselor and resource person for faculty and school staff members increase the relevance and applicability of these RDAs.

As an adjunct to the RDAs given in Table 7-4, Table 7-5 details the recommended energy (caloric) intake for persons of all ages, with corresponding mean ($\overline{X}$) heights and weights for each age group within the life span. It is significant to note that in comparison with the RDAs, heights, and weights included in the 1974 revision, the current recommendations (Food and Nutrition Board, 1980) generally represent *reductions* in daily caloric intake and in a number of suggested body weights, which may reflect the public's recent preoccupation with weight control and physical fitness. Again, it is important to remember that individual variations among persons must be considered when evaluating nutritional intake and body size (height and weight).

Ensuring consumption of a nutritionally adequate diet should not be a major problem if individuals discipline themselves to eat suggested quantities of foods from all four food groups. Unfortunately, in recent years many people have tended to use vitamin supplements to meet their RDAs, rather than simply trying to eat a nourishing, well-balanced diet. Too often the result of such daily use of vitamin and mineral supplements is an excessive intake of certain vitamins and/or minerals while the overall dietary intake remains inadequate.

Obviously, a more prudent approach to good nutrition would be daily consumption of foods from the four basic food groups as listed in Table 7-6. These food groups include milk and other dairy products like cheese and ice cream; meats such as beef, pork, and poultry, plus eggs and fish; vegetables and fruits; and breads, cereals, and other grain products like noodles (Williams, 1977). Quantities of foods from these basic groups suggested for daily intake vary according to the age and physiological state (such as pregnancy and/or lactation) of the individual. The differences in recommended intake based on age are shown in Table 7-7. Although Table 7-7 does not include preschoolers or adolescents, it does effectively illustrate the changes in size of servings or portions needed by children as they grow up and should therefore be a helpful guide in assessing daily food intake for school-age children.

Nutritional patterns and problems

While it should be relatively simple for health-conscious, responsible adults to obtain a

Text continued on p. 107.

Table 7-4. Recommended dietary allowances for children, youth, and adults (designed for the

	Age (years)	Weight		Height		Protein (g)	Fat-soluble vitamins				
		kg	lb	cm	in		Vitamin A (μRE)†	Vitamin D (μg)‡	Vitamin E (mg α TE)§	Vitamin C (mg)	Thia-min (mg)
Infants	0.0-0.5	6	13	60	24	kg × 2.2	420	10	3	35	0.3
	0.5-1.0	9	20	71	28	kg × 2.0	400	10	4	35	0.5
Children	1-3	13	29	90	35	23	400	10	5	45	0.7
	4-6	20	44	112	44	30	500	10	6	45	0.9
	7-10	28	62	132	52	34	700	10	7	45	1.2
Males	11-14	45	99	157	62	45	1000	10	8	50	1.4
	15-18	66	145	176	69	56	1000	10	10	60	1.4
	19-22	70	154	177	70	56	1000	7.5	10	60	1.5
	23-50	70	154	178	70	56	1000	5	10	60	1.4
	51+	70	154	178	70	56	1000	5	10	60	1.2
Females	11-14	46	101	157	62	46	800	10	8	50	1.1
	15-18	55	120	163	64	46	800	10	8	60	1.1
	19-22	55	120	163	64	44	800	7.5	8	60	1.1
	23-50	55	120	163	64	44	800	5	8	60	1.0
	51+	55	120	163	64	44	800	5	8	60	1.0
Pregnant						+30	+200	+5	+2	+20	+0.4
Lactating						+20	+400	+5	+3	+40	+0.5

*Reproduced from: Recommended Dietary Allowances, Ninth Edition (1980), with the permission of the National Academy
as they live in the United States under usual environmental stresses. Diets should be based on a variety of common foods in
†Retinol equivalents: 1 retinol equivalent = 1 μg retinol or 6 μg β carotene.
‡As cholecalciferol: 10 μg cholecalciferol = 400 international units (IU) vitamin D.
§α tocopherol equivalents: 1 mg d-α-tocopherol = 1 α TE.
‖One NE (niacin equivalent) = 1 mg of niacin or 60 mg of dietary tryptophan.
¶Folacin allowances refer to dietary sources as determined by *Lactobacillus casei* assay after treatment with enzymes
**The RDA for vitamin B-12 in infants is based on average concentration of the vitamin in human milk. The allowances after
factors such as intestinal absorption.
††The increased requirement during pregnancy cannot be met by the iron content of habitual American diets nor by the
lactation are not substantially different from those of nonpregnant women, but continued supplementation of the mother for 2

maintenance of good nutrition of practically all healthy people in the U.S.A.)*

Water-soluble vitamins					Minerals					
Ribo-flavin (mg)	Niacin (mg NE)‖	Vitamin B-6 (mg)	Folacin¶ (µg)	Vitamin B-12 (µg)	Calcium (mg)	Phos-phorus (mg)	Mag-nesium (mg)	Iron (mg)	Zinc (mg)	Iodine (µg)
0.4	6	0.3	30	0.5**	360	240	50	10	3	40
0.6	8	0.6	45	1.5	540	360	70	15	5	50
0.8	9	0.9	100	2.0	800	800	150	15	10	70
1.0	11	1.3	200	2.5	800	800	200	10	10	90
1.4	16	1.6	300	3.0	800	800	250	10	10	120
1.6	18	1.8	400	3.0	1200	1200	350	18	15	150
1.7	18	2.0	400	3.0	1200	1200	400	18	15	150
1.7	19	2.2	400	3.0	800	800	350	10	15	150
1.6	18	2.2	400	3.0	800	800	350	10	15	150
1.4	16	2.2	400	3.0	800	800	350	10	15	150
1.3	15	1.8	400	3.0	1200	1200	300	18	15	150
1.3	14	2.0	400	3.0	1200	1200	300	18	15	150
1.3	14	2.0	400	3.0	800	800	300	18	15	150
1.2	13	2.0	400	3.0	800	800	300	18	15	150
1.2	13	2.0	400	3.0	800	800	300	10	15	150
+0.3	+2	+0.6	+400	+1.0	+400	+400	+150	††	+5	+25
+0.5	+5	+0.5	+100	+1.0	+400	+400	+150	††	+10	+50

of Sciences, Washington, D.C. The allowances are intended to provide for individual variations among most normal persons order to provide other nutrients for which human requirements have been less well defined.

("conjugases") to make polyglutamyl forms of the vitamin available to the test organism.
weaning are based on energy intake (as recommended by the American Academy of Pediatrics) and consideration of other

existing iron stores of many women; therefore the use of 30 to 60 mg of supplemental iron is recommended. Iron needs during to 3 months after parturition is advisable in order to replenish stores depleted by pregnancy.

Table 7-5. Mean heights and weights and recommended energy intake*

Category	Age (years)	Weight		Height		Energy needs (with range)	
		kg	lb	cm	in	kcal	MJ
Infants	0.0-0.5	6	13	60	24	kg × 115 (95-145)	kg × .48
	0.5-1.0	9	20	71	28	kg × 105 (80-135)	kg × .44
Children	1-3	13	29	90	35	1300 (900-1800)	5.5
	4-6	20	44	112	44	1700 (1300-2300)	7.1
	7-10	28	62	132	52	2400 (1650-3300)	10.1
Males	11-14	45	99	157	62	2700 (2000-3700)	11.3
	15-18	66	145	176	69	2800 (2100-3900)	11.8
	19-22	70	154	177	70	2900 (2500-3300)	12.2
	23-50	70	154	178	70	2700 (2300-3100)	11.3
	51-75	70	154	178	70	2400 (2000-2800)	10.1
	76+	70	154	178	70	2050 (1650-2450)	8.6
Females	11-14	46	101	157	62	2200 (1500-3000)	9.2
	15-18	55	120	163	64	2100 (1200-3000)	8.8
	19-22	55	120	163	64	2100 (1700-2500)	8.8
	23-50	55	120	163	64	2000 (1600-2400)	8.4
	51-75	55	120	163	64	1800 (1400-2200)	7.6
	76+	55	120	163	64	1600 (1200-2000)	6.7
Pregnancy						+300	
Lactation						+500	

*Reproduced from: Recommended Dietary Allowances, Ninth Edition (1980), with the permission of the National Academy of Sciences, Washington, D.C.

The data in this table have been assembled from the observed median heights and weights of children, together with desirable weights for adults, for the mean heights of men (70 inches) and women (64 inches) between the ages of 18 and 34 years as surveyed in the U.S. population (HEW/NCHS data).

The energy allowances for the young adults are for men and women doing light work. The allowances for the two older age groups represent mean energy needs over these age spans, allowing for a 2% decrease in basal (resting) metabolic rate per decade and a reduction in activity of 200 kcal/day for men and women between 51 and 75 years, 500 kcal for men over 75 years and 400 kcal for women over 75. . . . The customary range of daily energy output is shown for adults in parentheses and is based on a variation in energy needs of ±400 kcal at any one age . . . emphasizing the wide range of energy intakes appropriate for any group of people.

Energy allowances for children through age 18 are based on median energy intakes of children these ages followed in longitudial growth studies. The values in parentheses are tenth and ninetieth percentiles of energy intake, to indicate the range of energy consumption among children of these ages.

Table 7-6. Daily food guide—the basic four food groups*

Food group	Main nutrients	Daily amounts†
Milk		
Milk, cheese, ice cream, or other products made with whole or skimmed milk	Calcium Protein Riboflavin	Children under 9: 2 to 3 cups Children 9 to 12: 3 or more cups Teenagers: 4 or more cups Adults: 2 or more cups Pregnant women: 3 or more cups Nursing mothers: 4 or more cups (1 cup = 8 ounces fluid milk or designated milk equivalent‡)
Meats		
Beef, veal, lamb, pork, poultry, fish, eggs	Protein Iron Thiamine	2 or more servings Count as one serving: 2 to 3 ounces of lean, boneless, cooked meat, poultry, or fish
Alternates: dry beans, dry peas, nuts, peanut butter	Niacin Riboflavin	2 eggs 1 cup cooked dry beans or peas 4 tablespoons peanut butter
Vegetables and fruits		4 or more servings Count as 1 serving: ½ cup of vegetable or fruit, or a portion such as 1 medium apple, banana, orange, potato, or ½ a medium grapefruit, melon
	Vitamin A	Include: A dark green or deep yellow vegetable or fruit rich in vitamin A, at least every other day
	Vitamin C (ascorbic acid)	A citrus fruit or other fruit or vegetable rich in vitamin C daily
	Smaller amounts of other vitamins and minerals	Other vegetables and fruits including potatoes
Bread and cereals		4 or more servings of whole grain, enriched or restored Count as 1 serving:
	Thiamine	1 slice of bread
	Niacin	1 ounce (1 cup) ready-to-eat cereal, flake or puff varieties
	Riboflavin	½ to ¾ cup cooked cereal
	Iron	
	Protein	½ to ¾ cup cooked pastas (macaroni, spaghetti, noodles) Crackers: 5 saltines, 2 squares graham crackers, etc.

*From Williams, S. R.: 1977. Nutrition and diet therapy, 3rd ed., The C. V. Mosby Co., St. Louis, p. 317.
†Use additional amounts of these foods or added butter, margarine, oils, sugars, etc., as desired or needed.
‡Milk equivalents: 1 ounce cheddar cheese, 3 servings cottage cheese, 1 cup fluid skimmed milk, 1 cup buttermilk, ¼ cup dry skimmed milk powder, 1 cup ice milk, 1²/₃ cups ice cream, ½ cup evaporated milk.

Table 7-7. Daily food guide for school-aged children*

Food group	Amounts recommended	Average (6 to 9 yrs)	Servings (10 to 12 yrs)	Foods included	Contribution to diet
Milk and cheese (1½ ounces cheese = 1 C milk) (C = 1 cup, 8 ounces, or 240 g)	4 servings per day	¾ to 1 C	1 C	Milk—fluid, whole, skim, evaporated; cheeses (natural or processed); ice cream	Calcium, magnesium, riboflavin, protein, phosphorus, vitamins A and B_{12}, and vitamin D, if milk is fortified
Meat group (protein foods) Egg Lean meat, fish, poultry (liver once a week) Peanut butter Dried beans	3 or more servings per day	1	1	Beef; veal; lamb; pork; variety meats such as liver, and sausages; poultry; fish; shellfish; eggs; alternates include dry beans, dry peas, lentils, nuts, peanut butter	Protein, iron, thiamine, riboflavin, vitamins B_6 and B_{12}, phosphorus, and niacin
Fruits and vegetables	At least 4 servings including:				Vitamins C, A, riboflavin, folic acid, iron, and magnesium
Vitamin C source	1 or more (twice as much tomato as citrus)	1 medium orange	1 medium orange	Citrus fruits, berries, tomato, cantaloupe, mango	
Vitamin A source Other vegetables Other fruits	1 or more 2	¼ C ⅓ C 1 medium	⅓ C ½ C 1 medium	Green or yellow fruits and vegetables Potatoes, legumes Apple, banana	
Bread and cereals (whole grain or enriched) Bread Ready-to-eat cereals Cooked cereal	At least 4	1 to 2 slices 1 ounce ½ C	2 slices 1 ounce ¾ C	Includes macaroni, spaghetti, rice, grits, noodles	Protein, iron, thiamine, riboflavin, niacin, vitamin E, and food energy
Fats and carbohydrates	To meet caloric needs				
Butter or margarine (1 tablespoon = 100 calories)		2 tablespoons	2 tablespoons	Mayonnaise, oils	Vitamins A and E
Desserts and sweets		3 portions	3 portions	100 calorie portion = ⅓ C pudding or ice cream, two cookies, 1 ounce cake, 1⅓ ounces pie, 2 tablespoons jelly, jam, honey, or sugar	

*From Pearson, G. A.: 1977. Nutrition in the middle years of childhood, MCN **2**(6):380. Adapted from Vaughan, V., and McKay, J. R., et al., editors: Textbook of pediatrics, Philadelphia, 1975, W. B. Saunders Co., p. 159. Originally from Four food groups of the daily food guide, Institutes of Home Economics, U.S.D.A., and Publication No. 30 Children's Bureau of the U.S. Department of Health, Education, and Welfare.

nutritionally sound daily diet, ensuring the adequacy of children's daily food intake can be difficult. Although parents (especially mothers, who research indicates are families' food "gatekeepers") can exercise control over their children's nutrition and food habits when the children are at home, parental control over nutrition (and all aspects of children's behavior) weakens once children begin to enter the world beyond their homes. Thus, when children are sent to babysitters, day-care centers, preschools, or formally begin school (kindergarten or first grade), other adults and children begin to exert influence on children's eating habits and behaviors.

Children from families with limited incomes, irregular meal patterns, and limited food selections due to parental biases, preferences, and/or lack of knowledge regarding nutrition may develop inadequate nutrition and food habits early in life (Pearson, 1977). If these children are entrusted frequently to the care of others (such as babysitters) who have similarly poor nutritional habits and beliefs, then the pattern of inadequate nutrition is further reinforced. Fortunately, the licensing requirements for day-care centers and preschools in most states are sufficiently stringent that children in those settings should be reasonably assured of receiving adequate meals. However, the same optimism cannot be voiced regarding public schools. Too often, even in a school that participates in federal school lunch and/or breakfast programs, there are also vending machines dispensing such "junk" foods as pop, candy, and potato chips. This becomes a double message for students, reinforcing the notion of balanced nutritious meals (the school lunch or breakfast), while at the same time providing ready access to nonnutritious, high caloric, additive-laden foods, which are typically decried by parents, teachers, nutritionists, and others as "junk."

Although parental influence and control over children's nutrition gradually gives way to the influence of peers, other adults, and the school, other more insidious influences begin to shape the food habits and preferences of children and youth: the mass media. With children spending increasingly lengthy portions of their days watching television and listening to the radio, the strength of the media's effect on nutritional behavior cannot be denied. Through television alone, children are virtually bombarded with clever, colorful commercials, often animated using popular cartoon characters and accompanied by catchy music, for products that are laced with sugar (cereals, pastries, candy), high in salt (potato chips and similar snacks), or cooked in large quantities of fat (french fried potatoes). These commercials often contain a direct appeal to the child to "go ask Mom to buy" whatever the product is. The result, of course, is increased pressure on parents, who may yield on occasion just to avoid an argument.

Another important influence on children's eating habits that should be noted here is the increased use of so-called convenience foods by many Americans, especially for families in which both parents (or the only parent) work. Convenience foods are those which can be prepared quickly, often having been cooked prior to packaging, whether they are canned, frozen, or in some other form. Because of the widespread use of convenience foods, Pipes and Rees (1977) advocate efforts to educate parents to help them select nutritious and economical convenience foods.

It seems appropriate at this point to also distinguish between convenience foods and "junk" foods, even though many people may argue that there *is* no difference between them. Rubin (1980) points out that "fast" foods are not necessarily "junk" foods. Research indicates that depending on a person's selection of foods from the menu at fast-food restaurants serving burgers, pizza, fried chicken, tacos, and the like, a meal can provide up to 90% of the RDAs for protein and one third of the RDAs for vitamins and minerals. A more appropriate definition of junk foods would be those foods (whether or not they are fast or convenient) which have little nutritional value, but are high in calories, sugar, fat, and other unnecessary— even harmful—additives and preservatives. While the debate concerning processed, convenience, and junk foods rages on, it is important to recognize that children, who lack the cognitive maturity to analyze the data and form their own conclusions, are often caught in the middle of this war between food producers and advertisers on one hand and parents and consumer activists on the other. Obviously, health education to help children sort out the conflicting messages they are sent from a variety of sources is in order.

As a result of the confusing and often conflicting messages children are sent regarding nutrition, their eating patterns may be less than ideal. Children may develop a preference for sweet, sugary foods, while refusing to even try unfamiliar foods like vegetables. In addition, perhaps as an imitation of their parents or because they do not allow enough time in the morning before leaving for school, many children skip breakfast, which may cause them to be sluggish, tired, and disinterested in their classroom activities at school. Yet another danger, resulting from the practice in many families of eating meals in front of the television, is that children who sit watching television during meals may become so engrossed in the program that they lose interest in their food altogether (Pipes and Rees, 1981).

During the school day, environmental and social factors may influence a child's nutrition. If the cafeteria is noisy, crowded, and largely unsupervised, it may be difficult for children to concentrate on their meals. Also, if students' lunch periods are too short, there may not be enough time to consume a nutritionally adequate meal, and much of a child's food may be wasted. As mentioned earlier, in those schools where vending machines stocked with junk food are close at hand, children may abandon the well-balanced lunch they brought from home or bought in the cafeteria in favor of pop, potato chips, candy, and other nonnutritious foods (Pearson, 1977). For older children and adolescents, the influence of peers at school cannot be discounted; peer pressure to conform to group norms is so strong that many children and youth would consider it socially devastating to eat, let alone to actually enjoy, a nutritious cafeteria meal in the presence of their disapproving friends and classmates.

In addition to problems of irregular meals, overconsumption of high calorie, nonnutritious foods, and lack of knowledge of appropriate nutrition, children may suffer from malnutrition and/or obesity. Malnourished or undernourished children are likely to become easily fatigued, have lessened resistance to infection, resulting in frequent absences, and may have "unacceptable patterns of growth . . . accompanied by scholastic underachievement" (Pipes and Rees, 1981:172). For those children who consume more calories than they need, which is a frequent consequence of snacking on "empty" calories in foods like pop and candy, childhood obesity may result (Pearson, 1977). Not only are there negative social consequences (such as taunting, isolation, and exclusion from peer clubs and groups) for the obese child, but there are also negative physiological and psycholog-

ical consequences as well. Obese children may understandably have low self-esteem and a poor body image; as a result, they may not participate fully in school activities and may therefore not learn as much as they could otherwise; too, their poor self-concept makes it difficult to form friendships, thus confirming their negative self-image and increasing their isolation. In this vicious cycle, then, food may become the only positive, rewarding aspect of their lives.

For adolescents, nutritional problems that may have surfaced during the preschool and school-age years may intensify. As teenagers become more involved with extracurricular activities, such as athletics and school clubs, as they begin part-time employment, or as their interest in and involvement with the opposite sex and dating increase, their daily schedules may become more hectic and erratic; consequently, teens may be even more likely than younger children to skip meals or to fill up on junk food (Lucas, 1981). In addition, adolescents of both sexes tend to be preoccupied with their body images. Girls may worry about being overweight and tend to eat sparsely or unwisely in attempts to lose weight; boys become obsessed with body building and may follow restrictive or skewed diets to attain their goals. For both boys and girls, the influence of both peers and the media is strong and may directly affect eating patterns, attitudes, and beliefs.

To conclude this discussion, it seems appropriate to reiterate the importance of nutritional education for young people. The kinds of nutritional deficits and problems prevalent among today's young people are not particularly different from those of previous generations; thus it seems painfully obvious that whatever nutrition education efforts have taken place in schools and other community settings have not been effective. Education of both students and their parents regarding nutritional principles needs to become a priority and should entail use of innovative, creative teaching strategies such as games and simulations, since the tried and true methods have had little discernible impact on the nutritional attitudes and behaviors of children *or* adults.

Assessing nutritional adequacy

Nutritional adequacy can be assessed both indirectly through assessment of growth and development and clinical laboratory values and directly through assessment of nutritional intake, eating patterns and behavior, and direct

Table 7-8. Physical indications of nutritional status of the school-aged child*

Physical aspect	Well-nourished child	Malnourished child	Deficiency
Height and weight	Within growth norms—steady gain and increase from year to year	Above or below growth norms—failure to gain or excessive weight gain each year	Protein, calorie, other essential nutrients
Skin	Clear, smooth, elastic, and firm Reddish pink mucous membranes	Rough, dry, scaly, xerosis Petechiae, ecchymoses, poor wound healing Depigmentation of skin Lesions Dermatitis, sensitivity of skin to sunlight Pallor	Vitamin A Vitamin C Protein, calorie Riboflavin Niacin Vitamin B_{12}, iron, folacin
Skeletal-muscular	Well-developed, erect posture Shoulder blades flat Arms and legs straight Skull and jaw well developed Firm muscles with good tonus Moderate amount of fat	Head sags, winged scapula, bowed legs, costochondral beading, cranial bossing Epiphyseal enlargement of wrists Small flabby muscles, muscle weakness Faulty epiphyseal bone formation Pretibial edema, bilateral	Calcium, vitamin D Vitamins D, C Phosphorus, protein Vitamin A Protein, calorie, thiamine
Head	Hair—smooth, good amount, lustrous Eyes—clear and bright Mouth—pink, moist lips; pink, firm gums; full set of teeth	Dull, dry, depigmented, abnormal texture, easily pluckable, thin Dull with dark circles and hollows; Bitot's spots, conjunctivitis, xerosis, night blindness (nyctalopia), light sensitivity (photophobia) Cracking and scaling lips, cheilosis, fissuring of mouth corners Spongy, swollen gums, bleed easily (gingiva) Irregular or missing teeth with cavities; defective tooth enamel Glossitis Tongue fissuring	Protein, calorie Vitamin A, riboflavin Riboflavin Vitamin C Vitamin D, A Folacin, B_{12}, niacin, iron Niacin
Neck	Normal size	Enlarged thyroid Enlarged parotids	Iodine Protein, calorie
Neurological		Listless Loss of ankle- and knee-jerk reflexes, motor weakness, sensory loss Headache Polyneuritis, motor weakness	Protein, calorie Thiamine Niacin, thiamine Thiamine
Abdomen	Flat	Distended, protrudes, hepatomegaly	Protein, calorie
Cardiac	Normal heart size and sounds	Cardiac enlargement and tachycardia	Thiamine, potassium

*From Pearson, G. A.: 1977. Nutrition in the middle years of childhood, MCN **2**(6):383.

observation of eating behavior and physical condition. Physical indicators of growth that indirectly measure nutritional adequacy include height, weight, head circumference, skinfold and fatfold tests, and bone growth tests (such as x-ray examinations) (Chapters 12 and 13). Certain laboratory tests may also be useful in evaluating nutritional status; they include hemoglobin, hematocrit, and serum/plasma levels of specific nutrients such as protein, ascorbic acid, vitamin A, and iron, among others. Specific criteria for using these laboratory values to judge nutritional adequacy are suggested by Christakis (1973).

More direct assessment of nutritional status requires investigation of personal and familial eating patterns, through use of 24-hour recall of intake, in which the client is asked to write down everything he eats for a 24-hour period. The nurse or nutritionist then compares the reported intake with recommended intake norms to determine dietary strengths and weaknesses. Inaccuracies in recall or reporting of intake are the major limitation of this method. Obviously, if the nurse or nutritionist has an opportunity to observe actual meals and eating behavior, a truer picture of the client's intake may be gained; however, such opportunities are rare, so the nurse must often rely on client recall. Client recall and report can also be obtained through use of structured interviews or nutritional history taking and through use of questionnaires that are filled out by the client. Questions typically include such areas as individual and family meal patterns and practices, food preferences and dislikes, estimation of the frequency, kind, and amount of foods eaten from each of the basic food groups, and activity level (Williams, 1977).

Table 7-8 provides guidelines for using physical assessment and direct observation of school-age children as a means of assessing nutritional status and indicates the probable source of dietary deficiency for each physical sign of inadequate nutrition. If any physical signs of possible malnutrition are noted, further evaluation should be done, including referral to a physician if necessary.

Thus there are a number of means for assessing nutritional adequacy in children and youth. It is important to remember that isolated eating behaviors or laboratory values are not conclusive indicators of overall nutritional status; rather, the child's eating *pattern* and *pattern* of growth and development and the consistency of certain laboratory values over time are more

reliable indicators of the adequacy of his nutrition. Therefore in any situation where the outcome of nutritional assessment is questionable or inconclusive, repeated or additional assessments should be done.

Life events and their effect on the adaptation of children and youth

In addition to considering a child's stage and rate of growth and development and nutritional status, the school nurse must likewise assess the child's stress level and his ability to cope with and adapt to the stresses in his life, since many researchers and lay people have come to recognize that health status and stress level are related (Blair and Salerno, 1976; Coddington, 1972a; Holmes and Rahe, 1967). In recognition of the relationship between stress and health, the remainder of this section will focus on the life stresses or events affecting children and youth and ways to assess their impact on adaptation of young people.

Development of the social readjustment rating scale

Interest in psychobiology, the study of the interaction between psychosocial phenomena and biological processes, was stimulated by the work of Adolf Meyer during the early 1900s. Researchers began exploring the relationship between environmental change and the onset of illness in an effort to scientifically document the observation of many people that individuals who experience multiple and/or prolonged emotional stresses are likely to become ill (Williams and Holmes, 1978).

In 1967, Holmes and Rahe published the results of a study that had attempted to *quantify* the magnitude of the life events or stresses believed to be related to illness onset. The major product of their study is the now widely known and used Social Readjustment Rating Scale (SRRS). As shown in Table 7-9 the SRRS includes forty-three life events that were "empirically derived from clinical experience." The life events included in the scale require some adaptive or coping behavior and require "a significant change in the ongoing life pattern of the individual" (Holmes and Rahe, 1967:217). In other words, these life events required varying degrees of social readjustment on the part of the affected individuals.

According to Holmes and Rahe (1967:213), *social readjustment* includes "the amount and duration of change in one's accustomed pattern of life resulting from various life events. As

Table 7-9. The social readjustment rating scale*

Rank	Life event	Mean value
1	Death of spouse	100
2	Divorce	73
3	Marital separation	65
4	Jail term	63
5	Death of close family member	63
6	Personal injury or illness	53
7	Marriage	50
8	Fired at work	47
9	Marital reconciliation	45
10	Retirement	45
11	Change in health of family member	44
12	Pregnancy	40
13	Sex difficulties	39
14	Gain of new family member	39
15	Business readjustment	39
16	Change in financial state	38
17	Death of close friend	37
18	Change to different line of work	36
19	Change in number of arguments with spouse	35
20	Mortgage over $10,000	31
21	Foreclosure of mortgage or loan	30
22	Change in responsibilities at work	29
23	Son or daughter leaving home	29
24	Trouble with in-laws	29
25	Outstanding personal achievement	28
26	Wife begin or stop work	26
27	Begin or end school	26
28	Change in living conditions	25
29	Revision of personal habits	24
30	Trouble with boss	23
31	Change in work hours or conditions	20
32	Change in residence	20
33	Change in schools	20
34	Change in recreation	19
35	Change in church activities	19
36	Change in social activities	18
37	Mortgage or loan less than $10,000	17
38	Change in sleeping habits	16
39	Change in number of family get-togethers	15
40	Change in eating habits	15
41	Vacation	13
42	Christmas	12
43	Minor violations of the law	11

*From Holmes, T. H., and Rahe, R. H.: 1967. The social readjustment rating scale, J. Psychosom. Res. **11**(2):216.

defined, social readjustment measures the intensity and length of time necessary to accommodate to a life event, *regardless of the desirability of this event.''*

Once the list of forty-three life events requir-

ing social readjustment was identified, the events were ranked according to the relative degree of social readjustment needed for an average person to cope with the particular life change. Following statistical analysis of data from their subjects, Holmes and Rahe (1967) assigned a numerical weight or *life change unit* (LCU); the greater the degree of impact of the life change, the higher the value of the LCU. For adults the most significant and therefore most highly weighted life event (LCU equals 100) is death of one's spouse, whereas the least significant and lowest weighted life event (LCU equals 11) is minor violations of the law, such as getting a traffic ticket (Table 7-9).

To determine the overall magnitude of the changes confronting an individual during a given time period, the LCUs for all reported life events are totaled; research indicates that the higher the total LCU score, the more likely it is that the individual will experience a change in his health (Williams and Holmes, 1978). As a general rule, a cluster of life changes totaling 150 LCU or more within 1 year is considered a *life crisis*. The degree of life crisis is then determined as follows: 0 to 149 LCU equals no life crisis; 150 to 199 LCU equals a mild life crisis; 200 to 299 LCU equals a moderate life crisis; and 300 or more LCU indicates a major life crisis (Williams and Holmes, 1978).

Use of the SRRS with children and youth

As originally developed by Holmes and Rahe (1967), the SRRS considered the life changes of adults only; in fact, during the preliminary research, subjects were asked to assign a numerical weight to their various life events by comparing them to the perceived stress involved in getting married, which was thus used as a comparative referent event (Blair and Salerno, 1976). Since comparatively few children and youth get married, obviously getting married and many of the other life events included in the original SRRS cannot be usefully applied in assessing the stress levels of children and youth.

In recognition of that fact, Coddington (1972a and b) applied the research method devised by Holmes and Rahe to the study of children and youth, deriving lists of pertinent life change events and establishing their rank order and relative value (LCU) for specific age groups. As adapted by Coddington (1972b), the revised scales appear in Tables 7-10 to 7-13.

It is important to remember that these scales are only guides to the assessment of environmental stresses and demands placed on a given

Table 7-10. Life change unit values for preschoolers*

Rank	Life event	Life change units
1	Death of a parent	89
2	Divorce of parents	78
3	Marital separation of parents	74
4	Jail sentence of parent for 1 year or more	67
5	Marriage of parent to stepparent	62
6	Serious illness requiring hospitalization of child	59
7	Death of a brother or sister	59
8	Acquiring a visible deformity	52
9	Serious illness requiring hospitalization of parent	51
10	Birth of a brother or sister	50
11	Mother beginning to work	47
12	Increase in number of arguments between parents	44
13	Beginning nursery school	42
14	Addition of third adult to family (i.e., grandparent, etc.)	39
15	Brother or sister leaving home	39
16	Having a visible congenital deformity	39
17	Increase in number of arguments with parents	39
18	Change in child's acceptance by peers	38
19	Death of a close friend	38
20	Serious illness requiring hospitalization of brother or sister	37
21	Change in father's occupation requiring increased absence from home	36
22	Jail sentence of parent for 30 days or less	34
23	Discovery of being an adopted child	33
24	Change to a new nursery school	33
25	Death of a grandparent	30
26	Outstanding personal achievement	23
27	Loss of job by a parent	23
28	Decrease in number of arguments with parents	22
29	Decrease in number of arguments between parents	21
30	Change in parents' financial status	21

*From Coddington, R. D.: 1972b. The significance of life events as etiologic factors in the diseases of children I—a survey of professional workers, J. Psychosom. Res. **16**(1):13-14.

person within a specified time period. Thus although life change scores (the sum of an individual's LCUs) can be interpreted as predicting no, mild, moderate, or major life crisis, they do not definitively predict or project the outcome of exposure to a particular stress level. Whereas a score of 200 LCU generally indicates *moderate* life crisis, individual variations in coping ability, maturity, and emotional supports may result in certain persons with a score of 200 LCU actually experiencing only *mild* life crisis. It is therefore important for school nurses and others to weigh the child's (youth's) coping ability, support systems, and other factors in addition to determining his life change score so that an accurate assessment of his adaptive level and needs can be made. Indeed, Blair and Salerno (1976:30) emphasize the importance of assessing an individual's *response* to stress-re-

lated events, because "it is not the event itself that may send an individual into turmoil, but the combined effect of the event, its meaning to the individual, and the point at which it bisects his developmental process."

Finally, it is recommended that school nurses and other health care providers reassess the life change events of their clients (both children and adults) annually, so that supportive and/or preventive strategies can be initiated for those clients whose LCU scores and other situational factors indicate increased stress levels and increased probability of a change in health status. In addition, especially with older children, youth, and adults, the SRRS can be used as a counseling tool to help individuals understand the kinds of stresses they have in their lives and to help them identify coping strategies for the present and future. No doubt for many, merely

Table 7-11. Life change unit values for elementary school children*

Rank	Life event	Life change units
1	Death of a parent	91
2	Divorce of parents	84
3	Marital separation of parents	78
4	Acquiring a visible deformity	69
5	Death of a brother or sister	68
6	Jail sentence of parent for 1 year or more	67
7	Marriage of parent to stepparent	65
8	Serious illness requiring hospitalization of child	62
9	Becoming involved with drugs or alcohol	61
10	Having a visible congenital deformity	60
11	Failure of a grade in school	57
12	Serious illness requiring hospitalization of parent	55
13	Death of a close friend	53
14	Discovery of being an adopted child	52
15	Increase in number of arguments between parents	51
16	Change in child's acceptance by peers	51
17	Birth of a brother or sister	50
18	Increase in number of arguments with parents	47
19	Move to a new school district	46
20	Beginning school	46
21	Suspension from school	46
22	Change in father's occupation requiring increased absence from home	45
23	Mother beginning to work	44
24	Jail sentence of parent for 30 days or less	44
25	Serious illness requiring hospitalization of brother or sister	41
26	Addition of third adult to family (i.e., grandmother, etc.)	41
27	Outstanding personal achievement	39
28	Loss of job by a parent	38
29	Death of a grandparent	38
30	Brother or sister leaving home	36
31	Pregnancy in unwed teenage sister	36
32	Change in parents' financial status	29
33	Beginning another school year	27
34	Decrease in number of arguments with parents	27
35	Decrease in number of arguments between parents	25
36	Becoming a full-fledged member of a church	25

*From Coddington, R. D.: 1972b. The significance of life events as etiologic factors in the diseases of children I—a survey of professional workers, J. Psychosom. Res. **16**(1)14.

learning that these life events are generally stressful for most people may help relieve some of the tension and anxiety these events may generate. In our increasingly complex and stressful world, periodic assessment of stress, life changes, and adaptive level and potential are important primary and secondary prevention strategies.

Family development and assessment

Up to this point, this chapter has concentrated on understanding and assessing the adaptation of *individuals,* particularly children and youth (adolescents). Although that is certainly a relevant and important emphasis for a textbook about school nursing, it is equally relevant and important to consider the adaptive needs and concerns of *families* as well, since all children and youth are the products of some type of family.

The importance of a family focus

As noted in Chapter 1, beginning with the appointment of the first American school nurses in the early 1900s, school nurses have included students' families in their health education and

Table 7-12. Life change unit values for junior high school age youth*

Rank	Life event	Life change units
1	Unwed pregnancy of child	95
2	Death of a parent	94
3	Divorce of parents	84
4	Acquiring a visible deformity	83
5	Marital separation of parents	77
6	Jail sentence of parent for 1 year or more	76
7	Fathering an unwed pregnancy	76
8	Death of a brother or sister	71
9	Having a visible congenital deformity	70
10	Discovery of being an adopted child	70
11	Becoming involved with drugs or alcohol	70
12	Change in child's acceptance by peers	68
13	Death of a close friend	65
14	Marriage of parent to stepparent	63
15	Failure of a grade in school	62
16	Pregnancy in unwed teenage sister	60
17	Serious illness requiring hospitalization of child	59
18	Beginning to date	55
19	Suspension from school	54
20	Serious illness requiring hospitalization of parent	54
21	Move to a new school district	52
22	Jail sentence of parent for 30 days or less	50
23	Birth of a brother or sister	50
24	Not making an extracurricular activity he/she wanted	49
25	Loss of job by a parent	48
26	Increase in number of arguments between parents	48
27	Breaking up with a boyfriend or girlfriend	47
28	Increase in number of arguments with parents	46
29	Beginning junior high school	45
30	Outstanding personal achievement	45
31	Serious illness requiring hospitalization of brother or sister	44
32	Change in father's occupation requiring increased absence from home	42
33	Change in parents' financial status	40
34	Mother beginning to work	36
35	Death of a grandparent	35
36	Addition of third adult to family (i.e., grandparent, etc.)	34
37	Brother or sister leaving home	33
38	Decrease in number of arguments between parents	29
39	Decrease in number of arguments with parents	29
40	Becoming a full-fledged member of a church	28

*From Coddington, R. D.: 1972b. The significance of live events as etiologic factors in the diseases of children I—a survey of professional workers, J. Psychosom. Res. **16**(1):15.

other nursing intervention strategies. Public health nurses have traditionally maintained a family-centered focus, so the fact that school nurses, as a subspecialty group within public health nursing, have also retained a family focus is not at all surprising. However, despite the fact that school nurses sustained a family focus based on tradition and on their nursing "roots," there are other reasons for continuing to focus on families.

One of the primary reasons why school nurses and all school personnel need to maintain a family-centered approach is that through family assessment, school personnel can better know and understand a child and his family, since family assessment provides information about the family's structure, functioning, interactions, and home and neighborhood environment. Through family assessment, the *family's* perception of the child and his needs can be ob-

Table 7-13. Life change unit values for senior high school age youth*

Rank	Life event	Life change units
1	Getting married	101
2	Unwed pregnancy of child	92
3	Death of a parent	87
4	Acquiring a visible deformity	81
5	Divorce of parents	77
6	Fathering an unwed pregnancy	77
7	Becoming involved with drugs or alcohol	76
8	Jail sentence of parent for 1 year or more	75
9	Marital separation of parents	69
10	Death of a brother or sister	68
11	Change in child's acceptance by peers	67
12	Pregnancy in unwed teenage sister	64
13	Discovery of being an adopted child	64
14	Marriage of parent to stepparent	63
15	Death of a close friend	63
16	Having a visible congenital deformity	62
17	Serious illness requiring hospitalization of child	58
18	Failure of a grade in school	56
19	Move to a new school district	56
20	Not making an extracurricular activity he/she wanted	55
21	Serious illness requiring hospitalization of parent	55
22	Jail sentence of parent for 30 days or less	53
23	Breaking up with a boyfriend or girlfriend	53
24	Beginning to date	51
25	Suspension from school	50
26	Birth of a brother or sister	50
27	Increase in number of arguments with parents	47
28	Increase in number of arguments between parents	46
29	Loss of job by a parent	46
30	Outstanding personal achievement	46
31	Change in parents' financial status	45
32	Being accepted at a college of his/her choice	43
33	Beginning senior high school	42
34	Serious illness requiring hospitalization of brother or sister	41
35	Change in father's occupation requiring increased absence from home	38
36	Brother or sister leaving home	37
37	Death of a grandparent	36
38	Addition of third adult to family (i.e., grandparent, etc.)	34
39	Becoming a full-fledged member of a church	31
40	Decrease in number of arguments between parents	27
41	Decrease in number of arguments with parents	26
42	Mother beginning to work	26

*From Coddington, R. D.: 1972b. The significance of life events as etiologic factors in the diseases of children I—a survey of professional workers, J. Psychosom. Res. **16**(1):15-16.

tained before there are any identified academic or health problems requiring corrective action. As Holt and Robinson (1979) point out, often the family has critically important information about the child, which may aid in his appropriate academic placement. Failure to elicit this information may result in placement of a child in a classroom setting that is not conducive to his learning needs or may result in development of a nursing care plan doomed to failure because the family's involvement and support have not been secured.

In addition to the importance of family assessment as a means of understanding the needs of a particular child, Satir (1967) points out that a family focus is essential because the problems, needs, and illnesses of any one family member affect the *entire* family, which responds as a *unit*. According to Satir, the "Identified Patient" (IP) in any family, the person who is labeled "sick" or "different" or who is used as the scapegoat and blamed for many misfortunes, is *not* himself the family's real problem; rather, his symptoms, whether physical, psychological, or behavioral, are a barometer of the family's function or dysfunction, an "SOS" about the pained marital relationship and/or dysfunctional parenting. Satir believes, then, that the Identified Patient's symptoms result from his distortion of his own growth in an effort to alleviate and absorb the pain of the husband/father and wife/mother. Because the Identified Patient's symptoms serve a function for the family, the family may unwittingly keep him in the sick role and sabotage his individual therapy to enable his illness to continue to meet their needs. Therefore, to solve his problems, the therapeutic focus must be on the *entire* family.

In summary, two of the most important reasons for retaining a family-centered approach to school nursing are (1) that such a focus enables the nurse and other school personnel to better understand and assess the needs and capabilities of individual children and to more appropriately plan for their academic and health needs and (2) that because the family behaves as a unit, the problems and needs of any one member, including the so-called Identified Patient, directly affect and are affected by the other family members. Therefore a child's family must *always* be regarded as a vital influence on his health, well-being, and achievement.

The family as a social system

Having established the legitimacy and importance of a family-centered approach to school nursing, it is appropriate to clarify what is meant by "family" and to elaborate on Satir's assertion that the needs of any one member affect the family as a whole, an idea which is best explained by viewing the family as a social system.

Numerous authors, including Blair and Salerno (1976), Murray et al. (1979b), and Whitley and Madden (1978), have proposed definitions of "family." However, as Whitley and Madden wryly observed, there are almost as many definitions of family as there are families.

Many definitions commonly encountered in the literature define "family" in terms of the tradiional nuclear family: mom, dad, and the kids. However, this popular conceptualization of the nuclear family is no longer the predominant family form in this country. Partly in response to the rapid tumultuous social change of the 1960s and 1970s, other family forms, including single parent families, married childless couples, homosexual families, communal families, and blended families (those formed through remarriage or cohabitation of divorced or widowed adults incorporating children from previous marriages or relationships), have become more prevalent. Therefore the task of defining "family" in a way that includes most existing family structures is more difficult, although not impossible. For the purposes of this chapter, the following definition of family incorporating nontraditional life-styles will be adopted. According to this definition, a *family* is a group of two or more persons related (or joined) by ties of marriage, blood, adoption, or mutual consent, who share a common history and culture, interact with each other in their respective familial roles, and who may or may not constitute a single household (Blair and Salerno, 1976; Murray et al. 1979b). Thus, as this definition indicates, a family may be any group that thinks of itself and functions as a family.

A family is also a *system,* more specifically, a *social system.* As defined by Lough et al. (1975:19), a *system* is "an entity consisting of definable interdependent parts that are in equilibrium." A *social system,* then, consists of "two or more people interacting together" (1975:19). A family clearly fits this definition of social system, although the family may also be part of a larger social system such as the community.

As a social system, the family has certain system characteristics (Aldous, 1972:26-27):

1. Elements that make up the family system, that is, the family positions, are to varying degrees *interdependent*. Therefore change in the behavior of one family member (system element) results in change in the behavior of other family members (system elements).
2. The family's unity and identity are established through *selective boundary maintenance*. Families set and maintain their boundaries by means of:
   a. Establishing and maintaining *separate residences* or households. This is the basis of the so-called *neolocal* pattern common in our cul-

ture, in which newly established families, such as young married couples, move out of their parents' homes and establish a separate residence elsewhere.

b. Use of *kinship terminology, nicknames, and other idiosyncratic forms of communication.* Examples include references to "the wife" or "hubby" or "Babe," as well as use of phrases or idioms handed down through the family, such as explaining an indirect route taken by a family member as "He went 'round by Hogan's barn," or explaining who mysteriously washed the dishes without being seen by claiming that "Reno [the magician] did it."

c. *Shared experiences and intimacies,* which are concealed from public scrutiny; for example, the fact that mom and dad have separate bedrooms because dad snores or the fact that big brother and his girlfriend live together without the sanction of marriage.

d. *Periodic family rituals,* such as the particular way the family celebrates birthdays, Christmas and other holidays, and their annual family vacation which is "always" spent fishing and canoeing up at their lake cabin.

The permeability of the family's boundaries is *selective;* the family decides which, if any, outsiders can permeate their boundaries and in what circumstances. Typically, families "close ranks" against outsiders, only gradually relaxing their boundaries to admit them.

3. To meet changing demands from within the family and from society, the family *modifies its structure* of interacting. To preserve its unity, the family must be able to counteract or amplify the changes necessitated by events leading to family formation (such as marriage), addition of family members (through birth, adoption, and so on), their passage through the educational system, and their eventual departure to establish their own family units, all of which require the family to "change existing interaction patterns to accommodate new personnel, to fill in the gaps of those gone, or to meet changing member and societal demands" (Aldous, 1972:53).

4. The family is a *task performance* group that is expected to meet society's demands as well as the demands of its own members. The specific tasks all families are expected to accomplish include:

a. *Physical maintenance of family members,* including adequate income to meet expenses, clothing and shelter, and food and nutrition. Families unable to meet this task without outside help (for example, poor families seeking welfare) are unable to maintain their boundaries, being forced instead to answer invasive questions regarding their income and living conditions, and to allow intrusions into their homes by government workers and other "helpers." It should also be noted that the

family's ability to carry out this physical maintenance task critically affects its ability to achieve its other tasks, including morale maintenance.

b. *Socialization of family members for roles in the family and other groups.* This includes teaching children about marital and parental roles, instilling values regarding adult employment, and so on. Although the school also has a role in socializing children, the primary responsibility rests with the family.

c. *Maintenance of social control within the family and between the family and society.* According to Aldous (1972:48), this entails family members' attempts "to avoid disruption of established behavioral patterns as well as destruction to property and person." Establishment of rules and disciplinary measures are ways the family can maintain social control and avoid conflict with law enforcement agencies.

d. *Morale maintenance,* or *maintenance of family members' motivation to perform familial and other roles.* Families can help achieve this by providing emotional support and encouragement to members as they attempt to meet the often conflicting demands of the family and other societal influences, such as school and work.

e. *Addition of family members through reproduction, adoption, remarriage or other means, and their release when mature.* However, due to present concerns about worldwide overpopulation, this task is no longer regarded as essential to the survival of the species and is therefore less emphasized. For those families who remain childless, such as heterosexual couples who choose not to parent or homosexual couples, *nurturance of family members* may become a substitute emphasis.

Before concluding this brief discussion of universal family tasks it should be noted that the family's relative emphasis on performance of specific tasks shifts during the family's life cycle. Thus, physical maintenance is especially important and difficult during both the childbearing years, when the family may have only one income and have not yet reached their peak earning power, and during the retirement years, when both wage earners are retired and living on fixed incomes from pensions. For families with adolescents, social control may become the central task, as adolescents struggle to emancipate themselves, and parents struggle to retain some control.

Family development: one approach to studying the family

Based on her review of available literature concerning the family, Logan (1978) describes a number of approaches to studying families and includes a bibliography identifying sources of additional information for interested readers. Rather than duplicating Logan's discussion, this section will focus on only one method of studying families: the family development approach. This framework has been chosen for discussion because its developmental emphasis is compatible with this chapter's earlier discussion of growth and development and because it is a systematic approach to family study and assessment that can be readily applied.

Family development is one approach to studying and assessing families. As defined by Aldous (1972:1), *family development* focuses on "the characteristics of families over the period of their existence beginning with the couple's cohabitation and ending with the death of family members or their departure into other family units." The emphasis of this approach, therefore, is on *longitudinal study*—the systematic analysis of expected family changes over time; that is, the family is studied over the course of its life cycle.

The family development approach has a systems theory base; that is, it regards the family as a social system in and of itself and also looks at the family as part of a larger social system such as the community. However, in addition to analyzing the family unit as a system and as part of a larger social system, the family development approach also assesses subsystems within the family, generally in terms of *dyads* (relationships between two people) such as husband-wife or mother-daughter, as well as considering the impact of change by one family member on the entire family unit.

Family interaction patterns. A key aspect of assessment using the family development approach is the family's interaction patterns, which directly and critically affect the family's ability to achieve its tasks. Within a family's interaction structure and patterns, three basic areas should be addressed: *communication* structure, *power* structure, and *affection* structure (Aldous, 1972).

COMMUNICATION STRUCTURE. Within the family, verbal and nonverbal communication serves three basic purposes: (1) to share with other family members one's knowledge and intentions, which serves to minimize and resolve family conflicts and problems; (2) to help set and maintain the family's boundaries by underscoring family solidarity (such as remarking on the "peculiar" ways of nonfamily members), and (3) to communicate feelings, which is vital-

ly important in allowing the family to set goals, establish a power structure and effective division of labor, avoid conflicts, and make and/or modify family roles. Aldous (1972) identifies the following three basic aspects of communication that should be assessed and analyzed:

1. *Direct communication* among family members. Do all family members communicate directly with each other, or are there some individuals who rarely or never communicate?
2. Prevalence of *two-way communication*. Is there give and take to family communication, implying mutuality and openness, or does one person tend to initiate most of the conversation?
3. *Openness of communication channels*. Are communication channels generally open, or are there particular areas of family life and functioning that are considered off limits and hence not discussed?

As Aldous points out, however, the answers to these questions regarding family communication structure and patterns may vary depending on the topic of communication. For example, although communication may *generally* be direct, two-way, and open, there may be sensitive or "touchy" topics of conversation that may lead to communication breakdowns or avoidance by two or more family members.

POWER STRUCTURE. As defined by Aldous (1972:76), *power* is "the probability that one family member will be able to exert his will despite resistance." The family's power structure becomes especially important when decisions must be made concerning (1) distribution of family resources, such as money, food, and space and (2) division of labor in such areas as meal planning and preparation, purchase and maintenance of clothing, and household upkeep.

Assessment of a family's power structure is based on direct observation of the following behaviors:

1. *Discussion participation*. Who tends to participate most?
2. *Idea adoption*. Following discussion of a topic or decision-making area, whose idea is ultimately adopted?
3. *Identity of the eventual decision maker*. Regardless of who may have originated the idea or solution, who ultimately decides that it will be adopted?
4. *Interpersonal deference*. Who receives

the greatest deference during discussion and decision making?

5. *Power in the face of conflict.* In case of disagreement, whose idea is finally adopted? (This may be a different person from the one identified in number 2.)

Again, as previously noted in this discussion, the identity of the power holder(s) may vary based on the area of decision making or conflict involved; while a child may be allowed to decide what clothing he will wear on a given day, his mother may well retain the decision-making power concerning purchase of clothing.

AFFECTION STRUCTURE. The manner and degree of affection (verbal and nonverbal) displayed within a family depends in large part on the family's cultural/ethnic heritage and values (Chapter 8), the age and sex of family members, and on the family's socioeconomic status. Thus the English and German people are reputedly more reserved than the French or Italians in their expression of emotion and affection, while research also indicates that among American families, the higher the social class, the more mother-child affection is observed (Aldous, 1972). Assessment of affection structure is accomplished through observation of the following:

1. *Touching:* amount and frequency of tactile contact between family members, including kissing, hugging, caressing, and explicitly sexual contact.
2. *Comfort measures:* Who gives and gets comfort, both verbally and nonverbally? Do certain members give small presents or other tokens of affection? Are special favors done?
3. *Terms of endearment:* Who uses them? What terms are used (such as "honey," "dear," and so on)?

Affection structure and patterns are subject to change over the family's life cycle because family members' needs and involvement with each other are affected by the growth, development, and aging of each member (Aldous, 1972).

Developmental stages and the family life cycle. As noted earlier, the family development framework or approach looks at the family's life cycle over time. The concept of *developmental stage* is used to indicate separate divisions within the family life cycle based on changes in the *role complex,* which is "the total complement of positions, roles, and their associated norms that define a social system such as

the family at one particular time" (Aldous, 1972: Glossary p. 3). Thus, like individuals, families change and develop over time, and, like individuals, families have developmental tasks to accomplish at each stage throughout the life cycle.

Associated with each stage is a *critical role transition point* or "point of no return," a point at which there is a significant change in behavior of individual family members and, hence, in the family system and its role complex as a whole. Examples of critical role transition points are getting married for the first time, birth of the first child, and death of a spouse. Although these events, especially marriage and childbirth, may occur more than once in an individual's life and may be planned, the *first* occurrence of each is invariably met by the persons involved with some measure of uncertainty and requires significant change in their behavior and their family role. This change in the individual is irreversible, so that even if he becomes divorced, he can never regain the status of a never-married bachelor, and even if the child subsequently dies, the mother and father have been permanently affected by their parenthood experiences, no matter how brief (Aldous, 1972).

Therefore these critical role transitions affect the communication, power, and affection structures of the family, propelling the family into a new developmental stage. The stages of family development are established based on three criteria (Aldous, 1972:96-98):

1. *Change in plurality patterns.* This includes the number of family members and the number of possible interpersonal relationships in the family at any one time; the major cause of change in plurality patterns in the family is the arrival (birth or adoption) of children and their eventual departure into new family units due to marriage or emancipation and establishment of a separate residence.
2. *Age and school placement of the oldest child.* School entrance (kindergarten or first grade) of the oldest child disrupts the family's previous interaction patterns and requires both the child and his family to conform to new expectations from the outside world.
3. *Occupational retirement of the wage earner(s).* This is a critical role transition point because the couple now faces lower income and the accompanying disruption

in daily routine. The couple is likely to have more leisure time together, which requires changes in division of labor, daily routine, and communication patterns.

When all three criteria are applied, the stages of the family life cycle are as follows (Aldous, 1972; Duvall, 1971):

Stage I: Childless-married families
Stage II: Childbearing families
Stage III: Families with preschool children
Stage IV: Families with school-age children
Stage V: Families with adolescents
Stage VI: The family as a launching center
Stage VII: Families in the middle years
Stage VIII: Aging families

Although *most* families are believed to develop through these stages in the sequence given, Aldous (1972:102) emphasizes that the stages are "neither prescriptive or descriptive of all family life cycles" and that they are *not* invariant *or* irreversible, nor do they always occur in the order given. Thus unlike individuals, whose development tends to follow an invariant and predictable sequence, families may (1) progress through the developmental stages in a sequence different from that previously given; (2) skip one or more stages altogether, as in the case of childless families; (3) appear to be in more than one stage at a time, such as families with adolescents in which the adolescent becomes a parent and keeps the infant; (4) repeat a stage, for example, families whose first (oldest) child dies in early childhood; or (5) have their development abruptly halted during an early stage due to divorce, death of a spouse, death of a child, and so on. Due to the recent trend toward formation of nontraditional, alternative family structures and life-styles (Chapter 8), the number and frequency of the kinds of developmental variations just described have increased. Therefore in applying family development concepts and stages to particular families, it is important to consider the impact of the families' life-styles on their developmental progress and to avoid making value judgments about those variations.

Associated with each of the eight developmental stages identified by Duvall (1971) are certain *stage-critical developmental tasks,* which may be defined as growth responsibilities arising at a certain stage in the family's life cycle, which, if successfully accomplished, lead to "satisfaction and success with later tasks." If *not* achieved, they may result in

Table 7-14. Duvall's eight family development stages with stage-critical tasks*

Family stage: number and label	Stage-critical tasks
I. Childless-married families	Establishing mutually satisfying marriage Adjusting to pregnancy and promise of parenthood Fitting into kin network
II. Childbearing families (oldest child: birth to 30 months)	Having, adjusting to, and encouraging development of infants Establishing satisfying home for both parents and infant(s)
III. Families with preschool children (oldest child: 30 months to 6 years)	Adapting to critical needs and interests of preschool children in stimulating, growth-promoting ways Coping with energy depletion and lack of privacy as parents
IV. Families with school-age children (oldest child: 6 years to 13 years)	Fitting into community of school-age families in constructive ways Encouraging children's educational achievement
V. Families with adolescents (oldest child: 13 years to 20 years)	Balancing freedom with responsibility as teenagers mature and emancipate themselves Establishing postparental interests and careers as growing parents
VI. The family as a launching center (first child gone until last child gone)	Releasing young adults into work, military service, college, marriage, etc., with appropriate rituals and assistance Maintaining supportive home base
VII. Families in the middle years (empty nest until retirement)	Rebuilding marriage relationship Maintaining kin ties with older and younger generations
VIII. Aging families (retirement until death of both spouses)	Coping with bereavement and living alone Closing family home or adapting it to aging Adjusting to retirement

*From Duvall, E. M.: 1971. Family development, 4th ed., J. B. Lippincott Co., Philadelphia, p. 151.

"unhappiness in the family, disapproval by society, and difficulty with later family developmental tasks" (Duvall, 1971:149-150). These are tasks the family is expected to carry out at particular stages of their development *in addition to* the five basic tasks that all families must accomplish throughout their life cycle. The stage-critical developmental tasks as defined by Duvall are presented in Table 7-14.

Family assessment

The value of the family development framework and other family-oriented conceptual frameworks lies in their usefulness for assessing nursing needs and planning appropriate interventions for selected family units. Although it is beyond the scope of this chapter to conduct an in-depth discussion of the many available family assessment frameworks and tools and to describe in detail how they may be applied in particular instances, the remainder of this discussion will identify and highlight selected frameworks that may be especially useful to the school nurse.

With regard to the family development framework previously discussed, Duvall (1971) suggests three basic areas to assess in determining whether or not a given family is successful:

1. *Achievement of short-term goals.* How well is the family meeting its own short-term goals and ambitions?
2. *Achievement of society's goals.* How adequately is the family performing its universal tasks such as physical maintenance and social control? What kinds of contributions to the community have been made by family members? Has the family managed to avoid disruption due to divorce and desertion and to avoid police intervention? Have they succeeded in obtaining a complete education for their children (that is, without members being expelled or dropping out of school)?
3. *Achievement of developmental tasks.* Does the family encourage and assist individual family members with their personal developmental tasks, or are there unresolved conflicts between individual and family tasks? Is the family reasonably successful in achieving its stage-critical tasks? (This is important in allowing for smooth transition to the next stage.)

Assessment of a family's relative success in these areas is important because for many families success tends to generate further success,

whereas failure increases the difficulty of future tasks. To encourage the likelihood that a family will succeed, the public health-oriented school nurse should (1) be aware of the family's current stage of development and their expected stage-critical tasks, (2) assist the *family* to understand their current stage and expected tasks, (3) provide support and encouragement to the family as they move through the various stages of the life cycle, and (4) provide anticipatory guidance to the family so that members know what stage is coming up next, what tasks will be expected, and can therefore begin to plan how they will manage upcoming developmental crises and challenges.

A tool that parallels the family development approach is the "Family Assessment/Nursing Intervention Identifier" developed by Meister (1977) based on the schema proposed by Tapia (1972). Meister's tool views family development as incorporating five family levels, which were named and described by Tapia (1972) using child development terminology; they are infancy, childhood, adolescence, adulthood, and maturity (Meister, 1977). Using these five family levels, Meister identified twenty-seven behavioral indices of family functioning, which are divided among the five levels. The indices include such areas as family organization, security/survival needs, community involvement, intrafamilial trust, absence of socially deviant behavior (as defined by both family and community), parenting adequacy and appropriateness, evidence of members' self- and family acceptance, awareness and use of community resources, future orientation, ability to meet members' needs, and need for nursing during severe crisis situations. Meister advocates careful assessment of families using the twenty-seven behavioral indices and recommends that findings be plotted on the graph incorporated in her tool, so that needed nursing interventions can be clearly identified. Her suggested nursing interventions parallel the family's level of functioning; thus, beginning with the "infancy" level and moving sequentially toward the "maturity" level, nursing interventions are categorized as trust, counseling, skills, prevention, and "none."

Although Meister's tool incorporates some meaningful areas of family assessment, it seems to be a somewhat complicated and confusing tool for the uninitiated to use. In contrast to the apparent complexity of Meister's tool, Robischon and Smith (1977:90-97) describe family assessment in terms of a limited number of general factors that they believe affect family health:

1. *Family boundary definition:* effectiveness, flexibility, and selective permeability
2. *Family roles:* role changes and conflicts, role behaviors, patterns, and stability
3. *Family arrangements:* degree of individual freedom and choice within the family, rights and duties of family members, division of labor, plans for use of leisure time, opinions regarding sex, religion, and politics
4. *Amount of available energy:* amount of psychic energy needed by the family to maintain its structure and carry out its functions
5. *Power structure:* who has decision-making power, exercises authority, or takes charge, who obeys whom, and who withdraws from leading or obeying
6. *Ability to change:* in what direction is the family moving and can they assume responsibility for initiating change; how effectively does the family problem solve
7. *Communication patterns:* clarity of information sharing, family members in direct communication with each other, identity of any family members left out of conversations, nonverbal behavior, congruence of verbal and nonverbal behavior, formation of alliances within the family
8. *Condition and use of physical environment:* safety, space adequacy, privacy
9. *Use of economic resources:* ability to purchase adequate supplies of food, clothing, utilities and shelter, and fiscal priorities and budgeting
10. *Incidence of family illness:* distribution, frequency, and nature of disease within the family, level of knowledge of health and illness conditions
11. *Parental behavior:* childrearing practices and philosophy, appropriateness of parent-child relationships, and inculcation of cultural values
12. *Family self-care ability:* family's ability to meet basic universal needs (physical maintenance, social control) to maintain health, to be self-sufficient; determination of the family's abilities and strengths, and available reserve resources for meeting its needs

Another approach to family assessment, which capitalizes on the kinds of self-care factors that Robischon and Smith identify, is Otto's (1973) framework for assessing family strengths. As defined by Otto, *family strengths* are "those factors or forces that contribute to family unity and solidarity and that foster the development of the potentials inherent within the family." Indeed, the focus on familial *strengths* rather than weaknesses is the unique feature of this framework, which makes it ideal to use by itself or in combination with some of the more deficit-oriented frameworks and tools. The basic categories of family strengths according to Otto (1973:88-91) are:

1. Physical, emotional, and spiritual needs
2. Childrearing practices and discipline
3. Communication
4. Support, security, and encouragement
5. Growth-producing relationships and experiences within and without the family
6. Responsible community relationships
7. Growing with and through children
8. Self-help and accepting help
9. Flexibility of family functions and roles
10. Mutual respect for individuality
11. Crisis as a means of growth
12. Family unity, loyalty, and intrafamily cooperation
13. Flexibility of family strengths

Before concluding this brief discussion of Otto's framework, however, it is important to note that Otto regards these strength factors as "clusters or constellations that are dynamic, fluid, interrelated, and variable at different stages in the family's life cycle" (1973:71) and *not* as isolated variables. Otto regards his framework as a means of getting away from a pathology orientation regarding families and suggests that the community [school] nurse address the following five questions in working with families:

1. What strengths does the family have?
2. Is the family *aware* of its strengths and resources?
3. Does the family have any latent strengths?
4. What kind of help does the family need in order to develop and utilize its strengths?
5. At the conclusion of the nurse's therapeutic involvement or contract with the family, what strengths and resources can family members identify within themselves?

Another useful tool for family assessment is the *Family Coping Index,* developed as a cooperative effort by the Johns Hopkins School of

Public Health and the Nursing Service of the Richmond (Virginia) Health Department (1964). The purpose of the *Family Coping Index* is to "provide a basis for estimating the nursing needs of a particular family" (1964:1). The *Family Coping Index* is predicated on the belief that nursing needs can be defined in terms of the nursing *interventions* required to meet them; thus the assessment areas incorporated into the tool are based on *nursing* diagnoses rather than *medical* diagnoses. The overriding purpose of this tool, then, is to enable nurses to tailor their care plans to fit the needs of particular families, thus avoiding provision of "ritualized" or "routine" nursing care.

The *Family Coping Index* defines *coping* as "dealing with problems associated with health care with reasonable success" (1964:1), with coping being rated on a scale of 1 (poor) to 5 (excellent). Again, the emphasis is on *family* coping, not individual coping; a child with paraplegia whose family is nonetheless able to maintain his hygiene, complete his grooming, and transport him to and from school without difficulty is coping well with "physical independence," even though the child himself may be physically dependent on the rest of his family. Families are assigned coping scores for each category on the tool according to the following scale: 1, no competence; 3, moderate competence; and 5, complete competence. It is expected, however, that some families will fall between these ratings (at 2 or 4 for example). Because of the simplicity and clarity of the index, it can be readily used for both initial and periodic estimates of family coping. Following are specific coping categories included:

1. Physical independence
2. Therapeutic competence
3. Knowledge of health condition
4. Application of principles of general hygiene
5. Health attitudes
6. Emotional competence
7. Family living
8. Physical environment
9. Use of community resources

As a postscript, it should be acknowledged that Holt and Robinson (1979) have developed a family assessment tool specifically designed for use by school nurses. Their tool is completed following a home visit by the school nurse to the family of a child about whom school personnel are concerned. In addition to the usual demographic data about the family, their tool includes (1) observation of the home

and neighborhood environments, (2) assessment of "significant sociocultural influences" (family attitudes and values), (3) observation of family members' interactions, and (4) interview of the family to determine the family's perception of the problem, solutions (both previously tried and those proposed), family reactions to the possibility of special education for the child, parental description of the child and his typical behavior (including antenatal, natal, and postnatal growth and development), behavior problems and/or developmental delays exhibited by the child, the child's medical history and present social, nutritional, sleep, and elimination patterns, and family health and social history.

Following assessment of the family using the preceding factors, Holt and Robinson (1979) define the problem mutually (with the family) and make a plan for a follow-up contact. The summary of their assessment is then used to set priorities for problem solving, identify the family's strengths and weaknesses, identify nursing interventions, and implement the nursing care plan.

With so many family assessment frameworks and tools available, selection of a particular framework or tool for personal use becomes primarily a matter of individual preference based on philosophical compatibility and/or ease of application. Regardless of which framework/tool or combination is selected, it is important for the school nurse to use some kind of systematic approach to assess the adaptation of the most significant others in the lives of the children in her schools: their families.

PROMOTING ADAPTATION: THE ROLE OF THE SCHOOL NURSE

Although specific suggestions for understanding, assessing, and promoting the adaptation of students and their families have been incorporated throughout this chapter, it is appropriate to conclude this discussion by summarizing the role of the school nurse in promoting adaptation.

Obviously, one of the school nurse's primary tasks in promoting adaptation is to thoroughly and carefully *assess* the individual's (or group's) energy, perception, integration, and adaptive level (compensation, mobility, or growth) as defined earlier in this chapter and to further assess his/their adaptation using concepts and principles of growth and development, nutrition, impact of life events and social readjustment, and family development and functioning.

Assuming that this assessment is thorough and accurate, it becomes the basis for development of an appropriate nursing care plan for an individual or family. The care plan (Chapter 14) should be developed collaboratively with the client (individual or family), using the contract-setting process to increase the client's commitment to the plan, thus improving the chances for achieving the stated nursing goals. The nursing care plan will likely include provision of counseling, health teaching, and other appropriate interventions as needed for those individuals and families requiring some assistance with adaptation. In providing these services, Levine (1966) notes that the nurse's interventions would be classified as either *therapeutic* if she is able to positively influence the client's adaptation and well-being, or *supportive,* if, despite her best efforts, the outcome can be no better than maintenance of the status quo.

However, the school nurse's role in promoting adaptation goes beyond her direct interventions with specific individuals or families. The school nurse must be concerned about the adaptation and well-being of the school population and community as well. For example, she may actively encourage availability of adequate nutrition at school by lobbying school administrators to ban vending machines containing junk food or by consulting with food service personnel to encourage optimal nutrition in the school lunch program.

In addition to her direct interventions with and on behalf of individuals, families, or other groups and her concern for the adaptation of the school and community population as a whole, the school nurse may also provide in-service education and one-to-one assistance for faculty and other school personnel regarding the adaptation of students. This in-service and one-to-one consultation may include discussion of the adaptive needs and potential of particular students, or it may focus on the needs of general groupings of students, such as adolescents or elementary schoolchildren, including assessment of adaptation and how to decide when and where to refer students for further assessment or intervention.

Finally, because of her abiding interest in and commitment to primary prevention, the school nurse's efforts to promote adaptation will undoubtedly include scrutiny of the existing health education curriculum in the school and recommendation of any indicated changes; such changes might predictably involve expansion or updating of the health curriculum in such areas as nutrition education, promotion of mental health and a positive self-concept, and general concepts for improving adaptation.

Because the role of the school nurse in health education is discussed at length in Chapter 15, details of her involvement in health education as it relates to promoting adaptation are not included here. However, because the adaptive level and status of students affect their ability to use and benefit from their educational opportunities, understanding, assessing, and promoting adaptation are critically important aspects of the school nurse's role and should therefore be high on her priority list. In recognition of the importance of this focus on adaptation, then, Chapters 8 and 9 will continue exploration of concepts affecting the adaptation of children, youth, and their families.

REFERENCES

Aldous, J.: 1972. The developmental approach to family analysis. Vol. 1, The conceptual framework, University of Minnesota, Minneapolis.

American Academy of Pediatrics: 1977. School health: a guide for health professionals, American Academy of Pediatrics, Evanston, Ill.

Barnes, M. J.: 1978. The reactions of children and adolescents to the death of a parent or sibling. In Sahler, O. J. Z.: The child and death, The C. V. Mosby Co., St. Louis.

Blair, C. L., and Salerno, E. M.: 1976. The expanding family: childbearing, Little, Brown & Co., Boston.

Boland, M., Murray, R., Nolan, N., and Grohar, M.: 1975. Application of adaptation theory to nursing. In Murray, R., and Zentner, J.: Nursing concepts for health promotion, Prentice-Hall, Inc., Englewood Cliffs, N.J.

Brower, E. W., and Nash, C. L.: 1979. Evaluating growth and posture in school-age children, Nursing '79 9(4):58-63.

Byrne, M. L., and Thompson, L. F.: 1978. Key concepts for the study and practice of nursing, 2nd ed., The C. V. Mosby Co., St. Louis.

Christakis, G., editor: 1973. Nutritional assessment in health programs, American Public Health Association, Washington, D.C.

Coddington, R. D.: 1972a. The significance of life events as etiologic factors in the diseases of children II—a study of a normal population, J. Psychosom. Res. 16(3):205-213.

Coddington, R. D.: 1972b. The significance of life events as etiologic factors in the diseases of children I—a survey of professional workers, J. Psychosom. Res. 16(1):7-18.

Combs, A. W., Avila, D. L., and Purkey, W. W.: 1978. Helping relationships: basic concepts for the helping professions, 2nd ed., Allyn & Bacon, Inc., Boston.

Dubos, R.: 1965. Man adapting, Yale University Press, New Haven, Conn.

Dunn, H. L.: 1961. High level wellness, R. W. Beatty, Ltd., Arlington, Va.

Duvall, E. M.: 1971. Family development, 4th ed., J. B. Lippincott Co., Philadelphia.

Erikson, E. H.: 1963. Childhood and society, 2nd ed., W. W. Norton & Co., Inc., New York.

Erikson, E. H.: 1968. Identity: youth and crisis, W. W. Norton & Co., Inc., New York.

Food and Nutrition Board, National Academy of Sciences—National Research Council: 1980. Recommended dietary allowances, revised 1980, Washington, D.C.

Frankenburg, W. K., Dodds, J. B., Fandal, A. W., Kazuk, E., and Cohrs, M.: 1975. Denver developmental screening test reference manual, rev. ed., University of Colorado Medical Center, Denver, Colo.

Fredlund, D. J.: 1977. Children and death from the school setting viewpoint, J. School Health **47**(9):533-537.

Getchell, E. L., and Howard, R. B.: 1975. Nutrition in development. In Scipien, G. M., Barnard, M. U., Chard, M. A., Howe, J., and Phillips, P. J.: Comprehensive pediatric nursing, McGraw-Hill, Inc., New York.

Ginsburg, H., and Opper, S.: 1969. Piaget's theory of intellectual development: an introduction, Prentice-Hall, Inc., Englewood Cliffs, N.J.

Grohar, M., Leonard, B., Murray, R., Smith, M., and Zentner, J.: 1979. Assessment and health promotion for the toddler. In Murray, R. B., and Zentner, J. P.: Nursing assessment and health promotion through the life span, 2nd ed., Prentice-Hall, Inc., Englewood Cliffs, N.J.

Grollman, E. A.: 1967. Explaining death to children, Beacon Press, Boston.

Grollman, E. A.: 1976. Talking about death: a dialogue between parent and child, Rev. ed., Beacon Press, Boston.

Hames, C. C.: 1978. A theoretical framework for pediatric care: adaptation-level theory. In Brandt, P. A., Chinn, P. L., Hunt, V. O., and Smith, M. E., editors: Current practice in pediatric nursing, vol. 2, The C. V. Mosby Co., St. Louis.

Holmes, T. H., and Rahe, R. H.: 1967. The social readjustment rating scale, J. Psychosom. Res. **11**(2):213-218.

Holt, S. J., and Robinson, T. M.: 1979. The school nurse's "family assessment tool," Am. J. Nurs. **79**(5):950-953.

Hostler, S. L.: 1970. The development of the child's concept of death. In Sahler, O. J. Z., editor: The child and death, The C. V. Mosby Co., St. Louis.

Johns Hopkins School of Public Health and Richmond IVNA-City Health Department, Nursing Service: 1964. The family coping index, Cooperative Nursing Study, Richmond, Va.

Jones, P. S.: 1978. An adaptation model for nursing practice, Am. J. Nurs. **78**(11):1900-1906.

Kaluger, G., and Kaluger, M. F.: 1979. Human development: the span of life, 2nd ed., The C. V. Mosby Co., St. Louis.

Kastenbaum, R.: 1967. The child's understanding of death: how does it develop?" In Grollman, E. A., editor: Explaining death to children, Beacon Press, Boston.

Kohlberg, L.: 1964. Development of moral character and moral ideology. In Hoffman, M. L., and Hoffman, L. W., editors: Review of child development research, vol. 1, Russell Sage Foundation, New York.

Kohlberg, L.: 1968. The child as a moral philosopher, Psychol. Today **2**(4):24-30.

Leonard, B., Murray, R., Zentner, J., Smith, M., and Nolan, N.: 1979. Assessment and health promotion for the schoolchild. In Murray, R., and Zentner, J.: Nursing assessment and health promotion through the life span, 2nd ed., Prentice-Hall, Inc., Englewood Cliffs, N.J.

Levine, M. E.: 1966. Adaptation and assessment: a rationale for nursing intervention, Am. J. Nurs. **66**(11):2450-2453.

Levine, M. E.: 1971. Holistic nursing, Nurs. Clin. North Am. **6**(2):253-264.

Logan, B. B.: 1978. The nurse and the family: dominant themes and perspectives in the literature. In Knafl, K. A., and Grace, H. K.: Families across the life cycle, Little, Brown & Co., Boston.

Lough, M. A., Murray, R. B., and Zentner, J. P.: 1975. Delivery of health care. In Murray, R. B., and Zentner, J. P., editors: Nursing concepts for health promotion, Prentice-Hall, Inc., Englewood Cliffs, N.J.

Lucas, B.: 1981. Nutrition and the adolescent. In Pipes, P. L.: Nutrition in infancy and childhood, The C. V. Mosby Co., St. Louis.

Maier, H. W.: 1969. Three theories of child development, rev. ed., Harper & Row, Publishers, Inc. New York.

Martin, H. W., and Prange, A. J.: 1962. Human adaptation: a conceptual approach to understanding patients, Can. Nurse **58**(3):234-243.

McClinton, B. S., and Meier, B. G.: 1978. Beginnings: psychology of early childhood, The C. V. Mosby Co., St. Louis.

Meister, S. B.: 1977. Charting a family's developmental status—for intervention and for the record, MCN **2**(1):43-48.

Murray, R. B., Haugk, J., Jenkins, R., Smith, M., Westhus, N., and Zentner, J. P.: 1979a. Assessment and health promotion for the infant. In Murray, R. B., and Zentner, J. P.: Nursing assessment and health promotion through the life span, 2nd ed., Prentice-Hall, Inc., Englewood Cliffs, N.J.

Murray, R. B., and Zentner, J. P.: 1979. Nursing assessment and health promotion through the life span, 2nd ed., Prentice-Hall, Inc., Englewood Cliffs, N.J.

Murray, R. B., Zentner, J. P., Brockhaus, J. P. D., Brockhaus, R. H., and Palermo, E.: 1979b. The family—basic unit for the developing person. In Murray, R. B., and Zentner, J. P.: Nursing concepts for health promotion, 2nd ed., Prentice-Hall, Inc., Englewood Cliffs, N.J.

Murray, R. B., Zentner, J. P., and Smith, M. D.: 1979c. Assessment and health promotion for the preschooler. In Murray, R. B., and Zentner, J. P.: Nursing assessment and health promotion through the life span, 2nd ed., Prentice-Hall, Inc., Englewood Cliffs, N.J.

Nagy, M. H.: 1948. The child's view of death, J. Gen. Psychol. **73**(1):3-27.

Nolan, N., Murray, R., Grohar, M., Leonard, B., Smith, M., and Zentner, J.: 1979. Assessment and health promotion for the adolescent/youth. In Murray, R. B., and Zentner, J. P.: Nursing assessment and health promotion through the life span, 2nd ed., Prentice-Hall, Inc., Englewood Cliffs, N.J.

O'Neil, S. M., McLaughlin, B. N., and Knapp, M. B.: 1977. Behavioral approaches to children with developmental delays, The C. V. Mosby Co., St. Louis.

Otto, H. A.: 1973. A framework for assessing family strengths. In Reinhardt, A. M., and Quinn, M. D., editors: Family-centered community nursing: a sociocultural framework, vol. 1, The C. V. Mosby Co., St. Louis.

Pearson, G. A.: 1977. Nutrition in the middle years of childhood, MCN **2**(6):378-384.

Piaget, J.: 1952. The origins of intelligence in children, International Universities Press, Inc., New York.

Pipes, P. L.: 1981. Nutrition in infancy and childhood, 2nd ed., The C. V. Mosby Co., St. Louis.

Pipes, P. L., and Rees, J.: 1981. Between infancy and adolescence. In Pipes, P. L.: Nutrition in infancy and childhood, 2nd ed., The C. V. Mosby Co., St. Louis.

Powell, M.: 1963. The psychology of adolescence, The Bobbs-Merrill Co., Inc., Indianapolis.

Robischon, P., and Smith, J. A.: 1977. Family assessment. In Reinhardt, A. M., and Quinn, M. D.: Current practice in family-centered community nursing, vol. 1, The C. V. Mosby Co., St. Louis.

Roy, C.: 1980. The Roy adaptation model. In Riehl, J. P., and Roy, C.: Conceptual models for nursing practice, Appleton-Century-Crofts, New York.

Rubin, B. M.: 1980. The great fast-food debate: the burger court in session, Minneapolis Tribune 113(210):15A, Jan., 23, 1980.

Ryden, M. B.: 1977. A crucial consideration in the nursing process, Nurs. Forum 16(1):71-82.

Sahler, O. J. Z.: 1978. The child and death, The C. V. Mosby Co., St. Louis.

Satir, V.: 1967. Conjoint family therapy, rev. ed., Science and Behavior Books, Palo Alto, Calif.

Selye, H.: 1976. The stress of life, rev. ed., McGraw-Hill, Inc., New York.

Shuler, S. N.: 1978. Death during childhood: reactions in parents and children. In Brandt, P. A., Chinn, P. L., Hunt, V. O., and Smith, M. E.: Current practice in pediatric nursing, vol. 2, The C. V. Mosby Co., St. Louis.

Siemon, M. K.: 1978. Mental health in school-aged children. MCN 3(4):211-217.

Smart, M. S., and Smart, R. C.: 1972. Children: development and relationships, 2nd ed., Macmillan, Inc., New York.

Sutterley, D. C., and Donnelly, G. F.: 1973. Perspectives in human development, J. B. Lippincott Co., Philadelphia.

Tapia, J. A.: 1972. The nursing process in family health, Nurs. Outlook 20(4):267-270.

University of Minnesota: 1979. Unpublished course syllabus for N 5-203 "Adaptation I," University of Minnesota School of Nursing, Minneapolis.

Wallinga, J. V.: 1973. The physician and his adolescent, Minn. Med. 56(2):91-93.

Whitley, M. P, and Madden, L.: 1978. Encountering dysfunction in the family system. In Longo, D. C., and Williams, R. A., editors: Clinical practice in psychosocial nursing: assessment and intervention, Appleton-Century-Crofts, New York.

Williams, S. R.: 1977. Nutrition and diet therapy, 3rd ed., The C. V. Mosby Co., St. Louis.

Williams, C. C., and Holmes, T. H.: 1978. Life change, human adaptation, and onset of illness. In Longo, D. C., and Williams, R. A., editors: Clinical practice in psychosocial nursing: assessment and intervention, Appleton-Century-Crofts, New York.

SUGGESTED READINGS

Aldous, J.: 1971. The developmental approach to family analysis. Vol. 2, Selected readings by family life cycle category, University of Minnesota, Minneapolis.

Alfin-Slater, R. B.: 1974. Fats, essential fatty acids, and ascorbic acid, J. Am. Diet. Assoc. 64(2):168-170.

Bieri, J. G.: 1974. Fat-soluble vitamins in the eighth revision of the recommended dietary allowances, J. Am. Diet. Assoc. 64(2):171-174.

Brandt, P. A., Chinn, P. L., Hunt, V. O., and Smith, M. E.: 1978. Current practice in pediatric nursing, vol. 2, The C. V. Mosby Co., St. Louis.

Bruhn, J. G., and Cordova, F. D.: 1977. A developmental approach to learning wellness behavior. Part I: Infancy to early adolescence, Health Values: Achieving High-Level Wellness 1(6):246-254.

Calloway, D. H.: 1974. Recommended dietary allowances for protein and energy, 1973, J. Am. Diet. Assoc. 64(2):157-162.

Casey, R. L., Masuda, M., and Holmes, T. H.: 1967. Quantitative study of recall of life events, J. Psychosom. Res. 11(2):239-247.

Combs, A. W., and Snygg, D.: 1959. Individual behavior: a perceptual approach to behavior, rev. ed., Harper & Row, Publishers, Inc., New York.

Daniel, W. A.: 1977. Adolescents in health and disease, The C. V. Mosby Co., St. Louis.

Eggert, L. L.: 1978. Family subsystem: the therapeutic process with adolescents experiencing psychosocial stress. In Longo, D. C., and Williams, R. A., editors: Clinical practice in psychosocial nursing: assessment and intervention, Appleton-Century-Crofts, New York.

Erickson, C. J., and Friedman, S. B.: 1978. Understanding and evaluating adolescent behavior problems, J. School Health 48(5):293-297.

Erickson, M. L.: 1976. Assessment and management of developmental changes in children, The C. V. Mosby Co., St. Louis.

Galligan, A. C.: 1979. Using Roy's concept of adaptation to care for young children, MCN 4(1):24-28.

Graves, H. H., and Thompson, E. A.: 1978. Anxiety: a mental health vital sign. In Longo, D. C., and Williams, R. A., editors: Clinical practice in psychosocial nursing: assessment and intervention, Appleton-Century-Crofts, New York.

Gyulay, J-E.: 1978. The dying child, McGraw-Hill, Inc., New York.

Harper, A. E.: 1974. Recommended dietary allowances: are they what we think they are? J. Am. Diet. Assoc. 64(2): 151-156.

Harsh, C. M., and Schrickel, H. G.: 1959. Personality development and assessment, 2nd ed., The Ronald Press Co., New York.

Hoeffer, B. M.: 1978. Single mothers and their children: challenging traditional concepts of the American family. In Brandt, P. A., Chinn, P. L., Hunt, V. O., and Smith, M. E., editors: Current practice in pediatric nursing, vol. 2, The C. V. Mosby Co., St. Louis.

Hott, J. R.: 1977. Mobilizing family strengths in health maintenance and coping with illness. In Reinhardt, A. M., and Quinn, M. D., editors: Current practice in family-centered community nursing, vol. 1, The C. V. Mosby Co., St. Louis.

Kaluger, G., and Kaluger, M. F.: 1979. Profiles in human development, 2nd ed., The C. V. Mosby Co., St. Louis.

Knafl, K. A., and Grace, H. K.: 1978. Families across the life cycle, Little, Brown & Co., Boston.

Labuza, T. P.: 1975. The nutrition crisis: a reader, West Publishing Co., St. Paul.

Larson, M. L.: 1978. Violent behaviors. In Longo, D. C., and Williams, R. A., editors: Clinical practice in psychosocial nursing: assessment and intervention, Appleton-Century-Crofts, New York.

Lipkin, G. B.: 1978. Parent-child nursing: psychosocial aspects, 2nd ed., The C. V. Mosby Co., St. Louis.

Longo, D. C., and Williams, R. A., editors: 1978. Clinical practice in psychosocial nursing: assessment and intervention, Appleton-Century-Crofts, New York.

MacElveen, P. M.: 1978. Social networks. In Longo, D.

C., and Williams, R. A., editors: Clinical practice in psychosocial nursing: assessment and intervention, Appleton-Century-Crofts, New York.

Masuda, M., and Holmes, T. H.: 1967. Magnitude estimations of social readjustments, J. Psychosom. Res. **11**(2): 219-225.

Mertz, W.: 1974. Recommended dietary allowances up to date—trace minerals, J. Am. Diet. Assoc. **64**(2):163-167.

Mills, G. C.: 1979. Books to help children understand death, Am. J. Nurs. **79**(2):291-295.

Monea, H. E.: 1979. Psychosocial development of children: holistic care-giving approaches. In Burnside, I. M., Ebersole, P., and Monea, H. E., editors: Psychosocial caring throughout the life span, McGraw-Hill, Inc., New York.

Murray, R. B., and Zentner, J. P.: 1975. Nursing concepts for health promotion, Prentice-Hall, Inc., Englewood Cliffs, N.J.

Murray, R. B., and Zentner, J. P.: 1979. Nursing concepts for health promotion, 2nd ed., Prentice-Hall, Inc., Englewood Cliffs, N.J.

Palmer, B. B., and Lewis, C. E.: 1976. Development of health attitudes and behaviors, J. School Health **46**(7): 401-402.

Reinhardt, A. M., and Quinn, M. D.: 1977. Current practice in family-centered community nursing, vol. 1, The C. V. Mosby Co., St. Louis.

Satir, V.: 1972. Peoplemaking, Science and Behavior Books, Palo Alto, Calif.

Scipien, G. M., Barnard, M. U., Chard, M. A., Howe, J., and Phillips, P. J.: 1975. Comprehensive pediatric nursing, McGraw-Hill, Inc., New York.

Selye, H.: 1965. The stress syndrome, Am. J. Nurs. **65**(3): 97-99.

Siemon, M. K.: 1978. Family subsystem: working with school-age children experiencing psychosocial stress. In Longo, D. C., and Williams, R. A., editors: Clinical practice in psychosocial nursing: assessment and intervention, Appleton-Century-Crofts, New York.

Sobol, E. G., and Robischon, P.: 1975. Family nursing: a study guide, The C. V. Mosby Co., St. Louis.

Stendler, C. B.: 1964. Readings in child behavior and development, 2nd ed., Harcourt Brace Jovanovich, Inc., New York.

Swaiman, K. F.: 1978. Brain development in the middle childhood years, J. School Health **48**(5):288-292.

Taft, L. T.: 1978. Child development: prenatal to early childhood, J. School Health **48**(5):281-287.

Thompson, J.: 1977. Human growth and development: a basis for nursing assessment. In Steele, S., editor: Nursing care of the child with long-term illness, Appleton-Century-Crofts, New York.

Timnick, L.: 1978. Child suicides, The Minneapolis Star, July 26, 1978, p. 18A.

CHAPTER 8

Structural variables: factors affecting adaptation

JOANNE GINGRICH-CRASS

Chapter 7 described the adaptation framework and its application to school nursing. This chapter describes the use of more specific factors, structural variables, to help the nurse apply adaptation theory. Structural variables are factors, such as race, religion, and age, which affect how individuals adapt to life events by influencing personality, self-image, and lifestyle. This chapter will describe the following:

1. Definition and application of structural variables
2. Influence of structural variables on health and illness behaviors
3. Guidelines for the school nurse to identify the effect of structural variables on her students and to intervene appropriately

STRUCTURAL VARIABLES: DEFINITIONS AND INTERACTIONS
Defining structural variables

Byrne and Thompson define structural variables as "those factors common to all men that will direct attention to the particular generalizations likely to be applicable to a specific individual" (Byrne and Thompson, 1978:40). In other words, structural variables are factors, such as age, race, religion, culture, education, occupation, family, and health, which significantly influence behavior; therefore knowledge of them assists the observer to assess and predict responses. "Structural" connotes factors that shape all people's reactions and interactions; they are called *variables* because they affect individuals in different ways and to different degrees (Byrne and Thompson, 1978). An example concerns the child's occupation: school. School affects children differently; thus one child may be intellectually stimulated, another bored, and a third fearful. Even children who react to school in the same way, for example, with symptoms of school phobia, may do so with varying degrees of intensity; one child may cling to his mother and refuse to attend school at all, while another child may simply withdraw to a corner and not participate.

Knowledge of structural variables and how they affect behavior can improve the nurse's ability to assess her impact on a child's lifestyle and health and can improve the appropriateness and effectiveness of her interventions as well. The purpose of this chapter, then, is to discuss some of the structural variables affecting children and the application of that knowledge to school nursing.

Interaction among structural variables and impact on the client

Before discussing specific structural variables, it is necessary to describe the theoretical interaction among structural variables and their impact on individuals. Because individuals are influenced by many structural variables, the ultimate adaptive response is partially the result of the specific combination of variables and the intensity of each variable. For example, a child focuses on a stimulus such as entering a new school; how he chooses to respond to that stimulus will depend on the combination of structural variables he possesses. If he is 8 years old (structural variable: age), the effect of family structure may influence him more than if he were 16, since adolescents are more influenced by peers than family. In other words, structural variables form a matrix, interacting with one another and interpreting the meaning of the stimulus for the individual (Fig. 8-1). Each individual also has a self-concept, which may alter his perception and thus precipitate a unique response to that stimulus. The nurse therefore needs knowledge in two areas: (1) structural variables and (2) the client's self-concept and previous coping patterns.

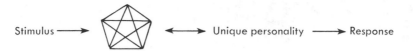

Stimulus ⟶ ⟷ Unique personality ⟶ Response

Fig. 8-1. Interaction among structural variables. Each point in the star signifies a structural variable. Personality includes self-concept and previous experience.

Relationship of structural variables to adaptation theory

Structural variables make up several of the parts that fit together to build the adaptation framework. (Other parts of the framework such as energy, perception, and integration are discussed in Chapter 7). By analyzing structural variables, the nurse is able to better understand the meaning of a response for an individual and predict likely future responses. Both of these abilities are important for nurses. Understanding the meaning of and being able to predict responses allows the nurse to (1) assist the client to choose more appropriate responses, (2) prevent unhealthy responses, (3) provide holistic care, (4) motivate clients, (5) teach appropriately, and (6) practice a high level of nursing.

The following example illustrates the assessment of structural variables and client's self-concept in predicting client responses.

15-year-old Clara is offered a cigarette. How she responds will be determined by the following:
1. Structural variables
   a. Age: since at 15, peer approval and independence are very important
   b. Sex: 25 years ago women did not smoke as much as men, whereas women today smoke almost as much as men
   c. Religion: Clara's Baptist church preaches against smoking
   d. Culture: smoking has not been a tradition in her family and is, in fact, frowned on
   e. Family composition and stability: Clara's family includes her parents and younger brother; she has just moved here from another state; she is anxious to become part of a new group
   All these factors will interact, perhaps leading Clara toward the decision to accept the cigarette.
2. Self-Concept
   Clara's self-concept is that she is a non-smoker. She teaches Sunday school and considers herself a role model for the younger children, so it is possible that she will refuse the cigarette.

Suppose Clara smokes the cigarette, a response the nurse may initially classify as inappropriate. Unless the nurse is aware of all the variables influencing Clara's decision, her interventions may be vague and unrelated to Clara's unique situation. If the nurse is unaware of these kinds of structural variables affecting a child, not only will her interventions tend to be ineffective and irrelevant, but she may also be completely bewildered by the child's behavior and reactions.

Although Byrne and Thompson (1978) identify seven structural variables (age, sex, religion, ethnic or cultural group, education and occupation, relational, or social, roles, and health), to limit the scope of this chapter, only the following structural variables will be discussed: age, family structure, culture, religion, and income. For each structural variable discussed, the following information will be supplied: (1) how the variables might influence a child's adaptation, (2) some guidelines for assessing adequate adaptation, (3) suggestions for interventions, and (4) bibliographical sources for further information.

STRUCTURAL VARIABLES AFFECTING ADAPTATION OF CHILDREN
Effect of age on adaptation

As discussed in Chapter 7, age and developmental stage affect the way in which children cope with their environment. By knowing the age-appropriate behaviors and developmental tasks for an age group and the coping patterns of individual children, the school nurse can identify inadequate coping. Methods of coping or adaptive responses appropriate for one age group may be inappropriate for another age group. For example, temper tantrums are appropriate for toddlers but not for school-age children. A child is not adapting adequately when the level of his coping responses is not within the limits expected for his age and developmental stage.

Inadequate coping may be due to stress. Specific stressors for school-age children include (1) loss of and separation from a parent, for example, through death or divorce; (2) being "different" from other children, for example, being handicapped; (3) unmet needs, such as not receiving affection; and (4) loss of self-esteem, which may occur when a student fails a grade (Siemon, 1978). A child who is not coping successfully with one problem may, however, proceed at a normal developmental level in other areas. The school-age child is in the stage Erikson (1963) calls "industry versus inferiority." If, in one of the previous three developmental stages (trust versus mistrust, autonomy versus shame and doubt, initiative versus guilt), a stress is encountered that remains unresolved, the effect may still be evident to the careful observer. For example, a child who was immobile due to need for a body cast during the developmental stage of initiative versus guilt may later be fearful when asked to try new behaviors because he was not able to successfully complete the tasks of that developmental stage.

Table 8-1 describes effects of unsatisfactory outcomes for each developmental stage and common events that may have interrupted successful completion of that stage. Although not every child will respond in the same way, the table is presented as an assessment guide.

The role of the school nurse includes promoting emotional health and modifying unsatisfactory coping mechanisms. Intervention to improve unsuccessful completion of an earlier develomental stage by a school-age child may be done either by a qualified school nurse, another professional, or through their joint efforts. A major part of such intervention is the helping relationship (Chapters 10 and 11). Other more specific approaches are shown here with necessary changes to adapt the information to the school setting (Tables 8-2 to 8-4).

Table 8-1. Assessing inadequate coping in school-age children*

Developmental stage	Behaviors showing unsuccessful completion of stage	Events stressful for stage
Trust versus mistrust (infancy to 1 year)	Craves dependence: clinging, whining or fearful of new situations Refuses all forms of dependence: aloof, refuses cuddling, refuses to admit to illness	Frequent prolonged separation from parents Emotional and/or physical abuse and neglect Variety of caretakers, that is, foster homes, lengthy hospitalizations
Autonomy versus shame and doubt (1 to 3 years, toddler)	Has no sense of cooperative relationships, that is, giving up, being compliant Acts in ways that give child sense of power, that is, aggressiveness	Rigid rules of right and wrong Punishment for assertiveness Discouragement when tries something new
Initiative versus guilt (3 to 6 years, preschool)	Afraid to try new things Will not perform tasks when asked Frequently asks for help from adults Waits to begin until told	Overly solicitous parents Lack of environmental stimulation Immobility, such as bedrest
Industry versus inferiority (6 to 13 years, school age)	Shuns social interaction Inhibited, apologetic Noncompetitive or must always win; unable to compromise	Emphasis on perfection Frequent comparison with siblings Lack of appreciation expressed for child's individuality and uniqueness

*Modified from Siemon, M.: 1978. Family subsystem: working with school-age children experiencing psychosocial stress. In Longo, D. C., and Williams, R. A., editors: Clinical practice in psychosocial nursing: assessment and intervention, Appleton-Century-Crofts, New York, pp. 289-318.

Table 8-2. Examples of specific approaches for unmet trust needs*

Structure	Toys	Activities
Retain sameness with respect to time and place for meeting	Allow child to bring familiar objects from home for transition in adjusting to new situation: blanket, toy, comics, clothing, pictures	Send a card during vacation to help maintain relationship during physical absence
Be consistent in limit setting, so that child knows what to expect and can feel secure		Play games of predictability: hide and seek, catch, peekaboo. (This can be done with child 6 to 8 years old by ducking into doorway and surprising child while walking down hallway)
Display appropriate affect with expression of feelings, so that messages are clear and consistent	Make it clear child is accepted: "Whatever toy you choose is OK"	
Follow through on promises made		
Physical comfort is important; consider things that will enhance comfort of child, such as sitting on chair, on floor, or on pillows; going to park; having snack		
Offer help if it is needed: "Would you like me to hold that for you?"		
The closer a relationship becomes, the more child will check out caring by testing limits or refusing to talk, to see if you will stay close anyway		

*Modified from Siemon, M.: 1978. Family subsystem: school-age children. In Longo, D. C., and Williams, R. A., editors: Clinical practice in psychosocial nursing: assessment and intervention, Appleton-Century-Crofts, New York, p. 311.

Table 8-3. Examples of specific approaches for unmet autonomy needs*

Structure	Toys	Activities
Allow child to have choice of time and day to meet (between alternatives acceptable to nurse)	Have many toys available from which child can choose	Give alternative list of activities from which child can choose
Do not make decisions a power struggle ("I'm bigger than you"); when deciding which exercises to do first or what game to play, flip coin or draw straws	Use toys that allow for control: guns (6 to 9), marbles (6 to 12), billiards (9 to 12), puppets (6 to 9), darts (9 to 12), pounding pegboard (6), beanbags (6 to 9), "Bozo" punch clown (6 to 8)	Use activities that allow child to push things around: games in which objects, not people, get pushed around: checkers, chess (9 to 12), knocking down block tower (6 to 7), pushing dolls around (6 to 9)
Give verbal reinforcement and praise for something done by child		Use games that involve being in control or gaining territory: Monopoly (9 to 12), captain, may I? (6 to 9), king of the mountain (6 to 9), tug-of-war (6 to 9)
Respect decisions child makes		
Give verbal reinforcement and praise for something done by child		Encourage child to claim territory and assert rights by making signs for his room or desk, "Do not disturb," "Joe's room"
Let children finish projects on their own, no matter how long it takes		Allow for modeling by child without getting into power struggle; when meeting is over, say, "I'm going now"; child is free to go on his own
Allow many choices: not if something will be done, but when ("Now or 5 minutes from now?"), or how ("This dressing first, or that one?"), or what ("Your blue jacket or your red jacket?")		Side-by-side activities allow child to follow without adult demanding that child do something; this is good for teaching; let child know, "I'm going to add this much water to my paint mix"; child will follow
Allow child to do as much for himself as possible; this requires patience and freedom to move at child's pace, not adherence to rigid schedule		Tell child that keeping secret diary is way of having some territory that no one else knows about

*Modified from Siemon, M.: 1978. Family subsystem: school-age children. In Longo, D. C., and Williams, R. A., editors: Clinical practice in psychosocial nursing: assessment and intervention, Appleton-Century-Crofts, New York, p. 312.

Table 8-4. Examples of specific approaches for unmet initiative needs*

Structure	Toys	Activities
Give child permission to explore, "It can be whatever you want it to be"	Use toys that can be taken apart and put together in new way: paper dolls (6 to 9), Tinkertoys (6 to 8), Lincoln Logs (6 to 9), Erector set (9 to 11), blocks (6 to 8), clay (6 to 9), Mr. Potato Head (6 to 8)	Encourage activities that evoke curiosity and risk: treasure hunt (6 to 8), find the hidden toy (6 to 8), dramatics (6 to 12), guessing games (twenty questions) (9 to 12), charades (9 to 12)
Offer encouragement to try things in new way: "Let's try to do things in a different way today!"		
Structure new experiences in stages, so that they are less threatening		
Express interest in task, without intruding on it and defining it, "Looks like you're having fun with that!" not, "That looks like a new belt for your Grandpa!"	Use toys that can change shape and form and be manipulated: paints (6 to 9); scissors, paper, and paste (6 to 12); soap bubbles (6); models, (9 to 12)	Recognize that speech is tool for exploration, not commitment to action; encourage fantasy exploration; act out different endings for stories; encourage talking through: "What if I do this? What will happen?"; focus on emotion, not absolute content
It is not fair to ask child what he is producing; he does not know what he will end up with; imposing such boundaries discourages experimentation		
If there is struggle about trying things out, find ways in which trying is safe at first: have puppets or dolls act out, fantasize with story character		Encourage exploring environment and making collections of rocks or leaves or making scrapbook
When child asks for answer to question, indicate where to look up information, but let child find answer		

*Modified from Siemon, M.: 1978. Family subsystem: school-age children. In Longo, D. C., and Williams, R. A.: editors: Clinical practice in psychosocial nursing: assessment and intervention, Appleton-Century-Crofts, New York, p. 313.

Effect of family structure on adaptation

In addition to age, family structure is another important structural variable affecting the adaptation of children. Family structure refers to the persons who make up a family and the roles they perform; size of the family is another aspect of family structure. The family has a significant influence on children because it teaches them how to cope with emotions, stresses, life, health and illness, loss, and other people, in addition to helping them develop a general outlook on life. Some of these learned coping responses are inadequate, others are adequate, but all are unique to that child. A greater knowledge of the effect of family structure on children will assist the school nurse in her efforts to optimize children's adaptive potential.

Before discussing the effect of specific family structures on children, a few selected statistics validate the assumption that an increasing number of children live in "nontraditional" families. According to Sussman (1978:35), (1) in 16% of households both parents work; (2)

37% of families are headed by a single parent; and (3) many children live in foster or adoptive homes or are a part of a combined family. As noted in Chapter 7, the nursing definition of family is slowly evolving to include types other than the traditional, two-parent, "married" family. These family structural changes have been incorporated into children's books and other literature (Merriam, 1961; Miles, 1971; Zolotow, 1971). There is a serious lack of research in the nursing literature, however, concerning the effect of various family structures on the adaptation of children. This is an area which school nurses are well qualified to study and on which they could have significant impact.

Effects of parental employment on children

One study by Miller (1975) on the effect of parental careers on children demonstrates that the effect does not depend on the number of *hours* parents spend working and away from their children, but rather on the parents'*feelings* about working; thus if parents feel negatively about their jobs or guilty about leaving the children, the children will have more difficulty adapting to their parents' absence (i.e., may do poorly in their schoolwork) than if the parents are fulfilling a career goal or feel positively about their work. Another study (Kanter, 1978) revealed that if parental employment obligations interfere with leisure time, the entire family is more likely to show irritability and stress. Examples include lower income families in which one parent assumes two jobs to pay the bills, as well as families headed by professional workers whose jobs demand well over 40 hours per week.

Children's coping is affected not only by attitude and numbers of hours worked, but also by the specific hours that are worked. Shift workers are confronted with unique adaptation problems that go beyond their expected frequent schedule changes (Mott, 1965). Among night-shift workers, for example, greater frequency of marital discord has been documented, while evening-shift workers have a higher frequency of parenting difficulties compared with daytime workers. In addition to the effects of parents' working hours, Kohn (1959) reports that the type of parental employment correlates with parental expectations of children. Kohn documents that white-collar parents value creativity, self-direction, and initiative in their children, while blue-collar workers value conformity and obedience. In addition, according to Kanter (1978), workers with low-autonomy jobs are more likely to be severe and hostile parents. Obviously, much more research is needed in this area. Likewise, as more and more children begin living in families in which both parents work or the only parent works, more information about the effect of parents' employment will be needed to help explain how children adapt to their own work, namely, school.

Alternative family life-styles

During the 1960s, alternative life-styles such as communal living, cohabitation of heterosexual couples, and open acknowledgement of homosexual couples became more widespread. Although group living such as the Israeli kibbutz has been common in other parts of the world for many years, the long-term effects of group living on children in our society have not yet been determined. In 1974, Eiduson began a study evaluating the effects of six different lifestyles on the growth and development of chil-

dren; after 4 years of testing, no significant differences could be found.

Experimental families. Sussman (1978) labels the communal and cohabitation lifestyles as "experimental" families, which make up 4% of American households. He identifies the advantage of communal living as being a larger support system for its members. This support system is especially important for families in transition, such as a mother and child recently separated from their husband/father or families recently moved to a new location. On the other hand, one disadvantage of communal living is the difficulty in organizing and defining roles. It is hypothesized that many caretakers and disorganization of roles within the communal family may result in role confusion for the maturing child. Research to support or reject the hypothesis is rare; many more studies are needed. The effect of experimental families on adaptation of children is therefore undetermined.

Blended families. "Blended families" is a new term and has been used by Satir (1972) and Levine (1974) to refer to any combination of parents and children that occurs with the marriage of people at least one of whom has had children before; 11% of all households are blended families (Sussman, 1978). This type of family requires special adaptive energy of the children, who are presented with the change by their parents without benefit of the love that motivates their parents. Children need the consistency of unchanged rituals and customs to help conserve their energy. They must spend energy on developing new relationships and coping with new and differing expectations and fears about losing the love and attention of a parent (Satir, 1972). This is not to say that blended families are too stressful for children, but rather that they present unique adaptation needs.

Foster families. Even the term "foster child" is a stigma to which the child must adapt. Foster children may change families often and must adapt and readapt to many settings. Both they and their foster parents may be hesitant about forming relationships because of their uncertain future. Jacobson and Cockerum (1976) describe some of the problems that former foster children reported experiencing. The first issue foster children identified was lack of information. They recalled experiences such as being taken away from their parents' home with no explanation or being moved from one foster home to another, sometimes in the middle of the night, without explanation. Other foster care problems described by Jacobson and Cockerum (1976) were (1) "double standards" for foster and biological children in the same home, that is, the favoring by foster parents of their own children; (2) misuse of funds provided for the foster children, usually for food or clothes for the biological children or parents; and (3) sexual advances toward foster children made by siblings or foster parents. Certainly this family structure requires skilled adaptation by the children. Although not all foster homes are unhealthy, even in the best of situations special adaptive demands are placed on the child who "doesn't belong."

Adoptive families. The family with an adopted child is yet another structure that will affect the child's adaptation. Most sources (such as Barnard, 1977; Murray and Zentner, 1975a) recommend telling children at an early age that they are adopted. The facts of their adoption should be explained to them in a way they can understand. The school-age child may be dealing with feelings of rejection by his biological parents. The adoption issue can also affect adaptation during adolescence. The adolescent identity crisis may spur the youth's interest in seeking information about his background and biological parents. As they develop plans for independence, many adolescents think about running away. Understandably, adoptive parents may become quite upset if a child threatens to run away to find his biological parents. Coping with these and other issues requires adaptive energy for the adopted child. The adoptive family structure is unique, and how each child copes with it will affect his future adaptive responses.

Single-parent families. Single-parent families make up 37% of all families (Sussman, 1978). They may result from death of a parent or divorce (Chapter 9) or may occur because a person chooses to parent alone. Examples include a single woman or man who adopts a child and a woman who either intentionally or unintentionally becomes pregnant and chooses to continue the pregnancy and raise the child herself. Because dual parenting is still considered the norm, single parents often face isolation and lack of support. Many times, significant others, such as family and friends, advise against the single parenting choice. Support groups are available, but much more help is often needed. Therefore the appropriate first effort in helping children adapt may be to support the parents.

One of the characteristics of single-parent families is that 85% of them are headed by women (Horowitz and Perdue, 1977). Since women's salaries are generally significantly lower than men's (Jenkins, 1978), many single-parent families experience financial difficulties. Therefore children must adapt to both the lack of financial and emotional resources of their parents.

Because the number of single-parent families is increasing, school nurses should develop an awareness and understanding of the special adaptive needs of children from these families and be prepared to help them adapt. Jack and Grinstead (1978) advise helpers to approach the single-parent family nonjudgmentally. They point out that helpers often assume that the single-parent family is a temporary state and therefore focus on changing the single parent's status. Instead of trying to alter the family structure or concentrating on the "missing" parent, school nurses and other helpers should identify and promote the strengths of the family.

Birth order, family size, and intergenerational families

Other aspects of family structure affecting adaptation are birth order, family size, and intergenerational families and are described here briefly. Birth order is important to development (Lidz, 1968; Messer, 1970). The oldest child receives more attention from parents while he is the only child, resulting in emphasis on intellectual achievements and a greater sense of responsibility. Younger children have the advantage of their parents' experience with parenting and can learn from their older siblings. The only child may suffer from lack of peer involvement and too many responsibilities at home. He also has the advantage of full adult attention in the development of creative and intellectual skills.

Family size can affect methods of childrearing. In a very large family, for instance, each child receives less individualized parental attention, and emphasis is placed more on individual conformity for the welfare of the family as a whole. In contrast, children from small families may have more individual freedom and attention than children from large families.

Mobility is a third factor that affects family structure. Increased mobility of families results in many people living long distances from their relatives; therefore more emphasis is placed on self-reliance within the nuclear family. Only 6% of families have a resident member of a third generation (Sussman, 1978). The support of kinship ties assists families to adapt to rapid change, and lack of kinship ties is therefore related to inadequate coping responses such as alcoholism and divorce (Messer, 1970).

The school nurse should be aware of these and any other variables within family structure because of their impact on the health of children.

Application of family structure as a structural variable to school nursing

As noted earlier, the school nurse should not attempt to change family structure, but instead should help children and families work within their structure. She can promote optimal coping with life events by individualizing her general knowledge of a particular family structure to a specific family. One method is to provide anticipatory guidance by informing the families and children of problems that have been experienced in other families and discussing various alternative methods of adapting. She can also use this knowledge for primary prevention by identifying which children are likely to have difficulties and taking preventive action, such as leading a group in which troubled adopted school-age children can express their feelings. Secondary prevention of adaptation problems related to family structure can be done in much the same way. An example is helping children in blended families to form new patterns of behavior to adjust to their new family and thereby decrease wasteful energy use. Another area in which school nurses can contribute is research. Much research is needed about the effects of various family structures on children.

Effect of religion, culture, and income on adaptation

Religion, culture, income, and age as structural variables affecting adaptation are summarized in Table 8-5. The intent of the table is to help the reader become acquainted with the effects of some beliefs regarding health on the adaptation of persons in various cultural, religious, and income groups. The beliefs selected reflect areas pertaining to health and are not intended to be comprehensive; however, they do present guidelines from which the study of an unfamiliar group can be approached and provide basic information about the effect of

that group's belief system on health practices. However, before the table is presented and examined, definitions for some key terms should be provided.

Culture. The first term is *culture,* which Murray and Zentner (1975b:273) define as "a complex integrated system that includes knowledge, beliefs, skills, art, morals, laws, customs, and any other acquired habits and capabilities of man. All provide a pattern for living together." *Subculture* is defined as a group of persons within a culture with something in common, such as ethnic origin, occupation, or physical characteristics. A culture provides a frame of reference for individuals; it is a structure within whose rules and customs the individual chooses an adaptive pattern. Cultures are stable, with customs that are learned and passed from generation to generation. Culture can determine not only the health of a population, but also how people react to illness. A well-documented example is the reaction of people in various cultures to pain; in one study (Zborowski, 1952) Jewish and Italian people responded verbally to pain; "American Yankees" were fairly stoic; and Irish people tended to ignore the pain.

Religion. Religious groups are a kind of subculture that can have a profound effect on health. The Random House dictionary defines religion as "a specific and institutionalized set of beliefs and practices generally agreed upon by a number of persons or sects." Many religions have rules directly affecting health that are vigorously followed by the believers. Some examples of these are the dietary laws followed by Jewish persons, birth control and abortion laws in the Roman Catholic religion, laws against accepting blood transfusions for Jehovah's Witnesses, and Christian Scientists' laws against any medical care other than faith healing.

Income level. Income level is another variable affecting adaptation. Statistics show that persons of lower income become ill and suffer from chronic diseases limiting function at a rate four times the national average (Fromer, 1979). *Low income* is defined as those people living at or below poverty level, a subculture characterized by a value system based largely in the present and with a fatalistic attitude toward health (Murray and Zentner, 1975b; Spector, 1979). Lack of future orientation makes illness prevention for low-income persons a rare practice, and their lack of money creates problems

Table 8-5. Comparison of health-related factors and subcultures

	Definition of health	Cause of illness—is prevention possible, if so, how?	Name of healer, healing practices
Navajo Indian	Harmony between individual, earth, and supernatural, as well as the ability to survive difficult circumstances[1,2]	Disease is disharmony and can be caused by violating taboo or attack by witch; illness prevented through elaborate religious rituals; do not believe in germ theory[1,2]	Medicine man, who is more than average human being, is therefore influential figure; medicine man diagnoses and treats problem; treatments include yucca root, massage, herbs, and chanting; his chant states person will get well, and person believes him[1,2]
Hispanic-American	Gift from God, also good luck; can tell healthy person by robust appearance and report of feeling well[1,3,4]	Illness is punishment from God for wrongdoing, to be suffered; it can be prevented by eating well, praying, being good, and working; wearing medals may help; physically, illness is an imbalance between "hot" and "cold" properties of body[1,3,4]	Healer called curandero; cures hot illness with cold medicine and reverse; classification of hot and cold diseases varies; penicillin is hot medicine; massages and cleanings are common[4]
Traditional black	Harmony with nature, no separation of mind and body[4]	Disease is disharmony caused by spirits and demons; it can be prevented through good diet, rest, cleanliness, and laxatives to clean out system; some use of copper and silver bracelets for prevention[4]	Some belief in voodoo still prevalent; religious healing practiced; geophagia (eating of clay) and pica (eating of starch) practiced[4,6]
Chinese-American	Balance of yin and yang (negative and positive energy forces); healthy body is gift from parents and ancestors[4,7,11]	Illness caused by imbalance of yin and yang, which may be due to overexertion or prolonged sitting; disease is prevented through better adaptation to nature[4,7]	Acupuncture and moxibustion (which is a therapeutic application of heat to skin) restore balance of yin and yang; herbal remedies such as ginseng used for many illnesses; healer is called physician[4,7]

[1]Data from Brownlee, A. T.: 1978. Community, culture, and care: a cross-cultural guide for health workers, The C. V.
[2]Data from Wood, R.: 1976. The American Indian and health. In Ethnicity and health care, NLN publ. no. 14-1625, pp. 29-
[3]Data from Gonzales, H.: 1976. Health care needs of the Mexican American family. In Ethnicity and health care, NLN publ.
[4]Data from Spector, R.: 1979. Cultural diversity in health and illness, Appleton-Century-Crofts, New York.
[5]Data from Murray, R., and Zentner, J.: 1975. Nursing assessment and health promotion through the life span, Englewood
[6]Data from Martin, B.: 1976. Ethnicity and health care: Afro-Americans. In Ethnicity and health care, NLN publ. no.
[7]Data from Wang, R.: 1976. Chinese Americans and health care. In Ethnicity and health care, NLN publ. no. 14-1625,
[8]Data from Eggert, L.: 1978. Family subsystem: the therapeutic process with adolescents experiencing psychosocial stress.
    Appleton-Century-Crofts, New York.
[9]Data from Kertzer, M.: 1955. What is a Jew? In Rosten, L., editor: A guide to religions of America, Simon & Schuster,
[10]Data from Rotkovitch, R.: 1976. Ethnicity and health care—the Jewish heritage. In Ethnicity and health care, NLN publ.
[11]Data from Channing, G.: 1955. What is a Christian Scientist? In Rosten, L., editor: A guide to religions of America, Simon
[12]Data from Fromer, M.: 1979. Community health care and the nursing process, The C. V. Mosby Co., St. Louis.

Problems of entry to health care system	Communication patterns	Sexuality and family life	Beliefs about death
Language; will first visit medicine man; general beliefs are not compatible with health care system and structure; problems also include money and past experiences of disrespect; fear of spirits of dead may influence decision to leave hospital early[1,2]	Time of silence after each speaker to show respect and reflection on what they said; little eye contact; time orientation not very strict; recording of conversation invasion of privacy[1,2]	Family, extended family, and tribal ties strong; cooperation emphasized; consider children as individuals as soon as they can talk, therefore can make own decisions[1,2]	Fear of spirits of dead; children and family should be with dying person[1]
Language; will first go to woman for advice, then if needed, to "señora," then to curandero, then to physician; many migrant workers are Hispanic, and frequent moves may make access to medical care difficult; belief that hospital is place to go to die causes underuse of system; modesty may result in woman bringing friend to physician with her[1,3,4]	Confidentiality and modesty important; too many questions are insulting; it is more acceptable to make tentative statement to which they can respond; time orientation not strict; politeness essential[1,3-5]	High degree of modesty, may prefer home births for this reason; men are breadwinners, women homemakers; women are healers, men make all decisions[1,3-5]	Afterlife of heaven and hell exists
May seek folk or religious healer first; money and type of service affect decision; emergency room frequent entry point; black women have high "noncompliance" rate[4,6]	Racism toward blacks still prevalent; common names for symptoms should be known by health worker; time orientation not strict[4]	Matriarchy prevalent; almost 30% of black families have woman head of household; therefore women make decisions[1,6]	Death is passage from evils of this world to another state; blacks have shorter life expectancy than national average[6]
Language; traditional Chinese physicians were paid to keep their patients well and cared for sick without fees because illness indicated they had failed in their job; Chinese physicians are available in community and may encourage	Open expression of emotions not acceptable; therefore might not complain about pain or symptoms; may smile when does not understand[1,7]	Women subservient to men; patriarchal family; ancestor worship and respect and obedience for parents observed; divorce considered disgrace[1,4,5]	Reincarnation[7]

Mosby Co., St. Louis.
35.
no. 14-1625, pp. 21-28.

Cliffs, N.J.
14-1625, pp. 47-55.
pp. 9-18.
In Longo, D. C., and Williams, R. A., editors: Clinical practice in psychosocial nursing: assessment and intervention,

New York.
no. 14-1625, pp. 37-46.
& Schuster, New York.

Continued.

Table 8-5. Comparison of health-related factors and subcultures—cont'd

	Definition of health	Cause of illness—is prevention possible, if so, how?	Name of healer, healing practices
Adolescents	Feeling well and looking good; body image important[5]	Future orientation unimportant; family and peers are strongest influence, and prevention is aligned with their beliefs; feelings of omnipotence lead to infrequent preventive practices[8]	Subject to advice from friends; may be superstitious; any illness affecting body image causes great concern[5]
Judaism	No formal definition of health[9]	Illness not caused by God who wants people to live happily; Jewish history contains much suffering; Jews do not believe God wants them to suffer; preventive practices include eating well, cleanliness, some fasting, and blessing of food[9,10]	Jews are required to visit the sick, placing emphasis on their emotional as well as physical needs; birth control is allowed, abortion prohibited unless necessary for health-threatening reasons; circumcision for infants is ritual[1,4,9]
Church of Christ, Scientist	Health is spiritual reality and is eternal[11]	Diseases are delusions of mind; they can be cured by prayer and spiritual understanding; do not believe in germ theory[11]	Practitioner prays for sick to be healed; practitioner is taught and tested before "being licensed," and can cure the sick from hundreds of miles away; beliefs include no one should be forced to obtain inoculations; nursing homes staffed by practitioners and traditional workers now being federally funded[5,11]
Low income	Functional definition; if you can work, you are healthy[5,12]	Belief that illness is not preventable; fatalism common; future orientation minimal because present problems are too great[1,5,12]	Will often rely on folk healers and remedies because of belief and problems gaining access to health care system[5]
High income	No data available	General belief in prevention of illness through diet, exercise, and good health habits; motivators such as previous experience or family tradition are influential in actual practice of prevention[5]	Combination of traditional practices of religion and culture, frequent use of health care system and self-help information[5]

Problems of entry to health care system	Communication pattern	Sexuality and family life	Beliefs about death
patients to use Western physician; family spokesman may accompany patient to Western physician[4,7]			
May fear that family physician will not maintain confidentiality; lack of funds and knowledge about health care system; may use specialty clinics; school nurse accessible resource	Open communication and contracting are useful; may be confrontive and mistrustful of adults as way of asserting independence; group milieu works well; use of slang common[5,8]	Sexual development; youth may be uncomfortable with bodily changes[5,8]	Cognitive understanding of death as final
Some religious affiliated hospitals; these are frequently preferred if available[5]	Emotions and physical complaints freely expressed[4]	Family ties are important; elaborate marriage ritual; divorce acceptable only as last resort[9]	Most do not believe in afterlife; dying person should not be left alone; honor and respect are due lifeless human being; concern is for the well-being of mourners; autopsies prohibited[4,9]
Refuse medical treatment; will ask for physician for childbirth because untrained in that area; if member has not achieved level of spiritual understanding necessary to be healed, he may use physician, especially in case of broken bone[11]	Prayer of high value[11]	No position on divorce or birth control, left to family[11]	Do not believe in death as finality; mind never dies; Bible service may or may not be held[11]
Use of public funding may limit access and type of care; present time orientation and beliefs about prevention may cause delay in obtaining care; inability to afford health insurance; may lose day's pay to go to physician[5,12]	May use slang and language of subculture; may view providers as authoritarian; time orientation not strict[5]	Many single-parent families with woman head of household[12]	Depends on culture and religion
Access not too difficult, usually through private physician; most have health insurance through employer[5]	Most like health care culture; cannot be expected to understand jargon	Women more likely to have career by choice than financial necessity	Depends on culture and religion

Continued.

Table 8-5. Comparison of health-related factors and subcultures—cont'd

	Definition of health	Cause of illness—is prevention possible, if so, how?	Name of healer, healing practices
Health care culture	Optimal level of functioning; more than absence of disease; physical, emotional, social, and mental health included[5]	Scientific approach to cause of illness; prevention involves periodic physical examinations, laboratory studies, inoculations, as well as avoiding smoking and overeating, etc.[4]	Healing done by physician, usually takes place in office or hospital; treatments based on scientific knowledge and are frequently embarrassing or uncomfortable; often emotional component of disease is ignored[4]

in getting adequate care. In addition, low income is often accompanied by low educational level, the combination of which often results in dependence on ''quacks'' who charge less but provide inadequate services.

Adolescents. A fourth subculture included in Table 8-5 is adolescents. Adolescents are considered a subculture because they have in common the physical characteristics of puberty, as well as common developmental tasks to achieve, such as making important decisions regarding career, marriage, and life-style, common communication patterns, and other characteristics of subcultures.

Health care provider culture. The last category in Table 8-5 is the health care culture. It is important for health care workers to remember that they have been acculturated into a unique specialty with rules, customs, and a language all its own. The health care culture's value system affects the type of care given. For example, cleanliness is valued and therefore workers wash their hands and equipment often and bathe hospitalized patients daily. In addition, this entire subculture operates with unwritten rules that can make entry and interaction with the system difficult for those unfamiliar with it. The health care provider culture is included in Table 8-5 to increase readers' awareness of the health care system as a subculture and the ways it interfaces with other subcultures.

As previously mentioned, Table 8-5 describes specific subcultures based on their frequency of occurrence in the population. Table 8-6 provides population statistics for the described subcultures, according to 1970 census data. All of the numbers are assumed to be low estimates because members of minority groups are often not accurately counted due to mobility

and other factors. The religions of Judaism and Church of Christ, Scientist, were chosen for their membership numbers and beliefs relating to health.

Although the chart format adopted for Table 8-5 allows for only limited data, it does illustrate, as intended, a variety of responses to the same stimuli; for an in-depth examination of any subculture, including those presented, the reader is referred to other sources, such as those in the reference list at the end of the chapter. Brief discussion of subcultures requires use of generalizations; however, the discussion is not intended to imply that all individuals are affected by their subculture in the same way. Such stereotyping can lead to erroneous assumptions, and the reader is urged to be cautious in this regard.

Definitions of health among various subcultures

The first assessment area, shown in column one of Table 8-5, considers how the subculture views health. Other relevant questions are as follows:

How does one obtain good health?

What importance is placed on health?

What are common beliefs about the body?

This is extremely important information to have in order to understand the basic health practices and daily routines of subcultures. All of the subcultures identified in Table 8-5 place some importance on health, but they vary greatly in their definitions. Two subcultures perceive health as a balance of forces; Navajos regard health as a balance between themselves and two external forces (earth and the supernatural), whereas the Chinese regard health as a balance between the opposing energy forces called yin

Problems of entry to health care system	Communication pattern	Sexuality and family life	Beliefs about death
Physician is main access to system; focus is basically curing illness rather than prevention; encouragement given to population to seek care as soon as symptoms appear; consider health care system as only provider	Widespread use of jargon and specialized language; large percentage of workers from middle class; often expect gratitude for care given; time orientation strict; written records kept[4]	Hierarchy, with physicians making decisions	Death usually means workers have failed to do their job; elaborate means are used to keep people alive; ethical and legal questions are being discussed and tested

Table 8-6. Numbers of subculture groups in population*

Group	Approximate total number	Families below poverty level (%)
Asian-Americans	1,500,000	8.8
Black Americans	25,000,000	29.9
Hispanic Americans	9,000,000	21.2
American Indians	500,000	33.3
Jews	5,000,000†	Unknown
Christian Scientists	300,000†	Unknown

*Modified from Spector, R.: 1979. Cultural diversity in health and illness, Appleton-Century-Crofts, New York. Data from the 1970 U.S. Census.
†Modified from Rosten, L.: 1955. A guide to religions of America, Simon & Schuster, New York.

and yang. Hispanic-Americans regard health as a gift from God; low-income persons are likely to define health functionally as the ability to continue working. The health care culture, in contrast, has standardized definitions of health, including optimal wellness and something more than the absence of disease.

The health care culture definition is broad enough to include the other definitions. It is different, however, in that it places responsibility for health with the individual, whereas other definitions hold external (sometimes uncontrollable) factors partially or totally responsible for an individual's health. This difference is important in practice; the school nurse must know what the client believes about health before she can plan appropriate interventions. A student may not follow a prescribed rest regimen for a sprained ankle if he believes God intends for him to suffer as punishment or if a folk healer advises a different treatment. Carefully planned teaching by the school nurse will probably not change the student's beliefs. Instead, the school nurse should identify the individual's beliefs

and shape her interventions to fit within his cultural norms. In doing so, it is also important that she not threaten his values. In this case, perhaps a contract could be arranged to combine treatments suggested by the folk healer with those medically recommended. In this way the nurse demonstrates respect for the individual's beliefs and the potential positive effect of the folk healer, while at the same time promotes medically recommended treatments.

Beliefs concerning disease causation and prevention

Another pertinent area to explore is the subculture's beliefs regarding cause of illness. Assessment questions include the following:
What causes illness?
Is illness preventable?
How can illness be prevented?
Given the belief of several subcultures that illness is caused by bad luck or spirits, prevention is, logically, aimed at pleasing the spirits. The health care culture does not adhere to this common belief, however, but places emphasis on

the "omnipotence of technology" (Spector, 1979:79). Thus instead of encouraging ritualistic dances and wearing of good luck pieces as various other subcultures do, the health care system recommends scientific methods of prevention such as inoculations. Both health care workers and members of subcultures may regard the practices expounded by the other as slightly foolish and not really helpful. Many times a stalemate results, since neither person is willing to forfeit his beliefs. It is not necessary for either to forfeit his beliefs; on the contrary, this in itself creates problems. The health care provider has the responsibility of bridging the gap created by different belief systems. This task requires delicate communication skills, a sense of respect for the client and his beliefs, as well as comprehensive knowledge of the belief system of the subculture, particularly regarding causation of illness.

Prevention of illness "correlates with an ability to control the future and . . . poverty makes such control impossible" (Bullough and Bullough, 1972:86). Adolescents also maintain a present orientation; Murray and Zentner (1975a) identify achieving interest in the future as one of the tasks of adolescents. For members of subcultures without future orientation, the school nurse should carefully define priorities. Immediate needs, as defined by the student, must be met before undertaking long-range planning. Assisting him to meet immediate needs will help the student reallocate his adaptive energy to either a higher level of adaptation or a more long-range focus. This procedure is also advantageous because the student will feel accepted by the school nurse, thus setting the scene for future cooperative relationships. The school nurse, then, should align her priorities (to the fullest reasonable extent) with the student's priorities.

Illness behavior

The third assessment area of Table 8-5 includes people's behavior when illness occurs; specific questions to consider are as follows:

Are folk healers sought? Are they available?

What are the specific illness-curing practices?

What type of relationship exists between the healer and ill person?

What symptoms are and are not reported?

Navajo Indians consult both a diagnostician and a medicine man when symptoms arise. The former decides what bodily part is out of harmony, and the latter treats it. As noted in Table 8-5, herbal drinks and chanting are two commonly used treatments. The medicine man, like folk healers from other cultures, takes special interest not only in the symptoms, but also in the ill persons. His belief and interest in their recovery is an important element of his treatment.

For many people, the folk healer is the initial source of treatment. Reasons for consulting the folk healer first include tradition, religious beliefs, established relationship with healer, previous favorable experience, belief in his healing powers, congruency with other cultural beliefs, and difficulty of access to the health care system. The practice of consulting a folk healer first may delay or entirely cancel entry into the health care system. It is important for health care workers to be aware that clients may have visited other healers first.

The school nurse has the opportunity to help shape future illness behaviors of students. The school health office may be one of the few contacts a child has with the health care system; if he feels comfortable, can establish a relationship with a nurse who respects and understands his values, and is accepted and assisted by her, he may use the health care system as an adult, assuming that he can identify the same characteristics in other parts of the health care system. The nurse can also teach children which situations and problems are best helped by the health care system (i.e., emergency or serious symptoms) and by the folk healer (i.e., routine problems).

The current American health care system places emphasis on technology to cure illness. This has led to an especially physiological and impersonal orientation, which is very different from the orientations of the folk healers. Folk healers may help their clients feel better psychologically, which provides increased energy resources to assist physiological adaptation. Lower income groups (who make up a large portion of minority cultures) must often resort to using clinics for medical care and may see a different physician each time they visit; this lack of continuity is an emotional energy drain, reinforcing their behavior of consulting folk healers. Higher income persons, on the other hand, often have personal physicians who remember them. Because of the lack of continuity for some consumers and for philosophical reasons, an increasing number of health care workers are becoming interested in holistic health care (treating the entire person and not only the disease), a trend which may eventually alter some of the present practices.

Thus far, only the effect of culture on the type of health care sought has been discussed. Whether or not a symptom leads an individual to seek care is also culturally determined. According to Brownlee (1978), women in some low-income subcultures accept low back pain as part of life and do not report this symptom. Culture may also determine who has "permission" to be ill. For instance, the role of the Hispanic-American man is vital to family functioning; he is therefore less likely to report symptoms than a child, whose role is less important to the family's well-being.

How symptoms are perceived is another culturally determined factor. Navajo Indians, for example, may respond with joy to a baby born with congenital hip dislocation because the family was strong enough to fight the evil spirits, resulting in a minor rather than major deformity (Brownlee, 1978). Adolescents, on the other hand, tend to perceive symptoms emotionally. Adolescents are particularly prone to illnesses and conditions that affect their body image, such as obesity, acne, accidents, venereal disease, and pregnancy. Body image is very important to adolescents because they are establishing their identity, hence, the emotional reaction. This, in turn, may lead to desperation and a willingness to follow advice, however inappropriate it may be. The adolescent is therefore susceptible to quack "cure-alls" and foolish health "fads" such as extreme or "crash" diets. As described in Chapter 9, the school nurse can be influential in preventing inappropriate responses.

Access to health care system

As described in Table 8-5, culture may influence how accessible the health care system is for individuals. In determining accessibility the following information is helpful:

Do language barriers exist?

Is money a limiting factor?

Is location and/or transportation a problem?

Is knowledge about the health care system available to consumers, providing more efficient use?

What entry points exist other than physicians?

The problems adolescents face regarding access to the health care system are fairly typical of other subcultures. They may fear that their family physician will not maintain confidentiality, but lack knowledge of other health care resources and the money to pay for them. Members of other subcultures may have language difficulties, leading to even further difficulties interacting with the health care system. For a low-income person to take a day off work without pay to spend a morning waiting at a clinic to be told something he does not understand, to have medicine prescribed of which he is suspicious, and to have to pay for all this, is, to say the least, a frustrating experience.

One method of decreasing difficulty of access to the health care system is the development of specialty clinics to meet the unique needs of particular client groups; examples include bilingual clinics and teenage clinics. The school nurse can ease access to the health care system through careful and knowledgeable referrals. Referrals with unfortunate outcomes will reflect negatively on her care. School nurses need to be aware of the entry points to the health care systems in their locale and of the difficulties specific subcultures are likely to encounter. The additional health assessment skills taught in school nurse practitioner programs enable these graduates to eliminate the need for some referrals, which also benefits students.

Communication patterns within subcultures

Communication patterns differ greatly from one subculture to another. This is of special significance to the school nurse in developing relationships with children and families of different cultures. Some pertinent questions to answer before communicating with members of other subcultures are as follows (Brownlee, 1978):

How important are greetings and goodbyes? Example: Native-Americans commonly leave without saying goodbye.

How much time is spent on chitchat before beginning an interview?

What can be done to increase another's comfort level? Example: Swedes talk more freely over shared food.

What is the normal tempo of a conversation? Example: Most cultures converse slower with more pauses than the dominant American culture.

Are any topics taboo? Example: One African tribe does not mention the name of a recently deceased person.

What are the norms of confidentiality?

Are feelings expressed? If so, how?

Are the following acceptable: profanity, raising of voice, disapproval, affection?

How do people ask for help?

What rules govern nonverbal behavior, such as touch?

Children are especially attuned to nonverbal behavior, making this an important part of communication for the school nurse. Nonverbal behaviors about which the nurse should be knowledgeable include common hand signals and knowing what kind of eye and body contact is acceptable. In some Indian cultures it is impolite and insulting to look into another's eyes; yet in other cultures it is equally insulting *not* to look directly at someone. Seemingly insignificant behaviors such as this can make a great difference in the establishment of a helping relationship.

Adolescents present unique communication challenges. Because they are asserting their independence, they may be initially mistrustful of adults (Eggert, 1978). Open, honest communication is imperative; any rules or restrictions should be stated as positive expectations during the first meeting or visit. Contracting is especially useful with adolescents because of its emphasis on mutual responsibility and clearly stated goals and expectations. The school nurse may also find that adolescents respond positively to small group experiences because acceptance by peers is important at this age. These methods of communication with adolescents are also useful in prevention of specific problems, such as substance abuse and obesity (Chapter 9).

Health care workers communicate extensively by using jargon of their own creation. They frequently use lengthy, scientific words when simple ones could be substituted. Some examples are "prioritizing" a client's needs, "negative" results of a test (which, although it sounds ominous, is *good* for the client), and "medication" instead of medicine or pills. In addition to jargon, abbreviations the client does not understand are often used, such as OD, QID, PRN, CBC, NHNF. All of this has the effect of increasing the distance between the caregiver and the recipient. It creates "turf" that serves as a safety zone for the caregivers, a somewhat illogical reverse of circumstances. One other common practice that often alienates clients (and students) is record keeping. It may be necessary to record specific data such as screening results, but it is usually not necessary to write while the client is speaking; in fact, some groups such as Navajo Indians regard recording while the client is talking as objectionable. As a nonverbal behavior, this practice can detract from trust formation; therefore when it can be avoided, it is best to do so.

Culturally-determined sex roles and family living

Questions for further data collection in this category include the following:

Are family roles assigned according to sex?

What are the roles each individual performs?

Who makes family decisions?

How flexible are the roles?

What are the beliefs and practices concerning birth control?

What types of family structures are common?

What is the role of children in the family?

Because the variable "family structure" was discussed previously, the focus here is to determine how the norms of the subculture affect the roles and life-style within the family and how that affects the health of individuals. One example is the Hispanic-American family, in which, traditionally, men have been the breadwinners and decision makers. Women may often wait several days for their husbands to make a decision regarding, for instance, whether or not a child should be taken to a physician. The school nurse should be aware of who makes decisions and on what basis, so that she can communicate more effectively.

Knowledge about sexual norms is especially important for the school nurse working with adolescents. Adolescents are becoming familiar with their sexuality and obtain information about how to behave from many sources, including friends, media, family, and the school nurse. The school nurse should remain nonjudgmental, which requires awareness of her feelings about sexuality and sex roles, as well as knowledge about practices within other cultural groups. Cultural norms are quite variable in this regard; in some subcultures any bodily contact and/or display of affection before marriage is prohibited, in others it is encouraged (Brownlee, 1978). Birth control is another aspect that varies widely. If she has accurate information and a reasonable comfort level with these topics, the school nurse can assist students to identify and discuss issues regarding sexuality and family roles, thus assisting them in the task of defining their future life-styles.

Cultural beliefs about death

The beliefs an individual holds about death influence the way in which he lives and the manner in which he adapts to his own death and the deaths of others. Issues to assess include the following:

What are the beliefs about death and after-life?

What is done for a dying individual?

What rituals are performed for the dead?

What, if anything, is done for the mourners?

Beliefs about death include belief in heaven and hell, reincarnation, no afterlife, and young children's belief that death is reversible. These beliefs fulfill the human need to explain death, thereby helping to ease the pain of loss and guide the individual toward acceptance. Similarly, the health care culture includes people with many beliefs about death and dying. The provider culture itself, however, invariably works toward preventing death; because health care providers view death as a failure of their preventive efforts, they may have difficulty accepting their clients' deaths.

Each culture has defined rituals surrounding the death of its members, allowing survivors to grieve effectively and continue their own lives. Navajos and Jewish persons, for instance, like dying persons to be surrounded by the whole family (Brownlee, 1978). When working with seriously ill children in school or with children who have had a death in the family, an understanding of the child's beliefs and family customs regarding death is essential for the school nurse. It is only with this knowledge that she can assist the child and family to adapt to the death in the best possible way for them.

SUMMARY

Structural variables are part of the adaptation framework and affect how people perceive and respond to their environment. Structural variables discussed in this chapter include age, family structure, culture, religion, and income. Information regarding the effect of these variables on health and illness behaviors is summarized in Table 8-5. Further assessment guidelines for the practitioner working with subcultures have been presented for each health-related data category. Suggestions and examples of application of theory and information provided are also in-cluded for each category. The intent of this chapter is not to provide comprehensive information, but rather to discuss structural variables and their usefulness in application of adaptation theory to school nursing.

REFERENCES

Barnard, M. V.: 1977. Supportive care for the adoptive family, Issues Comprehensive Nurs. **2**(3):22-29.

Brownlee, A. T.: 1978. Community, culture, and care: a cross-cultural guide for health workers, The C. V. Mosby Company, St. Louis.

Bullough, V., and Bullough, B.: 1972. Poverty, ethnic identity, and health care, Appleton-Century-Crofts, New York.

Byrne, M. L., and Thompson, L. F.: 1978. Key concepts for the study and practice of nursing, 2nd ed. The C. V. Mosby Co., St. Louis.

Channing, G.: 1955. What is a Christian Scientist? In Rosten, L., editor: A guide to religions of America, Simon & Schuster, New York.

Eggert, L.: 1978. Family subsystem: the therapeutic process with adolescents experiencing psychosocial stress. In Longo, D. C., and Williams, R. A., editors: Clinical practice in psychosocial nursing: assessment and intervention, Appleton-Century-Crofts, New York.

Eiduson, B. T.: 1978. Child development in emergent family styles, Child. Today **7**:24-31.

Erikson, E.: 1963. Childhood and society, 2nd ed., W. W. Norton & Co., Inc., New York.

Fromer, M.: 1979. Community health care and the nursing process, The C. V. Mosby Co., St. Louis.

Gonzales, H.: 1976. Health care needs of the Mexican American family. In Ethnicity and health care, NLN publ. no. 14-1625, pp. 21-28.

Horowitz, J. A., and Perdue, B. J.: 1977. Single parent families, Nurs. Clin. North Am. **12**(3):503-511.

Jack, M. S., and Grinstead, L. N.: 1978. The single-parent family: an issue in nursing, Issues Comprehensive Pediatr. Nurs. **2**:(3)30-39.

Jacobson, E., and Cockerum, J.: 1976. As foster children see it: former foster children talk about foster family care, Child. Today **5**:32-36.

Jenkins, S.: 1978. Children of divorce, Child. Today **7**:11-15.

Kanter, M.: 1978. Jobs and families: impact of working roles on family life, Child. Today **7**:11-15.

Kertzer, M.: 1955. What is a Jew? In Rosten, L., editor: A guide to religions of America, Simon & Schuster, New York.

Kohn, M. L.: 1959. Social class and parental values, Am. J. Sociol. **44**(4):337-351.

Kosa, J., and Zola, I. K.: 1976. Poverty and health: a sociological analysis, 2nd ed., Harvard University Press, Cambridge, Mass.

Levine, M.: 1974. New family structures: challenge to family casework, J. Jewish Communal Services **L**(3):238-244.

Lidz, T.: 1968. The person: his development throughout the life cycle, Basic Books, Inc., Publishers, New York.

Martin, B.: 1976. Ethnicity and health care: Afro-Americans. In Ethnicity and health care, NLN Publ. no. 14-1625, pp. 47-55.

Merriam, E.: 1961. Mommies at work, Street & Smith Publications, Inc., New York.

Messer, A.: 1970. The individual in his family: an adaptational study, Charles C Thomas, Publisher, Springfield, Ill.

Miles, M.: 1971. Annie and the old one, Little, Brown & Co., Boston.

Miller, S.: 1975. Effects of maternal employment on sex role perception, interests, and self-esteem in kindergarten girls, Dev. Psychol. **11:**405-406.

Mott, P. E.: 1965. Shift work: the social, psychological, and physical consequences, University of Michigan Press, Ann Arbor, Mich.

Murray, R., and Zentner, J.: 1975a. Nursing assessment and health promotion throughout the life span, Prentice-Hall, Inc., Englewood Cliffs, N.J.

Murray, R., and Zentner, J.: 1975b. Nursing concepts for health promotion, Prentice-Hall, Inc., Englewood Cliffs, N.J.

Rotkovitch, R.: 1976. Ethnicity in health care—the Jewish heritage. In Ethnicity in health care, NLN publ. no. 14-1625, pp. 37-46.

Satir, V.: 1972. Peoplemaking, Science & Behavior Books, Inc., Palo Alto, Calif.

Siemon, M. K.: 1978. Family subsystem: working with school-age children experiencing psychosocial stress. In Longo, D. C., and Williams, R. A., editors: Clinical practice in psychosocial nursing: assessment and intervention, Appleton-Century-Crofts, New York.

Spector, R.: 1979. Cultural diversity in health and illness, Appleton-Century-Crofts, New York.

Sussman, M.: 1978. The family today, Child. Today **7:**32-36.

Wang, R.: 1976. Chinese Americans health care. In Ethnicity and health care, NLN publ. no. 14-1625, pp. 9-18.

Wood, R.: 1976. The American Indian and health. In Ethnicity and Health Care, NLN publ. no. 14-1625, pp. 29-35.

Zborowski, M.: 1952. Cultural components in response to pain, J. Soc. Issues **8:**16-30.

Zolotow, C.: 1971. A father like that, Harper & Row, Publishers, New York.

SUGGESTED READINGS

Abril I.: 1975. Mexican American folk beliefs that affect health care, Ariz. Nurse **28:**14-20.

Allen, J. R.: 1973. The Indian adolescent: psycho-social tasks of the Plains Indian of Western Oklahoma, Am. J. Orthopsychiatry **43:**368-375.

Bauwens, E.: 1978. The anthropology of health, The C. V. Mosby Co., St. Louis.

Belgum, D.: 1967. Religion and medicine, Iowa State University Press, Ames, Iowa.

Bermann, E.: 1973. Scapegoat, University of Michigan Press, Ann Arbor, Mich. (Role of culture in dealing with death.)

Brunswick, A. F., and Josephson, E.: 1972. Adolescent health in Harlem, Am. J. Public Health **62**(suppl.):2, Oct.

Campbell, T., and Change, B.: 1973. Health care of the Chinese in America, Nurs. Outlook **21:**245-249.

Daniel, W. A.: 1977. Adolescents in health and disease, The C. V. Mosby Co., St. Louis.

Davis, K. S.: 1969. The paradox of poverty in America, H. W. Wilson Co., New York.

Donin, H. H.: 1972. To be a Jew, Basic Books, Inc., Publishers, New York.

Gardner, F.: 1972. Stories about the real world, Prentice-Hall, Inc., Englewood Cliffs, N.J.

Ginsburg, H.: 1972. Poverty, economics, and society, Little, Brown & Co., Boston.

Glaser, W. A.: 1970. Social settings and medical organization. A cross-cultural study of the hospital, Atherton Press, New York.

Humphrey, P.: 1974. Learning about poverty and health, Nurs. Outlook **22:**441-443.

Kluckhohn, C., and Leighton, D.: 1962. The Navajo, Doubleday & Co., Inc., New York.

Landy, D.: 1977. Culture, disease and healing, Macmillan Inc., New York.

Leacock, E. B.: 1971. The culture of poverty, Simon & Schuster, New York.

Leininger, M.: 1967. The cultural concept and its relevance to nursing, J. Nurs. Educ. **6:**27.

Lore, A.: 1973. Adolescents: people, not problems, Am. J. Nurs. **73:**1232-34.

Luckcroft, D.: 1976. Black awareness: implications for black patient care, American Journal of Nursing Co., New York.

Lynch, L. R.: 1969. The cross-cultural approach to health behavior, Fairleigh Dickenson University Press, Rutherford, N.J.

Mead, M.: 1950. Sex and temperament in three primitive societies, The New American Library, Mentor Books, New York.

Nall, F. C., and Speilberg, J.: 1967. Social and cultural factors in the responses of Mexican-Americans to medical treatment, J. Health Soc. Behav. **8:**302.

Palos, S.: 1971. The Chinese art of healing, Herter & Herter, New York.

Queen, S. A., and Habenstein, R. W.: 1974. The family in various cultures, 4th ed., J. B. Lippincott, Co., Philadelphia.

Ramey, J.: 1978. Experimental family forms—the family of the future, Marriage Family Rev. **1**(1):1-9.

Reinhardt, A. M., and Quinn, M. D.: 1977. Current practice in family-centered community nursing. Vol. 1, The C. V. Mosby Co., St. Louis.

Scott, W. R., and Volkhardt, E. H.: 1966. Medical care readings in the sociology of medical institutions, John Wiley & Sons, Inc., New York.

Segal, J., and Yakruees, H.: 1978. Protecting children's mental health, Child. Today **7:**23-25.

Suchman, E.: 1964. Socio-medical variables among ethnic groups, Am. J. Sociol. **70:**319-331.

Weaver, J. L.: 1976. National health policy and the underserved: ethnic minorities, women, and the elderly, The C. V. Mosby Co., St. Louis.

Woods, N. F.: 1979. Human sexuality in health and illness, 2nd ed., The C. V. Mosby Company, St. Louis.

CHAPTER 9

Stress and crisis: specific problems of adaptation

JOANNE GINGRICH-CRASS

Chapter 7 discussed adaptation of school-age children to life events, and Chapter 8 discussed factors that influence the adaptive process, such as age, religion, income, culture, and family structure. This chapter focuses on adaptation that occurs as a response to stress. The first discussion describes a theoretical framework of stress, crisis, and adaptation, which provides structure for nursing care of children and adolescents experiencing stress. The discussion includes the following:

1. Factors that influence adaptation to stress
2. Guidelines for assessing adaptation to stress
3. Suggested school nurse interventions to improve adaptation
4. Primary, secondary, and tertiary prevention of inadequate adaptation to stress

Ten specific stressful situations for school-age children are discussed using the format just presented to provide information and guidelines for working with children experiencing stress. The specific stressors discussed were chosen because they affect significant numbers of children. The ten topics are as follows:

1. Separation from a significant other through death or divorce
2. Seriously ill children in the school setting
3. Suicide in school-age children
4. School refusal and health-related absenteeism (including school phobia)
5. Delinquency and violence
6. Chemical use and abuse
7. Maltreatment of school-age children
8. Crises resulting from adolescent sexuality
9. Learning disabilities
10. Chronic diseases

STRESS AND CRISIS: THEORY AND APPLICATION
Definition and characteristics

Much has been written about stress and crisis, and many definitions have been proposed; the Random House dictionary definition is inclusive, but not concise: "Stress is: (a) the physical pressure, pull, or other force exerted on one thing by another, (b) any stimulus such as fear or pain that disturbs or interferes with the normal physiological equilibrium of an individual, (c) physical, mental, or emotional strain or tension." Popular use of the word stress connotes a negative overwhelmed feeling; however, stress as defined here is continually present in man. According to Byrne and Thompson (1978), stress is essential for life; for example, various self regulatory processes are constantly adjusting to stressors, although the individual may be unaware of their functioning. The following operational definition is based on a combination of those in the literature (Martin and Prange, 1962; Boland et al., 1979):

Stress is a physical and emotional state always present in a person, which is altered when the environment threatens or does disturb equilibrium.

Environment refers to both internal (for example, thirst) and external (for example, school) environmental stimuli. *Equilibrium* implies steady state or "optimal energy balance between utilization and conservation" (Boland et al., 1979:228). The steady state is altered when demands are made by stressors such as physical or psychological change, challenges, threats, conflicts, goals, expectations, boredom, or inadequate stimulation (Selye, 1974). Stressors, therefore, alter the state from one of balance to one of imbalance. A state of *imbalance* exists when a person cannot meet the demands placed on him by the stressor. Usually, through adaptation, a person deals with the demand successfully and rebalance results because each person has qualities and capabilities for dealing with stressors that function as *counterbalances*. Examples of counterbalances include (1) realistic perception of the event, (2) adequate support system, and (3) previous successful coping mechanisms.

Three methods of dealing with stressors are (1) successful overcoming of the stressor, (2) avoidance, and (3) coexistence, or "learning to live with it." Imbalance and rebalance occur daily, stimulating growth and new behaviors; for example, a child and family move from one town to another. The challenge of identifying the expected academic standards and a social niche for himself in the new classroom is a stressor that creates a temporary imbalance, during which the child assesses the situation and gathers his counterbalances together. Examples of counterbalances in this situation might be previously learned ways of making friends, perception of the new environment as a friendly place, and previous education level. After a period of time, the child adapts to the new environment, feels comfortable in the new

environment, makes friends, and soon has regained a steady state, or rebalance. The adaptation process has resulted in new learning that can be applied to future situations.

Not all stress results in adequate adaptation, however. Excessive stress is called *distress*. Distress occurs when the demands on an individual are (1) severe or too numerous, (2) chronic, (3) unexpected, or (4) ambiguous (Jasmin and Trygstad, 1979). When the individual's capabilities cannot counterbalance the stressor, an imbalance results. Imbalance is characterized by a nonspecific physiological response, described by Selye (1965) as the general adaptation syndrome (GAS). The GAS consists of three stages (Table 9-1): (1) *"alarm" reaction,* in which the body activates itself for defense against the stressor (also known as the "fight or flight" response); (2) *resistance stage,* during which adaptation occurs; and (3) *exhaustion stage,* which follows if adaptation reserves are depleted. Selye states the GAS is nonspecific; that is, it does not vary with differing types of stressors.

Each individual can tolerate limited amounts of stress. If the stressors remain within tolerable limits, adaptation and growth result. Dubós (1965) reports that a sheltered life (that is,

Table 9-1. The general adaptation syndrome*

	Stage one: alarm	Stage two: resistance	Stage three: exhaustion
Physiological responses	Total sympathetic nervous system response only: "fight or flight" reaction Epinephrine released to target areas Tachycardia and hypertension Shallow respiration Dilated pupils Skin pale and cool Reduced urinary output Increased metabolism as seen by perspiration, dry mouth Muscle tension	Hypothalamus instructs pituitary gland to secrete adrenocorticotropin, which increases blood sugar level, suppresses inflammation, blocks some allergic responses and mineralocorticoids, resulting in increased blood volume; overall results: increased endurance and strength, antibody production, blood sugar levels, and hormone secretion assists in "fight" response for self-preservation	Self-regulation no longer possible: potassium depletion causes slow respiration, irregular pulse, and lowered blood pressure; eventually weakness, fainting, and death may occur
Behavioral responses	Restlessness, irritability Feelings of heightened energy Problem solving Increased alertness	Diminished clarity and problem-solving skills Any emotion possible: ambivalence, helplessness, depression	Panic Disorganized and distorted thinking Impaired perception

*Based on data from Jasmin, S., and Trygstad, L. N.: 1979. Behavioral concepts and the nursing process, The C. V. Mosby Co., St. Louis; Murray, R., and Zentner, J.: 1979b. Nursing concepts for health promotion, Prentice-Hall, Inc., Englewood Cliffs, N.J.; Selye, H.: 1965. The stress syndrome, Am. J. Nurs. **65**(3):97-99.

without stress) weakens one's adaptability and that human potential can only be reached by continually meeting new challenges. However, when individual adaptive limits are exceeded, crisis results.

Crisis is defined as a turning point or situation that cannot be handled by previously acquired coping mechanisms (Aguilera and Messick, 1978). That is, new ways of adapting are necessary to resolve the situation. Caplan (1964) identifies two types of crises: developmental and situational. *Developmental crises* are "transition points that every person experiences in the process of biopsychosocial growth and development that are accompanied by changes in thoughts, feelings and abilities" (Murray et al., 1979a:294). Examples of developmental crises are school entry, marriage, and parenthood; developmental crises of school-age children in particular are discussed in Chapter 7. A *situational crisis* is an "external event or situation, not necessarily a part of normal living, often sudden, unexpected, and unfortunate, which looms larger than the person's immediate resources or ability to cope and which demands a change in behavior" (Murray et al., 1979a:294). Examples of situational crises for school-age children are death of a parent, change of residence, and illness.

Fink (1967) defines four phases through which the person in crisis moves: (1) shock, (2) defensive retreat, (3) acknowledgment, and (4) adaptation. The phases and their accompanying feelings and behaviors are described in Table 9-2.

Individuals progress through the phases at their own pace and may be in two phases simultaneously or may move "backward" and "forward"; each person acquires his own patterns of adjusting to crisis. The outcome of a crisis is considered successful if new coping mechanisms are learned; growth and maturity result. If the crisis situation is not fully resolved, when another crisis occurs, new coping mechanisms are not available because they have not been previously learned.

The relationship between crisis and stress is demonstrated in Fig. 9-1; crisis results when the person's counterbalances to stress are not sufficient for rebalancing. The stress reaction is a nonspecific reaction to a stressor; a crisis follows if equilibrium is not restored. The presence of excessive or chronic stress may increase anxiety, resulting in difficulties with daily functioning and failure of previous coping mecha-

Table 9-2. Psychologic phases of crisis*

Time	Phase	Self-experience	Reality perceptions	Emotional experience	Cognitive structure	Physical disability
↓	Shock (stress)	Threat to existing structures	Perceived as overwhelming	Panic, anxiety, helplessness	Disorganization; inability to plan or to reason or to understand situation	Acute somatic damage requiring full medical care
	Defensive retreat	Attempt to maintain old structures	Avoidance of reality, "wishful thinking," denial, repression	Indifference or euphoria (except when challenged, in which case anger), low anxiety	Defensive reorganization, resistance to change	Physical recovery from acute phase; functional return to maximum possible level
	Acknowledgment (renewed stress)	Giving up existing structure; self-depreciation	Facing reality; facts "impose" themselves	Depression with apathy or agitation; bitterness, mourning, high anxiety, if overwhelming, suicide	Defensive breakdown: (1) disorganization, (2) reorganization in terms of altered reality perceptions	Physical plateau: gradual slowing of improvement until no change is experienced
	Adaptation and change	Establishing new structure; sense of worth	New reality testing	Gradual increase in satisfying experiences (gradual lowering of anxiety)	Reorganization in terms of present resources and abilities	No change in physical disability status

*From Fink, S. L.: 1967. Crisis and motivation: a theoretical model, Arch. Phys. Med. Rehabil. **48**:593. Reproduced with permission of the Archives of Physical Medicine and Rehabilitation.

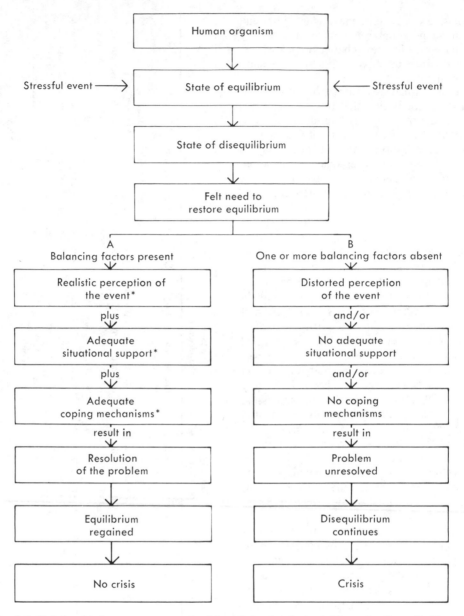

Fig. 9-1. Relationship between stress and crisis. *Balancing factors. (From Aguilera, D. C., and Messick, J. M.: 1978. Crisis intervention: theory and methodology, The C. V. Mosby Co., St. Louis.)

nisms (crisis), which in turn may lead to panic, increased stress, and further decreased ability to function (Fromer, 1979).

Factors affecting the outcome of stress and crisis situations

Factors influencing the result of a stressful event include (1) the developmental stage, (2) previous experience, (3) perception of the problem, (4) culture, (5) the support system, and (6) the number and chronicity of stressors (Caplan, 1964). These factors are similar to structural variables in that they affect all people to varying degrees. The school nurse can assess how each of these factors is influencing a student's adaptation.

Developmental stage

Developmental stages have been defined as one type of crisis, and although they are expected parts of life, each requires new behaviors. For this reason, an imbalance of equilibrium occurs, making the individual especially vulnerable to other stressors. As described in Chapter 8, if a stressful situation coincides with a developmental crisis, the outcome may be incomplete learning of the expected developmental tasks. Because children pass through many developmental stages, they are particularly sensitive to environmental stressors.

Previous experience

The previous experiences of a child also affect the outcome of stress and crisis situations. Although children's previous experiences are somewhat limited because of their young age, children do learn new coping mechanisms by experience. For example, children whose families move frequently learn how to adjust to new environments and can apply their adjustment skills to future moves. If an experience had special meaning for a child, that meaning will affect future adaptation to similar circumstances. For example, if a child is punished at home for creative new behaviors, such as playing a musical instrument, he may fear demonstrating creativity in other settings.

Perception of problem

School-age children may perceive their circumstances differently from the adults who observe them, which is due in part to cognitive development. For example, children at the stage of preconceptual thought are unable to understand the permanency of death. Developmental level also strongly influences children's perceptions of events; for instance, the self-consciousness of adolescence might influence a teenager to believe a laughing group of peers are laughing at him, whereas a younger child would react with curiosity. The objectivity with which one views an event also influences one's perception of it; the less objective one is, the more likely is unrealistic perception.

Perception significantly affects adaptation to stress because one's perception of an event determines one's response to that event. Perception is highly individualized; thus one child might view a family move to California as exciting, another, as frightening, a third, anger producing. For all three the perception will affect adaptation: the first child might pack toys in preparation for the move, the second might be more likely to cling to his parents and avoid the new school and classmates, while the third might act out. The school nurse must therefore determine whether the child views his circumstances as threatening or challenging.

Another characteristic of perception is that it changes. The three examples just given could characterize one child's perception as it varies over time—at first fearful, later, angry, and finally, excited. The school nurse can use this dynamic quality by assisting children to adopt realistic, healthy perceptions in life events, through accepting and encouraging children to express their feelings. For example, the fearful child may feel better when he talks about his fears, because they are less frightening when put into words.

Perception applies not only to external environment, but also to the internal environment, or self-concept. The child who perceives that he is capable of adapting to a stressor is not wasting energy on a stress reaction because he does not perceive the stressor as threatening. Although self-concept is discussed in more detail in Chapter 7, it is important to note here that one's self-concept influences one's perception of events.

Culture

Definition of stressful events and expected reactions to them are largely culturally determined. Japanese men, for instance, perceive events such as making mistakes in public as humiliating and therefore more stressful than other cultures. Hispanic-American children learn more expressive and even volatile reactions to stress, whereas Chinese children learn more subdued responses (Jasmin and Trygstad, 1979). Culture also includes religious beliefs and family traditions, both of which affect how one reacts to and perceives stressful situations. The school nurse must be very knowledgeable in these areas to effectively intervene and prevent crisis situations among students. Guidelines for gaining knowledge about culturally determined health-related behaviors have been presented in Chapter 8.

Support system

The support system is that group of people who are closely involved with an individual and on whom the individual depends for assistance and from whom he derives a self-image, sense of belonging, love, and approval. The school-age child's support system includes family, peers, friends, and readily available professionals, such as teachers and school nurses. Other professionals, such as school psychologists, social workers, and counselors provide important support when necessary but otherwise usually do not interact daily with students. When functioning well, support systems assist individuals to adjust favorably to life events; their absence or malfunction increases the risk of inadequate adaptation.

MacElveen (1978) provides several guidelines for assessing support systems. First, determine the size and "connectedness" of the system; that is, how many people within the system know each other. Second, assess entries and exits from the system; that is, has the child lost or gained a member through death or marriage. A change in residence may mean loss of the whole system and formation of a new one. At this time, MacElveen states that the child is vulnerable because energy is required to build a new support system; children whose families move frequently are in this category. Third, assess the phase MacElveen labels "construction," during which new relationships are formed. For children, the construction phase may be difficult because (1) acceptance into a new group partially depends on the group members, and other children tend to make the new child "prove" his worth and (2) forming new relationships involves identifying others with common interests, and children do not have a well-developed sense of self. Fourth, assess maintenance, which requires mutual give and take among the members. Fifth, assess if and how repair of the relationship is accomplished when a member withdraws temporarily. Both departure and return of the supportive person can be stressful for children. The school nurse therefore needs to assess not only the student's support system, but also the child's use of available supportive persons.

Number and chronicity of stressors

Both stress and crisis are additive phenomena; that is, the greater the number of stress factors present, the more difficult it is to cope with them. Jasmin and Trygstad (1979:52) document that chronically stressed persons are in a state of "sustained activation" during which physical responses to stress continue as demonstrated by blood levels of dopamine-beta-hydroxylase (DBH) in chronically stressed people, such as prisoners. One of the most demanding factors

on adaptive energy is physical illness. The child who has a chronic disease therefore has fewer energy reserves for other normal childhood stressors such as entrance to school and death of a pet. Tables 7-10 to 7-13 are useful for assessing the amount of stress a child is experiencing. Six factors affecting adaptation have been identified; knowledge of them provides the groundwork for assessment of the child experiencing stress.

Assessment of the child experiencing stress and crisis

Accurate assessment of the child who is experiencing stress and crisis is essential because if the helper can rapidly identify the problem and interrupt maladaptive behaviors, establishment of maladaptive patterns or physical damage can be avoided. Four areas of assessment of the child experiencing stress are (1) current reactions to the stressor, (2) significance of the stressor, (3) availability of help, and (4) previous coping strategies (Murray et al., 1979a). Specific assessment questions are suggested for each category.

Current reaction to the stressor

1. What is the child feeling?
2. What is the child's anxiety level? A child in crisis is likely to be open about his feelings of anxiety and dread when confronted with a trustworthy helper (Chapters 10 and 11).
3. Are symptoms present? If the child has symptoms, the school nurse should be alert for initial signs of stress response: muscle tension, perspiration, nausea, pallor, and tachycardia (Table 9-1). Illness sometimes indicates a psychosomatic response to anxiety. Children have little control over their environment, and illness is one method by which they can exert control (Jasmin and Trygstad, 1979).
4. Is the child suicidal or homocidal? The school nurse should ask clear, direct questions if she suspects suicide or homocide as a possibility; for example, "Are you considering suicide?" If the child communicates specific, realistic plans for committing either suicide or homocide, immediate action and referral are necessary.
5. What changes have occurred in his usual activities? When under stress, a child's pattern of activity may change; he may become withdrawn, for instance, because more and more energy is required by the stressor and unavailable for play or schoolwork. One stressor that is commonly known to result in a change in daily activities is chemical substance abuse.
6. Are verbal and nonverbal behaviors congruent?

Since children communicate largely through non-verbal behavior, any incongruence between what they say and how they act should alert the school nurse to possible conflicts. The first area of assessment therefore is the child's current reaction to his situation; the second area to assess is the significance of the stressor.

Significance of the stressor

1. How will the event affect the future? Death of a parent, for instance, will have a more profound effect on the child's future than temporary hospitalization of a parent.
2. How does the child interpret the stressor? A feeling of anxiety can distort perception; the child may misunderstand simple events, be unaware of his own abilities to solve the problem, demonstrate narrowing of the perceptual field by focusing on one detail or aspect of the problem, or may be unable to focus on any aspect of the problem.
3. Is the child's perception realistic? To determine if the child's perception is realistic, it is important to know what effect the change has already had and how it might affect future adaptation. The stressor may be causing problems for the child that are not readily apparent. Each child will place different importance on a stressor, depending on his perception of it.

Availability of help

1. Which family members and friends are available to help the child? It cannot be assumed that because a child has two parents that they are both available to the child in crisis. In highly mobile families, for example, parents are also affected by the move and may be temporarily unable to provide their usual support to the child because their own energy reserves are depleted.
2. What relationships exist between the child and his helpers? The quality of the relationship between the child and his support systems determines whether or not the child perceives them as available to help. A child whose older sibling continually hits him may not perceive him as a helpful support during a crisis.
3. What professionals are available and/or involved? The school-age child has many professionals available to assist him throughout the school system, such as teachers, nurses, counselors, psychologists, and social workers. The school nurse and teacher are responsible for appropriate referrals to these and other sources, making available to the student the professional help needed.

Previous coping strategies

1. What other problems has the child experienced? Before the school nurse can assess previous reactions to stress, she must determine what stresses the child has experienced. Some stressful experiences that most children encounter are entering school, death of a pet, and routine childhood illnesses.
2. How did the child solve previous problems? The school nurse can discuss with the child how he felt during a previous stressful event and what he did to make himself feel better. By building ongoing relationships with students, she can also learn through observation the child's approach to problem solving.
3. What does the child plan to do to solve the problem? Asking the child about his plans to solve the problem assists him to reorganize his thoughts, identify his strengths, increase his self-esteem, and begin the process of problem solving.

Intervening in stress and crisis

The goals of crisis intervention are twofold: (1) resolution of the crisis and return to the previous level of functioning and (2) improvement in the level of functioning and prevention of future similar crises (Fromer, 1979). The first goal is short term and the second is long term (and is more thoroughly covered in the discussion of prevention). The school nurse therefore helps students to adapt to their situation, either by altering the stressor or the child's response.

To assist the child in returning to his former level of functioning, the school nurse must first help alleviate some of the child's anxiety. One way to do that is to form an accepting, relaxed relationship with the student. Genuine expression of confidence and hope facilitates anxiety reduction. Children may feel better to know that their reactions are ''normal'' and expected in their situation. False reassurance, however tempting, should be avoided, since it increases anxiety. Coping mechanisms that students may use include denial, hostility (directed at the school nurse, others, or inwardly), and blaming others. Although sudden removal of these coping mechanisms increases anxiety, denial and blaming should not be reinforced. The emphasis of the helping relationship during the crisis phase is to reduce the child's anxiety. Within the context of this anxiety-reducing helping relationship are four basic steps of intervention: (1) identification of stressors, (2) identification of adaptive behaviors, (3) alteration of stressors and responses, and (4) evaluation of outcomes (Jasmin and Trygstad, 1979).

Identification of stressors

Step one, identification of stressors, allows the school nurse to determine what the student perceives as stressful. The real advantage of this step, however, lies in the student's increased self-awareness. His perception of the stressor may change from a vague concept to a specific, manageable problem. During this and the other steps of intervention, the student should also be encouraged to verbalize feelings because this may make the problem seem more manageable and reduces tension. When helping children to confront and identify their problems, it is important to allow them to set a pace at which they feel comfortable; forcing them to cope too rapidly increases anxiety feelings.

Identification of adaptive behaviors

Identification of adaptive behaviors includes previous coping behaviors, potential responses, and strengthening current appropriate responses. This step might include a brainstorming session. Both the child's internal and external resources should also be considered. A young child may need much direction during this step of the process. The school nurse can ask specific questions about previous coping behaviors, but since children are oriented toward the present time, they may have difficulty applying information about previous situations to current ones. Stories about children experiencing a similar problem, or playthings such as puppets and dolls are essential aids in communication.

Small children are not alone in their need for direction during a crisis. All people are open to suggestion at this time, and the school nurse who provides suggestions during the immediate crisis is a help to her students. Once the student's organizational capabilities return during the acknowledgment phase, the helper again facilitates the student's own problem solving. At this time it is also helpful if the school nurse identifies the student's current strengths, which might include seeking help, self-awareness, or previous successful problem solving. Identification of strengths increases self-esteem and thus releases adaptive energy for problem solving. After many possible solutions are identified, the nurse assists the child to choose which solutions are most likely to solve his problem.

This planning stage is most effective when all the consequences of each potential action are examined. An action will have consequences not only for the child, but also for his family, peers, and others. Predicting possible consequences and identifying unexpected outcomes help children make decisions.

In the process of identifying adaptive responses, it becomes necessary to determine if a given response is adequate. This requires the nurse and student to make an objective judgment. To reduce the subjectivity of judgments about the adequacy of adaptive responses, the University of Minnesota (1979) uses the following six criteria:

1. Is the response appropriate to the stressor situation?
2. Is the response appropriate to the individual's capacities?
3. Is the response likely to meet the individual's needs and goals or likely to conflict?
4. Is the response economical or wasteful of adaptive resources?
5. Is the response likely to precipitate other problems?
6. Is the response compatible with the welfare of others?

Using all of these criteria does not guarantee an objective judgment, but does provide a rationale for the decision. For individual situations additional criteria might be useful.

Alteration of responses or stressors

The third step of crisis intervention is to alter responses or stressors. This step may or may not require a change in life-style and/or values, but because it does require new behaviors, it is the most difficult step for the student. It is essential for the school nurse and student to agree on specific behavioral goals to accomplish. The child may need encouragement to accept help from others. The more support available to him during this time, the more likely he is to adapt successfully. During this step the child begins to gain control over his problem, a factor that motivates problem solving.

In addition to support, some general interventions for stress that involve relaxation have been identified in the literature. Because relaxation is the opposite physiological reaction to stress, its presence precludes the stress reaction. Several methods of achieving relaxation are meditation, biofeedback, and relaxation response. Benson (1975) found the relaxation response method results in decreased metabolic rate, decreased respiratory and pulse rates, and lowered blood pressure. Relaxation response is described here briefly as an example of altering responses to stress. To achieve the relaxation response as Benson describes it, the individual is instructed to (1) sit quietly and comfortably, (2) close eyes, (3) deeply relax all muscles, (4) breathe through the nose and say ''one'' at each exhalation, (5) continue for 20 minutes. A school nurse who uses any of these methods should be familiar with them and is referred to other sources for in-depth explanations.

Evaluation of school nurse intervention with stress and crisis

During evaluation, the whole intervention process should be reviewed. This reinforces problem solving, assisting the student to apply learning to the next situation he encounters. The goals and contract are reviewed at this time, and changes are made if necessary.

This approach to crisis intervention is based on a one-to-one relationship between the school nurse and student, but it can also be effectively applied to groups of students. For older school-age children the advantages of groups are that group members meet other children with similar problems, receive support from peers, offer suggested solutions, and are in an atmosphere in which verbalizing feelings is the norm (Fromer, 1979). Groups are especially helpful for dealing with specific problems such as alcohol abuse and dealing with loss through divorce.

Levels of crisis prevention
Primary prevention

The goal of primary prevention is to prevent a serious crisis from occurring. One method of primary prevention widely applied in the schools is health education (Chapter 15). By teaching children good health habits and maintenance of healthy bodily functions, poor health is avoided.

Another method of primary prevention is anticipatory guidance, helping a child with an expected developmental stage or situational crisis by discussing and planning for it before it becomes a problem. Timing is an important aspect of anticipatory guidance; children have little future orientation and if given too much advance warning of an event the child may waste adaptive energy on "false alarms." For example, a child is told that his mother will be entering the hospital for a few days and that when she does, he can visit her each evening; but he is told about the event 3 weeks in advance. Every time she leaves home, the child thinks she will stay away for a few days and experiences the fear of separation. When she finally does enter the hospital, his energy to adjust to the separation is at a low level. Through anticipatory guidance, the individual learns to adapt to life's events with growth and a minimal amount of "wear and tear," which is the goal of optimal adaptation (Selye, 1965).

Secondary prevention

Secondary prevention involves early detection of a crisis and assisting the child to adjust to the crisis, thereby preventing maladaptive behaviors. Therefore the school nurse must be aware of early symptoms of stress and crisis in children and observe children carefully for these symptoms. School nurses and teachers need to communicate frequently to detect problems before they become severe. Secondary prevention also includes early intervention with children experiencing stress, such as described in the discussion of intervention. Early intervention prevents complications of illness and promotes resumption of healthy adaptive patterns.

Tertiary prevention

Tertiary prevention occurs when the crisis has already precipitated maladaptive behaviors, such as school phobia, alcohol abuse, or depression; and its goal is to prevent further mal-

Table 9-3. Guidelines for school nursing of children experiencing stress or crisis

Factors affecting outcome	Data categories for assessment	Intervention	Prevention
Developmental stage	Current reactions to stressor	Identify stressors	Primary
Previous experience	Significance of stressor	Identify adaptive behaviors	Secondary
Perception of event	Availability of help	Alter stressors and responses	Tertiary
Culture	Previous coping strategies	Evaluate	
Support systems			
Number and chronicity of stressors			

adaptation and to restore adequate adaptive behaviors. Prevention of the following specific maladaptive behaviors is described in detail later in this chapter: school phobia, the seriously ill child, suicide and depression, substance abuse, problems of adolescent sexuality, delinquency, chronic diseases, and learning disabilities.

Table 9-3 summarizes guidelines for working with children experiencing stress and crisis.

THE EFFECT ON CHILDREN OF SEPARATION THROUGH DEATH AND DIVORCE
Definition and scope of the problem

Jasmin and Trygstad define separation as "a voluntary or involuntary, temporary or permanent situation in which the attachment figure becomes inaccessible" (1979:84). Separation is more difficult to resolve if it is involuntary and/or permanent. The most important attachment figures or loved ones for school-age children are their parents; therefore the most significant separations for them are parental divorce and death.

The incidence of divorce continues to increase. In 1973, 1 million children were in families involved in divorce action; by 1976, the number of children under age 18 whose families were not intact had reached 20 million (Jenkins, 1978). It is estimated that one third to one half of marriages in the United States end in divorce (Fromer, 1979; Gordon, 1979) and that 60% of divorces involve children. Death of a parent, on the other hand, affects fewer children than divorce; Fredlund (1977) estimates one in twenty school-age children experience death of a parent. To put these statistics into perspective, of 600 students in a hypothetical elementary school, approximately 30 will experience loss of a parent through death before they reach age 18, and about 100 will experience loss through divorce. These staggering figures indicate the

need for school nurses to help students adjust to losses in a healthy way.

Many authors have identified a predictable pattern of reacting to separation, whether through death or divorce (Kubler-Ross, 1969; Bowlby, 1973). Jasmin and Trygstad (1979) summarize this pattern by identifying three stages of reaction to separation: resistance, realization, and resolution. The stages are fluid, overlap at times, and are experienced differently by each individual, according to personality. The relationship of these stages to those of other theorists is outlined in Table 9-4.

The resistance stage is characterized by feelings and behaviors of denial, shock, and disbelief, a "this can't be happening to me" reaction. This stage is usually short, and sad realization begins to surface. The individual realizes it *is* happening to him, and reacts with depression and despair. Finally, resolution is reached. Adults may take a year to reach acceptance of the death of a loved one; children, on the other hand, grieve more sporadically and thus may take longer to resolve their feelings of loss (Sahler, 1978). It is only after this acceptance and resolution have been accomplished that the individual can form new relationships and thus experience growth.

The guidelines in Table 9-5 apply to children experiencing separation through either death or divorce. When necessary, distinctions between loss through death and divorce are noted.

Factors affecting adaptation to separation
Developmental stage

As discussed in Chapter 7, the child is only able to understand his loss at his current level of cognitive development. Some misconceptions about death that can be disturbing to children are that it is the child's fault, he might die next, sleep and death are related, and if the child wishes the parent to return, he will. The child who is separated from a parent through divorce

Table 9-4. Patterns of response to separation and loss*

Separation process	Bowlby	Kubler-Ross	Engel
Resistance	Protest	Denial Isolation Anger Bargaining	Shock Disbelief
Sad realization	Despair	Depression	Developing awareness
Resolution	Detachment	Acceptance	Restitution

*From Jasmin, S., and Trygstad, L.: 1979. Behavioral concepts and the nursing process, The C. V. Mosby Co., St. Louis.

may experience the same misconceptions (Moller, 1967).

Previous experience

Several authors (Sullivan, 1953; Bandura and Walters, 1963) believe that children learn to deal with separation from their early experiences of separation from their parents. For instance, the child who is given familiar toys and left with a loving caretaker for a short period of time will interpret separation as less distressing than a child left in a strange environment for several days. They believe that positive separation experiences help children with the separation-related task of entering school. The death of a pet may be the first time a child experiences loss through death; the nature of this experience will affect his future adaptations to loss.

Perception of event

The extent of the child's dependence on the lost parent also determines how he perceives his loss. Young children are highly dependent and react with concern about how they can meet their own needs without the help of the parent. Adolescents may feel much the same way, but are learning to be independent and are therefore less likely to openly display these dependency feelings (Nolan et al., 1979). If an event is expected, such as divorce and terminal illnesses, the child may begin to anticipate the separation before it occurs. This anticipatory grief can facilitate adaptation by helping the child achieve a realistic perception of the event.

Culture

Most religions and cultures have beliefs and rituals concerning death that facilitate mourn-

Table 9-5. Guidelines for nursing children experiencing separation

Factors affecting separation	Assessment	Intervention	Prevention of inadequate adaptation
Developmental stage Child's concept of death changes with maturity; may have many misconceptions Previous experience Likely to be limited to death of pet or short absences from parents Perception of event School-age children worry about how they will be cared for in future; adolescents are less dependent on parents; whether loss is expected or not and preparation also affect perception Culture Religious and cultural rituals assist adaptation to loss Support system Loss affects stability of entire family; child experiences loss of major source of support Number and chronicity of stressors Separation from parent results in many changes in child's daily routine	Current reaction to stressor At what stage of grieving is child? How does child relate to remaining parent? Is child experiencing physical symptoms or behavioral changes? Significance of stressor Loss of parent is most significant stressor for children Availability of help Family may be unable to help child because of their feelings of loss Previous coping strategies Due to inexperience, may imitate parental coping strategies; children depend on adults for accurate knowledge	Identify stressors Loss may not be only stressor for child; other stressors such as increased responsibility, fear of death, as well as child's perception of stressor should be assessed Identify adaptive behaviors Assess how child's behaviors are working for him; being sick may allow child not to attend school and to gain attention Alter stressors and responses Teach about event, encourage verbalization, mobilize resources, and answer questions Evaluation Must be continuous throughout entire process and based on specific goals	Primary Death education, acceptance of variety of life-styles, factors associated with divorce Secondary Early identification and intervention including teaching as necessary and crisis groups Tertiary Avoid continued inadequate coping, that is, suicide and antisocial behavior, by referral and counseling

ers' adaptation. Schowalter (1976) asserts that children over age 7 should be allowed to participate in funerals to the extent that they desire. In this way, they too can benefit from the culture's adaptation mechanisms.

Support system

The school-age child's support system lies within the family structure. Events as traumatic as death and divorce affect the emotional stability of the entire family; the reaction of his parents partially determines the child's reaction to separation (Murray and Zentner, 1975a). If the surviving parent is unavailable to the child (due to emotional reaction or the belief that children are too young to understand), the child may experience loss of his entire support system.

Number and chronicity of stressors

The school-age child depends on routines for security; the loss of a parent upsets many of his routines, including mealtime, discipline practices, and personal responsibilities. This kind of change in patterns requires energy and is therefore an added stressor for the child. The child in crisis may react by blaming or rejecting the remaining parent. In addition, if death is the result of a long illness or divorce occurs after a time of family upheaval, the chronicity of the stress is additive and drains the child's adaptive energy.

Assessment of the child experiencing separation
Current reaction to stressor

The child who has been separated from a parent will experience many feelings. The school nurse may want to assess which of the three stages of separation (resistance, sad realization, or resolution) dominates his feelings. Behaviorally, children may (1) withdraw and appear sad, (2) become boisterous in an attempt to compensate for the loss, or (3) appear to have no reaction (Fredlund, 1977). Children having difficulty coping may temporarily regress to an earlier developmental stage, as in the school-age child who begins wetting the bed. Others may react with hostility or idealization of the lost parent; physical symptoms are also common. Other grief reactions of children are fear of further losses, violent behavior, loss of concentration resulting in poor schoolwork, and vacillation between happy and sad moods. Adolescents are more likely to feel depression and exhibit physical symptoms than are younger children. All of

these symptoms, plus any other changes in behavior are part of the school nurse's assessment of the child's reaction to loss of a parent.

Significance of loss

Coddington (1972) states that loss of a parent is the most stressful event a child can experience. When loss of a parent occurs through suicide, the child is at especially high risk for maladaptation (Sahler, 1978). Teenagers have been known to imitate the suicide act, and younger children have much difficulty understanding suicide. Children who have experienced a parent's suicide can be expected to need more help and take longer to adjust to their loss than children whose parents die after a long illness or divorce after much strife in the home.

Cline (1978) states that the most difficult aspect of divorce for children to accept is the bitterness of parents toward each other. Children who are exposed to fighting may have more difficulty adjusting to the separation than those who have not been exposed to parental bitterness.

Availability of help

As stated earlier, family members may be unavailable to help the child because of their own grief reaction. For adolescents, peers may be a source of support at this time. The school nurse should let the student know she is available to talk about the loss, if he so desires.

Previous coping strategies

Children may not have experienced loss before and therefore must depend on what they observe and are taught by adults. If no explanations are offered, they may feel responsible or guilty over the loss. Because children develop quickly, previous coping strategies are likely to be inappropriate for their present age level. It is important to assess what separations the child has experienced in the past and how he dealt with them.

Assessment should be a continual process because the child's reaction to separation is constantly changing. The school nurse and teacher should work together, offering observations from their areas of expertise. The school nurse's assessment will help determine whether the child attends school and what arrangements are necessary to implement that decision. For a comprehensive assessment, the school nurse can make a home visit. When her assessment is complete, she begins intervention.

Intervention with children experiencing separation

The goal of intervention is for children to resolve the loss and to grow as a result of the experience; to accomplish this, children need to progress through the stages of coping with separation. The first step is to identify the stressors affecting the child.

Identification of stressors

Loss of a parent is an obviously stressful event, although the meaning and outcomes of this event will be unique for each child. A child who fears that he will also die is dealing with more than one significant stressor. The nurse should therefore assess what "theories" the child holds about death. Loss may mean for an adolescent that he will become the "man of the house" when his father leaves; this tremendous responsibility is a heavy burden for a teenager. Loss of family support for a child may be another stressor, as previously described. The school nurse or other helper must understand the event as the child perceives it, or intervention will be ineffective.

Identification of adaptive behaviors

The meaning of coping behaviors for the child must also be assessed before alternative responses are identified. Many children who are grieving the loss of a parent do poorly in school (Moller, 1967); this may be a very adequate coping response, since by spending less time on schoolwork they may be conserving energy required for maintaining equilibrium. A student's adaptive responses should be supported unless they are self-destructive (for example, refusing to eat or attempting suicide). Physical symptoms such as stomachache and headache are also common adaptive responses; therefore the school nurse should assess for physical signs of stress as well. By discussing his stress and responses with the nurse, the child becomes more aware of his situation. He may feel relief to know that his reactions are normal and expected.

Alteration of stressors and responses

Once the school nurse understands the student's perception and reactions to his loss, she is able to intervene. If the child harbors misconceptions, the nurse can provide accurate, frank explanations at a level he can understand. Answering the children's questions about separation and loss is another method of modifying the stressful event. However, before answering questions, the school nurse should determine exactly what the child is asking; for example, by asking, "What happens when people die?" the child may be asking for a philosophical interpretation, a physiological account, or for reassurance that someone will take care of him. It is important that all information given to children be truthful; fairy tales and stories intended to soften the impact of loss only distort children's perceptions, making adaptation more difficult.

The school nurse may assist the child by helping him identify alternative responses and mobilize resources. She may also suggest that the child resume more of his usual activities (assuming the child has withdrawn socially) or that he take care of himself physically by eating and resting adequately. The therapeutic value of listening and encouraging the child to talk about feelings should not be underestimated. If the child finds it is acceptable to talk about feelings, the need for acting out and other disruptive behaviors will diminish.

Evaluation

The school nurse continually evaluates the child's responses and stage of resolution of the separation, adjusting her interventions to coincide with the student's needs. By collaborating with others, such as the teacher and parent, the most effective methods of intervention for this particular child are identified.

Prevention of inadequate adaptation to separation
Primary prevention

Numerous sources identify the school as the appropriate setting for death education (Moller, 1967; Fredlund, 1977; Sahler, 1978). The purpose of death education according to Sahler (1978) is to (1) teach the social, biological, and practical aspects of death; (2) teach various ways to deal with death; (3) prevent unnecessary fears through this knowledge; and (4) promote discussion about death. This expanded knowledge base will provide children with more resources to use when faced with a loss and will help them to perceive events realistically. Fredlund (1977) states that children handle death in the family more easily if they have had "previous educational conditionings," including learning to talk about death and accepting the fact that it happens to everyone. Sahler (1978) identifies ten objectives for death education in the school and provides an outline for establishing such a program. The school nurse should take an active role in death education, since it helps prepare children for separation and thus prevents inadequate adaptation.

Another aspect of primary prevention is prevention of divorce. Gordon (1978) identifies the following factors as being associated with a high divorce rate: marriage at an early age (15 to 19 years), short courtship, short engagement, mixed racial or religious backgrounds, disapproval of family and friends, dissimilar backgrounds, and unhappy parental marriages. She suggests that discussion of these factors be a part of high school family living classes. Another aspect of primary prevention regarding divorce is the stigma and resulting stress that single-parent families often face. Education and tolerance for a variety of life-styles should be established, beginning with elementary school-age children.

Secondary prevention

Secondary prevention involves intervening with children experiencing separation. They should be identified as soon as possible because anticipatory guidance can help facilitate the grief process. The group setting is often helpful to children experiencing separation and has the advantages of emphasizing the normalcy of their feelings and providing a support system at a time when withdrawal and isolation are likely. When a schoolchild suffers a loss, his classmates should be told about it. This may be the ideal time to talk about separation as a fact of life. The other children can be more empathetic and supportive if they understand what has happened. Because of her expertise, the school nurse can provide consultation for the teacher and help with the classroom discussion.

Tertiary prevention

Tertiary prevention focuses on the child having difficulty with a loss. The nurse should assess for the presence of additional stressors. Difficult adjustment can lead to other problems such as failing a grade, acting out behaviors, physical illness, and even suicide. The school nurse's role in tertiary prevention includes case finding, intervention, and referral for counseling.

SERIOUSLY ILL CHILDREN IN THE SCHOOL SETTING
Definition and scope of the problem

Seriously ill children are those with life-threatening, incurable diseases like cancer. Al-
though the actual leading cause of death for children under 14 is accidents, cancer is the leading disease causing death in children below age 14 (President's Committee on Heart Disease, Cancer, and Stroke, 1968). Recent advances in medical science have led to longer, more productive lives for many children with incurable diseases; as a result, they spend more time in school. Some are hospitalized and return to school several times throughout the course of their illness. The goals of professionals working with these children should include assisting them to live as "normally" as possible; that is, they should be encouraged to do what they would normally do: attend school and participate in activities as their health allows. Cyphert advises that they be treated "as if they were going to live forever" (1973:215). For many children, remaining in school with a serious illness would not be possible without the creative interventions of a school nurse.

A serious illness creates many specific stresses for the school-age child: not feeling well, frequent hospitalizations, changing body image; even the medical regimen may be stressful. The school nurse intervenes as individual stressors arise, but must also consider the total effect of a chronically high stress level. This requires a wider scope than specific crisis intervention and focuses particularly on prevention of unnecessary stress to maintain the student at a functioning level. The focus of this discussion is therefore on the entire stress configuration for seriously ill children rather than a single stressful event. Table 9-6 summarizes guidelines for nursing seriously ill children in school.

Factors affecting the seriously ill child in school
Developmental stage

Developmentally, the school-age child is learning industry or to be independently ambitious and accomplish age-appropriate tasks such as schoolwork and physical skills (Erikson, 1963). An incapacitating illness can significantly impair the child's opportunities and ability to perform in both these areas, resulting in feelings of inferiority. It is important, therefore, for the child to continue to accomplish the appropriate developmental tasks within the limits imposed by the illness. Adolescents are concerned about identity formation and the future; it is a time for them to make marriage and career decisions and set personal goals. Often, in their zeal to accomplish these tasks, they are so idealistic that they do not believe in their own mortality

Table 9-6. Guidelines for nursing seriously ill children in school

Factors affecting ill children	Assessment	Intervention	Prevention

Developmental stage
  Determine cognitive maturity; school-age children are in stage of industry versus inferiority; adolescents are planning for future
Previous experience
  Length of illness, previous history of seriously ill children in school
Perception of event
  Very ill children may know of impending death even if they have not been told; perception also depends on age, religion, and perception of significant others
Culture
  Culture influences attitudes toward illness and death as well as attitudes about role of children
Support system
  Family experiencing grief; many parents divorce after death of child; school can be support system for child
Number and chronicity of stressors
  Length of illness and other special problems such as divorce and adoptive status contribute to stress
	Current reactions to stressors
	  Assess both child and family, stage of grieving, nonverbal and verbal language, physical symptoms, basic health
	Significance of stressor
	  What changes has illness caused in family routine? Does child fear rejection as result of illness? Would attending school reduce or increase stress level?
	Availability of help
	  Parents, classmates, teacher, friends, extended family, role of school nurse
	Previous coping strategies
	  Physiological status, how child deals with setbacks, changes that have occurred due to illness, flexibility of family roles, how family deals with knowledge of illness, current stage of acceptance
		Identify stressors
		  Possible stressors include treatments, appearance, physical and cognitive abilities. Would school increase amount of stress?
		Identify adaptive behaviors
		  Current emotional and physical adjustment of student and family is considered; stage of acceptance determines type of intervention
		Alter stressors and responses
		  Include classmates in teaching, maintain support system, alleviate stressors in school as possible, facilitate coping with difficult aspects of illness, maintain liaison role with other professionals
		Evaluation
		  As needs of child change, constantly evaluate and alter as necessary
			Primary
			  Teach classmates about illness and death; allow them to ask questions and begin grieving; teacher and school nurse work together to recognize and deal with own feelings; team approach; teach faculty about health-related student needs
			Secondary
			  Identify stress reaction early to minimize unnecessary energy consumption and alternatives to school attendance
			Tertiary
			  Complete grieving; attend funeral; talk to students about death; communicate with public health nurse; make other appropriate referrals

and may take unnecessary risks, such as riding motorcycles and not using seat belts, to affirm their invulnerability. The adolescent cannot afford to think about his own death because he has much to lose if he should die. Strong use of denial is therefore common among teenagers faced with their own death (Jasmin and Trygstad, 1979).

Previous experience

The duration of a child's illness affects how well he adapts to it. Although not all children who experience a long-term illness reach the acceptance stage, a sudden, short disease course makes it more difficult for the child and family to reach acceptance because there is less time. On the other hand, for some adolescents, the frustration caused by a long-term illness makes acceptance impossible. Experience can help children cope with the changes they face; a young child will be less fearful about a second hospitalization if the first one was a pleasant experience.

A school nurse and faculty who have had

experience in working with seriously ill children in school can help students adjust to their illness. As the prevalence of seriously ill children in the schools continues to increase, the professionals involved will need to develop routines that can be individualized to meet the specific needs of these children. With experience, professionals will also be able to resolve their own feelings about this emotional issue. In these ways, professionals are becoming better prepared to help students who are seriously ill.

Perception of event

Students' perception of their illness also affects their adaptation. Waechter's (1971) study demonstrated that most seriously ill children know they will die, even when they have not been told. For school nurses, this emphasizes the need to assess the child's perception of his situation and his perception of death, not relying on what records show he has been told.

Parents' feelings regarding the child's illness influence how the child views his situation; for example, parents who react with fear may increase the fear of their children. The school nurse is also an influential person for the child; her accepting, matter-of-fact attitude can help children gain a realistic perception of their situation by decreasing anxiety. Other factors affecting children's perception are age, religion, and degree of illness. A very ill child may be in the exhaustion phase of stress and unable to perceive realistically due to lack of available energy.

Culture

Culture is another factor that strongly influences the adjustment of children and families to serious illness and death. The views of a few selected cultures and religions and their effect on adaptation are discussed in Chapter 8. Death of children involves more than cultural attitudes about death primarily because children are not expected to die. Cultural views about the importance of children, therefore, must also be assessed. Some cultures place a high value on children; for them the loss may be greater than for members of a culture that regard children as less valuable than adults. In cultures where children are expected to do a portion of the necessary daily family maintenance chores, for instance, the adjustment to a serious illness will involve a different focus than in a culture where children are considered dependents for whom parents take responsibility.

Support system

When children are seriously ill, the entire family experiences grief. Although parents honestly want to help their ill children, at times their own grief interferes. Perhaps their grief becomes overwhelming and they temporarily cannot cope, or their grief results in a distorted perception of the situation. Although other examples could also be described, the point is that the child's natural support system, the family, will not function optimally when experiencing grief. The school, including teachers, peers, and the school nurse, is an important support system for the seriously ill child. Children need the support of this network throughout all phases of illness, whether they are in school, hospitalized, or homebound.

Number and chronicity of stressors

Achievement of tasks of their current developmental stage is a stressor for seriously ill children. Length of illness is another stressor because illness requires energy. When the child is faced with an illness, other aspects of the environment such as divorced or adoptive parents may become stressors (Gyulay, 1978). A child of divorced parents must deal with feelings of rejection by a parent at a time when the child needs that parent very much. Even if the divorce happened in the past, the present crisis may reopen the previous crisis for the child. Adopted children may experience a repeat of the crisis of rejection by their biological parents. Older children may want to find their biological parents before they die, a wish that has potential for creating stress within the family. Twins are another factor that can become a stressor when illness ensues. It is extremely difficult for children to adjust to death of a sibling, but the emotions become even more complex for both parents and child when the sibling is a twin.

Any change in routine and/or environment is stressful for children. The cycle of moving from hospital to home to school and the differing expectations in each setting are stressful for a child. From an adaptation theory perspective, it is often less stressful for a child to remain in school than to stay at home. The seriously ill child has a complex of stressors at a time when his natural energy resources are low due to physical illness. The thoughtful school nurse will assess each situation individually and comprehensively, identifying the complex interactions of the many variables that affect each seriously ill child.

Assessment of the seriously ill child
Current reaction to stressor

Before intervening with seriously ill children and their families, the school nurse carefully assesses their current behaviors, including the stage of the grief process within which they are functioning. The school nurse should assess the grieving process of each family member individually because children tend to grieve more slowly and erratically than adults; therefore the child and his family may not be in the same stage of grief (Sahler, 1978). As mentioned in the previous discussion about loss, experiencing grief is not a linear process, so the nurse must continually assess the individual's reactions.

Children often express their concerns nonverbally, and the school nurse should carefully assess their behavioral messages. School phobia is a symptom that may appear in a seriously ill child, due to fear of the potential embarrassment his illness may cause (Gyulay, 1978); an example is a child whose drug therapy causes vomiting or alopecia. The parents in this case may overprotect the ill child, thus encouraging the school phobic response. Even the teacher may feel relief at not having to cope with the problem of the child in the classroom, thus indirectly contributing to the school phobia. The school nurse must carefully assess the needs of such children, including the need to have peer group support, to lead a normal life, to obtain adequate rest, as well as the need not to be different from the other children. In this example, one solution might be to alter the stressor by allowing the child to sit by the door and go to the bathroom when necessary. Teaching other children about the child's special needs can reduce stress because they can be supportive. This solution also allows the child to continue to learn to face and adapt to life events. The school nurse helps the family and other professionals decide whether or not the child can and should remain in school. In making this decision, the child's physical and emotional health and energy levels must be considered, in addition to the special arrangements that must be made.

Significance of stressor

A life-threatening disease is obviously a stressor of significance for school-age children and their families. Children may interpret their disease as a cause for parental rejection, a highly stressful event for children (Coddington, 1972). Therefore if a child fears parental rejection as a result of illness, the illness acquires a doubly stressful significance. A long-term serious illness also causes many changes in such daily routines as individual chores, roles, and mealtime, thus compounding the stress. For each student and family the school nurse must assess the particular stressors and their significance, but for any family, impending death of a child is one of the most traumatic events that can happen.

A seriously ill child attending school can also be a stressful event for teachers, administrators, the nurse, and the child's classmates. Extra time and special planning are necessary to assure the student a favorable environment. School-based professionals must also determine their values and state realistically at the beginning of the planning process what they are willing and able to offer to ill children. By discussion and team planning, the interdisciplinary team members are able to support one another as well.

Availability of help

The child's most likely resources are parents and family members, peers, teachers, and the school nurse. For the parents, resources such as friends, the extended family, and the community are vital. The school nurse can be a resource for parents through her frequent conferences with them for support and planning and by making home visits and assuming a liaison role. Many cities have various support groups, such as the Candlelighters, for families with a seriously ill child. These groups can provide a special type of support to parents because all members are experiencing similar problems. The larger and stronger the support system for the family and child, the more likely they are to make successful adjustments to their situation. The school nurse, therefore, should assess and mobilize all potential resources.

Previous coping strategies

In addition to support systems, previous coping strategies also influence the child with a serious illness. Previous coping strategies include the family's usual reaction to illness of a member. The school nurse should assess the following areas:

1. Are the family roles flexible, so they can accommodate an ill member?
2. How has the child responded to illness in the past?

3. Has the family or child experienced loss before?
4. A child with a serious illness experiences many setbacks; how has he handled them in the past?
5. What personality traits can be strengthened to facilitate coping?

It is also valuable to assess how the family and child reacted to the initial knowledge of the illness. Describing the sequence of events is often therapeutic for the family and helps the nurse determine usual coping mechanisms and their current stage of acceptance.

Intervention with the seriously ill child in school

Many of the factors about helping relationships discussed previously also apply to the seriously ill child. It is especially important when working with seriously ill children that the school nurse retain a natural affect; that is, that she not be overly cheerful or gloomy.

Another aspect of school nurse intervention for seriously ill children is determining whether or not they should remain in school. Many authors defend the position that children should stay in school as long as they are able to do so (Cyphert, 1973; Kaplan, 1974; Kirten and Liverman, 1977). The school nurse plays an important role in the accomplishment of this goal by helping to decrease the emotional and physical stress of the school setting. To accomplish this, the school nurse assesses the stressors the child has in his present setting and the potential effect of the school setting.

Identification of stressors

Some specific items to assess are as follows:
1. Physical strength. Can the child participate in physical activities? What changes in structure or schedule can be made to conserve energy?
2. Appearance. Does the disease affect the child's appearance and is this stressful?
3. Need for and effect of treatments. Does a particular medicine cause stressful reactions such as nausea or confusion? Is it possible to provide the treatments in the school setting?
4. Emotional aspects of school attendance. Does the child or parent view school attendance as stressful? On the other hand, is the isolation of not attending school stressful?

The child's needs will constantly change, and the school nurse and teacher must continually assess the stressors in the school environment. While some of this information can be gathered from careful observation, it is also appropriate for the school nurse to ask the child how he feels, how things are going, and to offer assistance. By being open to the child's perspective, the school nurse is more effective in reducing the child's perceived stressors.

Identification of adaptive behaviors

The school nurse should also assess the child for physical and nonverbal reactions to stress, such as pale, cool, clammy skin, palpitations, dilated pupils (Table 9-1), depression, decreased cognitive ability, and decreased frustration tolerance. If the school nurse or teacher identifies any of these or other adaptive behaviors, she then needs to assess which stressor is causing them.

In addition, the school nurse may wish to talk to the student and parents to determine potential adaptive behaviors. A child who is weak due to surgery, for example, may be able to attend a half day at school before attending all day; likewise, a child who has responded to past setbacks as a challenge has the potential to do so again.

Alteration of stressors and responses

The biggest task for the school nurse is to assist the student and family in dealing with stressors when possible. The child and family will cope best if their support system is functioning optimally. Since the school is part of that support system, it is important for the school nurse to stay in touch with the family even if the child is not currently attending school. During home visits, the school nurse can assist in planning for future school attendance, thereby offering anticipatory guidance as well as maintaining a supportive relationship with the family. Classmates of an ill child can provide peer support by visiting, calling, or sending cards to their friend. This helps the child feel like part of the group, makes reentering school easier, and maintains the child's support system.

Stressors can be altered by teaching classmates the nature of the illness; with this understanding, instead of teasing the ill child, they may offer their help. If physical activity is a stressor, the child might carry out another "special" task while the other children have gym class (Gyulay, 1978). Overprotection and too many special rules may cause stress by emphasizing the child's differences. Ill children should continue to follow the rules, unless the rules pose a health hazard for them. By maintaining rules and discipline, the child feels secure and part of the group. In addition, peers are not so likely to tease if the child is not overprotected by adults.

If attending school is a stressor, alternatives may be found. Cyphert (1973) suggests a combination of school and home study; under this plan, children can attend for a portion of the day, thus maintaining a routine and support system. Even if a child is completely homebound, schoolwork can be accomplished if teachers, parents, and other students cooperate.

In addition to altering stressors, the school nurse may assist the seriously ill student to alter his responses. After assessing the child's current reaction to his illness, the school nurse selects appropriate interventions. During the resistance stage of reaction to crisis, the student needs an empathetic listener to help sort out his feelings and begin to realize his circumstances. Privacy is an important aspect of the helping relationship at all times, but especially for the ill child. As emotions become intense, the student may express anger and protest. The school nurse can help by reflecting, clarifying, and summarizing feelings expressed. She can also confront the ill child when he is unrealistic, if the confrontation is done in a gentle kind manner. The school nurse should not feel personally attacked by the feelings expressed, but should remember that the student has a right to feel angry and does not intend to offend the helper. As the second stage, sad realization, is entered, the student will show signs of depression; he may lose his appetite, appear lethargic, and withdraw from friends. At this time, the emotional support of the helper is vital, since the student may not feel as overwhelmed if he knows someone will help him when he needs it. This support also facilitates his entry into the third stage: resolution. In this stage the student begins to solve his problems and needs the nurse to provide information, assist in decision making, and discuss the nature of the situation.

Another aspect of altering stressors and responses for the school nurse is assuming a liaison role between hospital caretakers and school administrators. She is uniquely suited to this role because she is knowledgeable about the possible health needs of the child and is situated in the school setting. This role requires interpreting medical needs and maintaining communication to reduce the total amount of stress to a level that permits optimal functioning.

Evaluation

The school nurse must continually evaluate both the student and her interventions because student's needs are specific and variable. Attending school may decrease stress at one time and increase it at another.

Prevention of problems of adaptation for the seriously ill child
Primary prevention

Prevention of unnecessary stressors for the seriously ill child in school requires the education and awareness of those who will work with him. The school nurse can teach faculty and students about the illness and about the child's likely feelings when returning to class: that is, the fact that he might tire easily or look different. Students should be able to ask questions and get clear answers, which may relieve their fears regarding their own potential for illness and death.

The school nurse, faculty, and others must be aware of their own feelings regarding seriously ill children. Impending death of a child is an emotional strain, seems "unfair," and emphasizes human mortality. Resolving these feelings helps professionals avoid two pitfalls: either becoming overinvolved or avoiding the ill child altogether. As a health care professional, the school nurse has had experience with and education about adjusting to grief and the dying patient. Teachers, however, may feel unqualified to deal with these issues. The school nurse can therefore be a resource for faculty, initiating anticipatory guidance and resolution of feelings, thus preventing the child from experiencing additional stress.

Secondary prevention

The school nurse practices secondary prevention by early identification of stress experienced by ill children in school. To do this, the nurse applies her knowledge about (1) stress and crisis, (2) the child's illness and treatment, (3) growth and development, and (4) the child's usual coping patterns. She can alert teachers to danger signals and confer with them frequently about the progress and needs of an ill child. Communication with the family is also an important part of secondary prevention and includes planning and educating them about symptoms. If the stress of attending school has become too much for the child, the school nurse can assist the family to plan alternatives. She may confer with the public health nurse regarding the family's needs.

Tertiary prevention

If a school-age child dies, the school nurse still has a role in prevention. She may be the one to talk to the classmates about death. Assessment and early identification of stress reactions among siblings and peers is another aspect of tertiary prevention. It is appropriate for school professionals to attend the child's funeral if they so desire and to maintain contact with the family. At this time, the school nurse with a public health background may refer family members to other professional helpers to help them reestablish their lives. Families need to know that the school nurse cares about them as well as their child. Although prevention of most serious childhood illnesses is not technologically possible, the school nurse has a vital role in the prevention of the unnecessary stress that often accompanies such illnesses.

SUICIDE IN SCHOOL-AGE CHILDREN
Definition and scope of the problem

Suicide is the act of killing oneself intentionally. This discussion includes attempted suicides and actual suicides. Children are most likely to commit suicide when they are experiencing depression following a crisis (Table 9-2). (Those few cases in which suicide is a response to a terminal illness are not discussed here.) In 1976, 2000 children committed suicide in the United States; of these, 200 (10%) were under age 14 (Timnick, 1978). Among adolescents, suicide is the third leading cause of death (Murray et al., 1979b). Adolescent suicide has been increasing; in 1957, the rate was 4 per 100,000, but by 1975 it had risen to 12.2 per 100,000 (U.S. Division of Vital Statistics, 1976). These figures are considered underestimates because many suicides are unreported, considered accidents (such as traffic deaths and drug overdoses), or are not reported as suicides by parents and physicians. Rohn's (1977) study found that a number of children who attempted suicide also had minimal brain dysfunction, a circumstance that puts further limits on potential problem-solving capabilities. The school nurse must not overlook these and other factors. Because of the scope and seriousness of this problem, the school nurse needs to identify potential suicide victims and be active in prevention. Table 9-7 summarizes guidelines for helping children considering suicide.

Factors affecting suicide
Developmental stage

As indicated in Chapter 7, developmental stage and age determine a child's ability to comprehend death and its permanence. Often a child commits suicide in an attempt to visit a loved one who has died (Siemon, 1978). Adolescence is characterized by change and conflict. Adolescents are striving to be like their peers, but also want the love and affection of their parents. Their need for belonging is so intense that perceived lack of acceptance can be unbearable (Hart and Keidel, 1979). Marthas-Sampson (1978) states that when an adolescent has many stresses in a short time, weakened impulse control may contribute to a disturbed thought process, leading to suicide.

Previous experience

The problem that leads a child toward suicide might be the first significant problem with which he has had to cope; therefore he has no previous experience with solving difficult problems. In addition, people who have attempted suicide have a higher risk of death by suicide than the general population, especially during the first 5 years after the attempt (Paeregaard, 1975). If the child's parent committed suicide, the risk of imitation exists, especially for adolescents (Sahler, 1978).

Perception of event

Often, children who commit suicide are depressed, and depression itself can distort their perception of their situation. Symptoms of depression in school-age children include anger, school avoidance, physical complaints, sadness, and withdrawal. Symptoms of depression in adolescents are more difficult to observe due to frequent mood changes; they include apathy and inactivity, loss of appetite or excessive eating, insomnia, tearfulness, withdrawal, as well as sudden behavior problems such as stealing (Renshaw, 1974). Poor self-image and helplessness accompany depression at any age and affect the objectivity with which stressors are perceived. Isolation is another feeling most suicide victims sense and is a danger signal. If a child feels isolated, he may believe that no one

Table 9-7. Guidelines for nursing suicidal children

Factors affecting suicide	Assessment	Interventions	Prevention

Developmental stage
  Child may be too young to understand that his death is final; may want to "visit" someone who has died
Previous experience
  Young age of child may indicate lack of experience dealing with significant stressors
Perception of event
  Depression may cause poor self-image and feelings of helplessness, leading to distorted perception of stressors
Culture
  Three times more boys than girls actually commit suicide; 70% of victims under age 15 are American Indians (Spector, 1979)
Support system
  Of victims in one study, 59% were from single-parent families (Rohn, 1977)
Number and chronicity of stressors
  Poor school work, alcoholic parent, and depression are associated with suicide
	Current reaction to stressors
	  Reactions may include truancy, disrupting class, behavior change; determine if suicide is imminent danger (if attempt has been made)
	Significance of stressor
	  Death of parent and divorce are common stressors
	Availability of help
	  If family problem exists, assess capacity of family to help child
	Previous coping strategies
	  History of self-destructive behavior, such as previous suicide attempt or alcohol or drug abuse, increases risk of future suicide; assess strengths to build on
		Identify stressors
		  Loss and separation are important stressors for children; identify stressors from child's perspective
		Identify adaptive behaviors
		  How are child and family currently coping and what potential do they have for future? Do not expect children under stress to cope as adequately as before stress began; in one study, many suicidal children also had minimal brain dysfunction (Rohn, 1977)
		Alter stressors and responses
		  Need for referral? Assist child to try new behaviors, provide hope, build self-esteem
		Evaluation
		  Is child free of suicidal intentions?
			Primary
			  Mental health education to promote adequate coping mechanisms; death education to improve knowledge about death; respond to minor clues of stress reaction
			Secondary
			  Crisis intervention; early detection and treatment of potential victims; coordinate helpers; provide support
			Tertiary
			  Assist children who have attempted suicide to reassimilate into school; focus on survivors of actual suicide victim

would mourn his death, and suicide becomes a possibility.

Culture

Suicide rates among races and cultures vary little, with a few exceptions. American Indian children commit an extremely high percentage (70%) of the suicides of children under age 15 (Spector, 1979). According to Shore (1975) the suicide rate among American Indians varies by tribe. Factors contributing to this high incidence include breakdown of traditions, unemployment, alcoholism, and unstable family relationships. In the general population, boys commit suicide at a rate three times that of girls, perhaps because it is more culturally acceptable for

boys than girls to demonstrate violence (Marthas-Sampson, 1978).

Support system

Unavailability of support systems was a significant factor in Rohn's (1977) data from a sample of sixty-five attempted suicides by children. In 59% of Rohn's cases, the children came from single-parent families. Others have demonstrated a relationship between attempted suicide and extreme family conflict (Lindsay, 1973). Jacobs (1971) concluded that parental loss itself does not have a cause-effect relationship to suicide, but when combined with other stressors, parental loss becomes a factor. Family disorganization also contributes to reduced support system for the child. For the adolescent whose family lacks adequate communication (one form of family disorganization), acting out may be the only way to obtain love and recognition. According to Lukianowicz (1968), most children do communicate their inability to cope, either verbally or behaviorally; if their support systems are scanty or unable to respond, the child is more likely to make suicide attempts. In cases where support systems are inadequate, the school nurse may be the only supportive adult available to the child.

Number and chronicity of stressors

The number and chronicity of stressors are usually intense when a child considers suicide. Rohn (1977) showed that 31% of children studied who attempted suicide had at least one alcoholic parent, which is a chronic stressor that may lead to other stressors such as inconsistent family life and maltreatment. In addition, 75% had poor school records, 19% had failed at least one grade, and 35% were truant. These and other possible stressors need to be thoroughly assessed because stress has a cumulative effect. Tables 7-10 to 7-13 are valuable to the school nurse in assessing a student's existing stressors. The more prolonged the stress, the more depleted will be adaptive energy resources, and therefore inadequate adaptation such as suicide is more likely to occur.

Assessment of the suicidal child
Current reaction to stressor

Children's behavior often changes drastically when they become presuicidal. The following patterns of presuicidal behavior have been identified by Lukianowicz (1968):
1. Anxiety
2. Agitation
3. Depression
4. Irritability
5. Sleep disturbances
6. Sudden outbursts
7. Substance abuse

Some children begin acting out (for example, sexual promiscuity or drug abuse) as a method of calling attention to themselves and their problem. These children need to be identified and helped, not punished. Presuicidal symptoms lasting more than 2 weeks are danger signals (Renshaw, 1974; Timnick, 1978). Imminent suicide and the need for immediate intervention are signaled by (1) giving away prized possessions, (2) increasing moroseness and isolation, (3) statements of suicide intent, and (4) unexplained mood elevation. Some children talk of death and suicide, others do not. In a few cases, suicide appears to be an impulsive act (Lukianowicz, 1968).

When children make suicide attempts (broadly defined by Greer and Lee (1967) as deliberate, self-destructive, nonfatal acts), it is necessary to assess the seriousness of the intent. The student who makes a gravely serious attempt requires close surveillance and perhaps hospitalization, whereas the ambivalent victim may need counseling. Beck et al. (1974:54-56) developed a scale to assess seriousness of intent, which is partially reprinted as follows:
1. Timing and isolation of attempt, likelihood that someone would find him
2. Precautions taken against discovery
3. Attempt to get help (either before, during, or after the attempt)
4. Plans well thought out or impulsive
5. Communication of intent
6. Purpose of intent: removal of self from environment or manipulation of environment

Significance of stressor

The significance of stressors is viewed differently by children than by adults; therefore the significance of a child's stressors must be viewed from his perspective. According to Marthas-Sampson (1978), the presuicidal personality is often characterized by a "primitive perception of events"; that is, an event that the average student would perceive as normal or uncomfortable is perceived by the presuicidal student as devastating and cause for loss of self-esteem. The actual stressor that precipitates a suicide attempt may in fact be a minor event; however, it serves as the "last straw" for the presuicidal student with a history of crises and stress.

Availability of help

Availability of help has already been discussed as a factor affecting suicide. However, it should be noted that although the child may have help available, he must perceive it as help and as available to him. The school nurse who is accepting of students who have frequent minor complaints and/or who appear emotionally troubled becomes an available resource.

Previous coping strategies

Assessment of previous coping strategies should include use of drugs and alcohol and any previous suicide attempts. If a history of any of these self-destructive behaviors is present, a serious threat exists. If previous coping strategies include an emotional disturbance, referral to the school counselor or psychologist is appropriate. This assessment should also include the strengths and positive coping mechanisms used in the past, so the nurse can assist the student to build on these skills during his current crisis. Principles of assessment of the suicidal child are the same principles of crisis intervention discussed in Tables 9-2 and 9-3.

Suicide intervention
Identification of stressors

Suicide intervention is a specific example of crisis intervention, which was discussed generally in the beginning of this chapter. It is especially important that the school nurse remain nonjudgmental about the problem and the student's proposed solutions; judgmental comments may alienate the student from the nurse, who may be his last resource for help. It is important to restore the self-esteem of a depressed child, to involve him with others, and to show hope. Discussing the child's specific stressors compels him to perceive his situation objectively and decreases feelings of being overwhelmed.

Identification of adaptive behaviors

To determine the student's current adaptive process, the school nurse must ask specific questions about possible self-destructive actions the student may be considering. The nurse should not feel that she is suggesting suicide by introducing the topic; on the contrary, a child may fear punishment as a result of verbalizing his thoughts. He may, therefore, actually be relieved to have the nurse approach the topic and may feel free to discuss his thoughts and plans in this accepting atmosphere.

When working with a presuicidal student, it is vital not only to assess current adaptive behaviors, but also to consider alternative solutions to his problem. The nurse must judge how realistic the child's proposed solutions are for him at this time. If he is coping with several significant stressors, for instance, his usual coping strategies, although realistic at another time, may not be realistic now. The nurse should not expect too much from a child under stress, since high expectations court failure and further damage to self-esteem.

Alteration of stressors and responses

If a student is seriously threatening suicide, immediate referrals and plans should be made for his protection. These plans may include hospitalization, referral to counselors, or contracting with the student to contact a specific individual when he feels depressed; the contract may specifically state that the presuicidal student will not hurt himself.

Suicide intervention by school nurses includes altering stressors as perceived by the student. The most common stressors are sense of parental rejection (for elementary school-age children) and parental or peer rejection (for adolescents). Altering the student's responses to his stressful situation is the second half of intervention in a crisis, which, in this case, means assisting the student to deal in nonsuicidal ways with the sense of rejection. The school nurse can decrease the child's feelings of isolation by demonstrating concern for him. Just knowing that one person cares is often influential in preventing suicide. Reversing isolation is a gradual process; as an initial step, the nurse can encourage students to become involved with family, peers, and classmates. The school nurse should involve parents and teachers of a suicidal child in the treatment process, to help decrease isolation.

Evaluation

Evaluation, the final step of intervention, takes place at several times throughout intervention: the school nurse evaluates presuicidal students, intent of a suicide attempt, need for referral, and outcome of treatment. She must also constantly evaluate the behavior of children being treated, to determine effectiveness of treatment. Because those who attempt suicide have a high risk of future successful suicide, long-term follow-up is essential. In fact, these students may need anticipatory guidance for future developmental and situational crises to prevent coping by suicide.

Suicide prevention
Primary prevention

Caplan (1961) emphasized education as a means of suicide prevention. By teaching students of all ages about good mental health and ways of coping with problems, including asking for help before the problem becomes overwhelming, students will learn healthy adaptation and eliminate the option of suicide. Faculty may also be interested in an in-service discussion about suicide and recognizing presuicidal behaviors; they should be encouraged to consult with the school nurse if they identify a student displaying sudden behavior changes or other presuicidal signs. When students, educators, and parents are aware of early warning symptoms and how to get help, early detection and assistance to potential victims can be better accomplished.

Secondary prevention

Secondary prevention is early recognition of potential suicide victims and prompt intervention. Stengel (1962) states that in most suicide attempts something is left to chance, so the possibility of prevention exists until the last minute. The school nurse must be constantly aware of symptoms of depression, isolation, anxiety, and other potentially self-destructive behavior. Persons involved with the student, including the teacher, counselor, parents, and school nurse, should meet to share information and discuss methods of treatment. Parents and teachers of a child who attempts suicide may feel guilt (Bloomquist, 1974), and the group can help to put these feelings into perspective and provide mutual support, allowing them to resume their helping relationship with the child. The peers of an adolescent who attempts suicide should likewise be involved in discussions about suicide and methods of coping. Adolescents tend to imitate each other; therefore one suicide may lead to others.

Often students who commit serious suicide attempts are treated in an inpatient setting. When they return to school, peers may react unkindly or suspiciously. The student must reestablish a peer group, as well as try new behaviors. The school nurse can be a liaison to the inpatient facility and provide support for the student during and after hospitalization.

Tertiary prevention

Hart and Keidel (1979) refer to activities after a suicide death as "postvention," the focus of which is on the survivors. Signs of disturbance in siblings and classmates should be assessed, and parents and friends will need support. Grief reactions can be facilitated through discussions and referrals if necessary.

SCHOOL REFUSAL AND HEALTH-RELATED ABSENTEEISM
Definition and scope of the problem

School refusal is a term that includes school phobia, which is a specific disturbance, plus other types of absences. School phobia is defined by Kahn and Nursten (1964:68) as, "a specific neurosis where anxiety is partly relieved by fixing it on to a single object [such as school], as an attempt to preserve intact the remainder of the personality." That is, the child wants to go to school, but cannot because he is afraid to leave home. The basis for this fear is varied and includes feelings resulting from magical thinking that his parents might leave or die while the child is at school. School refusal may also result when, due to the parents' insecurity and/or neurosis, children sense that their parents do not want them to leave home. Truancy, on the other hand, is not related to fear of leaving parents; in fact, often parents are not even aware of their child's frequent absences. Reasons for truancy may be that school is too difficult or not stimulating enough. Both truant and phobic children often malinger, exhibiting very real symptoms that bring them to the school nurse. The school nurse should be aware of the stressors that initiate these symptoms and direct her interventions toward alleviating the stress. The school nurse does not, however, have a role in monitoring attendance or in identifying nonhealth-related truancy.

Absenteeism is a large problem; in New York City alone, 200,000 children are absent from school each day (Fromer, 1979). Specific statistics regarding which of these absences were due to truancy are unavailable. Leton (1962) found an incidence of three severely school phobic children per 1000, and an additional seven per 1000 with mild forms of school phobia. In that survey, more girls than boys showed signs of school phobia, and a disproportionate number of the school-phobic children were from the upper socioeconomic levels. Absenteeism can cause long-term effects unless identified and treated early. Table 9-8 provides guidelines for the school nurse working with children who are frequently absent.

Factors affecting absenteeism
Developmental stage

Entering school is commonly defined (Duvall, 1971; Leonard et al., 1979) as a developmental crisis because it requires the child

Table 9-8. Guidelines for nursing children with frequent absences

Factors affecting school refusal	Assessment	Intervention	Prevention

Developmental stage
  Magical thinking may intensify fears
Previous experience
  Both child's experience and that of others are experiences for children; illness is viewed as only valid reason for not attending school; time away from parents helps children learn successful separations
Perception of event
  May have fears about leaving parents; may acquire parent's fears; may be bored or overwhelmed by school
Culture
  Affects perception of school: Mexican Americans, for example, place low priority on education; separation: some cultures encourage more independence than others
Support system
  Family patterns may encourage absence
Number and chronicity of stressors
  Absenteeism more common when combined with other stressors such as change in schools, parents ill at home, parental conflict
	Current reaction to stressors
	  Range may include no symptoms, pattern of repeated illness, panic attacks, vomiting, and generalized anxiety
	Significance of stressor
	  If related to fear, may be very intense; if patterns continue into adulthood, may cause employment problems
	Availability of help
	  Professional support services such as social workers, educators, counselors as well as nurses can be helpful to child; parents should be involved in treatment; child guidance clinics may also be available
	Previous coping strategies
	  Did crisis of school entrance lead to new and adequate adjustment?
		Identify stressors
		  Fear of school, other; discussion and identification of problem helps decrease anxiety level
		Identify adaptive behaviors
		  Assess both student and family; refer to "current reaction to stressors" for common adaptive behaviors
		Alter stressors and responses
		  May remove child from school for part of day or treat in boarding school; encourage peer relationships; alter responses gradually
		Evaluation
		  Long-term follow up of students is portant
			Primary
			  Educate population regarding normal growth and development and identification of problems in adjusting; prepare children for school; teach other professionals (educators, truant officers) about symptoms and prevention of school refusal, to increase number of referrals
			Secondary
			  Early recognition; distinguish fear-caused from social-caused absence; encouragement to stay in school and accepting attitude is important
			Tertiary
			  Prevent future complications such as absenteeism from work and job jumping

to use new behaviors to adapt. For the first time, the child must spend most of the day away from home, interact with a group of peers, meet the expectations of another influential adult (the teacher), and become a part of a social group. The age at which children first attend school varies; for some, the experience starts with nursery school at age 2½, whereas for others it begins with kindergarten or first grade at age 5 or 6. The age and developmental stage at which children first enter a school situation affect how they adapt to school; for example, although older children can cognitively understand that

their parents will return, younger children may not. A young child's magical thinking may intensify fears about separating from his parents. The natural ambivalence children have regarding their parents leads to occasional feelings of anger toward them; magical thinking results in the belief that these feelings could actually come true. Since children depend on their parents to a great extent, a conflict results, leading to an intense fear of separation or an inability to go to school or anywhere without their parents. The adolescent developmental stage in our society requires accomplishment of many tasks, including becoming independent from family; therefore if previous separations were not adequately handled, the adolescent crisis may lead to absenteeism problems.

Previous experience

In a case reported by Moller (1967), a child who had experienced the death of other children's parents developed a fear of his own parents' death and refused to attend school. The experience of another child was a factor in school refusal. Children learn at an early age that illness is the most acceptable reason for not attending school. Most often the symptoms that result are very real and therefore demand a comprehensive approach.

Another aspect of previous experience to be assessed is separation from parents prior to school entry. Some children are prepared for school separation by past experiences with successful separations; they have learned that their parents will return for them. For others, school entry may be the first experience away from their parents and is therefore a threatening experience.

Perception of event

As part of gaining a realistic perception of separation through experience, the child must perceive objectively both leaving his parents and entering the school environment. Some children, as noted, are afraid to leave their parents, while others may take on their parents' fears of separation. Some parents actually unconsciously encourage their children not to attend school by saying things like "you'll get hurt and then have to come home" (Davis, 1977). These parents have problems separating and may appear overprotective or dependent. Children's perceptions of school also affect their attendance. Thus children who are not sufficiently challenged at school may become bored and seek ways of avoiding school, including skipping classes and feigning illness. Children who are overwhelmed by school stimuli are also likely to avoid it; examples of this category include children with learning disabilities or a combination of other stressors.

Culture

Culture significantly affects school attendance. Some cultures highly regard education, whereas others, such as Hispanic Americans do not (Brownlee, 1978). Cultural beliefs about the importance of education may affect the child in several ways. For example, if a child from a culture that values school is unable to do well in school, he will experience a great deal of pressure and stress and may therefore avoid school. On the other hand, if education is not important to the child's significant others, it may not seem important to him either. The culture also creates the norms about separation of parents and children; in some cultures children must fend for themselves and be independent; in others their dependency on parents is encouraged. Thus culture as well as personality affect children's adjustment to school.

Support system

Davis (1977) states that families of school phobic children tend to show a similar pattern; the mother is often the dominant parent, and both parents may contribute to keeping the child at home. Often, neither of the marriage partners feels independent; they are therefore unable to meet each other's needs, with the result that the child is viewed as integral in keeping the family together. In this case, the child's support system encourages him to stay home, which may cause difficulty for the child in forming a peer support group. Children who skip school often cannot get help from their family because they are unaware of the problem.

Number and chronicity of stressors

The number and chronicity of stressors significantly affects the outcome of any crisis situation, especially school refusal. Several factors identified by Kahn and Nursten (1969) as commonly accompanying school refusal are (1) a change in schools, especially changing from junior high to high school; (2) parents' illness, during which children may stay at home to care for their parents; (3) susceptibility to emotional disturbances; and (4) failure of adolescents to work through problems of school and separation. If children who are having difficulty adjusting to school are not identified, the symptoms will continue and the child's stress reaction may reach the exhaustion stage.

Assessment of school refusal
Current reaction to stressor

School refusal can manifest itself in many different symptoms, ranging from no obvious symptoms at all to severe panic and anxiety reactions. Most common are patterns of absences, often related to psychosomatic illness. When school absence becomes a pattern, the school nurse needs to be alert to the possibility of school refusal.

Significance of stressor

Truant students who participate in antisocial activities instead of attending school may let those deviant behaviors become a life-style. Children who have a phobia about attending school, on the other hand, may develop a severe neurosis or psychosis if untreated. For these untreated school phobic children, avoidance of their problem becomes their coping mechanism, an obviously inadequate adaptation.

Availability of help

Assessment of availability of help includes the services within the school system such as counselors, social workers, and educators with whom the school nurse can consult and refer. The parents, of course, are a logical support system for the child and should be included in any treatment program. Many communities have specialty clinics for children having difficulty attending school. This is an ideal resource. The nurse should also determine what help is available within the classroom. Is the teacher responsive to the special needs of these children or do time and working conditions create too many barriers for the teacher to take an active role?

Previous coping strategies

The final area of assessment in previous coping strategies. For young children, experiences of separation from parents such as nursery school attendance and occasional use of babysitters can be assessed. If the school setting stimulates a fear response, previous coping with fearful situations should be assessed. For older children, strengths and weaknesses (such as whether or not they cry when their parents leave and degree of social interaction) in their adaptation to school entrance is an area for assessment. A pattern of illness is a coping strategy with serious consequences, because physical damage can result from psychosomatic illnesses. A thorough physical examination is necessary to determine the child's physical health. Children without real illnesses should be discouraged from using illness as a coping mechanism. Assessment includes considering all of the discussed items, as well as assessing the way in which each factor affects the child's adaptation to school.

Intervention for children with frequent absences
Identification of stressors

Two stressors have been identified as leading to school refusal: fear of leaving parents and fear or trouble with the school setting. The stressor may appear to be a superficial stimulus (Kahn and Nursten, 1964) such as undressing for a physical examination or fear of a class pet. Children might give verbal clues such as "Do I have to go to school today?" well in advance of a severe fear reaction. Anxiety, by definition, is a vague response to nonspecific stimuli (Freedman et al., 1972), which makes the school nurse's task of identifying the stressor difficult, but nonetheless important. Kahn and Nursten (1964) documented that in school phobic children with physical symptoms who were treated only for their physical complaints, the pattern of nonattendance increased. Therefore, quick, accurate assessment and referral are vital to successful treatment of school refusal. Identifying the stressor through discussion with the child is part of the first intervention step because it allows the child to verbalize feelings. Verbalization helps children to separate fact from fantasy, making the stressor more specific and real to them, thus decreasing the anxiety level and mobilizing adaptive energy from fear and anxiety to problem solving.

Identification of adaptive behaviors

The second step of intervention, identification of adaptive behaviors, assists the child and family to recognize the responses they have chosen to alleviate stress, such as refusing to go to school. This recognition may help (1) reduce the need for inadequate coping responses like malingering and (2) identify other, more adequate, solutions. As soon as school phobia is diagnosed, treatment should begin. Allowing the stress to become chronic also allows more time for children to form behavior patterns, increasing the difficulty of changing them.

Alteration of stressors and responses

Treatment of school phobic children is best accomplished through a team approach, each professional contributing her or his expertise and increasing the range of services available to children. The school nurse may be especially active in identifying school phobic children, referring and assessing physical and psychological development and illnesses.

Initial treatment may involve conserving

adaptive energy by removal of the stressor—school. A child might go to school only for counseling, with the promise that if he becomes anxious he will be taken home. Under this plan, time spent in school is gradually increased and the success experience is part of the motivation for the child (Moller, 1967; Clarizio and Mc-Coy, 1970). Others attempt to deal with the fear of separation by removing the child from the home for treatment, thus forcing as well as assisting him to deal with the fear (Davis, 1977). As a result, peer relationships are developed, often for the first time, and become an incentive to stay in school. Changing children's responses to school is a gradual process; the school nurse and other professionals must be patient and allow the child to progress at a comfortable pace because rushing the process destroys the established trust and increases anxiety.

Evaluation

The school nurse should collaborate with other health team members in evaluation of each student. This evaluation will provide information to improve future care for the child and for other children. Long-term follow-up is necessary to observe for psychosomatic illnesses and for difficulty adapting to future developmental or situational crisis.

Intervention for other types of school refusal largely depends on the cause. If a child is found to have a learning disability, individualized education programs may be useful. For adolescent truancy problems, the causes can be as variable as the number of truants. Truancy as part of a delinquency pattern is discussed on pp. 174 to 180.

Prevention of school refusal
Primary prevention

Primary prevention of school refusal involves preparing children for school before they enter. Some suggestions are teaching children their name and address, independence in self-care, and basic safety rules (Leonard et al., 1979). Parents may also need some preparation for this change in their daily patterns; the school nurse can discuss with parents, individually or in groups, their feelings about loss of control and the influence of school on their children. The group setting has the advantage of allowing interaction among parents with similar problems. Both parents and educators can be taught more about normal growth and develop-

ment to assist them in identifying children who are having problems adjusting to school. Other professionals, such as truant officers, might benefit from periodic in-service programs to assist them in recognizing school adjustment problems and referring them early.

Secondary prevention

Secondary prevention includes early detection of children with problems and distinguishing phobic children from others. When children with problems are detected early, they are more amenable to treatment. For some, encouragement may help them to stay in school and cope with their problems.

Tertiary prevention

Complications during adulthood of untreated school refusal are agoraphobia (fear of going out in open places), frequent absences from work, and frequent job changes (Kahn and Nursten, 1964). These complications can be prevented through treatment of the school-age child. When complications such as these begin during adolescence, referral to a counselor is appropriate.

THE SCHOOL NURSE AND THE DELINQUENT STUDENT
Definition and scope of the problem

Fredlund defines delinquency as "antisocial behavior that is beyond parental control and therefore subject to legal action" (1970:57) and discusses the difficulty of defining the line between social and antisocial behavior because society and its norms are constantly changing. The following discussion will define as delinquents those children and youth who behave in ways that are or will be likely to cause society to take action to stop them; these actions may include stealing, truancy, and violent acts such as murder.

The incidence of juvenile delinquency appears to be increasing, but statistics are imprecise because although many agencies collect information, a variety of definitions are used as the basis for data collection. In 1965, 697,000 cases were brought to juvenile courts (Clarizio and McCoy, 1970); in 1970, 70,000 teachers were assaulted in United States' high schools, and the cost of vandalism in the schools was $600 million (Fromer, 1979). Clarizio and McCoy (1970) report that 60% of delinquents commit their first offense by age 10 and that the incidence of juvenile delinquency increases with age until age 17 when it levels off. Juvenile delinquency has serious ramifications in the areas of safety within schools, costs to citizens, future health and life-styles of delinquents, and child abuse potential. Table 9-9 provides guidelines for the school nurse.

Factors affecting delinquency

Developmental stage

Most delinquents begin antisocial acts at an age when future orientation is minimal; thus their developmental stage has the effect of allowing them to be aware of only their present needs, which may include securing love and attention or being part of a group. The incidence of delinquency among girls is increasing, but the majority of delinquents are boys (Clarizio and McCoy, 1970). Adolescents are involved with the developmental task of sex-role identification; the traditional role for men is to be brave and daring, which encourages boys more than girls to achieve the developmental task in antisocial ways. Adolescents' rebellious attempts to achieve independence may lead

Table 9-9. Guidelines for nursing delinquent students

Factors affecting delinquency	Assessment	Intervention	Prevention
Developmental stage Lack of future orientation; sex-role identity occurring; adolescent rebellion against parents and/or society Previous experience Maltreatment by parents; school problems at early age Perception of event Personality characteristics may include impulsiveness, aggressiveness, and irresponsibility; emotional disturbance theory widely accepted Culture Violence may be part of subculture; urban areas have higher rates of delinquent youth; acceptability of aggression is culturally determined Support system Parental support usually rejected; peer group important Number and chronicity of stressors Unstable family, previous experience, poor school performance, physiological predisposition, and others serve as stressors for children	Current reaction to stressors Feelings of helplessness and powerlessness lead to loss of control, which causes anxiety; may control feelings of anger until tolerance limit is reached; evidence of chemical abuse, physical stress reaction Significance of stressor Depends on student's perception; may be real or imagined; violence may be result of buildup of many stressors Availability of help Predelinquent and delinquent children need professional help, support from family, and positive peer group affiliation Previous coping strategies Delinquent children may not have learned adequate coping strategies	Identify stressors School performance, unstable family, maltreatment Identify adaptive behaviors Direct: argumentative, verbal assaults, demanding, belligerent, manipulative, physically controlling, combative, violent (fighting, rape, homocide, suicide); indirect: forgetting, misunderstanding, procrastinating, lateness, failure to learn* Alter stressors and responses Chronicity of stressors creates difficulty in alteration, although individualized stressors or perception of them can be altered; responses can be altered through contracting, behavioral learning, modeling Evaluation Review of contract, evaluate perception of stressors, team collaboration	Primary Prevent child maltreatment; teach problem solving (decreases feelings of helplessness); anticipate student needs and assist in meeting them; nonaggressively, teach others about school nurse role in mental health; involve students socially Secondary Use prediction tests for early detection; teach and experiment with alternative responses to stressors; avoid labeling; provide crisis intervention centers Tertiary Group therapy, institutionalization, peers judge behaviors, former delinquents work with students who return to school

*List from Jasmin, J., and Trygstad, L. N.: 1979. Behavior concepts and the nursing process, The C. V. Mosby Co., St. Louis.

some to antisocial behavior. Delinquent juveniles fail to satisfactorily achieve the developmental tasks of their age group.

Previous experience

Although the adolescent developmental stage can precipitate delinquency, previous experience with violence is another factor that influences children's proclivity toward antisocial behavior. Statistics show that many children who commit delinquent and violent acts have been maltreated by their parents. King (1975) reports on nine boys who committed homicide before the age of 14; as children they had all either been beaten or lived in homes that condoned violence. In studies of adult murders, a high proportion (between 66% and 100%) had experienced constant and cruel abuse by their parents (Helfer and Kempe, 1976). Steele (1976) found 82 of 100 juvenile delinquents had a history of maltreatment—fully one half of these juveniles could remember severe maltreatment in the form of being knocked unconscious by a parent (Helfer and Kempe, 1976). In a 12-year follow-up study of maltreated children, 19% became juvenile delinquents (Alafro, 1976). According to Helfer and Kempe, parents of juvenile delinquents "showed more lax, unkind, inconsistent discipline with far greater resort to physical punishment" compared to parents of nonjuvenile delinquents (1976:20). Children learn through imitation, and aggressive children are "identifying with aggressive parents" (1976:21).

Another common factor in the previous experience of many delinquents is problems with school at an early age. The research of Glueck and Glueck (1952) compared 500 delinquent and 500 nondelinquent boys and found that many of the delinquent boys had had problems in early school grades. Clarizio and McCoy (1970) found that 90% of juvenile delinquents were truant, 70% had repeated two or more grades, and 67% were reading below the sixth-grade level.

Perception of event

Perception of environment is largely influenced by personality, and personality types of violent and aggressive people have been identified. Clarizio and McCoy (1970) state that the personality characteristics of impulsiveness, aggressiveness, and irresponsibility as demonstrated on the Minnesota Multiphasic Personality Inventory are associated with violence.

The youth may be rebellious, hostile, or unable to postpone pleasure. Emotional disturbance is a widely accepted theory of the causation of antisocial behaviors (Fredlund, 1970). The aggressive youth may therefore be misperceiving events or distorting reality (Jasmin and Trygstad, 1979).

Culture

Many authors describe the cultural influence on antisocial behaviors (Fyvel, 1962; Rubenfeld, 1965; Helfer and Kempe, 1976). Helfer and Kempe (1976) attribute the violent atmosphere of ghetto life to many violent acts, but according to Clarizio and McCoy (1970) the commonly held belief that violence is a lower class problem is debatable because middle class delinquency is largely unreported. Their studies demonstrate a higher rate of delinquency in urban settings than in rural areas. In addition, the cultural groups of Jews and Japanese have a low delinquency incidence compared to blacks, Mexicans, and American Indians. Clarizio and McCoy (1970) attributed the higher rates of delinquency among blacks to lack of male role models, emphasis on physical combat, and poverty. Breen (1968) has described the black subculture as "aggressive-expressing." It should be emphasized that the norms defining standards of acceptable and unacceptable aggression are culturally determined. Thus, aggressive behaviors, when viewed from the perspective of a street gang may not only be acceptable but also provide status. Kaplan (1972) has stated that persons raised in an environment accepting or condoning aggression are more likely to act aggressively when under stress; these people have learned through experience that aggressive behavior results in satisfaction of personal needs such as self-esteem or financial gain.

Support system

For the adolescent and preadolescent, peer group acceptance is important. Peers become the support group, parental support becomes secondary. Antisocial acts are often committed in groups. For some children, the need to belong is so intense that they participate in delinquent group acts to satisfy their need for belonging.

Number and chronicity of stressors

Clarizio and McCoy (1970) found that 50% of juvenile delinquents come from unstable or broken homes. Glueck and Glueck (1952) confirm these figures. Factors identified in unstable families that might lead to delinquent behaviors included (1) inadequate supervision, (2) erratic or overly strict discipline, and (3) lack of cohesiveness within the family unit. All of these factors may be stressors that contribute to inadequate adaptation in the form of aggressive behavior.

Other factors that increase the likelihood of delinquency include a poor school record and meaningless educational curricula. It has been documented that many delinquents have poor school records and high truancy rates; Clarizio and McCoy (1970) and others have considered the effect of the curriculum on these factors. Adult learning theory states that adults need to understand the potential application of material to be motivated to learn (Redman, 1980). However, in many cases, students remain unmotivated. It is postulated that life preparation classes such as budgeting and parenting would be motivating for some students.

Genetic factors might also be stressors, predisposing individuals to violent acts. Montagu (1969) discusses the theory that an abnormality of chromosome 47 is associated with antisocial behavior. These men have an extra Y chromosome, resulting in the XYY scheme. Another theory suggests higher than normal levels of androgen in delinquents, but the study is inconclusive (Helfer and Kempe, 1976). Organic brain disorders and seizures have also been associated with antisocial behavior (Johnson, 1972).

Many researchers have theorized about the causes of antisocial behavior, but most authorities tend to favor a combination of theories (Rubenfeld, 1965; Clarizio and McCoy, 1970; Fredlund, 1970). The school nurse therefore must be aware of the many factors that influence antisocial behavior.

Assessment of the delinquent and potentially delinquent child
Current reaction to stressors

It is important to assess not only juveniles who are already delinquent, but also those who have potential for becoming delinquents. Predicting delinquency is advantageous to the school nurse because it provides a basis for prevention. The school nurse should assess the feelings and actions of the student in a stressful situation, through interviews, direct observation, and role playing. Feelings that may result

in aggressive behaviors include a sense of helplessness and powerlessness in controlling one's environment. This perceived lack of control may cause an intense overwhelming anxiety, and the crisis reaction ensues, in an effort to control the environment, an impulsive student may use aggressive or violent behavior.

The young school-age child might show potential for violence by being easily provoked, appearing to seek confrontation, offering simple explanations for violent behavior and not seeming to understand why others are upset about it (Larson, 1978). Larson defines behavior patterns such as enuresis, fire setting, and cruelty to animals as potentially violent due to emotional disturbance.

The opposite reaction—not expressing anger—is also potentially violent. Students who tend to be controlled may suddenly become violent when their tolerance limit has been reached. Another common but inadequate reaction to stressors is abusing drugs and/or alcohol. Students who turn to drugs or alcohol when they are stressed have the potential for addiction, which is discussed separately. Violent behavior may result in abuse of these substances (Larson, 1978). Symptoms of the stress reaction, tachycardia, increased respiration, perspiration, pallor, and muscle tension (Table 9-1), indicate physically that the student is experiencing stress and should be considered a danger signal.

Significance of stressors

A delinquent student may behave violently at an unexpected time, seemingly with little provocation. His perception of his stressor may be distorted due to several factors: (1) buildup of several stressors, (2) cultural norms regarding aggression, (3) effect of drugs or alcohol, (4) impulsive personality or emotional disturbance, and (5) lack of security and warmth in family relationships. Whether the stressor is real or imagined is immaterial if the individual perceives it as threatening. When delinquency becomes an established behavior pattern, it is significant for society because of its antisocial character.

Availability of help

In exploring resources to help the delinquent and predelinquent child, the school nurse must assess whether or not the family is aware of the problem, and their feelings and responses to it. Ideally, the family would respond positively to seeking and participating in professional help; however, adolescents might not accept parental help. Peer group affiliation is another support system to assess. The student whose only friends are juvenile delinquents suffers potential isolation is he changes behavior patterns and therefore has no peer incentive to change. More professionals are needed within school systems to assist teachers to identify and work with predelinquent children.

Previous coping strategies

Children who behave antisocially are not able to respond in socially acceptable ways; this may be because (1) they have not previously learned adequate coping mechanisms, (2) the usual coping mechanisms do not work for them, or (3) antisocial behavior has been reinforced and therefore learned. The school nurse can assess how children have coped with stressors in the past and determine if previous methods of coping were appropriate. Perhaps for a delinquent child the stressors are too great for previously learned coping mechanisms to work, or perhaps the child learned that aggressive behavior was successful. According to social learning theory, aggression is learned through reinforcement (Bandura, 1973).

School nurse interventions for delinquent students

Identification of stressors

To assist students who behave delinquently, the school nurse must identify stressors as students perceive them. For many, emphasis by teachers and family on excellent performance in school is a stressor (Clarizio and McCoy, 1970). If a student feels unable to meet the expectations others place on him, stress may result. For others, constant worry about family stability may be stressful. The family is the main source of emotional support and identity formation for a young child; if his family is unstable, extreme stress is the result. The child may fear that no one will care for him in the future or that he is the cause of the family instability. Any disruptions in family relationships can produce a high degree of stress for children. Children who are maltreated withstand continual stress; they must always consider whether their actions will produce punishment. Many commonplace events may prove stressful to children with continual stress factors such as the three described. Other stressors are, of course, important to individual children. The three described (high expectations, family instability,

and maltreatment) have been demonstrated in the literature as common stressful factors experienced by delinquent children. It is important for the school nurse to determine what the student views as stressful before she begins identifying adaptive behaviors and patterns.

Identification of adaptive behaviors

Jasmin and Trygstad (1979) list behaviors of aggressive behavior as either (1) direct, such as arguing, verbally assaulting, demanding, being belligerent, manipulating, physically controlling, combating, and being violent or (2) indirect, such as forgetting, misunderstanding, procrastinating, being late, and failing to learn. When the school nurse observes a pattern involving these behaviors, inadequate adaptation is occurring, and it may be helpful to talk to the student about his behavior, of which he may be unaware. Awareness of inadequate responses is the first step toward identifying adequate responses. The nurse and student can together discuss alternative responses and their possible consequences. The delinquent student usually begins behaving antisocially in an effort to gain attention and recognition; if he can identify more acceptable ways of achieving this attention before it becomes an established pattern, treatment is more likely to be successful. Discussion of alternative solutions to aggressive behavior is especially successful in a group setting because students are not threatened and can learn from each other. Also, since adolescents are so influenced by their peers, the group is a powerful intervention approach.

Alteration of stressors and responses

Alteration of the stressors of unstable family life and maltreatment is a difficult and long-term process. Unless the school nurse has expertise in dealing with the identified stressors, referrals and the team approach are most valuable. If school performance is a stressor, the school nurse can help to alleviate the stress through discussions and consultation with educators and counselors. Perhaps the required course work is too strenuous for the student and should be changed. In conclusion, many chronic stressors are difficult to alter and are best treated through prevention.

Although many chronic stressors cannot be altered, the school nurse can assist the student to alter distorted perceptions of daily stressors. If the student views a particular teacher, for example, as threatening, two options are available. The student can be removed from the class or the student's perception can be changed through discussions and reinforcing reality.

The responses students make to the stressors they perceive can be influenced by the school nurse. In assisting students to try new responses, it is important to maintain the student's self-esteem because if self-esteem is threatened, he may return to aggressive behaviors that have enhanced self-esteem previously.

Aggressive behaviors are learned, and behavioral therapy is one way for the student to learn different responses. The school nurse and student may contract for a mutual goal, such as the student discontinuing physical fighting behaviors. Within the contract, the student identifies rewards and punishments for his behavior. The contract gives the student control and responsibility to change behaviors and can be used with other methods. Control and responsibility are not only motivating but appeal to the adolescent's sense of independence, helping him to achieve this important developmental task.

Modeling, or observing others, is another way new behaviors are learned (Bandura, 1973). Observation of others can occur when members of a group describe their behaviors, during direct peer observation, through movies and books, or in a number of other creative ways. If the school nurse assesses modeling to be an effective learning method for a student, she can incorporate it into her intervention.

Evaluation

Periodically the school nurse and student and other involved persons (family, teachers, counselors) review the contract and the progress made, discussing reasons for reaching or not reaching goals. This evaluation time is a learning experience for the student, and review of progress is a positive reinforcement for him. If methods used are not effective, new methods are tried; some students work better in groups than others, for instance. If, during evaluation, progress is not evident, consultation and referral should be considered. Because delinquency is a far-reaching problem, the team approach has been demonstrated to work well (Fredlund, 1970). The school nurse may be the one to initiate interdisciplinary case conferences. Her open communication with other team members is vital for comprehensive care.

Prevention of juvenile delinquency
Primary prevention

The most significant role of the school nurse regarding delinquency lies in prevention. Methods of prevention relate to multifactorial theories of causation; a combined approach is presented here. The most basic aspect of primary prevention is preventing child maltreatment, which is highly associated with antisocial behavior. A detailed discussion about preventing maltreatment of children is given on pp. 187 to 193. Another aspect of primary prevention involves curriculum additions such as teaching problem solving, teaching parents about care of and expectations for their children, and providing a variety of meaningful classes for older students such as vocational, family living, and sex education classes. Although the school nurse may not actually teach these classes, she can contribute valuable knowledge to the formation of curriculum objectives and be a resource person for faculty. Fredlund (1970) asserts that school nurses should see themselves and be viewed by others as an active member of the faculty. With this in mind, the school nurse can also teach the other faculty about her role in promoting the mental health of students. The school nurse should present herself as a concerned knowledgeable professional and attend meetings of parents and teachers and participate in other activities that will result in improved care and education for students. If teachers consult frequently with the nurses, together they can anticipate student needs and assist students to meet their needs without aggression. In accordance with social theory, prevention of juvenile delinquency includes involving the students in activities and preventing isolation. This involvement with others can be accomplished within the curriculum through creative means such as group projects.

Secondary prevention

Secondary prevention involves early detection of delinquency-prone students. Several tests are available to predict delinquency, none of which has impeccable validity due to the individuality of the problem. Three of the best are the Glueck Prediction Tables (Glueck and Glueck, 1950), the Minnesota Multiphasic Personality Inventory, and the Kvaraceus Delinquency Scale (Kvaraceus, 1953, 1956); on a less formal basis, children identified as troublemakers can be referred to the school nurse, who is perceived as a helper. Referral to the nurse helps maintain the child's self-esteem as opposed to punishment, which carries a negative connotation. Labeling a young child as a troublemaker can be a self-fulfilling prophecy. The school nurse can intervene early by assisting children to develop healthy methods of dealing with stress and can also work with teachers for early case finding.

By educating the faculty, parents, students, and general public about delinquency-prone behaviors, the school nurse encourages those who know individuals who need help to refer them before their actions become antisocial patterns. In addition to education, crisis prevention centers need to be available.

Tertiary prevention

Once a student has been identified as delinquent, the focus of tertiary prevention is to prevent delinquency from becoming a permanent way of life. Treatment of delinquency includes institutionalization, psychological therapy, behavior modification, and group therapy, to name a few. Recently it has become popular to include former delinquents in the treatment to add information about the realities of a life of crime. Although this is effective on a short-term basis, it has not been documented to have a long-term effect and is therefore used in combination with other treatments. Several states have decreased juvenile deliquency rates by using juries composed of teens for juvenile offenders. The school nurse becomes involved in tertiary prevention by assisting students to reassimilate into the school environment. She might maintain communication with them during treatment and participate on the team of helpers to ensure a smooth transition into the school environment.

CHEMICAL USE AND ABUSE
Definition and scope of the problem

Three of the most commonly used chemicals will be discussed here: alcohol, drugs, and tobacco. A *drug* is "a substance other than food that, when taken into the body, produces a change in it" (Barnhart, 1956:150). For the purposes of discussion, alcohol, cigarettes, and other drugs are considered collectively. *Drug use* includes both occasional and experimental use. *Drug abuse* has been defined as "the frequent use of any drug in excess or for the feeling it arouses" (Nolan et al., 1979:241) and as "the nonmedical use of drugs" (Henderlich, 1977:209). *Drug dependence* or habituation is the physical or psychological desire for continued use of the drug. *Addiction,* a more severe problem, refers to a state of drug dependence in which withdrawal symptoms occur if the drug is discontinued. Addiction is characterized by

drug tolerance, that is, "having to take increasingly larger doses to get the same effect" (Nolan et al., 1979:241). In the past, treating the individual as a criminal was common; however, this discussion will not include the legal issues, but will focus on the treatment and prevention of drug abuse, dependence, and addiction.

Society has standards and norms regarding drug use; cigarette smoking—even dependence on and addiction to nicotine—is acceptable. Alcohol is also an acceptable drug, but addiction to it is not. Most other drugs, such as barbiturates, amphetamines, cocaine, and heroin are not at all acceptable, even for occasional use; with the possible exception of marijuana and sleeping pills. Because most of these drugs are illegal and not acceptable by society's standards, users are considered deviants. This label often affects the care they receive. The difference in cultural attitudes toward these three categories of chemicals (alcohol, nicotine, other drugs) creates the need for and results in varied treatment (prevention) of addiction, and they are discussed separately as necessary.

Our society has been called "drug oriented" because widespread use of drugs exists. It should not be surprising, then, that teenagers and younger children also use drugs. Available statistics on the number of young people using and abusing drugs are only estimates because some students do not answer surveys accurately, and others, such as dropouts, are not included in surveys. The available statistics do provide an estimate of the scope of the problem. Most sources (Notaro, 1976; Estes and Heinemann, 1977) agree that 93% of twelfth graders have used alcohol, with the percentage of boys being slightly higher than the percentage of girls. The incidence decreases for younger children; by the seventh grade, 63% of students had used alcohol in 1974. These figures include those who tried it only once; according to Finn (1977), 25% of all seventh graders get drunk one or more times per year, 23% of all high schoolers get drunk four or more times per year, and 5% of high school students get drunk once a week. In addition, 18.5% of high school students reported riding in a car with a heavily drunken driver 12 times a year.

Alcohol consumption among adolescents is increasing in proportion to the increase of alcohol consumption in the general population (Lee, 1978). Califano, former Secretary of Health, Education, and Welfare, estimated that about 3 million teenagers a year have problems related to alcohol and that alcohol-related accidents are the leading cause of death in the 15- to 24-year-age group (The Nation's Health, 1979). According to Notaro (1976), these and other figures indicate that alcohol usage among teenagers is of a significant nature.

Alcohol use appears to be more widespread than use of other drugs. According to Finn (1977), 20% of junior and senior high school students reported using marijuana at least once in 6 months. The National Commission on Marijuana and Drug Abuse concluded that alcohol is a bigger problem than marijuana and that most marijuana users do so in social settings and in moderation. Yankelovich (1975) reports that almost half of all high school students have experimented with drugs once or twice, and one third consider themselves regular users.

Table 9-10. Guidelines for nursing students who use and abuse chemicals

Factors affecting use of chemicals	Assessment	Intervention	Prevention

Developmental stage
  Adolescents must make many adjustments and become independent; rebellion may be seen as independence from adult world; drugs may provide needed status in peer group; altered consciousness may fulfill dependency needs
Previous experience
  Alcohol is usually introduced to children in home; children of alcoholics are at high risk
Perception of drug usage
  Escape, tension relief, status boost, excitement, rebellion, crutch, etc.
Culture
  Dominant culture is drug-oriented; norms vary but society as whole labels abusers as deviants; deviant individuals may be deviant in more than one behavior; peer drug culture may encourage abuse
Support system
  Many abusers are runaways and have poor bonding to others and society
Number and chronicity of stressors
  Family disturbances common among drug addicts; drug abuse is stressor; many changes of adolescence are stressful
	Current reaction to stressors
	  See p. 184 for general signs and symptoms of drug abuse; three stages of addiction are (1) knowledge of drug, (2) gradual dependence, (3) physiological dependence and tolerance
	Significance of stressor
	  Physiological and psychological effects of drug abuse require much adaptive energy
	Availability of help
	  Family may contribute to abusing behaviors; school professionals, community organizations can be called on for emergencies and rehabilitation
	Previous coping strategies
	  Preaddiction coping mechanisms might include indifference, withdrawal, poor relationships with others, dependency, and fear of loss; for addict, drug taking becomes coping mechanism
		Identify stressors
		  In addition to drug-induced stresses, addicted student may feel stress from poor school performance, ineffective personal relationships, decreased family functioning, legal problems, and poor health; it is more important to deal with current behaviors than reasons for initial dependence
		Identify adaptive behaviors
		  Tell student if you believe he is chemically dependent; be accepting, help to motivate, and reassure to decrease paranoia
		Alter stressors and responses
		  Provide role model, specialized setting; recovery process similar to separation process; encourage to become involved; include family; set realistic goals; assist to be responsible; focus on present; improve self-concept
		Evaluation
		  Long-term follow-up with student and family
			Primary
			  Educational approaches include (1) "scare" tactics, (2) factual data, and (3) attitudinal approach; studies favor combining facts with attitudes; teach about drugs separately from alcohol and smoking; begin teaching in early grades; examine own attitudes; group approach and including students in planning appear to be successful
			Secondary
			  Treat early before addiction becomes adult life-style; be alert to early symptoms of abuse and potential abuse; work closely with other school personnel
			Tertiary
			  Include family in treatment; establish new behaviors within families; treat behavior rather than focusing on reasons for addiction

Finn's statistics are more specific: 1.8% of teen-agers use hallucinogens, amphetamines, or barbiturates more than twelve times per year (1977). The statistics are underestimates, but the message is clear: drug abuse is widespread in the adolescent population and has reached significant enough proportions to warrant the attention of school nurses.

In the study of smoking habits of 343 high school students in England, about 44% called themselves nonsmokers, 49% said they had tried smoking, and 6% said they were smokers. Of the nonsmokers, 13% said they smoked occasionally, that is, less than one cigarette per week (Dale, 1978). Department of Health, Education, and Welfare statistics demonstrate a rising trend in the numbers of adolescent smokers. From 1968 to 1974 the percent of girls under age 18 who smoked increased from 19% to 26%; the percentage of boys increased only slightly, 30% to 31%. According to recent statistics, the trend of increased use of alcohol and tobacco among teenagers leveled off in the mid-1970s, but marijuana use has continued to increase (Kovar, 1979).

Smoking, drugs, and alcohol are critical health problems and can lead to serious, long-term consequences; yet increasing numbers of young people consume these chemicals. For the school nurse to fulfill her role of promoting the health of young adults, she must become involved in and knowledgeable about this serious problem. Table 9-10 provides some guidelines for the school nurse working with students who abuse chemicals.

Factors affecting use and abuse of chemicals
Developmental stage

The adolescent developmental stage is characterized by the need to make many adjustments: to a new body image, to adult status, and to making decisions regarding careers. As discussed earlier, adjustments require energy, and maladaptation may result. Some adults use drugs to help them adjust to their environment. Feelings of self-confidence and euphoria often associated with drug use may mislead adolescents into believing that the drugs help them to adjust when actually the opposite is true. Uncertainty regarding one's self-esteem often accompanies the adolescent developmental task of achieving independence. The need to appear independent and self-confident when feeling the opposite can lead to rebellion against the standards of society, including the norm against drug abuse. By using drugs as a form of rebellion, the adolescent gains a sense of satisfaction and power (Blades, 1976). Drug use can also provide a sense of belonging to a peer group and even status within that group. Drug use is therefore appealing to many adolescents because of their developmental stage.

Previous experience

Most children are introduced to alcohol at home. Here they may become familiar with the effects of the drug, but most students report they drink in cars. Children who have alcoholics and/or smokers for parents are at higher risk of following the same pattern (Estes and Heinemann, 1977). Students who find the altered consciousness of drugs or alcohol to be an escape mechanism build experiences that confirm their perception. On the other hand, youths who have a bad experience with a drug may learn that they do not enjoy the sensations or circumstances surrounding drug ingestion.

Perception of event

Drugs are taken for many different reasons, partially depending on the individual's perception of what the drug will do for him. For some, drug consumption reduces fear of loneliness by making them part of a group; for others, altered consciousness makes socialization easier. Teenagers often experiment with drugs because of the aura of excitement or relaxation drugs create. Smoking is often considered relaxing, as are drinking and using chemicals. By using drugs to avoid tensions, one can escape from reality; however, the more one escapes from reality, the more difficult it is to deal with reality, which is the beginning of psychological addiction. Drug consumption may also be an aggressive act, because it hurts both the individual and his significant others. Aggression was covered in detail in the previous discussion on delinquency; among the personality characteristics of aggressive persons cited are low frustration tolerance, passive dependency, and impulsiveness.

Culture

Often, children who abuse drugs have parents who abuse drugs (Chafetz et al., 1970). These children are raised in an environment that may not condone abuse but accept it as a fact of life. Chemical abusers are often referred to as part of the "drug culture," a subculture with unique norms, standards, language, and life-style. Being a member of this culture actually encourages one to abuse drugs.

The "drug culture" is not the only culture that encourages drug abuse. The dominant American culture also condones the use of many drugs such as sleeping pills, tranquilizers, and analgesics, until addiction results—then the individual is labeled as deviant. Given society's drug orientation, it is not surprising that young people experiment with drugs; they may not view it as different from adult pill taking. Another cultural factor influencing adolescents is the media, in which alcohol and cigarettes are associated with romance, good times, and sexuality.

Support system

Studies have shown that drug abusers often have a negative self-image and depend on drugs for psychological support (Goldhill, 1971). More drug abusers than users run away from home and feel isolated from others. They, like delinquents, have deficient socialization and feel apart from society (Estes and Heinemann, 1977). The drug-dependent juvenile generally does not identify a support system, feels isolated from and unacceptable to others, and relies on drugs and a drug-oriented peer group for psychological support.

Number and chronicity of stressors

Klimenko (1968) states that family disturbances are a major influencing factor in the life of a drug addict. When the disturbance is parental drug abuse, the parents are usually unreliable, disorganized, and argumentative. Statistics show that 9 million Americans are alcoholics and that each of these 9 million directly and seriously affects the lives of four to six others, many of whom are children (Triplett and Arneson, 1978). Children of alcoholics are likely to feel rejected and confused as a result of their parents' illness. Cork's (1969) study showed that of 115 children of alcoholic parents, all were affected by the disease in some way; the most common problems were relationships within and outside of the family, feeling unwanted by parents, and lack of self-esteem. These stresses are both chronic and multiple and create a serious potential for adaptive difficulties. The adolescent who uses drugs to escape daily problems does not really escape problems, but merely postpones them. The longer the problems are postponed, the longer the stress affects the individual.

Drug abuse in itself is a stressor. For example, cigarette smoking results in decreased lung capacity, a physiological stress. Another stressor associated with drug use is the illegality of many drugs.

Assessment of the student who uses drugs
Current reaction to stressors

Behaviors indicative of drug abuse are given on p. 184. They involve changes in personality or daily activities as well as behaviors oriented toward obtaining drugs. Often the drug user is malnourished and in poor health.

Becoming addicted is described as a disease process beginning with experimentation with the drug (Huberty and Malmquist, 1978). *Experimenting* increases the individual's awareness of how drugs affect him. He also realizes that the drug-induced state can be obtained at will and may begin to anticipate the altered state as a method of relieving tension. At this point, the individual enters the second stage of becoming addicted: *gradual dependence* (Fromer, 1979), during which a pattern of drug use as a coping mechanism is established. The repeated consumption of drugs for assistance in coping results in a feeling that the user could not cope without the help of the drug. The third stage, *addiction,* follows when the individual becomes physiologically dependent; the body adjusts to the drug and begins developing a tolerance to it. Characteristics of addiction include withdrawal symptoms and an overwhelming craving for the drug so that obtaining the drug becomes more important than anything else.

Significance of stressors

Consuming chemicals creates a significant physical stress on the body. For example, nicotine causes a release of epinephrine from the adrenal medulla, similar to that previously described in discussion of the stress reaction, causing an increase in heart rate and blood pressure. Other physiological effects of nicotine that mimic the stress response are excitation of the central nervous system, antidiuretic action, and increased respiration. After this stimulant phase, a depressant phase follows. Nicotine is a highly toxic drug; a fatal dose for an adult is 60 mg (a cigarette contains 6 to 8 mg) (Goodman and Gilman, 1975). Symptoms of nicotine toxicity occur rapidly and include nausea, salivation, abdominal pain, vomiting, diarrhea, cold sweat, headache, dizziness, and weakness.

GENERAL SIGNS AND SYMPTOMS OF DRUG ABUSE*

Changes in school or work habits, attendance or work output.
Changes in personality and attitudes, outbursts of temper.
Takes little or no responsibility.
Shows little interest in physical appearance and grooming.
Uses secretive behavior regarding activities and possessions.
Wears sunglasses most of time to conceal pupil changes.
Wears long-sleeved garments continuously to conceal needle marks.
Associates with known drug abusers.
Borrows money inappropriately from anyone in vicinity.
Shoplifts or steals items from home, work, or school.
Tries to appear inconspicuous in behavior and manner.
Frequents unusual places at any time, such as basement, storage cabinets, closets, or attics.
Seems susceptible to suggestion.
Loses weight; may show decreased coordination.

*From Nolan et al.: 1979. Assessment and health promotion for the adolescent/youth. In Murray, R., and Zentner, J.: Nursing assessment and health promotion through the life span, Prentice-Hall, Inc., Englewood Cliffs, N.Y.

Therapy includes inducing vomiting. Death may result from respiratory failure.

The longer term chronic effects of nicotine and tobacco are also physiological stressors. According to Reports by the Surgeon General of the United States (1964, 1967), 360,000 people die annually in the United States due to cigarette smoking. The association of the chronic stress of cigarette smoking with lung cancer has been widely publicized. Other associated diseases are smoker's respiratory syndrome (an asthmalike condition), Buerger's disease, emphysema, peptic ulcer, and low birth weight.

Alcohol ingestion is also a physiological stressor because it depresses the central nervous system. According to Goodman and Gilman (1975), chronic ingestion of large amounts of alcohol has a deleterious effect on the heart, skeletal muscles, gastrointestinal tract, and liver function. Alcohol may create the illusion that the user is better able to perform tasks, but research shows that this is not so. Alcohol also causes euphoria and decreased inhibitions, which may cause an adolescent to attempt feats he would otherwise consider dangerous. In this way, alcohol is not only a physical stressor but is also life threatening.

Amphetamines, on the other hand, are central nervous system stimulants; their precise ef-fect depends on the drug, dose, and method of administration. The euphoric effects of cocaine and its toxic syndrome are the same as those of amphetamines. On ingestion of amphetamines, a "rush" or intensely pleasurable bodily sensation occurs. With drug dependence, toxic symptoms appear, including touching and picking of the face and extremities, suspiciousness, and a feeling of being watched. It is common for the user to consume amphetamines frequently for as long as 2 days while on a "run," during which time he will not sleep or eat much. The "run" is followed by a "crash" during which sleep may last 18 hours. Excessive doses of amphetamines may cause chest pain and unconsciousness; excessive doses of cocaine can cause seizures and death from respiratory failure. The physiological stress of drug ingestion needs no further emphasis.

Availability of help

Both Blades (1976) and Henderlich (1977) describe the family's contribution to addictive behavior. Because the family must retain equilibrium, the family gradually readjusts itself to drug-related behaviors, which then become an integral part of the family's adaptive patterns. Removal of these behaviors would upset the family equilibrium. Although the family often unconsciously encourages drug dependency behavior, they commonly use the addict as the family scapegoat. By emphasizing the inadequate coping of one member, they do not deal with the more basic and threatening problems within the family structure.

In addition to help from the family, specialized professional help is available in most communities. Adolescent chemical dependency is becoming a subspecialty for social workers, psychologists and others. Alcoholics Anonymous, a third resource, has developed many young people's groups throughout the country, which have had success in working with alcoholics (Notaro, 1976). Many "quit smoking" clinics are also available in most communities. School systems have a variety of helping professionals who are available to counsel students with drug-related problems. The school nurse should be familiar with the resources in her community.

Previous coping mechanisms

Particular types of coping mechanisms and personality traits have been associated with the tendency toward drug addiction, although studies are inconclusive because it is difficult to determine cause of addiction. Freedman et al. (1972) describe adaptive behavior of addicts as indifference and withdrawal. A school-age child who has low self-esteem and feels isolated from peers might adapt with indifference and withdrawal. A prealcoholic personality has been described by Freedman (1972) and Notaro (1976) as having difficulty with interpersonal relationships, resulting in loneliness and depression. For adolescent girls, real or imaginary fear of loss can be a precipitating factor in alcoholism (Lee, 1978). A study by DeLint (1964) showed that, compared to boys, a significant number of adolescent girls with drinking problems had experienced loss of a parent. Coupled with a fear of loss is dependency and a need for the approval of others. No data was found about coping behaviors of smokers versus nonsmokers.

Depending on drugs is itself a coping mechanism, and for addicts it is the major one used. The school nurse can help the student determine what coping mechanisms he used before drug dependency. According to Blades (1978), youth are more willing to talk about their drug-related behavior than their previous experiences because feelings prior to drug taking include low self-esteem and loneliness and are uncomfortable to remember. Therefore intensive interviews may be needed to identify previous positive coping strategies.

School nurse intervention with the chemically dependent student
Identification of stressors

The chemically dependent adolescent who seeks treatment probably has identified either the addiction or related behaviors as stressful. Discussing with the school nurse the various stressors he is experiencing can help him understand the effects of his behavior. In addition to the effect of the drug itself, drug-related behaviors that are stressful are the inability to perform at school, inability to meet family responsibilities and expectations, difficult interpersonal relationships, legal problems, and poor health. Huberty and Malmquist (1978) emphasize the importance of concentrating on the addiction and indicative behaviors rather than on the precipitating factors. For the adolescent who is not sure whether he is addicted, it is more therapeutic for the helper to take a stand and tell him that he is chemically dependent than to try to spare his feelings. Adolescents need limits and a helper who is willing to be kind yet firm. If they are denying their problem, gentle confrontation may help them to begin facing it. The school nurse, unless specially trained, will not be the only helper for chemically dependent students. Her role includes case finding, referral, and working together with other professionals.

Identification of adaptive behavior

The chemically dependent student may or may not feel that he is experiencing crisis. Identifying adaptive behaviors is useful for those who sense a crisis, because they feel unable to cope. Identifying his positive, adequate behaviors gives the student a foundation on which to build. Examples of adequate behaviors might be seeking help, identifying the problem, developing a trust relationship with the helper, and the desire for actual elimination of drug consumption.

In helping a chemically dependent youth, the school nurse must be accepting of the student and his problem. This may mean exploring her own attitudes regarding addicts. Her ability to motivate the adolescent to want to work on the problem and to seek further help is a vital skill. Increasing the self-esteem of drug users is often motivating for them. Drug users may be suspicious and paranoid and will need continued reassurance and demonstrated interest and concern to form a trust relationship.

Alteration of stressors and responses

One of the basic principles for helping chemically dependent people is to set realistic goals. The nurse might want students to abstain from drugs completely, but they may not be willing to do so. If goals are set too high, the student may feel discouraged from the beginning.

The school nurse can provide a supportive relationship with students who abuse drugs or whose parents abuse drugs. Specifically, this can mean providing specific, positive feedback for accomplishments, thoughtful referral, discussing alternative coping strategies, and being available and concerned.

Whenever possible, intervention for drug-dependent youth should include their families. Huberty and Malmquist (1978) describe drug recovery as progression through the grief reaction as theorized by Kubler-Ross (1969). During the denial stage, the family and adolescent believe they can control the addictive situation; this denial assists them to maintain their self-esteem. During denial the helper's goal is to establish an accepting relationship and to assist them to describe the chaotic changes that have occurred in their lives. Alcoholics Anonymous uses part of this theory in their approach to alcoholism, by encouraging addicts to admit that their lives have become unmanageable due to drugs. During the second stage, anger seems undirected; the parents may actually be frustrated with themselves for not being able to "fix" the addict's problem. At this point, the helper should assist the family to recognize their feelings of anger and responsibility. During the bargaining stage it is helpful for the family to recognize their powerlessness to change the addict. Once this occurs, depression follows. The helper's role at this time is to sustain hope, which leads the family to the final stage of accepting realistic limitations.

Evaluation

Long-term follow-up is necessary for chemical abusers. Huberty and Malmquist (1978) state drug addiction is an incurable disease, explaining that although persons can remain symptom-free for long periods of time, craving for the drug does return. The school nurse should periodically assess the recovered student's status.

Prevention of chemical abuse
Primary prevention

The goal of primary prevention is to avoid having students become dependent on drugs. Drug education is one important method of primary prevention. Many studies are currently being done to determine the effectiveness of different styles of drug education. Three styles that have been used are (1) "scare" tactics in which the horrors of the drug are described; (2) the factual approach, in which basic information about drugs and their effects are described, and (3) the attitudinal approach, which includes discussion about values and responsible decision making. In a study of a comprehensive smoking education program, which included both factual and attitudinal approaches, Dale (1978) found a decrease in smoking behavior only in the students who had reported being occasional smokers. Greenberg and Deputat (1978) did an experimental study on students who were smokers, comparing the three mentioned styles of education and a control group. The first group, receiving the "scare" approach, showed the greatest decrease in smoking immediately after the classes; however, 5 months later, students who received the attitudinal approach showed the greatest improvement. Stone's data (1978) confirms these results; she recommends an educational model that combines factual with attitudinal approaches, including decision-making practice. If education for primary prevention of smoking is to have long-term effects, it needs to provide facts as well as values clarification and other attitudinal approaches.

The same educational approach for primary prevention of drug and alcohol abuse has also been recommended. The emphasis in the attitudinal approach for drugs and alcohol often includes discussions with families and adolescents regarding living and communicating together in today's society (Notaro, 1976). To achieve this purpose, school nurses can teach parents about the adolescent developmental stage—what behaviors to expect from their teenagers and what role parents can assume in their development. Adolescents are encouraged to discuss and practice mental health principles: basic communication, self-acceptance, and problem solving. Other attitudinal aspects of drug education include discussing ways of achieving a sense of status, independence, belonging, and "natural highs" without drugs. The image projected by television and other media regarding alcohol and smoking should be discussed in school to assist students to separate fact from fantasy.

Primary prevention education can never begin too early. Most state departments of education recommend beginning alcohol education by the fourth grade. Curriculum models such as the one used by Stone (1978), entitled *School Health Education Study,* are available for grades kindergarten through twelve.

Information should be geared to the cognitive level of the students and can take a creative approach. Young students may put on a puppet show or do craft activities relating to facts and attitudes about drugs. For older students, drug education can be integrated into many aspects of the curriculum such as biology, physical education, health, and philosophy.

Finn (1977) believes that alcohol education should remain separate from drug education because of the behavioral, social, legal, and attitudinal differences surrounding the two types of drugs. He explains that alcohol is in common usage, and the goal of education might therefore be responsible use, whereas drugs are illegal and less commonly used, and goals might include total abstinence. The school nurse who participates in curriculum development has much to offer in the area of drug usage and prevention.

Some teaching methods that appear to be successful are peer group programs, homogeneous groups of students (that is, all smokers or all nonsmokers), and student participation in program development (Greenberg and Deputat, 1978). In the area of drug dependence, primary prevention may well be the school nurse's most significant contribution.

Secondary prevention

Early detection and treatment of drug abuse are also largely the responsibility of the school nurse. Early case finding includes identifying both potential and current drug users. Children with alcoholic parents, low self-esteem, who seem friendless, or who show signs of drug abuse need special attention. The school nurse can form a supportive relationship with these children and assist them to choose more adequate coping mechanisms. Teachers, students, families, and the general public also need to learn the early warning signs of drug abuse, so they can be case finders and assist others to seek help.

Tertiary prevention

Tertiary prevention is avoiding further complications or relapses into drug abuse. Including the family in treatment is highly recommended for this reason. The formation of new behavior patterns is also an important part of tertiary prevention. Students often associate pleasure and fun with smoking and drug consumption; the substitution of more healthful attitudes leads to new behavior patterns. The school nurse's role in tertiary prevention also includes assisting students in their reassimilation to school. For those who have been in another setting for treatment, reassimilation includes forming a new peer group, becoming involved with new classes and schoolwork, and avoiding students who encourage drug-related behavior. These changes can be stressful, and the school nurse and teachers can help the student in these new adjustments.

MALTREATED CHILDREN
Definition, history, and scope of the problem

P.L. 93-247 defines child abuse and neglect as follows:

Physical or mental injury, sexual abuse, negligent treatment or maltreatment of a child under the age of 18 by a person who is responsible for the child's welfare under circumstances which indicate that the child's health or welfare is harmed or threatened (Colucci, 1977).

The term maltreatment refers to both abuse and neglect. There are many types of maltreatment; Halperin (1979) describes nine categories: (1) physical abuse, (2) sexual abuse, (3) physical neglect, (4) medical neglect, (5) emotional abuse, (6) emotional neglect, (7) educational neglect, (8) abandonment, and (9) multiple maltreatment.

Recently, children's rights have been a widely publicized topic, culminating in the United Nation's designation of 1979 as the "International Year of the Child." Children have not always enjoyed rights; they have been considered the property of their parents, and therefore their treatment was a private matter. Abusive childrearing practices were accepted by society; excessive physical abuse as punishment is the most common example. Sexual abuse, such as incest, was also common and is still a serious problem. During the industrial revolution, child labor was the norm. Until recently, not much was done to stop cruel treatment of children, mainly because children were considered miniature adults and their parents' property. Although this proprietary attitude is no longer prevalent and the identification of developmental stages has disproved the "little adult"

theory, maltreatment is still a significant problem.

Maltreatment of children has been called an epidemic in American society. The available statistics are only estimates because much mal-

Table 9-11. Guidelines for nursing maltreated children

Factors relating to child maltreatment	Assessment	Intervention	Prevention

Developmental stage
  Children of all developmental stages are abused; their parents often have poor bonding, low self-esteem, and difficulty coping with activities of daily living
Previous experience
  Parents may have history of delinquency and maltreatment and little knowledge or skills regarding parenting
Perception of children
  Often parents have unrealistic expectations; children that are likely to be maltreated are foster, adopted, unwanted, hyperactive children and boys under age 12, and girls older than 12
Culture
  "Poverty" culture might be correlated with maltreatment; myths that children are happy and parenting is easy are predominant in American culture and contribute to child maltreatment
Support system
  Parents usually have few friends and difficulty establishing trusting relationships
Number and chronicity of stressors
  Correlations found between parents scoring high on *Social Readjustment Rating Scale* and abusive parents; other common stressors are financial problems, chemical dependency, large family, feeling overwhelmed
	Current reaction to stressors
	  During crisis: assess injuries and causes, note incongruency, lack of affection between parent and child, child who is stoic and reluctant to trust helper
	Significance of stressor
	  Physical and emotional injury affects child intensely, but also parent and possibly future generation
	Availability of help
	  Often team of professionals work together; often support system is lacking, so professional help is all that is available to family
	Previous coping strategies
	  Important for school nurse to keep accurate records to identify patterns and assist in determining treatment modality
		Identify stressors and adaptations
		  Parents-other crisis in home; may fail to meet other parenting responsibilities also; children-specific types of maltreatment are physical, sexual, emotional, medical, educational neglect, abandonment, or any combination; may adapt to maltreatment with aggressiveness, showing off, disobedience, stealing, poor relationships, listlessness, carelessness, being accident prone, tearfulness, shyness, withdrawal, emotional instability, or low achievement
		Alter stressors and responses
		  Promote sense of worth, acceptance of help, trust, social skills, modify inadequate parenting and emotional control of parents; for children promote sense of self-worth and modify inadequate adaptive responses
		Evaluation
		  Planned long-term follow-up and support
			Primary
			  Education in schools for family living, beginning with young children and including facts and attitudes; identification of high-risk students and providing education and promoting adequate coping
			Secondary
			  Work together with teachers to identify and treat maltreated children early; organize team efforts and perform liaison duties with other agencies
			Tertiary
			  Support for recuperating families and long-term follow-up

treatment is unreported; however, the American Humane Association estimates that more than 1 million children were abused in 1978 (Houston Chronicle, 1978). The National Center for Child Abuse and Neglect (1976) estimates that 1.7 million children suffer maltreatment each year. To put these figures in perspective, since there are 68 million children under the age of 18 in the United States, approximately one in forty children is maltreated. Because education is mandatory, most of these maltreated children attend school. Estimates indicate that from one half to two thirds of maltreated children are between the ages of 5 and 17 and are therefore enrolled in school (Broadhurst, 1978). The proportion of school-based reporting of maltreatment is only about one third (Broadhurst, 1978), well below what should be expected.

Most states require that educators report suspected abuse. Teachers and the general public have been educated about the problem and the number of reported cases is increasing; however, more case finding must be done in the schools. The other major responsibility the schools have regarding maltreatment is prevention. Table 9-11 provides guidelines for the school nurse working with maltreated children.

Factors affecting the maltreatment of children

Developmental stage

Abusive parents fit no stereotype; they are of all ages, cultures, and socioeconomic levels and about equally divided between men and women (Halperin, 1979). Characteristically, they demonstrate poor attachment to their children, have low self-esteem, and have difficulty coping with daily life events.

Previous experience

Often, parents who maltreat their children have been maltreated themselves as children and often have a history of delinquency during their teenage years. Lack of experience and knowledge about parenting is another predisposing factor to child maltreatment. Personality characteristics of maltreating parents include hostility, blaming, impulsiveness, and punitiveness. These traits and inadequate parenting skills are learned and used by their children, and the unhealthy cycle continues.

Perception of event

The way in which parents perceive their children can contribute to maltreatment. Parents who hold unrealistic expectations for their children may punish them when they do not measure up. A common example is the parent who expects the child to meet the parent's needs, often called role reversal. Another example is punishing children for activities that are normal for their age, such as a 2-year-old wetting the bed. If the child is hyperactive or handicapped, parental expectations may be accurate for an average child and therefore unrealistic for this particular child. When parents do not make adjustments for individuality among their offspring, unrealistic expectations result.

Certain groups of children are more likely than others to be perceived by their parents in ways that precipitate maltreatment, including foster children, unwanted children, adopted children, stepchildren, children born out of wedlock, firstborn or secondborn and youngest children, boys until age 12, and girls over age 12 (Justice and Justice, 1976).

Culture

Although maltreatment of children is found in all cultural groups, Helfer and Kempe (1976) state that statistics for the United States show a higher proportion of child maltreatment among nonwhites than whites; this is probably due to factors other than ethnicity, such as their overrepresentation in low-income status, resulting in stress. Culture does, however, affect childrearing practices. Cultures favoring an authoritarian family structure appear to be prone to abuse because this structure has been identified as a factor common among abusive parents. Some cultures are more likely to publically shame children than to punish them, which is a form of emotional abuse. It is interesting to note that Sweden passed a law in 1979 forbidding parents to spank their children.

According to Halperin (1979), the dominant American culture has several characteristics that contribute to maltreatment of children. One of these is the myth that childhood is a happy, joyful time. Belief in this myth perpetuates denial of the problems, fears, and frustrations that children face. Another myth Halperin reveals is the belief that parenthood is a joyful, fulfilling experience for all adults. This myth contributes to the frustration parents experience when parenting is not what they expected. Fortunately, the need for parenting education is being recognized, and the decision not to become a parent is also a more acceptable alternative.

Support system

Our highly mobile society also contributes to child maltreatment. Mobility has been shown by Holland et al. (1974) and McNeese and Hebeler (1977) to be stressful, producing isolation from support systems. ten Bensel and Berdie (1976) correlate poor support systems with maltreatment; they state that frequently the parent who maltreats a child feels alone, has no one to call on, and is not involved in the community. The picture is of a "loner"; one who has few close friends and has trouble developing trust in relationships. Frequently, the marriage relationship, a potential source of support, is unstable.

Number and chronicity of stressors

Unstable marriages also contribute to maltreatment because they are a source of stress. Justice and Justice (1976) found that parents who maltreat their children have a significantly higher rank on the *Social Readjustment Rating Scale* (Table 7-9) (Coddington, 1972) than those who do not. Therefore persons with chronic stress are more likely to maltreat their children than those experiencing minimal stress. Some examples of chronic stressors are abuse of drugs or alcohol, having a large number of children, job dissatisfaction, unemployment, and other economic stressors such as inadequate housing. Parents experiencing a large amount of long-term stress may feel overwhelmed by their children's needs. Often, maltreatment results from a specific minor crisis, such as spilled food; the parent overreacts to the minor crisis because of his chronically high level of stress. Justice and Justice (1976) and others postulate that maltreatment behaviors become part of a pattern and that removal of the stressors alone does not eliminate the abusive behavior.

Many factors regarding maltreating families have been identified. For the maltreated child, crisis is never far away. Maltreatment may be discovered by school personnel or disclosed to them by the student or parents. Often, the school nurse is called on to assess the situation.

Assessment of the maltreated child
Current reaction to stressor

Assessment of physical abuse begins with determining the extent of the injury and how it occurred. To assess the extent, it is important to undress the child and examine him carefully. Bruises and welts are about 50% of physical injuries and are often inflicted where clothes will cover them. If possible, the school nurse should determine by the nature of the injury whether it was inflicted intentionally. It is important to keep accurate records and to consult them to determine the frequency and nature of complaints. After assessing the actual physical injury, the school nurse assesses how it occurred; does the reason given match the actual injury? If not, she should begin assessing for other signals of maltreatment such as poor communication between parents, parental reluctance to leave the child with the nurse, lack of affection for the child, or a child who is overly stoic or seems suspicious rather than responsive to adults.

Children's reactions to the crisis of sexual abuse is different from their reaction to physical abuse. Sexual abuse is most commonly inflicted on girls over the age of 12; 75% of the abusing adults are from the child's family (DeFrancis, 1965). Since society has strong taboos against incest, the family often tries to hide it from outsiders. Halperin (1979) states that frequently the student can be identified by a sudden behavior change when the abuse begins or when she learns not all children are treated that way. Behaviors might include withdrawal, crying for no apparent reason, sudden hostility and acting out, and anxiety about undressing.

Significance of stressor

The effects of maltreatment are so far-reaching they are immeasurable. Parents who maltreat their children suffer from guilt, shame, and low self-esteem. Physical injury to children may be mild or fatal. Sexual abuse can cause physical injuries, pregnancy, and psychological damage. Both physical and medical neglect have long-range effects on the child's health. In addition to physical sequelae, all forms of maltreatment have a serious emotional impact on children. The intense emotional pain children experience is in itself traumatic, but unfortunately, instead of ending there the pain often results in other problems, such as behavior problems that may become lifelong patterns, difficulty establishing and maintaining relationships, and maltreatment of the next generation. The significance of this problem is great; its ramifications affect not only children, but the future of American society.

Availability of help

Because most schools require teachers to report maltreatment, and because most maltreated children attend school, it appears that help is readily available for maltreated children. Unfortunately, this is not necessarily true; reporting of maltreatment by school personnel is increasing, but remains at about one half the number of maltreated children estimated to be attending school (Broadhurst, 1978). The school nurse plays an instrumental role in assisting school systems to perform their identified responsibility to report maltreated children.

Once maltreated children have been identified, many professionals and agencies are available to help them. The currently preferred team approach for correcting maltreatment has the advantage of providing a comprehensive, organized service. Members of a team might include the school nurse, public health nurse, social worker, physician, psychologist, lawyer, law enforcement officer, and hospital representative. The school nurse often organizes the team and is the liaison among the school, hospital, and family.

Previous coping strategies

The school nurse should keep records of students' physical complaints, emotional status, and health-related problems because accurate record keeping is important in case finding and in defining treatment modalities. For example, children who consistently come to school hungry or inappropriately dressed should be thoroughly assessed for parental neglect. Accurate, comprehensive records assist the school nurse to identify patterns indicative of maltreatment.

School nurse intervention for maltreated children

Identification of stressors and adaptive behaviors

Identification of stressors and adaptation to the stressors are discussed together for clarity. Identification of stressors includes both stress felt by the parents and the student. If the parents are available, the school nurse should assess stressors in their lives; very often they are experiencing crisis unrelated to the child. If this is true, the school nurse can work with them to alleviate the crisis or refer them to another qualified professional. Very often the best adaptation the parent can make is inadequate. Areas of parenting in which maltreating parents often show inadequate adaptation include failure to stimulate the children, play with them, individualize the needs of their children, provide a good adult role model, and instill a sense of morality.

The maltreatment itself provides a stressor for the child. The school nurse must carefully assess which type of maltreatment or combinations thereof the child is experiencing. This task requires expertise and a long-term relationship with the child to develop trust and assess patterns. It is important to remember that different children may have opposite reactions to the same stimulus and that all children occasionally display inadequate adaptive behaviors; the school nurse should observe for patterns of inadequate behaviors. Following are fourteen behavior patterns that Halperin (1979) lists as guidelines for identifying maltreated children:

1. Aggressiveness: tries to get attention and releases emotion by starting fights and other physical assaults.
2. Show-off: attempts to get recognition by calling out in class.
3. Disobedience: purposefully breaks rules, believes that even anger directed at him is better than indifference.
4. Lying, cheating, and stealing: often lies are fantastic and grandiose; child lives for today and may not have learned sense of morality.
5. Unlikeable: sullen, depressed, bragging, unable to establish peer relationships.
6. Unkempt: dirty clothes, poor manners, poor hygiene, no sense of self-pride; parental neglect probable.
7. Listlessness: low energy, daydreamer, fatigued; may be lacking energy resources such as food and sleep or may attempt to avoid failure and the resultant parental anger.
8. Carelessness: messy appearance, sloppy schoolwork; parents neglectful in these areas.
9. Accident prone: may feign injury to avoid failure or has low self-esteem leading to carelessness.
10. Fearfulness: afraid to take risks, of being criticized; may ''cling'' to esteemed adults and be skeptical of strangers.
11. Shyness: soft voice, lowered head, few friends, afraid of contact with people; may be afraid of failure.
12. Withdrawn: isolated, easily frustrated, tense, unhappy; may lack affection; parents may be unpredictable.
13. Emotionally unstable: defensive, hypochondriacal, unpredictable; parents may not be meeting emotional needs.
14. Low achiever: short attention span, developmental lag; could be many causes, such as brain damage or poor nutrition.

Alteration of stressors and responses

Following are some of the goals that might be identified by the family and professional team:

1. Promote self-worth of parent and child. The parent may have been maltreated as a child and may feel incompetent as a parent.
2. Promote parental acceptance of help. The school nurse must be flexible and adapt to the needs of the family, encouraging them to work with helpers. The school nurse may want to make home visits to ensure privacy.
3. Promote understanding of the child's needs and behaviors. Teach normal growth and development, as well as interpret the child's behaviors to promote realistic expectations of the child by his parents.
4. Promote trust. Parents and child may have difficulty forming a trust relationship. If the school nurse is available, caring, and an advocate for the family, their trust relationship becomes a model for future relationships.
5. Modify inadequate parenting. Confront parents with their inadequate parenting, discuss the problem openly, problem solve for alternative methods based on child and parent needs, and be a role model. It may also help to ease the parent into new behaviors, such as beginning to play with the child for 5 minutes a day.
6. Modify emotional control. Lack of control can lead to overpunishment. Teach alternative methods of expressing anger, including seeking a supportive person.
7. Promote social skills. This goal helps to decrease isolation and improve future adaptive potential. A group of parents with similar problems can be socially motivating as well as supportive of each other.

Because of her expertise and school-based practice, the school nurse is in an excellent position to work with children who have been maltreated. As the maltreatment stops, the child's behavior may also change. If the child's adaptive behaviors to maltreatment have become longstanding patterns, he may need some assistance to develop new behavior patterns. According to Helfer and Kempe (1976), not enough research is available to advise health professionals about the special needs of children adjusting to a parent who has stopped maltreating them. They advise that treatment should be individualized according to the child's assessed behavior pattern. If, for example, the child has become fearful of new experiences, the goal of intervention is to modify that fear and associated behaviors. Most school nurses are not educationally prepared for such intense counseling, but can offer the child an emotionally supportive relationship with a concerned adult. Through this relationship, the student learns that an adult respects and cares about him. One way for the school nurse to initiate a supportive relationship is to ask the student to be a "nurse's helper" once or twice a week.

Other intervention roles for the school nurse include participating in physical therapy, medical treatment plans, and other rehabilitative programs. The school nurse might also work with the teacher. Perhaps the expectations for the child's schoolwork need modification; the teacher and nurse can align their approach for a student to better meet his needs. The school nurse is knowledgeable about helping relationships and may also be able to facilitate the teacher-parent relationship.

Evaluation

Evaluation of interventions is continual and is performed by the team members during case conferences. The school nurse should also plan long-term follow-up with students and families. She can follow the child's school progress, meet with the child, and be available to the family by phone or home visit.

Prevention of child maltreatment
Primary prevention

School nurses are in the ideal setting to do primary prevention of child maltreatment because they can contribute to education of future parents. Of the educators responding in favor of child abuse education in a survey (Riggs and Evans, 1978), 71% indicated they thought this subject should be taught before the sixth grade. Presentation of the subject will vary for different age levels, but young children can learn about parenting and family life even through animal stories (Riggs and Evans, 1979). The topic can be taught as a special class or can be incorporated into the present curriculum. Various suggested curriculum guidelines have been published (Helfer and Kempe, 1976). Some pertinent topics to include are marriage, parenthood, child growth and development, discipline, divorce, sex roles, and dealing with stress. As with drug education, the curriculum should contain both factual data and attitude discussion. In this way, older students can discuss dilemmas of child maltreatment, such as privacy rights, reporting, and how to help the family. Riggs and Evans (1979) give many specific suggestions for school personnel planning maltreatment education, such as use of role playing and value clarification statements.

Many schools currently provide "family living" courses; the school nurse should actively participate in planning these courses and, in some circumstances, teach specific classes. If the school has no program, the school nurse, as a health professional, is responsible for initiating changes that facilitate program development. To accomplish this, the school nurse needs change agent skills (Chapter 19).

Two other forms of primary prevention are discussed in the literature: use of health visitors and licensing for parenthood. Helfer and Kempe (1976) suggest the "health visitor plan." Under this plan, each family with a new baby is visited by a health visitor, who is trained to assess families for potential maltreatment. This plan is carried out in several European countries, and its goal is to identify and help potentially abusive parents before they abuse their children. The plan has many ethical, practical, and financial considerations, but school nurses could apply it in principle to their pregnant students. Teenage mothers are at a high risk for maltreating their children because of lack of knowledge and experience, a number of other stresses, and developmental immaturity. The school nurse can identify them as a population at risk and provide education for their special needs, both individually and in groups.

Justice and Justice (1976) advocate another form of primary prevention: licensing for parenthood. They postulate that society requires licenses for less important jobs and should require licenses for parents as well. Again, the ethical questions are far reaching. This seemingly radical suggestion emphasizes that education is required for a difficult, lifelong job of parenting. The school nurse role includes responsibility for helping educate the future generation for what might be the most important job they ever do: parenting.

Secondary prevention

Secondary prevention is another school nurse activity. To facilitate early detection of maltreatment, the school nurse might provide refresher programs for faculty in the school, as well as teach students to identify victims and seek help. Coordination within the school for each detection and treatment is essential, as is external coordination with community agencies, and the school nurse may be the logical liaison person. The care children receive depends on open communication between agency and school personnel. The school nurse should also be active within the school's child abuse team and initiate such a team if one is not already functioning.

Other aspects of secondary prevention include day care before and after school for maltreated children to allow the child and parent less time together (excess time together increases the potential for maltreatment in some families), and formation of support, social, and educational groups for both children and parents.

Tertiary prevention

An example of tertiary prevention is a hotline that parents can call if they are losing control and feel they may harm their children. Special support systems, removing a child from home, and long-term, frequent follow-up all help to prevent the recurrence of abusive incidents.

STRESS AND CRISIS ASSOCIATED WITH ADOLESCENT SEXUALITY
Definition and scope of the problem

During the adolescent years physical development of secondary sex characteristics occurs, accompanied by a change in body image. Some of the many developmental tasks adolescents face are adjusting to their new body image, defining a masculine or feminine social role, and establishing a sexual identity. Consequently, many adolescents are sexually active. Graf (1976) estimates 40% of adolescent women and about twice as many men are sexually active. For some, sexual activity leads to a crisis, such as pregnancy, parenting, abortion, and/or venereal disease. This discussion will include these and other problems (birth control and peer pressure) associated with adolescent sexuality.

Statistics show that the number of adolescent pregnancies continues to increase, while pregnancies in other age groups are decreasing. Approximately 17% of all live births are to 15- to 19-year-old women (Zelnick and Kantner, 1974); in 1973, approximately 250,000 women under the age of 18 gave birth. The 10- to 14-year-old age group showed a 30% increase in births from 1968 to 1973 (Jekel, 1977). Along with the rising teenage birthrate is the rising

Table 9-12. Guidelines for nursing adolescents in sex-related stress

Factors affecting adolescent sexuality	Assessment of sexuality in adolescents	Intervention with sex-related problems	Prevention of sex-related problems

Developmental stage
  Physical sexual maturity is reached, accompanied by turbulent emotional adjustment
Previous experience
  Most lack knowledge about anatomy and physiology; may have misinformation about sex-related problems such as venereal disease
Perception of event
  Sexual activity can be associated with feelings of pleasure, affection, guilt, rebellion; student may intend to get pregnant or may avoid birth control for other reasons
Support system
  Peer group may encourage or discourage sexual activity; loneliness may encourage it; pregnant adolescent is at risk of losing her support system
Culture
  "Sexual revolution"; media is sex laden; sex no longer taboo topic; however, teens are told not to be sexually active
Number and chronicity of stressors
  Adolescence is time of rapid change; many developmental tasks are stressful; pregnancy at this time can lead to chronicity of stressors and "syndrome of failure"
	Current reaction to stressors
	  Denial is common and leads to detrimental physical and emotional problems; students often have unrealistic expectations of pregnancy
	Significance of stressor
	  Physically, adolescents and their infants are at high risk for toxemia, prematurity, infant and fetal mortality; venereal diseases can have serious long-term sequelae
	Availability of help
	  Reaction of friends and family affects availability of support system; school nurse is important resource
	Previous coping mechanisms
	  Early sexual activity influences later behaviors; teens should be able to maintain reality, control impulses, reason, and plan
		Identify stressors
		  Physical needs, especially nutrition during pregnancy; lack of support; feelings surrounding problem
		Identify adaptive behaviors
		  Tasks of pregnancy identified; documented reactions of teens to pregnancy show inadequate adaptation; statistics show great many problems in future such as incidence of divorce twice national rate and increased incidence of child abuse
		Alter stressors and responses
		  Decrease high risk; mobilize resources, use group approach; school-based specialized programs; encourage family support
		Evaluation
		  Program evaluation and cost analysis needed; continual assessment of student
			Primary
			  Discuss healthy attitudes toward sexuality; plan and implement educational programs; provide easy access to birth control
			Secondary
			  Minimize health risks of adolescent pregnancy; encourage health care; provide emotional support; prevent isolation; prevent second pregnancy
			Tertiary
			  Reduce stress and avoid future crises; assist students to stay in school; maintain or regain health

abortion rate; teenagers account for one third of all legal abortions (Center for Disease Control, 1974).

The rate of venereal disease among adolescents is also rising; between 1960 and 1972 it quadrupled (Center for Disease Control, 1974). Although it is difficult to get accurate data about venereal disease because it often is unreported, these figures indicate that a significant number of adolescents experience problems related to sexuality. The school nurse is a central figure in the assessment, intervention, and prevention of these stressors (Table 9-12).

Factors affecting adolescent sexuality
Developmental stage

Physical development of secondary sex characteristics is accompanied by a change in body image, strong sexual urges, and feelings of conflict between society's admonition not to be sexually active and the need to form a sexual identity and gratify sexual drives. Adolescents must accomplish tasks related to sexual maturity, including understanding themselves as sexual beings, forming values related to sex, and accepting their sexual responsibility. Adolescence is characterized by ambivalence, during which teens are highly susceptible to peer pressure. According to Leese (1974), the younger the adolescent, the less likely he is to consider the possible consequences of sexual activity. Most adolescents participate in sexual behavior on some level, as a normal part of development.

Previous experience

According to Brown and Clancy (1976), most adolescents have an inadequate understanding of anatomy and physiology. This lack of knowledge results in sexual practices based on inaccurate information, such as the belief that ovulation occurs just before menstruation. Inaccurate knowledge about birth control, pregnancy, and venereal disease may also influence the teenager to delay seeking health care.

Because adolescents have little previous sexual experience, sexual activities of their peers are influential. It is important to the self-worth of adolescents that their sexual experiences be as good as their friends', who may even fabricate experiences (Graf, 1976). Feelings of inferiority during adolescence can have long-term effects because they occur during development of sexual identity. Graf (1976) states adolescents may have fears concerning homosexuality because many heterosexual adolescents participate in some pleasurable homosexual activity as part of their development. As adolescents become sexually active, they build up a reserve of experiences that influences future sexual adjustment.

Perception of event

According to Graf (1976) and Nakashima (1977), adolescents consider sexual activity as a way to obtain affection and peer approval, rebel, be self-destructive, or experiment. Although development of a sexual identity is an expected task, distorted perceptions can lead to stressful events; for example, 75% of sexually active teenagers use *no* birth control (Graf, 1976). Klerman (1975) proposes that a reason so many adolescents do not use birth control is that they perceive sexual activity as wrong.

Use of birth control implies planning for sexual activity; thus they would have to consciously plan to do something that is wrong. Brown and Clancy (1976) agree with this theory and add that adolescents do not want others to know about their activities; therefore they have difficulty asking for birth control advice. Others may believe that pregnancy could not happen to them.

Pregnancy may also be welcomed as proof of one's masculinity or femininity, or adulthood. The baby may be viewed as someone to love the parents (Anderson, 1976). Klerman (1975) states that the role of women in society is to be mothers, and teenagers who try to get pregnant are striving toward early attainment of that adulthood goal.

Culture

Some cultural factors appear to encourage adolescents to engage in sexual activity. The so-called sexual revolution has led to increased acceptance of nontraditional life-styles, a lessening of the double standard, and acceptance of open discussion about sex (Graf, 1976). Everyone, especially teenagers, is bombarded daily with sexually laden media and entertainment. Another cultural factor, Klerman (1975) states, is that teens often have no sense of purpose in society. Lack of stable family structure is a third variable considered by Nakashima (1977) to influence relaxing the restraints regarding acceptability of sexual activity. On the other hand, many states have laws that youth under 18 years old need parental permission to obtain birth control devices, in effect telling youth that they are too young to be sexually active. The dominant American culture thus delivers confusing messages to adolescents, contributing to their natural sense of conflict.

Support system

Because teens are so influenced by peers, the values of the peer group regarding sexual activity significantly influence individual decisions. The need for belonging to the peer group may be more important than differing values between an individual and the group. Once a pregnancy occurs, however, isolation from peers is common. Many times the pregnant adolescent is removed from the school, at least for the time surrounding parturition, if not for the entire pregnancy. She has less in common with her friends, and since sexual activity is considered "immoral," she may be ostracized. The father of the baby may be unable to help; if teens marry, their isolation is enhanced. Judgmental comments from professionals also contribute to feelings of isolation. There is some logic therefore to the following tragic statistic: for pregnant women under 18, the suicide rate is ten times greater than the rate in the nonpregnant population (Gabrielson et al., 1970).

Number and chronicity of stressors

The number and rapidity of adolescent developmental changes have been discussed in Chapter 7. The number and rate affect adaptation, so adolescents have an inherently high risk of inadequate adaptation. Klein (1975) reports a "syndrome of failure" that a pregnant adolescent might experience: poor health, low educational status, low self-concept, and poor parenting abilities. Often, pregnant teens do not return to school after delivering, which means they are not high school graduates, and employment is difficult to find. Low education and employment levels contribute to poor self-concept, a factor in child maltreatment. One stress leads to another, the stresses become chronic, and the youth experiences an inadequate adaptive cycle—a "syndrome of failure."

Assessment of sexually active adolescents experiencing stress

For the discussions of assessment and intervention, it is assumed that sexual activity has led to a crisis for the adolescent. As previously mentioned, not all sexual activity leads to a crisis situation, but when a crisis does occur, the most common is pregnancy and/or venereal disease.

Current reaction to stressor

When an adolescent becomes pregnant, her perception of her situation influences her reactions. As mentioned earlier, adolescents commonly use denial as a defense mechanism—one that can have serious physical consequences. Denial of a pregnancy can mean not seeking prenatal care, not telling parents or boyfriend, not gaining weight, or other seemingly negligent actions. Denial of venereal diseases delays treatment of self and others.

Some teenagers plan to become pregnant. Their reactions may include an unrealistic perception of the baby and the event of pregnancy, including perception of the baby as someone to love them or to improve a relationship. Assessment of the students' reactions should include how realistically they view their situation; unrealistic plans can lead to a more serious crisis when reality is finally faced.

Physical reactions to the stress of pregnancy also need assessment. The school nurse can assess nutritional status, weight gain, blood pressure, and drug ingestion and collaborate with other professionals who are responsible for obstetrical care.

Significance of stressor

Assessment of physical reactions to pregnancy is very important because women under age 17 are at greater risk for complications such as toxemia, anemia, and prolonged or premature labor and delivery (Shapiro et al., 1968). Pregnant teens also have a higher incidence of contracted pelvis, probably due to physical immaturity, resulting in a higher number of caesarean births (Battaglia et al., 1963). The infants of adolescent mothers are also considered high risk: low birth weights are common, and fetal death and infant mortality rates are higher than for the over 17 population (Shapiro et al., 1968). In addition, these infants are four times as likely to have neurological deficits and mental retardation (Oppel and Royston, 1971). The physiological problems of adolescent pregnancies are well documented and significant. Social and psychological ramifications are given in the discussion of intervention.

Untreated venereal disease also has serious physical sequelae. Syphilis can lead to, among others, cardiovascular and neurological deficits, and gonorrhea can result in arthritis, rheumatism, and sterility (Graf, 1976). These effects are long term and are therefore little deterrent for the shortsighted adolescent.

Availability of help

The reaction of the adolescent's friends and family to her pregnancy determines how much emotional support and other help she receives. The father of the baby may not be able to help financially or even emotionally, but should be included in decision making whenever possible. The active participation of the young woman's family can be very supportive for her. They may have difficulty accepting and dealing with the pregnancy, in which case the whole family will need external support throughout the pregnancy. If the adolescent feels that help is available to her, isolation and potential suicide may be prevented.

Professional help is also important for the adolescent with sex-related problems. The school nurse may be the first resource sought because of her availability in the school and previously developed trust relationship. She needs to provide students with accurate information, an accepting adult relationship, and thoughtful knowledgeable referrals. The atmosphere and tone of the initial interaction are important because adolescents are characteristically "touchy" about sexual topics. The school nurse should show respect for them and their feelings, remain nonjudgmental, provide confidentiality and privacy, and be an emotionally stable role model. This is a difficult task and requires self-awareness of one's feelings regarding adolescent sexuality. In addition, the school nurse should be able to supply accurate, clear answers to students' questions on topics such as birth control, reproductive anatomy and physiology, abortion, venereal disease, pregnancy, and sexual function. The school nurse must also be knowledgeable about community resources: where teens can obtain pregnancy tests, treatment for venereal disease, and birth control devices. She should know which of the available resources specialize in adolescent sexuality, since adolescents' needs are different from those of adults. The school nurse's role includes making professional help available to adolescents with sexual problems.

Previous coping strategies

Adolescents usually begin sexual behavior in the form of necking during their early teen years. According to Nolan et al. (1979), this experience not only results in sexual gratification but also in the realization that they are acceptable to others and the knowledge of how to control their sexual impulses. The adolescent who does not complete this developmental task may not learn control and/or of his acceptability to the opposite sex, resulting in irresponsible sexual behavior. Nolan et al. (1979) list some coping mechanisms expected of adolescents that the school nurse can facilitate, including (1) maintaining reality; (2) mediating between impulses, wishes and actions, and integrating feelings; (3) reasoning, judging, and planning; and (4) subsuming contradictory values and attitudes. The adolescent in crisis needs adult emotional support and guidance, but

should participate in problem solving and assume responsibility. As with any crisis, it is important to assess previous coping patterns in crisis situations.

Intervention with sex-related problems
Identification of stressors

As mentioned previously, the physical stress of pregnancy and venereal disease for an adolescent is significant, uses energy, and should not be overlooked. The increased nutritional demands of pregnancy and the average adolescent's inadequate diet result in poor nutrition for the mother and fetus. Lack of adequate nutrition may cause some congenital defects. For some adolescent women, the changing body image of pregnancy is stressful; they do not want to appear "fat" or pregnant. Therefore, to maintain their slender body image, some young women intentionally do not eat much. When body image results in such maladaptive behaviors, the baby is less of a priority to the mother than her own identity. One strategy to change her behavior is teaching her about the weight of the placenta and her own bodily fluids during pregnancy, in contrast with emphasizing the growing fetus (Anderson, 1976).

Many emotional stressors accompany sex-related problems, partially because of society's attitudes about sex. The adolescent with sex-related problems often feels guilty and ambivalent. Particular stressors differ for each individual, but are more intense if accompanied by loss of support systems, as is often the case for adolescents. The school nurse can assist the student by helping identify what is stressful about his or her situation and can determine the need for counseling.

Identification of adaptive behaviors

Tanner (1969) lists three psychological tasks of pregnancy, which ideally all pregnant women should accomplish: (1) acceptance, incorporation, and integration of the fetus as an integral part of the woman; (2) at quickening, perception of the fetus as separate and not an integral part of self; and (3) establishment of a caretaker relationship with the infant. The adolescent who is not coping well with those tasks may demonstrate some of the following behaviors identified by Richards (1972): suspiciousness and hostility, fear that may be expressed as anger, helplessness that may be camouflaged by contempt, and frustration. Inadequate coping leads to the "syndrome of failure," a bleak picture in which a teenager has a baby and drops out of school. Most never return. Repeat pregnancies are common in this population (Braen and Forbush, 1975). If the young couple marries, their potential for divorce is twice the national average (Nakashima, 1977). Schwartz (1975) reports an increased incidence of child abuse for unmarried adolescent parents. Obviously, not all pregnant adolescents will demonstrate such inadequate adaptation, but the statistics are not in their favor. They need knowledgeable and skillful intervention to prevent this "syndrome of failure."

Alteration of stressors and responses

The immediate goal of the school nurse when a teenager becomes pregnant is to reduce the risk to her physical health. Other goals include maximizing her coping mechanisms to prevent further problems; subgoals include increasing self-confidence and knowledge. To reduce the high risk, early maternity care is needed. Adolescents should be encouraged to seek medical attention as soon as they suspect pregnancy. In this way, the young woman increases her options: continue the pregnancy and keep the baby, continue the pregnancy and give the baby up for adoption, or abort the pregnancy. If abortion is chosen, it should be done as early as possible; the woman who waits to seek care may eliminate abortion as an option. The school nurse can discuss these options with the student, providing the information she needs to make a decision and encouraging clear, realistic problem solving. Whenever possible, the woman's significant others are included in these discussions. Following abortion, the pregnant adolescent and her family will need to be referred for further counseling. If adoption is chosen, the adolescent mother can be expected to feel a sense of loss; understanding support can help her to cope with those feelings.

Reducing the risks associated with teenage pregnancy is a comprehensive task; pregnancy affects adolescents emotionally as well as physically, and promotion of healthy adaptation requires a holistic approach. An important aspect of reducing risks of pregnancy is establishing a helping relationship with the adolescent and mobilizing her resources. The helping relationship assists the student to verbalize her fears, put them into perspective, and comprehend some basic teaching about pregnancy. By involving the teenager's significant others, the school nurse prevents isolation and the inadequate responses that can develop from isolation. If the pregnant student still has a relationship with the father of the baby, he should also be involved, both for the support he can provide to the mother and receive from her. Smith (1975) writes about facilitating the adolescent's relationship with her mother. She states that the school nurse can help to ease the normal conflicts between mother and daughter, resulting in an increased likelihood of the adolescent continuing her education, having her dependency needs met, and providing adequate mothering for her baby. The school nurse can also expand the adolescent's resources by involving pregnant teens in a group. Adolescents are especially responsive to the group setting because they can give and receive emotional support, feel a sense of belonging, and learn about pregnancy and related information.

Many schools have programs for their pregnant students; these programs work well when a variety of professionals, agencies, and community members are involved. The program should include (1) education about pregnancy, birth control, and parenting; (2) day care, perhaps on the school campus; (3) medical care; (4) family counseling; and (5) other components such as vocational counseling and small groups. One advantage of having such a program based in the school is that it encourages the young mother to continue her education while providing the emotional support and information she needs to adapt successfully to her new role. The school nurse has much to offer in the planning and implementation of such a program.

Jekel (1975) discusses the advantages and disadvantages of placing pregnant adolescents in special schools during their pregnancy. The strengths of such placements, as defined by Jekel, include the possibility of a 12-month flexible program, group teaching, small classes and individualized attention, flexible program design, and a school-prepared lunch. The weaknesses are extra distance from the adolescent's home, lack of extracurricular activities, limited staff and curriculum, transfer forms become part of the student's permanent record, and duplication of educational services. Arguments can be made for both sides of the issue and each woman has unique needs; however, considering the disruption of support systems resulting from transferring from one school to another and the extra motivation required to go to a more distant school, application of adaptation theory favors maintaining students in the same school. Both special programs within regular schools and special schools for pregnant adolescents provide assistance to the pregnant adolescent; however, the relative merits of each need further study.

Evaluation

Long-term comparisons of students in special and regular programs is needed to determine the effects of special programs. Cost analysis is also needed. Evaluation also determines the effectiveness of prevention strategies; is it possible to decrease the number of adolescent pregnancies, and, if so, what methods are effective? Evaluation of programs is more thoroughly discussed in Chapters 13 and 18. The school nurse must also continually evaluate her relationship with each student, the coping abilities of each student, and her approachability.

Prevention of sex-related crisis

Primary prevention

Promotion of healthy growth and development is a major component of primary stress prevention. Society's increasing openness regarding sexual issues is instrumental in promoting healthy adaptation. Changes occur slowly, however, and many adults are not comfortable with such topics. Adult discomfort will be detected by adolescents and may be interpreted by them in a variety of unhealthy ways. For many adolescents, the concept that sex is "wrong" leads to stressful situations, either because of a need to rebel or because it suppresses the need to plan for sexual activity and use birth control. An important aspect of primary prevention, therefore, is creating a healthy positive attitude regarding sex in adolescents and in adults working with them. Values clarification is one method of defining and changing attitudes. Desired outcomes include responsible problem solving, decision making, and participation in sexual activity.

Educating adolescents about facts is another important aspect of primary prevention. The consensus in the literature is that schools should be involved in sex education and that it should occur within the broad context of family living. Topics might include those contained in the family life classes previously discussed, as well as sex education, birth control, parenting, and responsible decision making. Some suggest an experiential component to education such as participation in child care at day care centers. Because students make decisions based on the information they receive, professionals have the responsibility to see that students' information is complete and accurate. The federal government's support of this approach is demonstrated by the establishment of an Education for Parenthood Program implemented in 500 school districts in 1973.

Easy access to birth control is a third aspect of primary prevention. Brann's study (1979) demonstrated that increased availability of publicly subsidized contraception can be expected to decrease fertility of teenage girls in low income areas. Easy access implies making contraception widely and readily available to adolescents, keeping the cost minimal, and making it available in a nonjudgmental, confidential atmosphere.

To have the greatest impact, primary prevention should consist of a full-scale educational program integrated into junior and senior high school curricula. The school nurse is in a position to contribute her expertise in the development of such programs. Many school districts are not financially equipped to institute full-scale programs. The school nurse can contribute to primary prevention without increasing the cost to the school district in several ways: maintaining a nonjudgmental atmosphere; providing information related to sexual development, growth, anatomy and physiology, functioning, and contraception; referrals for contraception and other problems; providing a good role model and resource; and participating in education by encouraging the inclusion of sexually related information into current curricula.

Secondary prevention

The goal of secondary prevention is to minimize both the physical and emotional risks of pregnancy. Methods of achieving this goal were described in the discussion of intervention. The school nurse can initiate services in her school to assist the pregnant student to stay healthy, such as appropriate educational strategies, emotional support through groups, and easy access to health care. Prevention of a recurrence of pregnancy and the "syndrome of failure" are other important aspects of secondary prevention.

Nearly one half of pregnant adolescents seek abortions (Jekel, 1977). The school nurse must collaborate with the family and medical team to provide counseling and education for the youth who chooses abortion. This population is also in need of reliable birth control information. Jekel (1977) states that it is more practical to concentrate available funds to assist students who have had pregnancies and to provide contraception and abortion education and services than to develop large expensive organized primary prevention programs.

Tertiary prevention

Tertiary prevention focuses on the pregnant student who has developed problems that could be physical, social, or emotional. The school nurse's goals with these students are to prevent further crises from occurring, reduce the stress related to the current crisis, and improve adaptation. Methods of achieving these goals include intervening to improve diet and exercise and general physical health of pregnant students, especially those with pathological conditions. Some of these students may need frequent rest or complete bedrest. The school nurse can assist them to find acceptable ways of regaining health as well as facilitate their return to school and their reintegration into a social network. Group therapy is especially motivating for these young mothers, because it contributes to social interaction, provides emotional support, and encourages group problem solving.

LEARNING DISABILITIES
Definition and scope of the problem

The literature contains many definitions of learning disabilities, most of which are consistent with Kirk and Bateman's (1962:1) definition:

A learning disability refers to a retardation, disorder, or delayed development in one or more of the processes of speech, language, reading, writing, arithmetic, or other school subjects resulting from a psychological handicap caused by a possible cerebral dysfunction and/or emotional or behavioral disturbances. It is not the result of mental retardation, sensory deprivation, or cultural or instructional factors.

The definition makes it clear that the term covers a variety of disorders; some examples are minimal brain dysfunction, dyslexia, brain injury, and aphasia. In the 1960s the label most frequently applied to these children was minimal brain dysfunction; however, the Association for Children with Learning Disabilities was formed and lobbied for the new name (learning disability) because it emphasized the symptoms rather than the etiology. In 1975, P.L. 94-142 was passed, stating that learning disabilities are classified as handicaps, and therefore learning disabled children deserve appropriate education and related services within the public school system at no extra fee. As a result, school districts are required to establish an interdisciplinary team, identify learning disabled children, and provide a special program if necessary to meet their learning needs.

Attitudes about children with learning disabilities are changing. As physiological dysfunction becomes the accepted cause, less blame is placed on the parents and children. It is important to remember that behavior is a function of the brain and that a behavior disorder may not be under the child's conscious control. Emphasis on the physiological origin of problems assists helpers to be more accepting of afflicted children.

The precise number of children with learning disorders is difficult to determine because of the variety of criteria applied by data collectors. Most authors agree that boys outnumber girls by about five to one (Binder and Butler, 1978). The reason more boys than girls are affected is unknown; however, sociologists have suggested that boys receive more pressure to achieve academically than girls, and the impact of failure to achieve is intense. Statisticians report that between 5% and 20% of school-age children have a learning disability, perhaps as high as one child in every classroom (Binder and Butler, 1978). School nurses are becoming increasingly involved in the care of children with learning disabilities. Intervention is very complex, requiring a team of specialists. Because this discussion is confined to the role of the school nurse, the reader is referred to other resources for a more comprehensive discussion. Table 9-13 outlines the guidelines for nursing the learning disabled.

Factors affecting the child with learning disabilities
Developmental stage

Some learning disabled children show developmental lag in one or more areas. Careful assessment is needed to determine their current developmental status in the skill areas of motor, language, and personal-social development. Most learning disabled children are identified in second and third grade, after which the incidence declines progressively (Connolly, 1978). Connolly explains that this is because those are

Table 9-13. Guidelines for nursing the learning disabled child

Factors affecting the learning disabled	Assessment	Intervention	Prevention
Developmental stage Lag in one area common; assess previous patterns and current status Previous experience Assess illnesses, trauma, stresses, etc., from prebirth to present Perception of event Disability may threaten basic needs for acceptance and competence of both student and family Culture Five times more boys than girls have learning disabilities Support system May be sparse due to delayed diagnosis; family needs support to alter life-style to meet child's needs Number and chronicity of stressors Stressors of school plus those caused by disability; school stressors include high achievement orientation, inflexible curricula, forced waiting periods	Current reaction to stressors Characteristics of learning disabled: hyperactive, impulsive, distractible, emotionally labile, poor motor coordination, perceptual deficits, and poor peer relationships; detailed developmental and physical assessment necessary Significance of stressor May lead to maladaptive life-style of delinquency, unemployment due to patterns of non-achievement, and isolation as child Availability of help P.L. 94-142 requires that interdisciplinary team of specialists such as school nurse, teacher, counselors, and physician be available to help students with learning disabilities Previous coping strategies May include delayed motor development, hyperactivity, poor coordination, and physical complaints	Identify stressors Diagnosis of learning disability may be stressor; parental perception of both child and self may also become stressors Identify adaptive behaviors Parental reaction to diagnosis may include grief, guilt, anxiety, and anger; child may use deviant behaviors to gain attention Alter stressors and responses Dispel fears; mobilize resources; provide factual information; promote healthy attitude among other professionals toward learning disabled children, refer to other resources as necessary Evaluation Various treatment modalities include behavioral therapy, family counseling, medical therapy, and educational therapy; all involve specific goal and frequent evaluation	Primary Prevent prenatal maternal and fetal complications of pregnancy; teach mental health in school curriculum through either incidental education, separate courses, or integration into current curriculum Secondary Early identification of children with characteristics of learning disability and early treatment to prevent inadequate adaptive patterns from developing Tertiary Participate in treatment provided by professional team; prevent illness by promoting good health habits

the grades that require the greatest adjustment, and have the greatest concomitant stresses. Various stresses of the classroom are described in the "number and chronicity of stressors" discussion. Unfortunately, because learning disability is so difficult to diagnose, it is rarely diagnosed when symptoms are mild.

Previous experience

It is important for the school nurse to assess the student's early experiences and adaptations to contribute to the diagnosis of a disabled child. Data collection begins with prenatal, perinatal, and postnatal information and continues through the years, obtaining information about childhood illnesses, emotional trauma, stresses, family dynamics, and academic performance.

Perception of event

Connolly (1978) describes two basic human needs that are threatened by learning disabilities: the need to be accepted and the need for competence. Because of the nature of the disorder, children and families may perceive the disability as a threat to accomplishment of these basic needs. The child who does not achieve well in one area of schoolwork may generalize the failure to other areas in a self-fulfilling prophecy. Failure to achieve can also mean failure to gain peer acceptance. Once the individual perceives a threat to fulfillment of basic needs, the possibility of a crisis exists. The family also may believe they have failed because they have produced a member who cannot achieve in all areas. Their life-style may have to change to allow for the special needs of a learning disabled child, and sacrifices are often necessary.

Culture

As noted previously, more boys than girls are affected by learning disabilities. It also appears that more children of lower socioeconomic levels are learning disabled, although it has not been clearly proven that their disabilities are due to an actual dysfunction as opposed to social and economic disadvantages. Data in this area is difficult to obtain and evaluate. Nothing in the available literature suggests that one cultural group is more or less prone to producing children with learning disabilities.

Support system

Unfortunately, until most children are diagnosed, their support systems are more likely to aggravate the problem, by punishing the child, than they are to alleviate it. Teachers and parents often punish children for seemingly inappropriate behavior, not realizing the child's needs and limited abilities. Learning disabilities are a family problem, and the parents need support, information, and guidance to accept and deal with the problem; otherwise, they cannot provide the support their child needs from them. Often the child's behavior in some way alienates him from his peers, a factor which school personnel are qualified to modify. The child's supportive resources are therefore largely within the control of the adults who care for him.

Number and chronicity of stressors

It is especially important that the child and family learn to adjust to the stress of a learning disability. Clarizio and McCoy (1970) describe some stressors of the school setting for all children, which are especially stressful for the learning disabled: high achievement orientation, inadequate provision within curricula for individual abilities, cultural differences, continued waiting (for the recess bell, to use bathroom, etc.), interruptions in the classroom, and occasional ignoring of students' questions and comments. Of course these are all normal occurrences, and elimination of such stressors would result in children poorly equipped to adapt to life situations. For learning disabled children,

however, each of these stressors is compounded by the disability. The number and chronicity of stressors therefore result in increased vulnerability of learning disabled children to other problems and illnesses.

Assessment of the learning disabled child

As a member of the professional team, the school nurse has much to contribute to the assessment of a learning disabled child. Most school nurses are not qualified, however, to diagnose the disorder. Diagnosis is not made until the following have been thoroughly assessed: history, physical examination including neurological, ophthalmological, and otological examinations as well as laboratory tests when indicated (electroencephalogram, genetic assessment), psychological evaluation, intelligence tests, linguistic evaluation, and educational evaluation (McCarthy and McCarthy, 1969).

Current reaction to stressors

Although the school nurse does not diagnose learning disabilities, she is qualified to assess many aspects of the child's adaptation, including his reactions to the present situation. Adler and Steinberg (1977) describe some characteristics of the learning disabled student: hyperactivity, impulsiveness, distractibility, labile emotions, poor motor coordination, perceptual deficits, difficulty with either expressive or receptive language, left-right confusion after age 9, reflex asymmetry, and poor peer relationships. These characteristics are often found in normal children, but when they interfere with learning or classroom interaction, they may signal a more serious problem. Approximately 80% of learning disabled children have a combination of these symptoms (Binder and Butler, 1978).

To assess children's behavior, the school nurse may observe in the classroom and visit in the home. Her observations should be recorded as specific behaviors, stating the time and frequency of the behavior, the child's ability to follow instructions, peer interaction patterns, and fine and gross motor coordination. In the home, the school nurse can complete a health history, including illnesses, medications, and developmental achievements, such as age when the child crawled and walked; history of learning problems with other family members; stress; and parent's perception of the problem. The school nurse's physical assessment may be the first indicator of a disability. The practitioner prepared school nurse has additional qualifications and can contribute a more in-depth assessment.

Significance of stressor

Learning disabilities can result in maladaptive life-styles if not treated. A student who does not perform well in school can become isolated from peers, and the combination of poor performance and isolation leads to a poor sense of self-worth. The student may become frustrated and lonely; he might drop out of school, turn to drugs, delinquency, and eventually to underemployment or unemployment. Special education and counseling can be effective in improving the adaptation of learning disabled children and their families, thus the potential for unfavorable sequelae is diminished.

Availability of help

P.L. 94-142 requires that an interdisciplinary team provide an individualized program for each student with a learning disability. Members of the team available to help the student might include the school nurse, teacher, and counselors. The school nurse is in a unique position to help families because she is not the primary professional dealing with the negative aspects of the child's problems and because nursing's image is traditionally that of a knowledgeable, concerned helper. The nurse can also be a liaison between specialists and between specialists and the family.

Teachers are also important resources for learning disabled students because they are qualified to observe and evaluate the child's cognitive learning patterns. As will be discussed in the intervention section, teachers may be called on to individualize the education process for these special children. Psychologists and other counselors are also influential resources; it is their responsibility to do educational and psychological testing and to contribute suggestions to the professional team for interacting with the child and family. Physicians are a fourth professional resource for learning disabled children; they are responsible for identifying any medically related cause of the disability and for prescribing a medical regimen if appropriate. Many professionals are available to most schoolchildren; if these professionals are not available in the school, the school district is likely to have available pupil personnel services such as those mentioned, once a problem has been identified.

Previous coping strategies

Accurate recording by the school nurse from the time children enter school and obtaining a history for high-risk children are crucial to early identification of learning disabled children. Areas of assessment include the following items:

1. Motor development. Delayed motor development may be related to future learning difficulties. These children should be referred to a physician for a more specific diagnosis. The *Purdue Perceptual Motor Survey* is a recommended instrument for measuring gross motor skills in young school-age children.

2. Hyperactivity. Hyperactivity is considered the most important characteristic suggestive of potential learning problems (Laufer and Denhoff, 1957; Werry, 1968). Although hyperactivity can be a symptom of learning disabilities, it is also a separate syndrome that causes difficulty in learning. Sources in the literature vary about whether or not hyperactivity syndrome is a learning disability or a separate category; legally it is considered separately.

3. Poor coordination. Poor coordination is also associated with potential learning disabilities (Reuben and Bakivin, 1968). Children who have difficulty in dressing, drawing, or play activities are included in this category. Poor coordination may also manifest itself as clumsiness and can be of either physical or emotional origin.

4. Physical complaints. The school nurse should review the frequency and nature of student complaints. Chronic complaints or long-term illnesses signal potential difficulties. Psychosomatic illnesses are also common among children with learning problems. Health history should include all illnesses and traumas the child has experienced, including maternal complications of pregnancy. Pregnancy complications are highly correlated with reading disabilities (Bogle, 1973).

5. Developmental history. The developmental history includes at what age the child accomplished specific tasks. A history of significant developmental lag in one or more areas warrants further consideration. The school nurse has much to contribute to the interdisciplinary team

regarding the assessment and early identification of learning disabled children.

School nurse intervention with the learning disabled child

Identification of stressors

The school nurse should consider the amount of stress a student is experiencing before initiating interventions. Normal classroom expectations, such as waiting to be called on before speaking, can prove stressful to the child with a learning disability. Other school-related stressors are described as part of the previous discussion on number and chronicity of stressors. Learning disabilities are of a chronic nature and so the stress is continually compounded. Holmes (1975) strongly advocates discussing the problem with the child, thereby helping him to understand his problem, particularly the singular nature of the disorder, thus decreasing the child's tendency to generalize the disability to other parts of his life. He uses the term "different kinds of brains" to explain learning disability to children and their parents.

Parents also need accurate information regarding the nature of their child's disability. Until they are given the facts, including diagnosis, etiology, and alternative solutions, they cannot deal realistically with the stressor. The school nurse who visits in the home can often identify additional stressors the family is faced with and can help by listening to and correcting (when necessary) the parent's perception of the problem.

Identification of adaptive behaviors

Connolly (1978) reports a typical pattern of parental reaction to the diagnosis of learning disability characterized by doubt, guilt, and anxiety regarding one's inadequacy as a parent. These feelings can result in anger, often directed toward the "imperfect" child.

Children with learning disabilities are at risk for developing deviant social behavior (Bogle, 1973). Because they cannot gain adult attention through the conventional means of accomplishing schoolwork, these children are likely to seek adult attention in other ways, such as through inappropriate behavior and psychosomatic illnesses. This type of adaptation is inadequate because it does not meet their needs and may interfere with the learning needs of their classmates. The goal of professionals is to modify inadequate adaptation before it becomes patterned behavior and to alleviate enough

stress to allow these children to learn by methods appropriate for them.

Alteration of stressor and responses

Treating learning disabilities requires a multidisciplinary professional team, and intervention should include the entire family. Connolly (1978) describes four aspects of intervention: (1) provide facts, (2) dispel unrealistic fears, (3) mobilize school and community resources, and (4) deal with residual problems, such as guilt. The school nurse can assist parents to interact with their learning disabled child by encouraging them to not be overprotective and to identify the relationship between problems they have at school and at home. Parents often need reassurance that they did not cause the problem through inadequate parenting. The school nurse can help parents understand their children, a necessary step toward helping their children, and can also function as a supportive professional and a resource.

In working directly with learning disabled children, the school nurse must collaborate extensively with the other professionals. The school nurse continues to monitor both the child's physical and emotional health, as the student participates in specially designed education.

The attitude of professionals working in this area is extremely influential. The school nurse can assess and emphasize the strengths of the student and family. She can deemphasize the importance of the skill with which the student has trouble to help reduce the stress related to learning that skill. Many times students can learn the skill, if provided enough time (Holmes, 1975). It is important to put the disability into perspective: because a person cannot read fluently does not make him less of a person, nor does it mean he has failed. It only means he does not read fluently. This type of matter-of-fact attitude is helpful for affected families in a society that is achievement oriented.

The school nurse does not directly involve herself in the education of children with special needs, but collaborates, supports, and helps children and their families to adapt adequately.

Evaluation

Several methods of special education for learning disabled children are currently advocated, including family counseling, behavioral and psychological therapy, medical therapy, and educational therapy. The choice of which method to use depends on the philosophy of the professionals involved as well as the individualized needs of the student. A combination of treatment modalities is also acceptable. Some aspects of each method are briefly described here. Family counseling assists the entire family to adjust to their situation. Problem solving for dealing with discipline is discussed, as well as methods of increasing the child's self-esteem. Family counseling not only focuses on the child, however, but also functions to meet the needs of other family members.

Binder and Butler (1978) state that behavioral therapy has had moderate success in modifying behavior patterns of learning disabled children. After behavior is changed through the use of external reinforcements, the children are taught self-control, which demonstrates that they have achieved internal control.

Medical therapy for learning disabled children, an area fraught with controversy, consists of predominantly using stimulant drugs to decrease temper outbursts and improve classroom behavior. Schain and Reynard (1975) have demonstrated significant results through this method. The school nurse needs to monitor children taking such drugs, continually evaluating drug effectiveness and perhaps managing administration as well.

Educational intervention can take one of two forms: total separation of education for the learning disabled from education of other students or a combination of regular education with special education only in specified subjects. Most authors favor keeping the learning disabled student with other students as much as possible.

Regardless of the treatment modality used, specific goals are made for each student. Progress toward the goals is evaluated periodically, and continual assessment by the school nurse is crucial to such evaluation.

Prevention of learning disabilities
Primary prevention

A large portion of primary prevention of learning disabilities involves attacking unfavorable maternal, fetal, and infant conditions. Retrospective studies show that more mothers of children with learning disabilities experienced complications of pregnancy than mothers of children without learning problems (Bogle, 1973). Pregnant teenagers are at greater risk of experiencing complications than are older mothers. The school nurse, by contributing to good care for the pregnant teenager, is therefore also preventing learning disabilities at the primary level.

Good mental health and a positive self-image are important attributes that are being incorporated into school curricula; they are especially important for children with learning disabilities who need to develop a positive self-image and satisfying peer relationships. Other students are also assisted by being aware of the problem and the fact that each person learns differently. Clarizio and McCoy (1970) discuss three ways mental health concepts can be incorporated into school curricula. The first is incidental education, discussing problems as they arise, when students are most motivated. The second is to use separate courses to teach values and attitudes, perhaps through the use of incomplete stories and group discussion. Their third suggestion is the inclusion of mental health "units" in regularly scheduled classes. All three of these methods lead to improved self-esteem for all children, including the learning disabled, as well as an increased awareness and ability to accept individual differences.

Secondary prevention

Early identification of children with learning problems is one focus of secondary prevention. Because schools are dedicated to the education of students, they are responsible for identifying any obstacles to the child obtaining that education. The school nurse and teacher can observe and assess children as they enter school, observing closely any children with characteristics placing them at high risk. Psychologists and physicians are usually available within the school system for consultation when necessary.

Another important aspect of secondary prevention of learning disabilities is early treatment, which can assist the child to learn and prevent secondary behavior problems. Binder and Butler (1978) describe a potentially maladaptive cycle that can occur when the child cannot learn the way other children do. The cycle includes poor self-esteem and poor peer and adult relationships and can result in school dropouts and deviant social behaviors.

Tertiary prevention

Tertiary prevention focuses on special education and family counseling for those affected by learning disabilities. The school nurse can be an active member of the professional team, contributing her expertise for the family's benefit. She can help the family to problem solve and to better understand their situation, thus preventing maladaptive behaviors. The school nurse can be instrumental in maintaining communication among the various professionals working with the family, a function vital to successful intervention.

Because intervention is stressful for children and families, they are more vulnerable to physical illness. The school nurse should promote good health habits, encouraging regular sleep patterns and adequate nutritional intake for all family members. Prevention of physical illness is an important aspect of tertiary prevention.

CHILDREN WITH CHRONIC DISEASES
Definition and scope of the problem

By definition, chronic diseases are of long duration; frequently the disease process is intermittent. Usually chronic diseases are not life threatening; instead, they demand continual small amounts of energy to adjust to the stress they create, leaving less energy for other life events. Frequently, children with chronic diseases require intermittent hospitalization, interrupting their school attendance. Their lowered energy level and poor attendance affect learning. Some chronic diseases, such as heart disease, are severely impairing; others are more subtle and perhaps not even diagnosed, such as allergies. Whether or not the disease is severe, it still has a significant impact on the life and adaptation of afflicted children.

The multiple problems and alterations of daily life when living with a chronic disease are discussed here. Three specific types of chronic diseases are used as examples: allergy, obesity, and handicaps. These examples demonstrate the application of adaptation theory and knowledge of chronic disease.

Allergy is defined by Rapaport and Flint (1976:139) as "a disease syndrome, denoting increased or excessive sensitivity to certain substances." This sensitivity can be either mild or severe and is considered chronic because it generally affects the individual for many years, if not throughout the life span. One estimate reports 1½ million children suffer from asthma alone (Weiss, 1975); others estimate that 25% of children suffer from some form of allergy (Rapaport and Flint, 1976). This serious problem is so widespread that it warrants the attention and intervention of school nurses.

Obesity is another type of chronic syndrome.

It has been defined as "an excessive accumulation of adipose tissue" (Anderson, 1972:560); 20% over the desired body weight is considered obese by insurance companies. Data for children indicates that 10% to 40% of adolescents are obese, a figure which parallels the percentages of overweight adults (Peckos, 1978). Obesity at any age is a serious, chronic problem in which the school nurse is qualified to effectively intervene.

The third category to be considered is handicaps among children, which may include heart disease, diabetes, and seizures as well as speech defects and crippling conditions. Estimating how many children are included in this category is nearly impossible; however, a few statistics follow. Gorwitz (1976) estimates that 86,000 children under age 17 have diabetes, which is about 1.3 per 1000 children. Seizures affect fewer children; about 0.5% experience nonfebrile seizures (Binder and Butler, 1978). Some children with severe handicaps are placed in special schools, but the recent trend has been for them to attend regular school. The school nurse must be ready to deal with a variety of handicaps. Guidelines for dealing with children who are chronically ill are given in Table 9-14.

Factors affecting the child with chronic illness
Developmental stage

As mentioned in Chapter 8, handicaps can influence a child's achievement of tasks for a particular developmental stage. An example is the child who is confined to bed for a chronic illness during the developmental stage of industry versus inferiority. Because the child is unable to be up and about, he may be unable to achieve the tasks of industry (such as cleaning his room, doing special projects). The illness does not need to confine the child to bed to interfere with task accomplishment; for example, an allergy may prevent a child from feeling well enough to do tasks by continually depleting energy sources.

Body image is another aspect of development; children define their body image as they mature. The child with obesity or a physical handicap may develop an unsatisfactory body image. One study demonstrated disturbed body images for physically disabled children as compared to healthy children (Fleming, 1972). Nathan (1973) found that obese children lacked detail and differentiation of body image, perhaps because they are often stigmatized in our

Table 9-14. Guidelines for nursing chronically ill children in school

Factors affecting children with chronic illness	Assessment	Intervention	Prevention
Developmental stage Illness can prevent accomplishment of developmental tasks; body image development is affected by illness Previous experience Heredity, early environmental experience such as amount of food given, types of developmental experiences all influence adaptation to life with chronic illness Perception of event Depends on child's ability to see dysfunctioning body part and on attitudes of significant others; obese adolescents are often discriminated against and appear passive and lack self-confidence Culture Cultural background affects not only care given by parents to ill child, but the meaning of the illness to the child (Chapter 8) Support system Family may lack energy resources to support chronically ill child; parents' emotional reaction to illness affects ability to be supportive; classmates can be supportive if child maintains school attendance Number and chronicity of stressors Long duration of illness contributes to amount and rate of stress to which children must adapt	Current reaction to stressors Poor schoolwork, emotional component of isolation, physical reaction to disease and treatments, other emotional reactions and coping patterns Significance of stressor May interfere with learning, as well as have serious physical and emotional sequelae Availability of help Most chronically ill children require care of specialists; school nurse is responsible for appropriate referrals Previous coping strategies Emphasize strengths; long-term relationships with child provide assistance in times of crisis; use family strengths and play therapy	Identify stressors Use life event scale; assess environment, perception of illness, emotional aspects such as deformity, and change in life-style Identify adaptive behaviors Assess physical status and emotional reaction to illness; see list of ten common emotional reactions in text Alter stressors and responses Alter stresses in environment to meet student's health needs; alter parental anxieties; group sessions for mutual support for students; monitor physical health Evaluation Must be continual because student's needs vary with time	Primary Difficult to prevent totally because cause unknown for many chronic diseases; promotion of good physical and mental health habits Secondary Early detection contributes significantly to reducing complications; teaching of family, student, and faculty can also prevent complications Tertiary Provide needed care to maintain health

society. Young children associate personal-social traits and abilities with body image, making it a very important aspect of their development (Staffieri, 1967).

Previous experience

Many chronic diseases such as diabetes and allergies tend to be hereditary. Early environment also affects health; for example, excessive weight gain during infancy has been associated with a high incidence of obesity in later childhood. Obese children often have hyperplastic obesity, a severe obesity problem associated with an excessive number of fat cells. Some researchers believe that the number of fat cells an individual has is determined and fixed before adulthood; thus obese children may become obese adults. It is difficult for hyperplastic obese persons to lose weight because of their extra fat cells (Peckos, 1978). Hypertrophic obesity is another type of obesity in which the size, not the number, of fat cells is increased.

Some physical handicaps alter the early experiences of children; for example, children with cerebral palsy cannot do the continual reaching and exploring that is normal for most babies. Children with sensory impairment also gain less information about the world around them. As the chronically disabled child develops, he may learn that he is different and may have trouble interacting with the outside world. These early experiences affect how he adapts to school, peers, and other life events. For example, during adolescence a disabled child may not be able to gain independence because a previous history of disability limits his experience. It is especially important, therefore, for schools and parents to build in success experiences for disabled children.

Perception of event

How children perceive their illness depends on (1) their cognitive capacity to understand and (2) the attitudes of those who interact with them, especially parents and peers. Many children assume that their illness is a form of punishment, which implies they are in some way responsible. Magical thinking may even convince children that their illness is the result of their own bad thoughts. It is difficult for school-age children to understand illnesses such as allergy and cardiac conditions, because they cannot see the dysfunctioning body part, but easier for them to understand a broken leg (Bergmann, 1965). Children who cannot understand their illness have a more difficult time adapting to it.

Parental responses to a child's illness strongly influence the child's perception. Arneson and Triplett (1978) found that children whose parents were accepting of a disfiguring illness were also more accepting, as compared to children whose parents did not accept the disfiguration. Juenker (1977) also discusses the phenomenon, stating that children incorporate their parents' emotions. Both authors suggest the best way to alleviate the child's fears and anxieties is to alleviate the fears and anxieties of the parents. Arneson and Triplett (1978) cite three examples of allaying fears, one in which a young girl with alopecia cheerfully wore a wig, showing positive adaptation to a difficult stressor.

Obese adolescents are discussed separately because they are a unique group; Peckos (1978) has found them to have common personality traits of passivity, dependency, lack of self-confidence, and distorted body image. Adolescence is a time when peer acceptance and body image are extremely important. Since obese adolescents commonly are not accepted by their peer group, they experience prejudice and often demonstrate personality characteristics and perceptions similar to ethnic and racial minorities (Peckos, 1978).

Culture

Because parents' attitudes have such a strong effect on their children, the cultural background of parents is an important factor affecting children with chronic illnesses. Illness means different things in different cultures; some illnesses are more readily acceptable in certain cultures than in others. The effect of culture on attitudes about illness is discussed in Chapter 8. The school nurse needs to be aware of the family's cultural background to effectively intervene with a chronically ill child.

Support system

The child's family, his most important support system, suffers from the continual stress of altering family roles to adapt to the needs of the ill person. The added energy required to meet the needs of an ill family member limits the energy available to provide adequate emotional support to that individual. Another factor affecting the family's ability to provide emotional support for an ill child is their perception of the illness. Parents may react with guilt when a child becomes ill, especially if he has inherited a disease, and their own reaction may interfere with their ability to be emotionally supportive.

Classmates and school personnel are another potential source of emotional support for chronically ill children. If school attendance is intermittent due to the illness, the continuity of school-based support systems can be interrupted. The school nurse can initiate contact with hospitalized and homebound children to maintain supportive relationships.

Number and chronicity of stressors

The child with a chronic illness must cope with many stressors over a long time. As the duration increases, new stressors are added to the current stressors; for example, the child with diabetes experiences the physiological stress of a lack of insulin production, the emotional stress of learning to inject himself, and the stress of peer pressure to eat like the other students. These stresses do not ever end, so the chronically ill child faces them in addition to the stresses of everyday life. Stress is not necessarily bad, and the student who learns to stand up to peer pressure may be learning adequate adaptation skills; however, at a certain unknown level, stress can demand more than the energy available to balance it. Chronically ill children are vulnerable to additional illness because of the rate and amount of stress to which they constantly adapt.

Assessment of the chronically ill child
Current reaction to stressor

The school nurse must be alert to various types of physical symptoms, especially when they affect the ability to do schoolwork. Rapaport and Flint (1976) report that the rising incidence of learning disabilities may in part be the result of allergies. Through anecdotal incidents they describe children who were labeled as learning disabled because of their normal intelligence and inability to perform but who were later found to have allergies. They believe those children could not perform well in school because physical symptoms affected their concentration.

Obesity seems to be an obvious problem to assess because it is apparent to all who look at a child that he is overweight. The school nurse should keep records and consult with the child and family; in fact, she may be the first professional to confront them with the tissue. She should not only observe the weight, but the child's reaction to his obese status. Even very young classmates might exclude the obese child from games, and the child must adapt to isolation at an early age.

Seizures are an example of an illness that may be diagnosed previous to school entrance. The school nurse carefully assesses children who have seizures, recording information about the seizures such as length of the seizure, type of seizure, behavior, appearance, and level of consciousness following the seizure, and the child's activities immediately prior to the start of the seizure. The school nurse may also observe the reaction of children to anticonvulsive drugs. She should be aware of all medications children are taking and possible side effects.

The emotional reactions of children to long-term illnesses are another important area for as-

sessment. Emotional reactions are based on various factors, some of which were just discussed. Children's emotional reactions are especially important because they can increase or reduce the stress a child experiences as well as form patterns of behavior that are difficult to change. Children should be observed to determine how they are coping and if the need for additional counseling exists.

Significance of stressor

Allergies have been described as having the potential to affect learning; for example, a child may have an allergy that creates nasal stuffiness to the point that it interferes with sight, hearing, and concentration. Any condition that interferes with learning is a very significant stressor. Allergies are not usually fatal, but can be in rare cases such as an anaphylactic reaction or status asthmaticus.

Obesity is stressful physiologically because it increases the cardiac load and emotionally because it tends to isolate individuals. Approximately 80% of all obese children remain obese as adults (Knittle, 1972). In adults, obesity is a risk factor for other diseases such as hypertension and heart disease; thus this seemingly innocent problem of children has lifelong consequences if untreated.

The significance of long-term and crippling diseases hardly needs reiteration. Diabetes and heart disease can lead to complications and eventual death. Cerebral palsy and physical disabilities result in altered life-styles, poor employability, and low self-esteem. The school nurse, because she is in the school, can have a significant impact on improving the child's adaptation to his illness.

Availability of help

The school nurse's expertise and unique setting allow for significant intervention with chronically ill children. By careful observation and application of her knowledge, the school nurse can do important case finding and make referrals. Most chronically ill children need the care of a specialist; some school districts employ specialists or have connections with municipal clinics. The school nurse must be aware of the specialty services available in her locale. The state-funded Crippled Children's Society is one such source of help. Many specialty clinics are also available, for instance, behavior modification weight-loss clinics. Teachers and classmates can be a source of help for a child who is temporarily out of school or who has special needs. The school nurse is also wise to inquire about support systems for the parents, assisting them to mobilize support as necessary.

Previous coping strategies

The school nurse who maintains a helping relationship with chronically ill students has assisted them through previous crises and is therefore better prepared to guide them through the future crises they will face. Students' strengths should be emphasized, and their diseases put into perspective. If the disease is lifelong, the school nurse can assist the school-age child to develop adequate coping strategies appropriate to his developmental age to adapt to his illness and the problems it entails. The school nurse who is working with the entire family can also assess and strengthen their coping strategies.

Intervention with chronically ill children
Identification of stressors

Chronically ill children may have such a high level of stress that activities of daily living are overwhelming. Tables 7-10 to 7-13 (Coddington, 1972) help the school nurse determine the amount of stress a chronically ill child is experiencing. In addition, the nurse can assess specific aspects of the child's illness that may be stress producing, such as environment, his perception of the illness, and direct consequences of the illness. An example of stress in the environment could be a class pet for a child who is allergic to animal dander. Perception can create stress for a cardiac patient who may worry about his heart rhythm because he cannot see or understand it. The school nurse should listen carefully to the child's interpretation of his illness to gain his perception.

Identification of adaptive behaviors

The school nurse constantly monitors the physical adaptation of chronically ill children to their diseases. She is cognizant of symptoms of inadequate adaptation and intervenes as necessary. For example, the school nurse might weigh children on a weight-reduction program each week to assess their progress. For schoolchildren who have chronic diseases, the school nurse has traditionally assessed their physical adaptation.

Because emotional adaptation strongly influences physical adaptation, the school nurse must also assess emotional adaptation. Juenker (1977:170) outlines ten methods children commonly use to adapt to long-term illnesses:

1. Children may choose one aspect of a stressful event that they feel they can handle and focus on it to reduce feelings of being overwhelmed.
2. The child may deny the existence of the crisis to allow more time to assimilate the stressful event.
3. The child may try to escape by running away or avoiding confrontation.
4. The child may consciously evaluate and accept the stress.
5. Children often seek reassurance and security.
6. Regression to a previous developmental level is another adaptation mechanism.
7. The child may transform the elements of a situation to deal with it more constructively; for instance, by reversing roles and playing "doctor."
8. Children who feel they are responsible for their illness may become depressed.
9. Hypochrondriacal symptoms are common among children who cannot understand their illness.
10. Sublimation, or substituting a realistic goal for an unrealistic goal, is another coping mechanism children may use.

The school nurse should assess these and other adaptive behaviors displayed by children with long-term illnesses and strengthen the most adequate ones.

Alteration of stressors and responses

The school nurse works with children's families and the school environment to reduce the stress experienced; for instance, a pet that arouses an allergic reaction can be replaced, or classmates who encourage consumption of food not allowed on the diabetic's diet can be discouraged. The school nurse must be an advocate for ill children, manipulating the school setting to make it a healthy one for all students.

When parent's anxieties are the source of stress for students, the school nurse can work to alter their perception of the illness, either counseling them herself or referring them to another professional.

The school nurse is also qualified to help students alter their responses to stressful stimuli; for instance, she may assist groups of students to find methods other than eating to relieve anxiety, thus reducing their weight. Behavior modification techniques have proved moderately successful toward weight reduction. The school nurse can initiate small groups and use this technique.

Children who acquire physical handicaps may need assistance to develop new responses to everyday situations, such as leaving class before the bell to allow extra time to get to the next class. Dealing with disfiguring illnesses requires that the child be prepared for the reactions of others, which is easier to do if he has determined his own attitude toward the disfigurement.

For many children physiological responses are altered through the use of medication. Most school-age children can take their own medicine if necessary during school hours; however, the school nurse should be informed about medication that students are taking and monitor them for side effects. The child may also need some teaching and discussion about the medicine to improve his reliability in taking it.

It is the job of the school nurse to ensure that students are adapting to life in as healthy a manner as possible. She is responsible for helping to make the school environment meet the health needs of a wide variety of students, including the special needs of the chronically disabled. This job requires creativity as well as effective communication with faculty and administration.

Evaluation

It is not enough to identify problems and provide appropriate interventions; children and their needs change, and a previously satisfactory plan may no longer meet the student's needs. The school nurse must therefore continually evaluate her interventions. Especially important in long-term care are goals and outcomes. The school nurse who arranges for a student to leave 2 minutes before the bell to get to the next class has set a goal of the student getting to class on time and without the problem of crowded hallways. If this student has a progressive disease, 2 minutes may eventually not be enough time to achieve the desired outcome. Evaluation allows the student to continue to meet the goal by changing the plan according to his needs. Setting actual time limits to reach goals is helpful in long-term care because it provides a specific time for evaluation.

Prevention of chronic illness
Primary prevention

Many chronic illnesses such as allergy and epilepsy cannot be prevented because their cause is unknown. Others such as diabetes appear to have a hereditary component. One method of primary prevention, therefore, is

genetic counseling for those with hereditary diseases. On the other hand, evidence suggests that obesity can be prevented through initiating good dietary patterns from birth. Although the school nurse can do little to prevent specific chronic illnesses, she can assist students in the general area of maintaining good health habits. Good mental and physical health can be promoted both through education and through the nurse's individual interactions with students.

Secondary prevention

Early detection of many chronic diseases reduces the potential for development of complications. Scoliosis, for example, if detected and treated early is easier to correct than if untreated until severe damage has been done. The school nurse's participation in screening is one method of early detection.

Teaching is an important aspect of secondary prevention. Not only the child can benefit by education; the faculty and family can contribute to secondary prevention when they learn the health needs of students. For example, parents can encourage proper eating habits, and teachers can prevent injuries secondary to seizures. Children who have been hospitalized have often been taught about their care by the hospital staff. The stress of hospitalization may necessitate review when these children return to school. In this case, it is most helpful if the school nurse has accurate information about what was taught so that she can build on it rather than confuse them with an entirely new approach.

Tertiary prevention

Whenever possible, the school nurse intervenes to stop progression of sequelae to chronic illnesses (Chapter 6).

SUMMARY

The adaptation theory was used as a framework to discuss school nursing of children experiencing common stressors. Use of this framework begins by becoming knowledgeable about factors that are likely to influence the child. Factors that have been systematically used here are developmental stage, previous experience, perception of the event, culture, support system, and number and chronicity of stressors. With this general knowledge base, the school nurse can then assess how the particular child is adapting to his circumstances. Items to include in assessment are current reactions to stressors, significance of the stressor for the child, availability of help, and previous coping strategies. At this point, the school nurse has determined whether she will refer the child and work with an interdisciplinary team, or whether it is a nursing problem. Intervention proceeds through four stages: identification of stressors, identification of adaptive responses, alterations of stressors and responses, and evaluation. The school nurse may wish to individualize this framework to her situational constraints and personal nursing philosophy. The emphasis is on using a framework that becomes an almost automatic system, allowing the school nurse to be comprehensive.

Prevention is an extremely important aspect of the school nurses' job. The 1970s were a time when the general public became more aware of the individual's responsibility for his own health. In addition, studies have demonstrated a significant correlation between life-style and health. Combined, these two facts demonstrate the need for teaching self-responsibility and prevention as a life-style to young children who are just forming their health habits. The school nurse can be instrumental in promoting a healthy future for the next generation.

Prevention is unique in that it promotes a healthy life-style, and often more than one stressor is avoided. For example, prevention of an unwanted teenage pregnancy may also prevent child abuse, chemical dependency, and learning disabilities. In this way, prevention is the most basic task for the school nurse, one which may make some of the problems children experience less severe.

REFERENCES

Adler, S. J., and Steinberg, R. M.: 1977. The pediatric examination of M.B.D., learning disabilities, and related disorders, Year Book Medical Publishers, Inc., Chicago.

Aguilera, D. C., and Messick, J. M.: 1978. Crisis intervention: theory and methodology, 3rd ed., The C. V. Mosby Co., St. Louis.

Alafro, J.: 1976. Report of New York State Assembly Select Committee on Child Abuse, Child Protection Report, vol. II, no. 1, Washington, D.C.

Anderson, C.: 1976. Adolescent pregnancy, Issues Compr. Pediatr. Nurs. 6(1):43-49.

Anderson, J.: 1972. Obesity, Br. Med. J. 1:560-563.

Arneson, S. W., and Triplett, J. L.: 1978. How children cope with disfiguring changes in their appearance, MCN 3(6):366-370.

Bandura, A.: 1973, Aggression: a social learning analysis, Prentice-Hall, Inc., Englewood Cliffs, N.J.

Bandura, A., and Walters, R. H.: 1963. Social learning and personality development, Holt, Rinehart & Winston, Inc., New York.

Barnhart, C. L., editor: 1956. Concise dictionary, Doubleday & Co., Inc., New York.

Battaglia, F., Frazier, T., and Hellegers, A.: 1963. Obstetric and pediatric complications of juvenile pregnancy, Pediatrics 32:902-910.

Beck, A. T., Resnik, H. L. P., and Lettieri, D. J.: 1974. The prediction of suicide, Charles Press, Bowie, Md.

Benson, H.: 1975. The relaxation response, Avon Books, New York.

Bergmann, T.: 1965. Children in the hospital, International Universities Press, Inc., New York.

Binder, F. Z., and Butler, J. E.: 1978. Children with learning disabilities, Issues Compr. Pediatr. Nurs. 3(3):1-14.

Blades, S.: 1976. Clinical notes on adolescent drug abuse, Issues Compr. Pediatr. Nurs. 6(1):59-64.

Bloomquist, K. B.: 1974. Nurse, I need help: the school nurse's role in suicide prevention, J. Psychiatr. Nurs. 12(1):22-26.

Bogle, M. W.: 1973. Relationship between deviant behavior and reading disability: a retrospective study of the role of the nurse, J. School Health 43(5):312-315.

Boland, M., Murray, R., and Nolan, N.: 1979. Application of adaptation theory to nursing. In Murray, R., and Zentner, J., Nursing concepts for health promotion, 2nd ed., Prentice-Hall, Inc., Englewood Cliffs, N.J.

Bowlby, J.: 1973. Attachment and loss: separation, vol. 2, Basic Books, Inc., Publishers, New York.

Braen, B. B., and Forbush, J. B.: 1975. School-age parenthood—a national overview, J. School Health 45(5):256-262.

Brann, E. A.: 1979. A multivariate analysis of interstate variation in fertility of teenage girls, Am. J. Public Health 69(7):661-666.

Breen, M.: 1968. Culture and schizophrenia: a study of Negro and Jewish schizophrenics, Int. J. Soc. Psychiatry 14:282.

Broadhurst, D. D.: 1978. What schools are doing about abuse and neglect, Children Today 7:22-24.

Brown, J. T., and Clancy, B. J.: 1976. Meeting the needs of teens regarding their sexuality, Issues Compr. Pediatr. Nurs. 1(4):29-42.

Brownlee, A. T.: 1978. Community, culture, and care. A cross-cultural guide for health workers, The C. V. Mosby Co., St. Louis.

Caplan, G.: 1961. An approach to community mental health, Grune & Stratton, Inc., New York.

Caplan, G.: 1964. Principles of preventive psychiatry, Basic Books, Inc., Publishers, New York.

Center for Disease Control (CDC): 1974. Abortion surveillance, 1972, Atlanta.

Chafetz, M. E., Blane, H. T., and Hill, M. J.: 1970. Frontiers of alcoholism, Science House, New York.

Clarizio, H. F., and McCoy, G. F.: 1970. Behavior disorders in school-age children, Chandler Publishing Co., New York.

Cline, F. W.: 1978. Adolescent suicide, Nurse Pract. 3:44-45.

Coddington, R. D.: 1972. The significance of life events as etiological factors in diseases of children, I: A survey of professional workers, J. Psychosom. Res. 16(1):7-18.

Colucci, N. D.: 1977. The schools and the problem of child abuse and neglect, Contemp. Ed. 48:98-100.

Connolly, C.: 1978. Counseling parents of school-age children with special needs, J. School Health 48(2):115-117.

Cork, M. R.: 1969. The forgotten child, Alcoholism and Drug Addiction Research Foundation, Toronto.

Cyphert, F. R.: 1973. Back to school for the child with cancer, J. School Health 43(4):215-217.

Dale, J. J.: 1978. An evaluation of a programme of school health education on smoking, Health Ed. J. **37:**142-144.

Davis, J.: 1977. School phobia in adolescence, Nurs. Mirror **144:**61.

DeFrancis, V.: 1965. Protecting the child victim of sex crimes, American Humane Association, Denver.

DeLint, S. C.: 1964. Alcoholism, birth rank, and paternal deprivation, Am. J. Psychiatry **120:**1062-1065.

Dubós, R.: 1965. Man adapting, Yale University Press, New Haven, Conn.

Duvall, E. M.: 1971. Family development, 4th ed., J. B. Lippincott Co., Philadelphia.

Erikson, E.: 1963. Childhood and society, 2nd ed., W. W. Norton & Co., Inc., New York.

Estes, N. J., and Heinemann, M. E.: 1977. Alcoholism: development, consequences, and interventions, The C. V. Mosby Co., St. Louis.

Fink, S. L.: 1967. Crisis and motivation: a theoretical model, Arch. Phys. Med. Rehabil. **48:**592-597.

Finn, P.: 1977. Should alcohol education be taught with drug education? J. School Health **47:**466-469.

Fleming, J.: 1972. Understanding children through drawings, Eighth Nursing Research Conference, Albuquerque, New Mexico, March 15 to 17, 1972, American Nurses Association, New York, pp. 133-147.

Fredlund, D.: 1970. Juvenile delinquency and school nursing, Nurs. Outlook **18**(5):57-59.

Fredlund, D. J.: 1977. Children and death from the school setting viewpoint, J. School Health **47**(11):533-537.

Freedman, A. M., Kaplan, H. I., and Sadock, B. J.: 1972. Modern synopsis of psychiatry, The Williams & Wilkins Co., Baltimore.

Fromer, M. J.: 1979. Community health care and the nursing process, The C. V. Mosby Co., St. Louis.

Fyvel, T. R.: 1962. Troublemakers, Schocken Books, Inc., New York.

Gabrielson, I. W., Klerman, L. V., Currie, J. B., and Tyler, N. C.: 1970. Suicide attempts in a population pregnant as teenagers, Am. J. Public Health **60:**2289-2301.

Glueck, S., and Glueck, E.: 1950. Unraveling juvenile delinquency, Commonwealth Fund, New York.

Glueck, S., and Glueck, E.: 1952. Delinquents in the making, Harper & Brothers, New York.

Goldhill, P. M.: 1971. A parent's guide to the prevention and control of drug abuse, Popular Library, New York.

Goodman, L. S., and Gilman, A.: 1975. The pharmacological basis of therapeutics, 5th ed., Macmillan, Inc., New York.

Gordon, V.: 1979. Women and divorce: implications for nursing care. In Kjervik, D., and Martinson, I., editors: Women in stress: a nursing perspective, Appleton-Century-Crofts, New York.

Gorwitz, K.: 1976. Prevalence of diabetes in Michigan school-age children, Diabetes **24:**122.

Graf, C. M.: 1976. Sex and the adolescent, Issues Compr. Pediatr. Nurs. **6**(1).31-41.

Greenberg, J. S., and Deputat, Z.: 1978. Smoking intervention: comparing three methods in a high school setting, J. School Health **48**(8):498-502.

Greer, S., and Lee, H. A.: 1967. Subsequent progress of potentially lethal attempted suicides, Acta Psychiatr. Scand. **43:**361-371.

Gyulay, J. E.: 1978. The dying child, McGraw Hill, Inc., New York.

Halperin, M.: 1979. Helping maltreated children: school and community involvement, The C. V. Mosby Co., St. Louis.

Hart, N. A., and Keidel, G. C.: 1979. The suicidal adolescent, Am. J. Nurs. **79**(1):80-84.

Helfer, R. E., and Kempe, C. H.: 1976. Child abuse and neglect: the family and the community, Ballinger Publishing Co., Cambridge, Mass.

Henderlich, J.: 1977. Health care of the heroin-dependent woman. In Lytte, N. A., editor: Nursing of women in the age of liberation, Wm. C. Brown Co., Publishers, Dubuque, Iowa.

Holland, J. V., Kaplan, D. M., and Davis, S. D.: 1974. Interschool transfers: a mental health challenge, J. School Health **44**(2):74-79.

Holmes, D. J.: 1975. Disturbances of the preschool and very young school child, J. School Health **45**(4):210-216.

Houston Chronicle, September 2, 1978, p. 2.

Huberty, D. J., and Malmquist, J. D.: 1978. Adolescent chemical dependency, Perspect. Psychiatr. Care **1**(6):21-27.

Jacobs, J.: 1971. Adolescent suicide, John Wiley & Sons, Inc., New York.

Jasmin, J., and Trygstad, L. N.: 1979. Behavioral concepts and the nursing process, The C. V. Mosby Co., St. Louis.

Jekel, J. F.: 1975. Appraising programs for school-age parents, J. School Health **45**(5):296-300.

Jekel, J. F.: 1977. Primary or secondary prevention of adolescent pregnancies? J. School Health **47**(8):457-461.

Jenkins, S.: 1978. Children of divorce, Children Today **7:**11-15.

Johnson, R. N.: 1972. Aggression in men and animals, W. B. Saunders, Co., Philadelphia.

Juenker, D.: 1977. Child's perception of his illness. In Steele, S., editor: Nursing care of the child with long-term illness, Appleton-Century-Crofts, New York.

Justice, B., and Justice, R.: 1976. The abusing family, Human Sciences Press, Inc., New York.

Kahn, J. H., and Nursten, J. P.: 1964. Unwillingly to school, Pergamon Press, Inc., Elmsford, New York.

Kaplan, D. M.; 1974. School management of the seriously ill child, J. School Health **44**(5):250-253.

Kaplan, H. E.: 1972. Towards a general theory of psychosocial deviance: the case of aggressive behavior, Soc. Sci. Med. **6:**605-615.

King, C. H.: 1975. The ego and the integration of violence in homicidal youth, Am. J. Orthopsychiatry **44:**134-145.

Kirk, S. A., and Bateman, B.: 1962. Diagnosis and remediation of learning disabilities, Exceptional Children **29**(2):73-78.

Kirten, C., and Liverman, M.: 1977. Special educational needs of the child with cancer, J. School Health **47**(3):170-172.

Klein, L.: 1975. Models of comprehensive service—regular school-based, J. School Health **45**(5):271-273.

Klerman, L. V.: 1975. Adolescent pregnancy: the need for new policies and new programs, J. School Health **45**(5):263-267.

Klimenko, A.: 1968. Multi-family therapy in the rehabilitation of drug addicts, Perspect. Psychiatr. Care **6:**220-223.

Knittle, J. L.: 1972. Obesity in childhood: a problem in adipose tissue cellular development, J. Pediatr. **18:**1048-1049.

Kovar, M. G.: 1979. Some indicators of health-related behavior among adolescents in the United States, Public Health Reports **94**(2):109-118.

Kubler-Ross, E.: 1969. On death and dying, Macmillan, Inc., New York.

Kvaraceus, W. C.: 1953. JD proneness scale and check list, World Book, New York.

Kvaraceus, W. C.: 1956. Forecasting juvenile delinquency, World Book, New York.

Larson, M. L.: 1978. Violent behaviors. In Longo, D. C., and Williams, R. A., editors: Clinical practice in psychosocial nursing: assessment and intervention, Appleton-Century-Crofts, New York.

Laufer, M. W., and Denhoff, E.: 1957. Hyper-kinetic behavior syndrome in children, J. Pediatr. **50**:463-474.

Lee, E. E.: 1978. Female adolescent drinking behavior: potential hazards, J. School Health **48**(3):151-156.

Leese, S. M.: 1974. Sexual urges in adolescents, Nurs. Times **70**(38):475.

Leonard, B., Murray, R., Zentner, J., Smith, M., and Nolan, N.: 1979. Assessment and health promotion for the schoolchild. In Murray, R., and Zentner, J.: Nursing assessment and health promotion through the lifespan, 2nd ed., Prentice-Hall, Inc., Englewood Cliffs, N.J.

Leton, D. A.: 1962. Assessment of school phobia, Mental Hygiene **46**:256-264.

Lindsay, J. S.: 1973. Suicide in the Auckland area, NZ Med. J. **77**:149-157.

Lukianowicz, N.: 1968. Attempted suicide in children, Acta Psychiatr. Scand. **44**:415-435.

MacElveen, P. M.: 1978. Social networks. In Longo, D. C., and Williams, R. A., editors: Clinical practice in psychosocial nursing: assessment and intervention, Appleton-Century-Crofts, New York.

Marthas-Sampson, M.: 1978. Adolescents who commit suicidal acts: suicidogenic factors, Issues Compr. Pediatr. Nurs. **1**(3):49-64.

Martin, H., and Prange, A.: 1962. Human adaptation: a conceptual approach to understanding patients, Can. Nurse **58**(3):234-243.

McCarthy, J. J., and McCarthy, J. F.: 1969. Learning disabilities, Allyn and Bacon, Inc., Boston.

McNeese, M. C., and Hebeler, J. R.: 1977. The abused child: a clinical approach to identification and management, Clin. Symposia **29**(5):1-36.

Moller, H.: 1967. Death: handling the subject and affected students in the schools. In Grollman, E. A., editor: Explaining death to children, Beacon Press, Boston.

Montagu, A.: 1969. Chromosomes and crime. In Readings in psychology today, Communications/Research/Machines, Inc., Del Mar, Calif.

Muehl, J. N.: 1979. Seizure disorders in children: prevention and care, MCN **3**(4):154-160.

Murray, R., Luetje, V., and Zentner, J.: 1979a. Crisis intervention: a therapy technique. In Murray, R., and Zentner, J.: Nursing concepts for health promotion, 2nd ed., Prentice-Hall, Inc., Englewood Cliffs, N.J.

Murray, R., Nolan, N., Zentner, J., and Smith, M.: 1979b. Assessment and health promotion for the young adult. In Murray, R., and Zentner, J.: Nursing assessment and health promotion through the life span, 2nd ed., Prentice-Hall, Inc., Englewood Cliffs, N.J.

Murray, R., and Zentner, J.: 1979a. Nursing assessment and health promotion through the life span, 2nd ed., Prentice-Hall, Inc., Englewood Cliffs, N.J.

Murray, R., and Zentner, J.: 1979b. Nursing concepts for health promotion, 2nd ed., Prentice-Hall, Inc., Englewood Cliffs, N.J.

Nakashima, I. I.: 1977. Teenage pregnancy—its causes, costs and consequences, Nurse Pract. **2**(7):10-13.

Nathan, S.: 1973. Body image in chronically obese children as reflected in figure drawings, English J. Personal Assessment **37**:456.

National Center of Child Abuse and Neglect: 1976. Child abuse and neglect reports, Department of Health, Education, and Welfare, No. 87-30086, Washington, D.C.

Nolan, N., Murray, R., Grohar, M., Leonard, B., Smith, M., and Zentner, J.: 1979. Assessment and health promotion for the adolescent/youth. In Murray, R., and Zentner, J.: Nursing assessment and health promotion through the life span, 2nd ed., Prentice-Hall, Inc., Englewood Cliffs, N.J.

Notaro, C.: 1976. Adolescents and alcohol, Issues Compr. Pediatr. Nurs. **6**(1):50-58.

Oppel, W., and Royston, A.: 1971. Teenage births: some social, psychological, and physical sequelae, Am. J. Public Health **6**:751-756.

Paeregaard, G.: 1975. Suicide among attempted suicides: a 10-year follow-up, Suicide **5**:140-144.

Peckos, P.: 1978. The treatment of adolescent obesity, Issues Compr. Pediatr. Nurs. **1**(3):17-29.

President's Committee on Heart Disease, Cancer, and Stroke: 1968. A national program to conquer heart disease, cancer, and stroke, U.S. Public Health Service, Washington, D.C.

Rapaport, H. G., and Flint, S. H.; 1976. Is there a relationship between allergy and learning disabilities? J. School Health **46**(3):139-141.

Redman, B. K.: 1980. The process of patient teaching in nursing, 4th ed., The C. V. Mosby Co., St. Louis.

Renshaw, D. C.: 1974. Suicide and depression in chilren, J. School Health **44**(9):487-489.

Report: 1964. Smoking and health: report of the Advisory Committee to the Surgeon General of the Public Health Service, Public Health Service Publication No. 1103, U.S. Government Printing Office, Washington, D.C.

Report: 1967. The health consequences of smoking; a public health service review, Public Health Service Publication No. 1696, U.S. Government Printing Office, Washington, D.C.

Reuben, R. N., and Bakivin, H.: 1968. Developmental clumsiness, Pediatr. Clin. North Am. **15**(31):601-610.

Richards, M. D.: 1972. Caught in conflict: the unmarried minor mother, Child Welfare **51**:391-395.

Riggs, R. S., and Evans, D. W.: 1978. The preprofessional elementary educator's knowledge and opinions regarding child abuse, College Student **12**:290-293.

Riggs, R. S., and Evans, D. W.: 1979. Child abuse prevention—implementation within the curriculum. J. School Health **49**(5):255-259.

Rohn, R. D.: 1977. Adolescents who attempt suicide, J. Pediatr. **90**:636-638.

Rubenfeld, S.: 1965. Family of outcasts, The Free Press, New York.

Sahler, O. J. Z.: 1978. The child and death, The C. V. Mosby Co., St. Louis.

Schain, R. J., and Reynard, C. L.: 1975. Observations on effects of a central stimulant drug in children with hyperactive behavior, Pediatrics **55**(5):709-716.

Schowalter, J. F.: 1976. How do children and funerals mix? J. Pediatr. **89**:139-141.

Schwartz, B. A.: 1975. Rock and "bye" baby, J. Obstet. Gynecol. Nurs. **4**(5):27-30.

Selye, H.: 1965. The stress syndrome, Am. J. Nurs. **65**(3):97-99.

Selye, H.: 1974. Stress without distress, New American Library, Inc., New York.

Shapiro, S., Schlesinger, E. R., and Nesbitt, R.: 1968. Infant, perinatal, maternal, and childhood mortality in the United States, Harvard University Press, Cambridge, Mass.

Shore, J. H.: 1975. American Indian suicide—fact and fantasy, Psychiatry **38:**86-92.

Siemon, M. K.: 1978. Family subsystem: working with school-age children experiencing psychosocial stress. In Longo, D. C., and Williams, R. A., editors: Clinical practice in psychosocial nursing: assessment and intervention, Appleton-Century-Crofts, New York.

Smith, E. W.: 1975. The role of the grandmother in adolescent pregnancy and parenting, J. School Health **45**(5):278-283.

Spector, R. E.: 1979. Cultural diversity in health and illness, Appleton-Century-Crofts, New York.

Staffieri, J. R.: 1967. A study of social stereotype of body image in children, J. Pers. Soc. Psychol. **7:**101-109.

Steele, B. F.: 1976. Violence within the family. In Helfer, R. E., and Kempe, C. H., editors: Child abuse and neglect: the family and the community, Ballinger Publishing Co., Cambridge, Mass.

Stengel, E.: 1962. Recent research into suicide and attempted suicide, Am. J. Psychiatry **118:**725-727.

Stone, E. J.: 1978. The effects of a fifth grade health education curriculum model on perceived vulnerability and smoking attitudes, J. School Health **48**(1):667-671.

Sullivan, H. S.: 1953. The interpersonal theory of psychiatry, W. W. Norton & Co., Inc., New York.

Tanner, L. M.: 1969. Developmental tasks of pregnancy. In Bergersen, B., Anderson, E., Duffey, M., Lohr, M., and Rose, M., editors: Current concepts in clinical nursing, vol. 2, The C. V. Mosby Co., St. Louis.

ten Bensel, R. W., and Berdie, J.: 1976. The neglect and abuse of children and youth: the scope of the problem and the school's role, J. School Health **46**(8):453-461.

The Nations Health: 1979. American Public Health Association **11:**0028-0496.

Timnick, L.: 1978. Child suicides, *Minneapolis Star,* Wednesday, July 26, 1978.

Triplett, J. L., and Arneson, S. W.: 1978. Children of alcoholic parents: a neglected issue, J. School Health **48**(10):596-599.

University of Minnesota: 1979. Unpublished course syllabus for N5203 "Adaptation I," University of Minnesota School of Nursing, Minneapolis.

U.S. Division of Vital Statistics: 1976. Annual summary for the United States, 1975, U.S. Government Printing Office, Washington, D.C.

Waechter, E.: 1971. Children's awareness of fatal illness, Am. J. Nurs. **71**(6):1168-1172.

Weiss, E. B.: 1975. Clinical symposia, bronchial asthma, CIBA-GEIGY Corp., Summit, N.J.

Werry, J. S.: 1968. Developmental hyperactivity, Pediatric Clin. North Am. **15**(3):581-599.

Yankelovich, D.: 1975. Drug users vs. drug abusers: how students control their drug crisis, Psychology Today **9**(5):39-42.

Zelnick, M., and Kantner, J. P.: 1974. The resolution of teenage first pregnancies, Fam. Plann. Perspect. **6**(2):74-80.

SUGGESTED READINGS

Adams, R. M.: 1979. Medication and hyperkinesis: a new concept, J. School Health **49**(4):226.

Algozzine, B., and Algozzine, K. M.: 1978. Some practical considerations of hyperactivity and drugs, J. School Health, **48**(8):479-483.

Bandura, A., and Walters, R. H.: 1959. Adolescent aggression, Ronald Press, New York.

Bandura, A., and Walters, R. H.; 1963. Social learning and personality development, Holt, Rinehart, & Winston, New York.

Chamberlain, N.: 1974. The nurse and the abusive parent, Nursing '74 **4:**72-76.

Chinn, P. C., Winn, J., and Walters, R. H.: 1978. Two-way talking with parents of special children: a process of positive communication, The C. V. Mosby Co., St. Louis.

Conway, B. L.: 1977. Pediatric Neurologic Nursing, The C. V. Mosby Co., St. Louis.

Court to use teen jurors in sentencing juveniles, *Minneapolis Star and Tribune,* Saturday, May 26, 1979.

Ferinden, W. E.: 1972. The role of the school nurse in the early identification of potential learning disabilities, J. School Health **42**(2):86-87.

Golden, G. S.: 1979. The effect of developmental disabilities on mental health, J. School Health **49**(5):260-262.

Gould, R. E.: 1965. Suicide problems in children and adolescents, Am. J. Psychotherapy **19:**228-246.

Greenberg, J. S.: 1976. Hyperkinesis and the schools, J. School Health **46**(2):91-97.

Greenberg, J. S., and Sullivan, R.: 1977. The need for prenatal health education, Health Ed. J. **36:**84-87.

Grollman, E. A.: 1971. Suicide. Beacon Press, Boston.

Haverkamp, L. J., 1970. Brain-injured children and the school nurse, J. School Health **40**(5):228-235.

Krager, J. M., Safer, D., and Earhart, J.: 1979. Follow-up survey results of medication used to treat hyperactive school children, J. School Health **49**(6):317-321.

Kruger, W. S.: 1975. Education for parenthood and school-age parents, J. School Health **45**(5):292-295.

Lindeman, C.: 1974. Birth control and the unmarried young woman, Springer Publishing Co., Inc., New York.

Marko, M. B.: 1974. Recognition of the allergic child at school: visual and auditory signs, J. School Health, **44**(5):277-284.

Matteson, D. R.: 1975. Adolescence today, Dorsey Press, Homewood, Ill.

McConville, B. J.: 1978. The effect of non-traditional families on children's mental health, Can. Mental Health **26**(3):3-10, supplement 1.

Muehl, J. N.: 1979. Seizure disorders in children: prevention and care, MCN **3**(4):154-160.

Peterson, M. L.: 1977. The pregnant adolescent in a primary care setting. In Lytte, N. A., editor: Nursing of women in the age of liberation, Wm. C. Brown Co., Publishers, Dubuque, Iowa.

Rapaport, H. G., and Flint, S. H.: 1974. Allergy in the schools, J. School Health **44**(5):265-269.

Reinert, H. R.: 1980. Children in conflict: educational strategies for the emotionally disturbed and behaviorally disordered, 2nd ed., The C. V. Mosby Co., St. Louis.

Robin, M.: 1973. How emotions affect skin problems in school children, J. School Health **43**(6):370-380.

Skellern, J.: 1979. The self-concept of children and adolescents and the effects of physical disability, Aust. Nurses J. **8**(6):36-38.

Steele, S.: 1977. Nursing care of the child with long-term illness, 2nd ed., Appleton-Century-Crofts, New York.

Thomas, J. E.: 1977. Adolescence and weight control, Health Educ. J. **36:**19-26.

Timmreck, T. C.: 1978. Will the real cause of classroom discipline problems please stand up! J. School Health **48**(8):491-497.

Washington, V. E.: 1975. Models of comprehensive service—special school-based, J. School Health **45**(5):274-277.

Weidman, W. H.: 1979. High blood pressure [hypertension] and the school-age child, J. School Health **49**(4): 213-214.

Wieczorek, R. R., and Horner-Rosner, B.: 1979. The asthmatic child: preventing and controlling attacks, Am. J. Nurs. **79**(2):258-262.

Woodard, P. B., and Brodie, B.: 1974. The hyperactive child: who is he? Nurs. Clin. North Am. **9**(4):727-745.

Woody, J. D.: 1973. Contemporary sex education: attitudes and implications for childbearing, J. School Health **43**(4):241-246.

PART IV

Helping relationship concepts in school nursing practice

CHAPTER 10

Defining and developing helping relationships

ELLEN D. SCHULTZ

Establishing a helping relationship is basic to all nursing care and is a vital component for the practice of school nursing. ''Professional helpers'' are individuals from various disciplines, including nurses, social workers, psychologists, and others. The purpose of this chapter is to provide information that the school nurse can apply to the development of helping relationships in individual practice. Included in this chapter are the following:

1. A description of the helping relationship
2. Identification of the participants in the relationship and their distinctive aspects and contributions
3. A description of stages and skills relative to the development of the helping relationship

DEFINING THE HELPING RELATIONSHIP
Description of helping

When defining a helping relationship, it is important to look at the process of helping as well as the end product, since it is only in the present, or through the process, that one individual can relate to another. The process of helping is an ''enabling act.'' It involves building a relationship that provides an atmosphere for exploration and a positive environment for growth and self-awareness. In addition, the helper attempts to facilitate a more satisfying exchange between the individual and his environment.

Although the helping relationship offers the helper rewards and satisfaction, the purpose of the relationship is to meet the client's needs. The relationship facilitates growth of the individual (or group) in a self-defined direction. This implies helping by agreement. A dilemma can be created if the nurse's sincere and honest desire to be helpful impels her to ''help'' before the client has agreed to the relationship. In this situation the helper must carefully examine whether she is meeting her own needs to ''care for,'' or if she is being directed by a perceived need of the client.

''To care for another person in the most significant sense is to help him grow and actualize himself'' (Mayeroff, 1971:1). In assisting another to grow, the helper uses the direction of the client's growth as a guide. Although helping is other directed, this does not mean it is a passive experience. On the contrary, helping is an active experience requiring a thorough assessment of the client, building of a trusting relationship, use of specific skills, investment of self, and evaluation of process and outcomes.

The client may enter into the relationship in a crisis state, during which he is unable to determine his own plan or solutions. In this situation a nondirective approach by the school nurse would not be appropriate. When the client is unable to problem solve, the nurse moves to a more directive approach, in which she jointly plans with the client or, in some cases, defines solutions for the client. This type of direction by the nurse is used only until the client is able to begin giving direction to the relationship.

Change is usually part of the relationship process. It is the responsibility of the helper to remove obstacles that might prevent change, but not to demand that a specific change occur. For example, a teenage girl may consult the school nurse because she wants to improve communications with her parents, but does not know how to begin in a constructive manner. The school nurse could provide the girl with information about useful communication skills, and she could arrange a family meeting in which the situation would be discussed and appropriate skills demonstrated. ''The helper enables the client to recognize, to feel, to know, to decide, to choose whether to change'' (Benjamin, 1974:xii).

Unlike some other professionals, the school nurse does not limit her clients to a select group. Her client system extends from students and their significant others to school personnel and the community. Although the participants may vary, the principles of helping remain the same. The primary adaptation is modification of language to meet the cultural, intellectual, and developmental needs of the client.

Professional and nonprofessional relationships

Helping exists as part of a variety of relationships and is not limited to professionals. Webster's definition of help, ''to make it easier for [a person] to do something, to give assistance, to be cooperative,'' supports the idea that most people are capable of helping. Why then is it necessary for the school nurse, as a professional, to learn about the helping relationship?

The professional helping relationship developed between the school nurse and her clients differs from one that is nonprofessional, even though they may share some common characteristics. In a friendship, people help each other; it is a give-and-take interaction. In a professional relationship, the helper is not looking for a friend, although at times this is an unexpected outcome. The helper receives satisfaction from the process, but does not expect to be ''helped'' in return.

The professional relationship is also more structured than one that is nonprofessional. Professional helping involves negotiation of a contract between the participants. This contract sets limits and goals for the relationship. Nonprofessional relationships rarely include this type of structure. Finally, in a helping relationship the helper uses specific behaviors and communication skills that have been learned through a formal educational process. These skills are described on pp. 224 to 226.

The humanistic framework

Before entering into helping relationships, the school nurse must examine her philosophical beliefs about fellow human beings. These beliefs are a frame of reference she uses to guide her actions. The humanistic framework is the basis for this chapter and has relevance for nursing. People operating from a humanistic orientation hold these three basic assumptions (Chapman and Chapman, 1975:29-30):

1. All people have a right to dignity.
2. To respect dignity is to look at people as they see themselves, as ''whole, conscious-experiencing persons.''
3. People have a ''satisfying, self-actualizing and committed existence'' as a life goal.

Humanism takes an optimistic view of man, focusing on his uniqueness and capabilities. Behavior is identified as purposeful; people are seen as being responsible and able to make their own decisions.

Professionals working from a humanistic framework demonstrate positive regard for their clients by respecting and accepting them. Genuineness is shown throughout the relationship, and the helper attempts to understand the client's perceptions accurately.

In summary, the helping relationship is a mutually agreed on interaction in which problems are not solved for the client; rather, the participants work together in the problem-solving process. The helper provides an atmosphere of acceptance and holds an attitude and set of behaviors that facilitate growth of the helpee.

PARTICIPANTS IN THE RELATIONSHIP
The helper

Actually, a helper can be anyone who gives aid or assistance to another. The focus here is not on any helper but rather on the highly skilled professional helper. Part of the following description may apply to nonprofessionals as well because the characteristics are not held exclusively by professionals.

Professionals working from a variety of theoretical frameworks and having differing personalities can be effective helpers. Therefore it would be nearly impossible to designate a list of adjectives that would appropriately describe all helpers. It is possible, though, to identify distinctive characteristics of helping professionals that facilitate the helping process. Six of the most significant characteristics will be described here.

1. *Self-awareness.* The helper must know and understand himself because ''. . . a fuller understanding of oneself seems to increase one's ability to appreciate more quickly who the person realistically is'' (Chapman and Chapman, 1975:49). Self-awareness includes perceptions, interpretations, feelings, intentions, and actions (Miller et al., 1975:30-31). For the helper to know and un-

derstand himself, the following questions may be useful:

a. *Perceptions:* Do I perceive my environment similar to the way that others do or are my perceptions frequently inaccurate?

b. *Interpretations:* Do my impressions, ideas, and beliefs facilitate the helping relationship?

c. *Feelings:* Am I able to recognize my feelings? Can I accept negative feelings?

d. *Intentions:* What do I want from the relationship? Can I accept a situation in which my goals differ from those of the client?

e. *Actions:* Do my behaviors facilitate the growth of the other?

2. *Involvement.* Glasser describes involvement as a necessary part of Reality Therapy, but its application extends to all helping relationships. "The therapist or helper must become involved with the person he is trying to help; the therapist, therefore, must be warm, personal and friendly. No one can break the intense self-involvement of failure by being aloof, impersonal or emotionally distant" (Glasser, 1972:107-108). The helper provides adequate involvement in the relationship to enable the client to develop new and lasting relationships. This requires that the helper be interested, human, and sensitive. Other aspects of the helping relationship are built on this basic foundation.

3. *Strength.* The professional helper must have sufficient strength to give of herself within the framework of the helping relationship. "Effective helping will be a function of the effective use of the helper's self . . ." (Combs et al., 1971:5-6). The helper does not mechanically use the necessary skills to achieve a goal; she invests some of herself in each relationship.

4. *Honesty.* Trust, which is basic to helping, is built on honesty. When one answers the client's questions in the best possible way, demonstrates a willingness to explore the client's concerns, and provides factual information and fair evaluations, one is being honest.

5. *Knowledge.* There are three areas of knowledge that are especially relevant for the professional helper: knowledge of oneself (self-awareness), knowledge of the other, and knowledge of the skills necessary to develop the relationship. Gaining knowledge about the client begins during the assessment process and continues throughout the relationship. The helper learns about the power and limitations of the client, his needs, and what is conducive to his growth. Knowledge of the appropriate helping skills will be discussed on pp. 224 to 226.

6. *Hope.* When the helper conveys hope, it is an expression of the "plentitude of the present, a present alive with a sense of the possible" (Mayeroff, 1971:26). Hope is based on the awareness of *this* person at *this* time and how present strengths can be used for future growth.

The helpee

The helpee is any person (or group) entering into a helping relationship for the purpose of receiving assistance in defining or achieving a goal. This definition could apply to most people at some time during their lives. Just as there are distinctive aspects of the helper that facilitate the process, there are also characteristics of the helpee that facilitate the process. Four characteristics will be discussed here.

1. *Self-disclosure.* In self-disclosure one makes oneself known to others. People disclose certain aspects of themselves to others daily, but the most personal aspects of the self can be kept well hidden. Jourard looks at self-disclosure as a means of achieving "personality health": ". . . a person who displays many of the other characteristics that betoken a healthy personality will also display the ability to make himself freely known to at least one significant human being" (Jourard, 1971:32). The professional helper is able to assist the client in self-disclosure through role modeling and positive reinforcement. Self-disclosure is most likely to occur when the helpee perceives the helper as trustworthy and/or willing to self-disclose in a similar manner. It is important to note here that the client should not be encouraged to disclose too much information too soon, since this may make the client reluctant to talk about himself later.

2. *Self-exploration.* Willingness to examine feelings and behaviors related to the current problem is an essential characteristic of the helpee. This process of searching leads to understanding and self-awareness. The helper plays a significant role in facilitating the client's explorative course through the use of facilitative communication skills.

3. *Honesty.* Honesty from the helpee is as necessary as from the helper. The client must maintain a commitment to providing the helper with accurate data as well as providing feedback related to the usefulness of the helping process. In helping relationships with children, the helper may have to rely on nonverbal communication for feedback and clarification.

4. *Cooperation.* The helping relationship is a collaborative effort between the participants; its effectiveness is greatly enhanced by mutual commitment. Cooperation means working together to achieve a common goal.

Significant others

The term significant other refers to any person having a special meaning or importance to the client and with whom the client has regular interaction. For the school nurse, the significant others involved in the helping relationship will usually be a client's parents, but may extend to include a friend or teacher.

Based on individual situations, the nurse decides whether inclusion of significant others is appropriate. I believe that inclusion of significant others in the helping relationship is, in most cases, appropriate and desirable. There are notable exceptions. The school nurse has frequent short interactions with many children, such as during an immunization clinic. In this instance there would be little rationale for inclusion of significant others. In some situations the client would refuse to enter into the relationship unless confidentiality and privacy were assured, for example, venereal disease counseling. Other instances in which the school nurse would not include family members in the helping relationship are as follows: inability of one or both parents to maintain an honest relationship, presence of a pathological condition that would make participation difficult, destructive motivations by family members, or significant prejudice by family members against participation in the helping relationship.

Studies have been conducted that show the interrelationship between family participation and alterations in physical or mental health of the identified patient. In the 1950s Sullivan wrote about the acute need to study not individual human beings, but rather the "interpersonal situation through which they manifest mental health or mental disorder" (Sullivan, 1953:18). Spitzer et al. (1969:159-181) reviewed several studies and concluded that the family plays a major role in identifying emotional problems, in deciding which course of action to take, and in influencing the outcome in terms of "recidivism" and "adjustment." The family also provides "socialization into the sick role." Following his observations of psychiatric patients, Albert (1960:684) made the following statement: ". . . the patient's presenting illness is always in some manner shared, shaped and supported by other members of the family, each for their own dynamic reasons." These studies cited, plus many others found in the literature, support the close relationship between the family and the illness process of the identified patient.

Significant others can also serve as informants, providing needed data about the client. Information from a relative or friend can be important in assessment, especially when the client, such as a child, cannot provide the necessary information. A study by Small (1965: 446) indicated that a "significantly greater amount of relevant material was contributed by the informants than by patients . . . [but that information is] usually limited to . . . information about present illness and current symptoms."

Significant others usually want to participate in the helping relationship. The nurse can initiate a therapeutic approach that uses the significant others' useful participation and collaboration. The school nurse makes this decision based on the individual needs of the client.

Summary

To summarize, the helper's power is based on the client's perception of her as a source of help. The success of the helper depends on her genuine concern for the client's welfare and on her knowledge, positive attitude, and willingness to participate with the client in the helping process. The helpee's part in the relationship is enhanced by exploring his feelings and behaviors and disclosing those aspects of himself that are relevant to the relationship. The helpee must cooperate in the relationship and provide accurate data. Significant others can provide valuable input into the helping relationship and usually are willing to participate. The school nurse must decide about including significant others based on evaluation of the client's individual needs.

DEVELOPING THE HELPING RELATIONSHIP
Stages of the relationship

The helping relationship unfolds in stages, each of which indicates a movement from one phase of the process to the next. Failure to identify the stages within the helping process may indicate that the relationship has not moved past the initial stage. There are three primary stages within the helping relationship, although substages have been identified.

Stage I: beginning phase

Initially both parties begin preparation for entry into the relationship. Mutual observation and assessment mark the beginning phase. The helper lays the groundwork for building trust throughout the relationship. She is also concerned with beginning the interview in a nonthreatening manner, which allows the client to request help in a relaxed way. The helper may use general leads that do not have a "problem" orientation, such as, "I'm interested in knowing what's on your mind."

The helpee's responsibility during the beginning phase is to define and state his concern or problem. Some people are better able to do this than others. The helper can help clarify and discriminate significant issues, enabling participants to identify the direction of the relationship. It is more useful to determine "what" the client is experiencing than "why" he wants help.

When the problem has been clarified, a contract is initiated to begin the problem-solving process. Contracts can range from an informal verbal agreement to a formal written document signed by the participants (Fig. 10-1). The contract provides structure, including limits and goals of the relationship, frequency and location of meetings, and fees.

Resistance may be encountered during the beginning phase, possibly due to reluctance to accept help, fear of change, inability to readily develop trust, or inaccurate perception of the problem. Cues to resistance observed by the helper are arriving late for appointments, poor posture, head down, shuffling gait, sitting away from the helper, and lack of verbal exchange.

Stage II: working phase

Following the contract agreement, the relationship moves to the working phase. It is during this stage that most of the "work" of problem solving is accomplished. If the groundwork has been properly laid during the first stage, the client will now feel secure in the relationship and will be more open for discussion.

Since the goals of the relationship have been previously determined, the participants can now take a more active role. A variety of methods may be used to increase client participation and accomplish the relationship objectives. Examples include, but are not limited to, using confrontation, giving "homework" assignments,

LET'S WORK TOGETHER

Date _____

This is a plan for _____ and _____
                (child's name)   (school nurse's name)

to work together. We will start working together on _____ and
                    (date)

end on _____.
     (date)

This is what we want to happen: _____

_____

_____

These are the things _____ will do: _____
           (school nurse)

_____

_____

These are the things _____ will do: _____
           (child)

_____

_____

We agree to work together:

_____ and _____
   (child's signature)   (school nurse's signature)

Fig. 10-1. Example of a working agreement suited to elementary schoolchildren.

and using behavior modification strategies. Selection of a specific method is based on the needs of the helpee and the skills of the helper.

Resistance may also be encountered during the working phase. The client may feel so much better after verbalizing his problems that he may want to discontinue the relationship without accomplishing the goals. When this occurs, the nurse reviews the original contract with the client, and a decision is made to either continue with this contract or to revise it. Some cues to resistance during the working phase are cancellation of appointments, refusal to take an active part in the relationship, and "yes, but . . ." statements from the client.

Stage III: terminating phase

Termination of the relationship is first considered when the contract is initiated and participants decide at what point the relationship will close. During termination, the events of the helping process are summarized and evaluated. No new material is introduced. Goals and objectives are reviewed. If they were not accomplished, the reasons for this are discussed.

Generally, closing is a positive phase because the participants feel good about the problem resolution and the learning that has taken place. However, if the helper has been meeting dependency needs of the client, the parting may provoke stress. Separation may also elicit anger

Table 10-1. Facilitative communication skills

Skill	Example: adult client	Example: student/child client
Remaining silent	Using nonverbal communication rather than verbal	
Giving client recognition	"Good morning, Miss _____."	"Good morning, Johnny."
Offering oneself to client	"I will be here with you."	"I'll stay with you, Mary."
Giving nonspecific openings	"I'd like to know what is on your mind."	"Tell me what you're thinking about now."
Giving nonspecific leads	"Go on."	"Go on."
Sequencing an event	"And what happened before that?"	"Can you remember what happened next?"
Asking open-ended questions	"How did that influence your thinking?"	"How did you react when your friend was suspended?"
Summarizing	"As I understand it, your son's problems in school began about the time that you and your husband separated."	"It sounds to me like you felt pretty happy until you moved to the new neighborhood and had to find new friends."
Reflecting feelings	"He makes you feel guilty about your behavior."	"You feel scared when your mom and dad fight."
Providing observations	"I noticed you've been wringing your hands."	"I see you're wiggling around a lot this afternoon."
Focusing	"Let's talk more specifically about how you react to your son's behavior."	"I know how you feel about most parents, how do you feel about *your* parents?"
Giving accurate information	"Moving to that part of the city will involve a rent increase for you."	"One of the rules here is that you must have a buddy to go swimming."
Identifying incongruencies in communication	"You said that you are feeling happier, yet your facial expression is sad."	"How can you feel happy with such a sad face?"
Encouraging comparisons	"Was it similar to your last experience?"	"Just like last time?"
Voicing doubt	"That is difficult for me to believe."	"I don't know if I can agree with that one."
Documenting reality	"Your sister is not in the room. I am your nurse."	"I'm not your mom, I'm your nurse."
Exploring	"Tell me more about your experience."	"Let's talk more about your sisters and brothers."
Assisting in verbalization of perceptions	"Describe what you are experiencing now."	"Tell me what you are thinking about right now."

and hostility from the client. The helper may observe cues to resistance in the following behaviors: regression of the client, introduction of new problems, or failure to appear for the last appointment.

Some of the negative aspects of termination can be reduced by periodically reviewing the terms of the contract with the client. For instance, the school nurse might say, "We agreed to meet six times to work on this problem. We now have two sessions left." If new material is introduced that seems to warrant attention or intervention, a new contract may be initiated to work on that issue.

Communication skills to facilitate the helping relationship

The school nurse uses many communication skills to facilitate the helping relationship. Communication techniques are listed as being facilitative (Table 10-1) or nonfacilitative (Table 10-2). It cannot be stated too strongly that the skills must be evaluated within the context that they are used. For example, ignoring the client is usually considered "nonfacilitative."

If a child is participating in a behavior modification program using extinction to decrease negative behavior, then "planned ignoring" is therapeutic. How a particular skill relates to a client's needs is more significant than the skill itself.

The school nurse uses facilitative communication skills to gain an increased understanding of the client's perceptions, to enhance the client's self-awareness, and to work toward accomplishing the relationship objectives. One of the most useful things the helper can do is to assist the client to improve his communication skills, for example, teaching a child how to express his thoughts and feelings.

Words used by the helper can have a powerful effect on increasing or decreasing the client's self-esteem, *if the client allows that to happen*. For instance, the helper may use several methods for communicating acceptance and positive regard, but if the client is discounting positive feedback because of low self-esteem, he will probably not internalize the helper's comments. The client holds the responsibility for how he responds to the helper,

Table 10-2. Nonfacilitative communication methods

Method	Example: adult client	Example: student/child client
Becoming defensive over issue	"What do you expect from the nursing staff under these conditions?"	"How else can I handle all you kids?"
Denying expressed feelings	"You couldn't be feeling *that* depressed."	"A tough kid like you shouldn't be making such a fuss."
Validating unrealistic statements	"It must be nice to be so wealthy" (to a grandiose patient).	"I'm sure you can lift 500 pounds with muscles like that."
Giving advice	"You probably should get a divorce."	"Tell your teacher that you won't do that homework."
Rejecting	"I have enough problems of my own; I don't need yours, too."	"Get lost."
Using inappropriate language, jargon	"Your son's inappropriate behavior could most favorably be eliminated through the human behavior management technique of extinction."	"Your profane language has become a source of anxiety for your second grade teacher."
Making tangential comments	TEACHER: "I am trying to figure out some way to cope with Mary's disruptive behavior in the classroom." NURSE: "I saw her mother in the principal's office; she looked upset."	CLIENT: "My mom and I had a bad fight before I came to school." NURSE: "What did your teacher say about the improvement in your speech?"
Making stereotyped statements	"We all have problems sometimes."	"That's life, kid."
Inappropriate self-disclosure	"That happened to me once, too. I didn't know how to handle it. I was really depressed."	"I certainly didn't raise my kids the way your mother raises you . . ."
Placing negative value	"You mean you are dating an exconvict?"	"That skinny little thing is your girlfriend?"

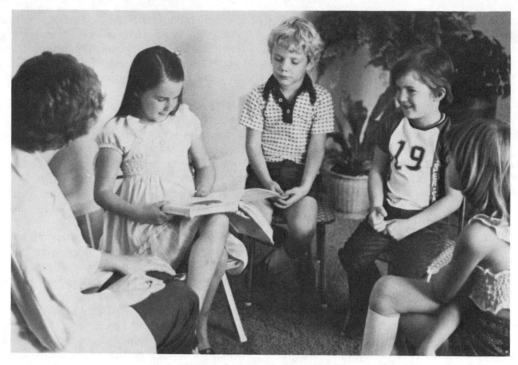

Fig. 10-2. The group approach in helping relationships provides needed peer associations and support.

but this does not relieve the helper of the responsibility to choose skills that will best facilitate accomplishment of the goals.

Special considerations for young children

Developing a helping relationship with young children requires some adaptations in approach. The principles and theoretical framework remain the same, but some communication skills require modification.

Preschool and early elementary school children may attach a particularly literal meaning to words. It is important to check out the correlation between what the school nurse said and what the child understood. There may be a tendency to joke with the child about a procedure or his state of health. Because of the child's stage of cognitive development, jokes may be taken literally and thus misinterpreted.

Children in the early elementary grades often experience anxiety about their bodies and fear bodily injury. The child may refuse to admit that he is ill because he anticipates negative consequences. It is helpful to use a nonthreatening approach, initially showing a broad interest in many aspects of the child and later focusing on the concern or illness.

The helping relationship must be geared toward increasing the child's self-esteem, building self-confidence, and allowing the child to be the decision maker when appropriate. Even though the child may not be able to describe the course of the helping process, he is able to guide the direction of the relationship if the nurse listens to verbal cues and observes nonverbal cues. "The therapist, to be effective, must have an inner faith in the child's ability to solve his problems" (Smith, 1977:1964). A child may be unaware that he is in some type of danger and needs help. For example, a child with diabetes may be in danger of an insulin reaction because he is not following his diet at school. The school nurse must take the initiative in such instances.

The use of play is an effective method for developing a helping relationship. Play allows the child to use inanimate objects to demonstrate thoughts and feelings he might otherwise be unable to conceptualize or verbalize (Smith, 1977:1963). The school nurse may have a playroom available for working with children. If not, she can provide materials that enhance expression, such as paints, crayons, clay, or dolls that represent family members. A text on play therapy should be consulted for more detailed information.

Another method of developing a helping relationship with children is a group approach. Children's needs for peer association can be met in this way (Fig. 10-2). Group sessions can be effective when working with children sharing a similar concern, such as children with separated parents, grieving children, or children having the same illness or handicap. Children are generally supportive and creative in their solutions.

SUMMARY

To summarize, the helping relationship passes through three predictable stages, and its development is facilitated by the nurse's use of the appropriate communication skills. Building a relationship with children requires some adaptations in approach, based on the various developmental stages. The use of play and groups can assist the helping process by providing a more effective way to communicate and by providing peer support.

The school nurse is identified as a helping person, and the development of helping relationships with clients is essential to school nursing practice. Because of the importance of helping relationships, the nurse must be aware that thoughts and techniques related to the helping process are not static. The school nurse must continually seek ways to improve her relationship skills.

REFERENCES

Albert, R. S.: 1960. Stages of breakdown in the relationships and dynamics between the mental patient and his family, Arch. Gen. Psychiatry **30**(3):130-138.
Benjamin, A.: 1974. The helping interview, 2nd ed., Houghton Mifflin Co., Boston.
Chapman, J. E., and Chapman, H. H.: 1976. Behavior and health care: a humanistic helping process, The C. V. Mosby Co., St. Louis.
Combs, A. W., Avila, D. L., and Purkey, W. W.: 1971. Helping relationships: basic concepts for the helping professions, Allyn & Bacon, Inc., Boston.
Glasser, W.: 1972. The identity society, Harper & Row, Publishers, New York.
Jourard, S.: 1971. The transparent self, Van Nostrand Reinhold Co., New York.
Mayeroff, M.: 1971. On caring, Harper & Row, Publishers, New York.
Miller, S., Nunnally, E. W., and Wackman, D. B.: 1975. Alive and aware, Interpersonal Communication Programs, Inc., Minneapolis.
Small, J. G.; 1965. The contributions of the informant in psychiatric evaluation, Int. J. Neuropsychiatry **1**(5):446-451.
Smith, L. F.: 1977. An experiment with play therapy, Am. J. Nurs. **77**(12):1963-1965.
Spitzer, S. P., Swanson, R. M., and Lehr, R. K.: 1969. Audience reactions and careers of psychiatric patients, Fam. Process **9**:159-181.
Sullivan, H. S.: 1953. The interpersonal theory of psychiatry. Perry, H., and Gawell, M., editors, W. W. Norton & Co., Inc., New York.

SUGGESTED READINGS

Brammer, L. M.: 1973. The helping relationship, Prentice-Hall, Inc., Englewood Cliffs, N.J.
Carter, F. M.; 1976. Psychosocial nursing, 2nd ed., Macmillan, Inc., New York.
Egan, G.: 1975. The skilled helper, Brooks/Cole Publishing Co., Monterey, Calif.
Landau, R., Harth, P., Othany, N., and Sharfhertz, C.: 1972. The influence of psychotic parents on their children's development, Am. J. Psychiatry **129**(1):38-43.
Shufer, S.: 1977. Communicating with young children, Am. J. Nurs. **77**(12):1960-1962.
Tubbs, S. L., and Moss, S.: 1974. Human communication: an interpersonal perspective, Random House, Inc., New York.

CHAPTER 11

Theoretical bases for implementing helping relationships within the school setting

SUSAN J. WOLD

Throughout this book the five strands of a conceptual framework for the practice of school nursing have been described. Specifically, public health, adaptation, tools, systematic processes, and helping relationships have been discussed. No weightings or ranks have been assigned to these strands based on their relative importance in school nursing practice because they are *all* vitally important for competent and responsible school nursing practice. Although all five strands are equally important, one is "primary" in applying the framework to actual practice. That primary strand is helping relationships. It is not enough for the school nurse to have a strong theoretical base in such areas as public health concepts, adaptation theory, tools, and systematic processes such as research, planned change, and the nursing process. To successfully *apply* such knowledge and skills, the nurse must be able to communicate effectively and establish goal-directed helping relationships. School nursing is a "people-centered" practice setting, and success in school nursing therefore depends on the adequacy of all the nurse's interpersonal helping relationships.

In Chapter 10, the helping process and relationship and the skills essential to helping were described. This chapter, building on that discussion, will describe the importance of helping relationships as tools in the school's mental health program, briefly describe some pertinent theoretical orientations to helping, and consider the kinds of settings (one to one, small groups, and classroom) in which the school nurse can apply helping relationship skills.

THE IMPORTANCE OF HELPING RELATIONSHIPS IN SCHOOL NURSING

As noted earlier, helping relationship skills are essential for the school nurse in contacts with school officials and staff, parents and other family members, and relevant community residents and agencies, as well as for involvement with students. Unfortunately, as Williams (1970) points out, helping professions have tended to be myopically preoccupied with helping clients solve or ameliorate problems, with little or no attention paid to *prevention* of problems.

This inattention to prevention of problems likewise occurs to some extent in school health programs. One explanation might be the fact that with reductions in the scope of school health programs (due to budgetary cutbacks), school health personnel (including nurses) have not been able to extent their efforts beyond immediate, identified problems and crisis intervention. Another possible explanation suggested by Williams (1970) is that because the educational and experiential orientation of many helping professionals (including social workers, physicians, and nurses) has traditionally been problem centered, they may not be equipped to deal with preventive efforts; Williams proposes that helping professions should emphasize the preventive dimension through modification of the academic programs which prepare helping professionals and through "reorientation" of helping professionals.

The need for preventive mental health in schools

As Siemon (1978) points out, all children experience stress in their lives in a variety of forms, including competition with siblings and peers, frustration, and unmet needs. How the child learns to cope with these stresses and the anxiety they produce may well affect his coping patterns for the rest of his life. Thus it is important that children learn to respond adaptively and rationally to stress and to cope with anxiety through problem solving. Because many of the stresses that confront children are direct or indirect consequences of the school environment, such as pressures to "achieve," emphasis on competition, and the struggle for recognition and acceptance within the school's peer social structure, and because children spend a great proportion of their waking hours at school, it seems only appropriate that the schools address children's needs in the area of preventive mental health and adaptive coping.

Although all children experience stress and need to learn healthy coping patterns, some children are especially vulnerable to mental health problems. According to available estimates (Joint Commission on Mental Health of Children, 1970), at least 1,400,000 American children and youth are in need of *immediate* psychiatric care; this is no doubt a conservative estimate. Of those children and youth who are mentally ill, the commission estimates that 0.6% are psychotic, 2% to 3% are "severely disturbed," and another 8% to 10% experience emotional problems and neuroses. Even more distressing is the commission's estimate that only 5% to 7% of children in need of professional mental health care are receiving it.

The literature and general media report that problems of delinquency, drug abuse, teenage pregnancy, depression and suicide, and venereal disease are steadily increasing among our nation's children and youth. Esty (1967) attributes these increases to what he calls "social pollution." According to Esty, social pollution results when a nation becomes so affluent that it begins to regard "things" with more consideration than people. He believes that highly affluent societies (such as the United States) view people as "natural resources" to be exploited and manipulated, resulting in social pollution of which escalating mental health problems are symptomatic.

Many factors can predispose a child to mental or emotional problems, including hyperactivity, learning disabilities, autism, and low socioeconomic status (Joint Commission on Mental Health of Children, 1970). Family and cultural living patterns and value systems may also contribute to a child's stress and anxiety levels. Siemon (1978) notes that children from mobile or transient families, such as those connected with the military or itinerant workers, have increased risks for mental health problems because of the lack of stability in their lives; such children may not live in one place long enough

to feel "at home" or to become part of their neighborhood and school communities. In addition, children whose home lives are unstable due to parental alcoholism, marital stress, verbal and/or physical abuse, low income or unemployment of parents, or other environmental stressors are especially vulnerable for development of mental health problems (Joint Commission on Mental Health of Children, 1970; Siemon, 1978). For these children, early and appropriate intervention can sometimes prevent long-term or permanent sequelae (Siemon, 1978).

Mental health needs of school-age children and youth
Definition of mental health

Mental health is a particularly elusive state to define and describe. Cook (1969) notes that mental health is an ideal state dependent on time, place, culture, and situational factors; thus behavior that is accepted and viewed as healthy in one culture or country may be unacceptable and unhealthy in another. Cook also points out that a person's mental health status varies from time to time—a person adapts better to stress and anxiety at some times than at others.

To define mental health, it may be most useful to identify the following behaviors that are associated with mental health (Cook, 1969; Joint Commission on Mental Health of Children, 1970):

1. Ability to understand and cope with reality
2. Development of mutually satisfactory interpersonal relationships
3. Ability to accept and control expression of sexual and aggressive needs
4. Ability to learn and apply learning
5. Self-confidence based on competencies
6. Development of a value system to guide one's life
7. Ability to cooperate with others and to consider others' needs
8. Ability to defer immediate gratification of needs for long-range satisfaction
9. Ability to love someone other than oneself

These behaviors emerge over time as the child/adult grows and matures. Again, depending on the specific stressors confronting the person at any one time, some of these ideal behaviors may not be present or may be temporarily diminished.

Children's mental health needs

In her excellent description of the mental health needs of school-age children, Siemon (1978) reiterates the child's need to learn to cope with stress and anxiety as a means of enhancing self-esteem. In other words, the child needs experience in dealing with stress—thus adults (parents, teachers, and others) who try to shield him by providing an "anxiety-free" environment are actually interfering with his development into a rational, adaptive adult with effective coping mechanisms.

As with all other aspects of growth and development, the child's emotional development builds on previous learning and experiences. If denied opportunities to make decisions for himself (within the limits of his maturity and experience) as a child, he will be handicapped as an adult. On the other hand, if he receives supportive acceptance and encouragement from his significant others (parents, teachers, etc.) plus reasonable, consistent (but not rigid) limits for his behavior, he should develop strong self-esteem and be relatively healthy mentally. In contrast, if he receives little or no recognition for his competencies and achievements and has no limits placed on his behavior, his development of self-esteem and a sense of right and wrong may be impaired (Joint Commission on Mental Health of Children, 1970; Siemon, 1978).

THEORETICAL AND CONCEPTUAL BASES FOR IMPLEMENTING HELPING RELATIONSHIPS
Helping relationships: tools for promoting positive mental health

As noted at the beginning of this chapter, effective helping relationship skills may well be the key to success for the school nurse's attempts to implement the school health program. Unquestionably, they are important tools for promoting and maintaining good mental health. Indeed, Rogers (1956), well-known for his "client-centered" therapy, believes that the helping relationship is the most important tool a therapist can offer the client. He acknowledges that after 25 years of questioning the adequacy of his skills, knowledge, and resources for treating, "curing," or "changing" his clients, he finally realized the important issue is how to provide a relationship that allows the client to grow and change. In other words, he discovered that "change in personality, attitude, and behavior appears to come about through experience in a relationship" (Rogers, 1956:994).

Promoting positive mental health among school-age children and youth requires that implementation of helping relationships, whether on a one-to-one basis, in a small group setting, or in the classroom, be based on application of adaptation theory and public health concepts. Specifically, this means that the school nurse or other professional helper must understand the student/client's expected and actual growth and development and what behaviors are age-appropriate. A behavior that is acceptable in a young child, for example, may not be appropriate when he is older. Thus to assist the student in improving his own mental health, the nurse must know what behaviors are healthy and acceptable for him at his stage of development.

Public health concepts are also important in implementing helping relationships within the school's mental health program. Specifically, levels of prevention (primary, secondary, and tertiary) can be readily applied to mental health program efforts. Indeed, the importance of prevention in school mental health programs has been emphasized resoundingly in the literature (Esty, 1967; Cook, 1969; Drake, 1970; Williams, 1970; Taintor, 1976).

At the primary prevention level, Taintor (1976) advocates that schools provide an environment conducive to positive mental health. This includes attention to the school's architecture and physical environment. Taintor reports that studies have shown the importance of a sense of "smallness," which probably contributes to students' feeling of "belonging." No doubt, schools designed with warm and colorful spaces also increase students' comfort (psychological as well as physical).

Another method for promoting mental health at the primary prevention level is health education, which can occur in formal or informal settings. Health education includes teaching children and youth about human relationships and feelings, problem-solving techniques, communication skills, and building self-esteem through self-acceptance of limitations and abilities and realistic goal setting. Health education efforts aimed at promoting positive mental health can be implemented by use of formal guidelines, such as those published in *Mental Health in the Classroom* (ASHA Committee on Mental Health in the Classroom, 1968) or through locally developed and/or published materials.

Role modeling is also an important health education tool, especially in the area of promotion of mental health. The classroom teacher is a powerful role model for students, whether she intends to be or not. If the teacher can be "genuine," honest, understanding, accepting, and respectful of the child, she can demonstrate how mentally healthy and responsible adults behave (Rogers, 1956; Siemon, 1978). However, Taintor (1976) warns that teachers who are unhappy or experiencing stress and problems in their personal lives may provide negative role modeling; children may conclude that growing up means having lots of problems and may thus resist growing up. In addition, teachers who are experiencing a great deal of stress and unhappiness may not be able to provide warmth, understanding, and positive feedback and recognition for their students because their energies will be consumed with their own coping behaviors. Thus the school should be concerned with the mental health of its faculty and staff, since it can directly affect the students.

Although teachers are the most available and usual adult role models in the school setting, school nurses can be important role models as well. Crosby and Connolly (1970) point out that the school nurse is in an ideal position to influence a child's mental health because she is accessible, supportive, and, most of all, nonjudgmental. The school nurse does not have the power of "grading" students or any day-to-day disciplinary functions. Thus she can be a nonjudgmental and trusted adult to whom students can turn for acceptance, understanding, warmth, and honest feedback, as well as for help with problems. Unfortunately, school nurses do not always find time and energy to be available for students' preventive mental health care, and many are not academically prepared for this role. In fact, for many school health professionals (including nurses) to competently assume responsibility for primary prevention in school mental health programs through teaching and role modeling, the "reorientation" described by Williams (1970) may be needed. This reorientation should include renewed emphasis on the importance of prevention as well as formal course work on personality development, normal growth and development (including cognitive, social, and emotional tasks), relevant child psychiatry concepts, and guidance and counseling techniques (Crosby and Connolly, 1970; Williams, 1970; Siemon, 1978).

At the secondary prevention level, the goal is early detection and prompt treatment of mental health and emotional problems to prevent disability. Unfortunately, because mental health is difficult to quantify and measure, there are no nice, neat screening tests to detect mental health problems (although at times various psychological tests have been misused for screening and predictive purposes). Thus early detection depends on astute observations of a child's behavior and interactions with others in a variety of settings. Generally, no conclusions can be drawn from one-time observations or incidents; the consistency and persistence of a given behavior pattern are more useful indicators of mental health or mental illness than are one-time observations.

As with other health problems, the role of the school's staff is *not* to diagnose and treat mental health problems; rather, the school's health team members and other special services staff can identify those students who probably need further study and evaluation and can facilitate implementation of the specified treatment plan within the limits of the school's program and resources. It is also appropriate and desirable for school nurses and other school personnel to use their helping relationship skills for counseling students and their families to help them accept and understand whatever mental or emotional problems confront them and to help them participate cooperatively in the established plan of care or treatment. Successful early counseling can prevent or minimize the long-range consequences or sequelae of the illness or problems.

Another method of secondary prevention in the area of mental health is the teacher-nurse conference. Such conferences are usually thought of as measures for early detection of a variety of physical problems. However, in addition to serving that function, teacher-nurse conferences can be an important source of data about children's usual behavior and general mental health. As previously suggested, the school nurse may use some kind of checklist (or structured interview guide) with teachers as preparation for these conferences. If the nurse incorporates some behaviors relevant to mental health into her tool, she can begin to identify high-risk children for further follow-up.

However, for that secondary prevention strategy to succeed, classroom teachers will need to know what behaviors they are looking for and how to recognize them. Since it is doubtful that most teachers are academically prepared to detect behavioral and mental health problems, some training will probably need to be provided (Taintor, 1976). The extent and nature of the training needed will depend on the background of the teachers; characteristics of the student population, such as age, developmental stage(s), and culture or ethnicity; and the types and numbers of mental and behavioral problems that exist in that population.

As previously noted, symptoms of mental health problems are not always easily recognized. Also, as mentioned earlier, behaviors that were considered ''normal'' at one age and developmental stage may not be acceptable or ''normal'' at another time. Thus in any attempt to list behaviors or symptoms that can indicate mental health problems, one must realize that the normality or abnormality of the behavior will vary by age, developmental stage, culture, and frequency and persistence of the behavior. Some of the ''symptoms'' of mental or emotional problems listed by Cook (1969) include jealousy, suspicion, aggression, stuttering, masturbation, crying, hyperactivity or lethargy, shyness, inattention, indecision, dishonesty, defeatist attitude, indecision, and constant talking. In addition, Taintor (1976) includes passivity, absenteeism, alcohol and drug abuse, depression, compulsiveness, inappropriate responses, and poor academic performance.

An early detection strategy that has been generally overlooked is *peer* detection. In their study of third graders who did and did not participate in their school's preventive mental health program, Cowen et al. (1973) found that peer judgment was the best predictor of later psychiatric problems. Their data further suggested that young children identify their ''troubled'' peers early *and* that those children who are singled out by peers as having problems are aware of their classmates' perceptions of them. This study not only points out another means of identifying children with problems (that is, by observing peer interactions), but it also shows the risks of early labeling of children by peers, which may result in self-fulfilling prophecies; thus children who are regarded as ''different'' or ''troubled'' may continue to behave in ways which reinforce that belief.

Successful secondary prevention will also require an effective referral system. Students who are identified as high risk and in need of further follow-up should be expeditiously referred to an appropriate resource. Thus some policy on who will handle referrals and to whom they will be sent should be developed; if appropriate re-

sources are not available or accessible within the community, the school nurse and other school staff should take whatever action necessary to correct the situation.

The goal at the tertiary prevention level is to prevent further deterioration. Specifically, Taintor (1976) urges schools to ensure that children who need treatment receive it. If students have needs or disabilities requiring special schools or classroom experiences, those needs should be addressed. Follow-up by the school nurse and/or other school staff should be continued to ensure the cooperation and continued participation of the students and their families.

Selecting theoretical bases for implementing helping relationships

As noted in the discussion of primary prevention in school mental health programs, many school health professionals and staff members are ill-equipped to take on this responsibility and are uncomfortable in the role of counselor. As also suggested, part of their uncertainty may be due to inadequate knowledge of personality development, psychological and psychiatric theories and concepts, and guidance and counseling techniques.

For school nurses and other school health professionals and staff members to most effectively implement helping relationship skills, some kind of theoretical or conceptual orientation to the process of helping is needed. It seems that too often nurses intervene with clients/patients by trial and error or custom, rather than on the basis of tested theories and approaches. For those school nurses who need an expanded knowledge base to intervene effectively as counselors at all prevention levels in the school's mental health program, additional course work plus guided field experience are requisite.

Although it is obviously beyond the scope and purpose of this book to fill that knowledge gap, as a means of illustrating the usefulness of such theories, concepts, and approaches, the remainder of this discussion will briefly present several theories and approaches that are appropriate for working with children. The theories and approaches included here have been selected solely on the basis of my preference. The list is not exhaustive, nor is it presented in order of preference or importance.

Although the school nurse may ultimately adopt one particular theoretical approach as her primary "style" of helping, she may alternatively choose an eclectic approach. In other words, the school nurse may prefer to use selected elements or techniques from two or more theories/approaches, combining them into a style or method that is workable and comfortable for her.

The Rogerian client-centered approach

One of the most widely respected and used approaches to helping is the "client-centered therapy" described by Rogers (1951). The basic premise of Rogers' theory is that the nature of the helping relationship itself is the most important factor in the counseling process. Rogers believes that all persons have the capacity and tendency to move toward self-actualization or self-fulfillment; that capacity may be latent or hidden in some individuals. Thus the goal of this therapy approach is to release the client's potential by providing a psychological climate conducive to personal growth.

The key to providing a growth-inducing psychological climate according to Rogers (1951; 1956; 1959) is to establish a helping relationship characterized as follows:

1. *Genuineness,* or "realness," which means that the counselor or therapist is willing to "be himself" and share his feelings and attitudes with the client even if they do not please the client. Only through the therapist's provision of his "genuine reality" is the client able to find his own reality.
2. *Unconditional positive regard,* or acceptance of the client as he is; the therapist accepts the person as an individual of worth, no matter what attitudes he expresses or how he behaves. By accepting the client unconditionally with his fluctuating attitudes and behaviors, the therapist provides the client with the safety of being liked; being liked, according to Rogers, is very important in a helping relationship.
3. *Accurate empathic understanding* of the client's feelings and thoughts as he perceives them at the time. Thus the therapist sees the client's "private world" through the client's eyes, which Rogers believes frees the client to explore himself and his inner experiences without fear of moral judgments.

Rogers (1956:995) admits that he is not always able to achieve this kind of relationship with others; however, he concludes that:

. . . When I hold in myself the kind of attitudes I have described, and when the other person can experience these attitudes to some degree, then change and constructive personal development will *invariably* occur.

The goal of the Rogerian approach is to help the client release his inner potential and move toward self-actualization. The client is helped to live in the present, accepting reality. To achieve this goal, the therapist or counselor relies on the self-directed self-disclosure of the client. The therapist encourages the client to verbalize his feelings, helping him clarify and state his feelings when necessary. The therapist may point out the client's nonverbal behavior and help him interpret that as well. The therapist encourages the client to live more fully in the present moment by concentrating on his immediate "phenomenal world" (Rogers, 1951; 1959).

In addition to his individually oriented client-centered therapy, Rogers has also been widely recognized for his work with groups (Yalom, 1975), which have included therapy groups, encounter groups, and class (student) groups. In his book *Freedom to Learn,* Rogers (1969) recounts his own development over time of a philosophy of education that apparently grew out of his group work. Rogers, like other contemporary therapists (Glasser, 1969), is deeply concerned about the educational environment in our schools and colleges. He believes that our schools do not trust students to be self-directed in learning, preferring to spoonfeed them and "check up" on them to be sure they "learn" the prescribed material. Rogers proposes that more attention be paid to his concept of "discovery learning" or "self-discovered learning," in which students learn by assimilating knowledge into their own experience, making it "theirs." In this philosophy of education the role of the teacher is like that of the client-centered therapist: facilitator of the student's growth by clarifying ideas and assisting him to assimilate his experiences.

Transactional analysis

Originated by Berne (1964) and publicized in his book *Games People Play,* transactional analysis (TA) was popularized through the writings of Harris (1969), author of *I'm OK— You're OK: A Practical Guide to Transactional Analysis.* Basically, TA analyzes the transactions or interpersonal messages people send one another as a means of understanding problems and freeing the "adult" portion of one's personality to choose or create new problem-solving options.

As a mental health tool, TA is based on the belief that an individual is responsible for his behavior, regardless of what happened to him in the past. Thus the past, which is "recorded" complete with accompanying feelings within one's memory, is looked at only as a means of understanding it and freeing oneself from it. Thus one of the goals of TA therapy would be to recognize the "old tapes" one plays back, so that they can then be shut off.

TA is also founded on the belief that each personality contains three "ego states," which are the Parent, Adult, and Child (P-A-C). These terms are defined differently from common usage. The Parent includes all the "do's, don'ts, and shoulds" internalized during one's childhood. As Harris (1969) points out, whether or not these are good or sound rules, they are recorded as "truth" in the Parent and are there forever, always available for "replay." In contrast to the Parent, which records *external* events, the Child records the young person's *internal* events or responses to what he sees and hears. Since the Parent and Child are both recorded early in life (usually during the first 5 years), during which time the young person's language skills are limited, the Child consists primarily of *feelings*. The feelings contained in the Child are both positive and negative. The negative feelings result from conflicting demands placing on him; his developmental urges to explore and express his feelings are at times in conflict with parental expectations and rewards—thus the child may feel bad or "not OK." On the other hand, the Child also includes happy, positive feelings, including creativity, curiosity, and the joys of first discoveries. Like the events recorded in the Parent, these reactions are indelibly recorded and available for replay.

The third ego state within the personality is the Adult. The Adult is the "data processing computer" (Harris, 1969:30) or decision maker for the individual. The adult collects data or information from the present situation and examines the data recorded in the Parent and the Child to see if it is still true and applicable. Although the Parent and Child recordings cannot be "erased," the Adult helps to update them; in this way the Adult decides what parts of the Parent are valid and which of the Child's emotions can be safely expressed.

TA is also based on the premise that there are four "life positions" underlying people's behavior. They are as follows:

1. "I'm not OK—you're OK," which begins early in life and is regarded as the "anxious dependency of the immature"
2. "I'm not OK—you're not OK," which is a position of despair or "giving up"
3. "I'm OK—you're not OK," which is the position adopted by criminals
4. "I'm OK—you're OK," which is the position of the mature adult who is at peace with himself

Harris (1969) points out that these are positions adopted early in life, usually by age 3. To change to another position, one makes a *decision* to change. Virtually all of us initially adopt the first position ("I'm not OK—you're OK") as infants. However, Harris emphasizes the fact that these life positions can be changed by conscious decision—no one is "stuck" forever with his initial life position.

The intent of TA, then, is to help clients become more *responsible* by strengthening and emancipating the Adult from the Parent and Child recordings. This should result in adoption of the ideal "I'm OK—you're OK" life position. This goal is achieved by helping the client understand his own transactions and those of others and by teaching him to recognize the P-A-C in himself and others. This requires a therapist-client relationship characterized by Adult-Adult transactions.

TA can take place on a one-to-one basis or in a group setting, although Harris (1969) believes the group approach is more effective. Because TA uses a jargon that is easily understood, it can be readily taught to clients as a tool for their own use; thus it is not just a treatment modality for "sick" people. In fact, TA can be readily used with children of all ages, as well as with adults. Freed has written an engaging series of books for children (the *Transactional Analysis for Everybody Series*), including: *T.A. for Tots* (1973), which is written about and for preschoolers and first graders; *T.A. for Kids* (1971), which is intended for school-age children in grades three through six; and *T.A. for Teens* (1976), which is written for adolescents. These books can be used to teach children about TA concepts and about their own personality and its development. They are written in terms that even adults can comprehend. For school nurses and other school staff interested in preventive mental health using a TA approach, these books can be invaluable teaching aids.

Reality Therapy

Another approach to preventive mental health and therapy that bears some resemblance to transactional analysis is Glasser's Reality Therapy. Both TA and Reality Therapy are founded on the belief that individuals are responsible for their behavior; they differ significantly, however, in the relative importance assigned to past events. TA proponents believe that the past helps one understand (through his P-A-C) the present, which thus enables the Adult to decide to change his behavior to be more responsible. Glasser believes, however, that the past is not important because it cannot be changed. Instead, he emphasizes the present and encourages the client to become more responsible by changing his behavior. Harris (1969) believes that Reality Therapy thus is more of a Parent-Child transaction than an Adult-Adult relationship. Regardless of this continuing controversy, both TA and Reality Therapy are accepted and widely applied methods of preventive mental health care that can certainly be (and, indeed, have been) applied in the school setting.

To describe Glasser's (1965; 1975) theory and approach as "controversial" is an understatement. Glasser's approach evolved from his dissatisfaction with the perceived inadequacies of traditional, psychoanalytically based psychiatry. As Glasser (1965) explains, traditional Freudians believed that the "patient" was "sick" because his conscience (superego) was too strong, forcing him to be "too good." Glasser's view of the client is quite different; as he sees it, the problem is not that the client's moral and behavioral standards are too high, but that his *performance* is too low (Glasser, 1965). Thus Glasser concludes that individuals do not behave irresponsibly because they are mentally "ill"; they are "ill" because they behave irresponsibly (Glasser, 1965).

Thus the premises for Reality Therapy are that there are no mental illnesses, but merely irresponsible persons, who have *chosen* to act irresponsibly to reduce their "pain." Pain is the result of the person's inability to fulfill his basic needs, which are to love and be loved and to feel worthwhile to himself and others (Glasser, 1965; 1975). Responsibility, as Glasser defines it, is the ability to meet one's needs *without* depriving others of the ability to meet their own

needs. Based on these premises, Glasser believes that *all* psychiatric patients/clients have the same basic problem: they are unable to meet their needs realistically and have therefore adopted some less responsible ways to do so. Thus the goal of Reality Therapy is to guide the client toward accepting reality and fulfilling his needs responsibly.

The actual practice of Reality Therapy is based on seven principles that have been carefully and completely described by Glasser (1975). The first principle is *involvement*. Similar to Rogers' "unconditional positive regard," involvement is a key element in Reality Therapy. Because the client's basic needs are to love and be loved and to feel worthwhile, acceptance by the helper or therapist is important. Thus Glasser admonishes helpers to "make friends" with the client and to be warm and understanding instead of distant and aloof. Involvement is seen as the "foundation of therapy," on which the remaining principles are built.

The second principle is the focus on *current behavior* and helping the client to become aware of his current behavior. Thus when the client identifies a problem such as depression, the helper does not focus on how the client *feels* or *why* he feels that way, but instead focuses on *what* he is doing about it; in other words, what is his current behavior? The reason for this focus on behavior is that behavior is the only thing the client can change, and that change can only occur if the therapist is involved and nonjudgmental (Glasser, 1975).

The third principle of Reality Therapy is *evaluating* one's *behavior*. The task for the client at this stage of the therapeutic process is to critically analyze his behavior and decide if it really represents his best choice (Glasser, 1975). The therapist or helper asks the client to evaluate his own behavior to decide whether it is good for him and for the other people he cares about and if it is "socially acceptable" in his community. Again, it is *not* the therapist's role to judge behavior or provide moral standards for the client—the client must evaluate his own behavior.

The fourth principle of Reality Therapy is *planning responsible behavior,* which entails developing realistic plans for action based on the value judgment made in the preceding stage (Glasser, 1975). The helper or therapist assists the client in planning responsible behavior by helping him recognize his options and encouraging him to make a plan that is *realistic*. Glasser believes that an overly ambitious plan is likely to fail, which would only increase the client's feelings of failure. Thus a child who is failing in school because he does not know how to study and does not spend any time at it should not plan initially to begin studying 2 hours per night. Glasser affirms that this is the stage at which reality is very important. Reality Therapy assumes that there *is* some behavioral solution that can be worked out, which is better than the behavior the client has been using. However, Glasser has also realized, based on his work with convicted felons serving lengthy prison terms, that there are some (fortunately rare) circumstances in which *no* reasonable plan can be made. In those situations, of which a life prison term without hope of parole is an example, Glasser admits that Reality Therapy will not work.

The fifth principle of Reality Therapy is *commitment* by the client to carry out the reasonable plan that he has made (Glasser, 1975). This commitment can be made verbally or in writing, to another individual (therapist, spouse, or friend), or to a group, but it *must* be made. Glasser believes that commitment increases the likelihood of the client carrying out the plan and provides him with additional motivation to do so. He acknowledges that successful people usually commit themselves and are self-directed; however, clients who generally have been "failures" need to make external commitments to another person as a means of getting started on a successful identity. This principle also signifies commitment of the client to the involvement with the therapist or other person; as Glasser (1975:96) describes it, commitment "binds the involvement."

The sixth Reality Therapy principle described by Glasser (1975) is to *accept no excuses*. Clients who have been behaving irresponsibly are likely *not* to honor their commitment to the therapist or other helper, at least initially. In fact, they may be expected to offer excuses for their failure instead. An excuse, according to Glasser, lets the client "off the hook" and reduces the pain of failure. However, an excuse does not lead to success and therefore the therapist must not ask for or accept any excuses, no matter how valid they may seem. Therefore the therapist should have the client recheck his earlier value judgment about his behavior and decide if it is still valid; if it is, the plan must be reassessed to see if it is still reasonable. If the plan is reasonable, the client

must then either reaffirm his commitment to it or state that he will no longer commit himself to the plan, in which case he is no longer responsible. Glasser emphasizes the importance of patience and persistence on the part of the therapist; he believes that if involvement is maintained and if the client and therapist continue to make plans and secure commitments to them, eventually the client will begin to fulfill them. Thus instead of saying to the client "You failed to keep your commitment—why?" the therapist's approach should be "You didn't do it when you said you would, so when *are* you going to do it?" Through his unwillingness to accept excuses, the therapist reaffirms his involvement and concern for the client and his unwillingness to "give up."

The seventh and final principle of Reality Therapy is *no punishment*. Quite simply, according to Glasser (1975), punishment does not work as a means of getting people to improve their behavior. Instead, punishment reduces involvement and leads "failures" to identify more strongly with their failure and therefore should not be used. Instead of punishment, Glasser advocates the use of logical and natural consequences of behavior, such as allowing a schoolchild who does not get up on time on school days to experience the consequences of being tardy, without parental "protection" or interference. Glasser also encourages use of praise and positive reinforcement for whatever successes the client does achieve.

In addition to its use in individual therapy, Reality Therapy can be applied in a group setting as well. Although in a group setting the extent of the therapist's personal involvement with each client may be reduced, the involvement of the group members with one another compensates for this; in fact, because group experiences increase a client's opportunities for involvement, Reality Therapy in a group setting tends to move along more rapidly than individual therapy (Glasser, 1965).

Probably the most controversial applications of Reality Therapy concepts are those detailed in *Schools Without Failure* (Glasser, 1969). Glasser's basic premise is that our educational philosophy in this country is failure oriented. As he points out (1969:26), "very few children come to school failures, none come labeled failures; *it is school and school alone which pins the label of failure on children.*" The problems created by our country's educational philosophy are "noninvolvement, nonrelevance, and limited emphasis on thinking'' (Glasser, 1969: xiv), and the solution is to move toward the opposite philosophy—that is, toward involvement, relevance, and thinking.

Among his many suggestions for achieving that shift in philosophy, Glasser discusses application of specific Reality Therapy principles, such as involvement on the part of classroom teachers (and school nurses!), teaching students to honestly evaluate present behavior and choose (plan) a more appropriate action if necessary, and securing students' commitment to their plans, accepting no excuses for failure and supplying no punishment. This shift in philosophy also emphasizes the use of praise for success and use of logical and natural consequences of behavior as a means of teaching students to behave responsibly. Furthermore, since the grading system is one more way that students are labeled as failures, Glasser (1969) suggests alternative systems (such as the "pass-superior" system) which do not incorporate the concept of failure. Finally, Glasser suggests further revolution of American contemporary education through incorporation into the regular school curriculum of "classroom meetings" of three types: problem solving, open ended, and educational diagnostic, which classroom teachers can (and should, he believes) be taught to conduct. These changes are needed to eliminate failure, prevent mental health problems, and help students attain a success identity.

Adlerian Psychology

Another theoretical frame of reference that has influenced theorists and therapists, such as Berne, Harris, and Glasser, is Adlerian Psychology, which was developed by Alfred Adler and popularized in this country through the writings of Dreikurs (1953; 1964; Dreikurs and Goldman, 1967).

Among the Adlerian Psychology concepts that have endured and been widely applied is the *family constellation*, which looks at how a child's ordinal position in his family based on birth order affects his role in the family (Dreikurs, 1953). Another popular element of Adlerian Psychology, especially as it applies to discipline of children within their families, is the use of *logical and natural consequences* (Dreikurs, 1953).

Dreikurs (1964; Dreikurs and Goldman, 1967) has developed and refined Adler's ideas and translated them into terms that lay persons can understand and *use*. Nurses and other help-

ing persons who work with children and their parents in the areas of preventive mental health and effective child discipline should find Dreikurs' books and pamphlets helpful.

"Peoplemaking" and conjoint family therapy

An approach to preventive mental health and therapy is the family systems orientation of Satir (1967; 1972). Satir's (1967) original book, *Conjoint Family Therapy,* is addressed to helping professionals and explains the importance of looking beyond the Identified Patient (IP) in a family to study the entire family system and its interactions. Satir believes that therapy can succeed only when the entire system (family) is included in the therapy, since in any system change in one part or element affects the functioning and homeostasis of other elements within the system and therefore the system as a whole.

To make these ideas available to the general public, who are, after all, charged with the ominous responsibility of bearing and rearing children, Satir (1972) rewrote many of her ideas in *Peoplemaking*. This book emphasizes techniques, including games and exercises that family members can practice together, for *preventing* problems in the family system. This prevention is achieved through the family's mastery and consistent application of principles of good communication, esteem building, and decision making. Satir's approach to helping can be readily applied by nurses in any setting after they have had adequate preparation and experience.

Parent Effectiveness Training

The final theoretical approach to be mentioned here is Parent Effectiveness Training (PET), which was developed by Gordon (1975a) in the early 1960s in California. PET is similar to TA and Reality Therapy in that it emphasizes responsibility for behavior. However, the methods used differ. Basically, PET teaches parents a method called "active listening," which is designed to encourage children to accept the responsibility to solve their own problems. PET is based on effective communication techniques and provides some excellent suggestions on communicating with children. These techniques could be very effectively taught to groups of parents under school sponsorship.

Gordon reports that he also has some concerns about the messages that children get from their "other parents," including scout troop leaders, relatives, and babysitters. Like Glasser, he is especially concerned about the messages children receive about themselves at school, from their teachers and other school personnel. Gordon (1975a; 1975b) also decries the "put downs" that children experience at school, agreeing with Glasser that such negative feedback does little to teach a child to feel good about himself and behave responsibly. Gordon likewise believes that our educational philosophy consequently needs to be changed. For that reason he has adapted his basic PET approach to Teacher Effectiveness Training (TET), and encourages educators and school administrators to use it.

SCHOOL NURSING SETTINGS FOR IMPLEMENTING HELPING RELATIONSHIPS
One-to-one relationships

One-to-one relationships have traditionally been the primary mental health therapy setting, dating back to Freud's early psychoanalytic school of thought. In nursing, medicine, and other helping professions, one-to-one relationships have predominated as well, probably because of the medical model's focus on the IP (Satir, 1967). That is, we have focused almost exclusively on the person who is obviously "sick" to the exclusion of his "significant others." However, that is not to say that one-to-one relationships are passé; there are indeed situations in which the one-to-one relationship is the appropriate setting, and even in therapy modalities like Satir's, in which the family group is the focus for therapy, establishment of a helping relationship with the IP(s) can provide the point of entry for the therapist.

The process of establishing a one-to-one helping relationship has been described by Schultz (Chapter 10) and will not be reviewed here. However, it is appropriate to consider the kinds of one-to-one helping relationships that the school nurse may wish to establish.

Obviously, the children and youth who comprise the school population are the primary source of "clients" for the school nurse. Some children may be referred to the nurse for vague or defined somatic complaints; others may refer themselves "just to talk." Using any of the theoretical approaches previously discussed, (or using other approaches with which the nurse may be familiar and comfortable), the nurse be-

gins to establish a relationship with the student in which the problem can be defined and clarified and some kind of plan or contract negotiated for its amelioration. It is important that the nurse take the time to truly "hear" the student, using techniques such as Gordon's (1975a) "active listening." No doubt, many children in today's busy society in which the majority of parents (both sexes) are employed outside the home feel lost at times and just need a caring adult to listen to them and reaffirm their worth as persons. As noted earlier, the school nurse is in an ideal position to offer this kind of supportive and encouraging relationship to schoolchildren, since she does not wield power over the child's academic success and because she is (or should be) highly skilled in the necessary helping relationship techniques.

The school nurse's relationships with individual children may lead to additional one-to-one relationships with their parents or other family members. If, for example, the nurse has been counseling a student about his adjustment to a diagnosis of diabetes, she may discover that part of the student's difficulty in accepting the limitations now imposed on him by the disease are due to pressures or problems his parents are experiencing; in that case, the school nurse may wish to meet with the parent(s) to help them cope. However, it is very important that the nurse discuss with the child her interest in meeting with the parents *before* she arranges a visit; failure to do so can irreparably damage the trust she has established with the child, thus preventing her from being able to help him again. This is especially important in working with adolescents, who often tend to believe that adults in general are highly suspect.

Another type of one-to-one relationship that the school nurse may establish is the teacher-nurse or school staff member–nurse relationship. This is not the collaborative, consultative day-to-day working relationship, however. This relationship is based on *helping* and goes beyond specific job- and performance-related concerns. Obviously, for teachers and other school staff persons to provide the best possible learning environment for students, they must be physically and mentally healthy themselves. Although the school is not and should not be responsible for the personal health of its staff and faculty, the school nurse can be a health resource person for school staff and can provide some individualized services. These services might include periodic blood pressure checks and other assessments for faculty or staff who have known or suspected health problems or concerns; the school nurse might also assist staff with health-related problem solving, referring them to various community resources as indicated. The services the school nurse provides for teachers and other staff members not only help ensure their physical and mental well-being for their jobs, but these services are also a way for the school nurse to establish credibility with them, thus increasing the likelihood that staff will accept and value her consultation and judgment regarding aspects of the school's health program.

The small group setting

Although, as noted earlier, "helping" and therapy have traditionally taken place within the context of one-to-one relationships, in recent years the use of small groups has become increasingly popular. One reason for this is the economy of the group approach; a small group of five persons provides "help" for five times as many persons as a one-to-one relationship. Thus one therapist or group leader can help more people in less time, which reduces the costs of the therapy or helping process. Another reason for the expanded interest in group work is the well-documented realization that "it works" (Pasnau et al., 1971; Bernstein, 1973; Garner, 1974; Bormann, 1975; Bormann and Bormann, 1976). Small groups provide a climate in which members can profit from the experiences of others, as well as from the actual sharing of those experiences and feelings with the group. Some clients are reassured by their realization in the group that other people have had the same experiences or problems.

In school nursing, groups can also be an effective means of implementing helping relationships. The clients in small groups initiated and conducted by the skilled school nurse group leader can include students, parents, other family members, or some combination of all three. The purpose of the group will determine its composition. If the purpose of the group experience is to *provide support* for individuals with a given problem or handicap, such as diabetes, low self-esteem, or chemical dependency, the group members would be drawn from those who have that particular problem.

Another type of small group experience that qualified school nurses could offer in their schools is the *growth,* or *self-development, group.* This type of group is an optimal primary

prevention strategy for promoting positive mental health. The focus of this kind of group is on self-improvement or self-actualization of its essentially healthy members through the experience of the group process. Thus members are encouraged to communicate honestly and directly, sharing their feelings with one another. The group develops a cohesiveness that allows members to trust one another, share their feelings, and grow from the experience.

Combs et al. (1971) describe a similar type of group they call a *discovery group,* for which there can be three purposes: sensitivity training, therapy, or learning of some specified content or theory. They also point out that for these groups (or the growth, or self-development, groups) to succeed, the group leader or therapist must create a climate in which self-disclosure is possible. This can be done through the techniques proposed by Rogers, Glasser, and others. The importance of creating this kind of open, trusting climate cannot be overstated; groups in which this climate does not evolve may not only prove to be of little benefit to the participants but may also actually harm some members. Therefore it is critically important for the school nurse or any other helping professional who plans to conduct this kind of group experience to ensure that she is academically and experientially prepared to guide the group responsibly, so that participants can learn and benefit from the experience and not feel devastated by it. Small groups can be an effective and powerful tool in school nursing if they are responsibly conducted by qualified nurse leaders.

The classroom setting

Another kind of group experience, although on a larger scale than the small groups of eight to ten persons previously described, is the classroom group. Classroom groups usually number about thirty students and have a learning or educational focus. Classroom groups offer an ideal opportunity (captive audience) for health education, particularly in the area of preventive mental health, which Glasser and others have already pointed out is an important need. The school nurse can be a resource to the classroom teacher in planning classroom meetings of the type described by Glasser (1969) and in helping the teacher incorporate esteem building, decision making, and interpersonal relationship skills into the classroom experience.

In addition to serving as a resource to the

teacher, the school nurse can participate directly in classroom teaching, using her helping relationship skills to teach students about mental health. The nurse can incorporate concepts and content from formal mental health curriculum guides, such as the one published by the ASHA (ASHA Committee on Mental Health in the Classroom, 1968), or she can base her group experience around some selected theoretical approach, such as TA, Reality Therapy, or PET/TET. Whatever approach she plans to use, however, must be consistent with the overall school curriculum and the goals and policies of the school health program. It is hoped that as school nurses expand their preparation level and skills, their abilities and opportunities for classroom involvement with students will increase.

CONCLUSION

A strong background in helping relationship skills is the cornerstone for the application of the other elements or strands (public health, adaptation, tools, and systematic process) of the school nursing conceptual framework. Preventive mental health is an important health need within contemporary society, and the school is in an ideal position to provide it. The school nurse, using a chosen theoretical or conceptual approach or an approach she has eclectically developed, can use her helping relationship skills and background to promote students' positive mental health, whether on a one-to-one basis, in a small group setting, or in the classroom. To further ensure an adequate emphasis on positive mental health, the school nurse can work within the school system to increase the priority assigned to preventive mental health within the school's health program and general curriculum and can encourage adoption of an educational philosophy that is oriented not to failure but to growth, responsibility, and self-actualization.

REFERENCES

ASHA Committee on Mental Health in the Classroom: 1968. Mental health in the classroom, rev. ed., J. School Health 38(5a):1-44, American School Health Association, Kent, Ohio.

Berne, E.: 1964. Games people play, Grove Press, Inc., New York.

Bernstein, S.: 1973. Explorations in group work: essays in theory and practice, Milford House, Inc., Boston.

Bormann, E. G.: 1975. Discussion and group methods: theory and practice, 2nd ed., Harper & Row, Publishers, Inc., New York.

Bormann, E. G., and Bormann, N. C.: 1976. Effective small group communication, Burgess Publishing Co., Minneapolis.

Combs, A. W., Avila, D. L., and Purkey, W. W.: 1971. Helping relationships: basic concepts for the helping professions, Allyn & Bacon, Inc., Boston.

Cook, L. W.: 1969. Mental health and the multiple roles of school nurses, J. School Health 39(9):614-617.

Cowen, E. L., Pederson, A., Babigian, H., Izzo, L. D., and Trost, M. A.: 1973. Long-term follow-up of early detected vulnerable children, J. Consult. Clin. Psychol. 41(3):438-446.

Crosby, M. H., and Connolly, M. G.: 1970. The study of mental health and the school nurse, J. School Health 40(7):373-378.

Drake, R. E.: 1970. The school as a locus of community mental health services, Nurs. Clin. North Am. 5(5):657-667.

Dreikurs, R. R.: 1953. Fundamentals of Adlerian psychology, Alfred Adler Institute, Chicago.

Dreikurs, R. R.: 1964. Children: the challenge, Hawthorn Books, Inc., New York.

Dreikurs, R. R., and Goldman, M.: 1967. The ABC's of guiding the child (booklet), Rudolf Dreikurs Unit of Family Education Association, Chicago.

Esty, G. W.: 1967. The prevention of psychosocial disorders of youth: a challenge to mental health, public health and education, J. School Health 37(1):19-23.

Freed, A. M.: 1971. T.A. for kids, Jalmar Press, Inc., Sacramento, Calif.

Freed, A. M.: 1973. T.A. for tots, Jalmar Press, Inc., Sacramento, Calif.

Freed, A. M.: 1976. T.A. for teens, Jalmar Press, Inc., Sacramento, Calif.

Garner, H. G.: 1974. Mental health benefits of small group experiences in the affective domain, J. School Health 44(6):314-318.

Glasser, W.: 1965. Reality therapy, Harper & Row, Publishers, Inc., New York.

Glasser, W.: 1969. Schools without failure, Harper & Row, Publishers, Inc., New York.

Glasser, W.: 1975. The identity society, rev. ed., Harper & Row, Publishers, Inc., New York.

Gordon, T.: 1975a. P.E.T.: parent effectiveness training, The New American Library, Inc., New York.

Gordon, T.: 1975b. T.E.T.: teacher effectiveness training, Wyden Books, New York.

Harris, T. A.: 1969. I'm OK—you're OK: a practical guide to transactional analysis, Harper & Row, Publishers, Inc., New York.

Joint Commission on Mental Health of Children: 1970. Crisis in child mental health: challenge for the 1970's, Harper & Row, Publishers, Inc., New York.

Pasnau, R. O., Williams, L., and Tallman, F. F.: 1971. Small activity groups in the school: report of a twelve-year research project in community psychiatry, Commun. Ment. Health J. 7(4):303-311.

Rogers, C. R.: 1951. Client-centered therapy, Houghton Mifflin Co., New York.

Rogers, C. R.: 1956. A counseling approach to human problems, Am. J. Nurs. 56(8):994-997.

Rogers, C. R.: 1959. A theory of therapy, personality and interpersonal relationships. In Koch, S., editor: Psychology: a study of a science, vol. 3, McGraw-Hill, Inc., New York.

Rogers, C. R.: 1969. Freedom to learn, Charles E. Merrill Publishing Co., Columbus, Ohio.

Satir, V.: 1967. Conjoint family therapy, rev. ed., Science & Behavior Books, Palo Alto, Calif.

Satir, V.: 1972. Peoplemaking, Science & Behavior Books, Palo Alto, Calif.

Siemon, M.: 1978. Mental health in school-aged children, MCN **3**(4):211-217.

Taintor, Z. C.: 1976. What the schools can do to promote mental health, J. School Health **46**(2):86-90.

Williams, R. B.: 1970. The helping professions: problems only? J. School Health **40**(1):24-27.

Yalom, I. D.: 1975. The theory and practice of group psychotherapy, 2nd ed., Basic Books, Inc., Publishers, New York.

SUGGESTED READINGS

Abrams, R. S., Vanecko, M., and Abrams, I.: 1972. A suggested school mental health program, J. School Health **42**(3):137-141.

Berne, E.: 1972. What do you say after you say hello? Bantam Books, Inc., New York.

Brammer, L. W.: 1973. The helping relationship: process and skills, Prentice-Hall, Inc., Englewood Cliffs, N.J.

Collins, M.: 1977. Communication in health care: understanding and implementing effective human relationships, The C. V. Mosby Co., St. Louis.

Glasser, W.: 1970. Mental health or mental illness? Harper & Row, Publishers, Inc., New York.

Kessler, J. W.: 1966. Psychopathology of childhood, Prentice-Hall, Inc., Englewood Cliffs, N.J.

Miller, S., Nunnally, E. W., and Wackman, D. B.: 1975. Alive and aware, Interpersonal Communication Programs, Inc., Minneapolis.

Missildine, W. H., editor: 1975. Interviewing techniques—children and adolescents, Feelings and Their Med. Significance **17**(6):1-4.

Oda, D. S.: 1974. Increasing role effectiveness of school nurses, Am. J. Public Health **64**(6):591-595.

Pazdur, H. C.: 1969. Innovation: the school nurse as a mental health specialist, J. School Health **39**(7):449-457.

Reinert, H. R.: 1976. Children in conflict: educational strategies for the emotionally disturbed and behaviorally disordered, The C. V. Mosby Co., St. Louis.

Ross, D. C., Meinster, M. O., and Gingrich, L. J.: 1978. A program for expanding the mental health function of the school nurse, J. School Health **48**(3):157-159.

Rubin, E. Z.: 1970. A psycho-educational model for school mental health planning, Commun. Ment. Health J. **6**(1):31-39.

Sellery, C. M.: 1973. The active role of schools in mental health as seen in retrospect and prospect, J. School Health **43**(7):455-457.

Singer, D. L., Whiton, M. B., and Fried, M. L.: 1970. An alternative to mental health services and consultation in schools: a social systems and group process approach, J. School Psychol. **8**(3):172-179.

Sundeen, S. J., Stuart, G. W., Rankin, E. D., and Cohen, S. P.: 1976. Nurse-client interaction: implementing the nursing process, The C. V. Mosby Co., St. Louis.

PART V

School nursing tools

CHAPTER 12

Systematic assessment

MARY LOU CHRISTENSEN

Assessment in the broad sense of the word has been a part of school nursing since the specialty began at the turn of the century. School nurses have looked at children from the viewpoint of physical appraisal; psychosocial-emotional adjustment in the context of their membership in families, peer groups, and individual classrooms; and within the spectrum of growth, development, and their varying placement along the health-illness continuum. This broad view of children continues to be important as school nurses expand on nursing judgments about the health status of children and youth in our schools.

While assessment practices have been ongoing and useful in the daily practice of school nursing, they have not always been systematic in nature. Recently, the emphasis on systematic assessment in the delivery of health care to people has been to increase the quality of care and improve their health status. School nursing is moving more and more in the direction of primary care, where health maintenance and promotion of wellness among the students/clients are priorities. This movement toward primary care demands greater skill and efficiency in health assessment of children and youth. Thus it is imperative that school nurses also incorporate systematic assessment skills into their practice of nursing.

This chapter focuses on definitions useful in systematic assessment, history taking, and physical assessment as these tools relate to comprehensive and acute complaints, and problem-oriented recording as a mechanism for organizing and communicating about health care given to the school-age child. The purpose of this chapter is to relate techniques of systematic assessment to the school setting, rather than to describe in detail the specific mechanism involved with health assessment. References on resources and formal school nurse practitioner programs for developing health assessment skills are given at the end of this chapter.

DEFINITIONS

The definitions presented here are basic to conceptualizing assessment practices within the school nurse's framework of nursing practice. Since words often have multiple definitions, it is important that the meaning of terms related to the school setting be clarified.

Systematic

In considering the term "systematic," the methodical aspect of the word needs to be recognized. In this context, the term can be used two different ways. It includes the usual, sequential manner a nurse uses in approaching the client. For example, when comprehensively assessing a student/client, the systematic approach proceeds in an orderly, cephalocaudal, or head-to-toe, manner. This methodical process ensures complete observation of the client, both as a functional whole and as a series of parts.

The use of the term systematic within the school system implies regular planning and implementation of similar health programs throughout the school district. The purpose of the systematic approach to health program planning is to include all students for whom the program or service is intended and to build sequentially on what has occurred previously. One of the mechanisms for assessing the health status of groups and, ultimately, individual group members is through screening programs. These programs occur periodically and are essential for continuous health appraisal and effective use of the ongoing epidemiological process (Hogue, 1977). In these ways the school nurse is systematic and responsive in her approach to students as individuals and as members of subpopulation groups.

Assessment

The term "assessment" as it relates to health is defined as an act or series of acts that are useful in identifying a student/client's health needs at a specific point in time. The acts of assessment differ from the assessment statement a nurse develops because these acts are the specific activities which lead the nurse to a conclusion in the assessment statement she records.

It is also useful to combine the terms systematic and assessment. In so doing, the student/client can be observed as a holistic being comprising more than the sum of his parts. He can be viewed as a complex, interrelated and interdependent being that is "influencing and being influenced by his environment" (Sills and Hall, 1977:24). Systematically assessing the student/client either in comprehensive or acute situations provides the school nurse with data regarding his level of physical and psychosocial-emotional function.

Continuous

In the school setting, the term "continuous" refers to ongoing screening and assessment data relating to individual students. The data collected is made a part of the student/client's cumulative kindergarten to twelfth grade problem-oriented health record (POHR), which in turn is part of the school cumulative record. The fact that the data is cumulative and made part of the POHR within the educational setting makes it continuous in nature throughout his school-age years.

Periodic

The term "periodic" refers to comprehensive health examinations occurring at regular intervals on a predetermined schedule. Periodicity means the "schedule is based on the fact that certain health threatening conditions have an increased incidence in an age/sex/time specific relationship" (Minnesota Department of Health, 1976:2). Thus the schedule is developed to coincide with peak periods of growth and development and subsequent health problems. The specific health maintenance schedule that is implemented in schools will be discussed later in this chapter. Furthermore, periodic is differentiated from the acute episodic complaint in that the interval health assessment has a wellness focus, and few, if any, acute complaints are anticipated.

Student/client

Throughout this chapter, reference is made interchangeably to the student and/or client. The term "student" is used as a means of identifying him as the health care consumer who happens to be of school age and located in a school setting. The term "client," as opposed to patient, is used to connote the contracting process that evolves between the school nurse and the student in decision making regarding his health care.

HISTORY TAKING

The most important aspect of health assessment is the history. Concrete information on which the school nurse identifies the student's physical and psychosocial-emotional problems is achieved through delineation of a thorough and accurate health history. Basically, history taking is gathering primarily verbal information from the student/client or other reliable informant for the purpose of identifying health needs and generating practical solutions for them. Often nonverbal observations also contribute to the health history and data base. Sometimes a self-administered or parent-respondent questionnaire is a valuable aid to eliciting a comprehensive health history.

Interviewing

The basic tool for obtaining a complete and accurate health history is effective interviewing. Skillful communication techniques are necessary to establish an effective therapeutic relationship with the student and to lay a firm foundation for physical assessment and future ongoing interactions. Sensitivity to client needs and allowing the student to talk freely in describing his health condition are imperative. A climate of trust, which allows for full expression of the student's needs, can be established through development of rapport. Building on mutual consideration, courtesy, and respect between the school nurse and student is one mechanism for establishing confidence in the interview process and the interviewer and ensuring continued trust and rapport.

There are several types of interviews, each with a different purpose to fit the situation (Brown and Murphy, 1975). First is the *comprehensive interview,* such as that which occurs at the preschool clinic when the school nurse takes the initial complete health history. Subsequent interval visits that have a wellness focus also fit this category. Pertinent past and family health history and developmental and nutritional information are obtained as part of the initial data base, which begins the client/student's cumulative POHR. This comprehensive interview takes time, approximately 30 to 45 minutes, and provides an opportunity for the school nurse to develop a meaningful relationship with the child and his parent(s) through sharing facts and feelings.

Another kind is the *problem-centered interview,* wherein the student refers himself for health services to meet an immediate physical or emotional need. Sometimes the problem presented is not of utmost concern to the student, but rather an excuse for seeking help for an underlying and more significant problem. It is of primary importance that the school nurse elicit the real problem through the use of clarifying techniques. The problem-centered interview can be difficult, demanding expertise in the use of therapeutic communication and the ability to effectively identify the complaint.

The third type to consider is the *therapeutic interview.* The format for this interview begins with problem identification and contract setting with the student for an ongoing health counseling relationship. Under the school nurse's guidance, alternative solutions to the problem are generated, and consequences of each potential solution are discussed. Through sharing resources and responsibility, trust evolves. The therapeutic interview is often used with students who have chronic disease such as allergies, hearing and vision deficits, obesity, and complex physical-psychosocial concerns such as pregnancy. This interview occurs over time, requiring technical nursing knowledge, organizational follow-up, and effective communication skills from the school nurse.

Assertiveness is one of the primary considerations of the school nurse in approaching the interview. Confidence is inspired by structuring the interview to allow free expression of feelings by the client as well as authoritative, as opposed to authoritarian, direction by the school nurse. Maintaining privacy within the interview is another consideration that will promote control and enhance free interaction between the student and nurse. Being warm, friendly, courteous, enthusiastic, and responsive also contributes to a successful approach to the client and results in a meaningful interview.

The school nurse's qualities are also important in achieving an effective interview. A nonjudgmental attitude is an essential quality for the school nurse to possess. Being nonjudgmental maintains one's own value system separate from that of the client's and allows for objectivity and caring in assisting the student with his concerns. Adaptability in the school nurse's interviewing style is necessary to communicate effectively with different ages and stages in children, youth, and their parents. Variety in the interviewing style to fit the situation is also important when working with clients who have significantly different cultural, ethnic, and socioeconomic backgrounds from that of the nurse.

To achieve the ultimate goal of data collection in the interview, questions are used. Generally, two types of inquiry, open ended and direct or closed questions, are pursued. Indirect or open-ended questions are used to elicit a description of the situation as the client sees it. Some examples of open-ended questions or suggestions are, "Tell me about how you are feeling" or "Tell me what that means to you." The advantage of this type of question is that the client volunteers his impression and can disclose the information the way he chooses without being clued or led by the nurse. The student's levels of mental-emotional functioning, attitudes, and beliefs are also observed in this way. Sometimes, however, the student may digress from relevant discussion about his situation, possibly due to anxiety and much difficulty with expression of more painful information. At these times a more structured approach to the interview is necessary (Malasanos et al., 1977).

The mechanism for clearly structuring the interview is through the use of direct or closed questions. This type of question elicits short words or phrases and forced responses. Some examples of direct questions would be, "How old are you?" "Did you have breakfast this morning?" "What kind of medication did you take?" Responses are limited by the very nature of these questions, which is desirable in some instances. On the other hand, when direct questioning is overused, the nurse may be seen as uncaring or uninterested (Malasanos et al., 1977).

There is a time and place for each of these types of questions. Most interviews contain elements of both, appropriately woven throughout in an effort to efficiently direct the interview while also effectively gaining the client's viewpoint.

In addition to questioning, communication within the interview also involves positive feedback. This mechanism is used to reinforce desired behavior. When a student has pursued a goal diligently, that behavior should be recognized. For example, when counseling an overweight teenager who has consistently followed a weight-reduction program, those efforts should be verbally and nonverbally rewarded. Whether intervening in an ongoing therapeutic or a comprehensive interview, client behaviors that have been performed well are elicited. The client deserves positive feedback for these behaviors, which will encourage their continuation.

The context of the interview is also appropriate for client teaching. Whether the contact with a student is brief and sporadic or building on previous ongoing visits, health teaching should take place with the student and/or his parent in relationship to his identified health needs. For example, preschool screening clinics offer an excellent opportunity to teach correct dental hygiene practices and good nutritional habits. When completing the Denver Developmental Screening Test (DDST), the school nurse can identify areas in which the child is developmentally deficient or immature. She can make suggestions to his parents for stimulating the child, anticipating his needs as they relate developmentally to school readiness in that specific school district. Teaching, whether it occurs with a planned format based on prior assessment or spontaneously at the "teachable moment," is a viable aspect of the interview. Effective client teaching will occur as the school nurse seizes these opportunities and develops strategies that fit with her personality and the teaching/learning situation.

Complete health history as a data base

The comprehensive health history is the baseline of information about the student. It provides the school nurse with the necessary data for problem identification and a working knowledge of the student as a unique individual. The significance of the health history as the most important aspect of health assessment and as a mechanism for problem identification is well documented. A pilot health assessment project was completed with 1151 preschool children (entering kindergartners and first graders) in a large city school district in Pennsylvania. Analysis of the data revealed that the history detected health problems 3.8 times the rate of the physical examination, excluding vision, hearing, dental, and overweight problems, which

were identified by other screening methods (Lynch, 1975). Thus the importance of obtaining a complete health history on children entering school and at periodic intervals thereafter cannot be overemphasized.

The student/client is viewed as a whole within the context of his own (or parents') perceptions of his health status and himself as a physical, psychosocial, and emotional being. The data base obtained through the health history is a useful tool in providing health maintenance, preventive care, and anticipatory guidance for the student's encounters in the school setting.

The entire health history can be obtained verbally through a predeveloped format designed to gather pertinent data using the interview process. The advantage in using this format is that with skilled interviewing, depth can be achieved on a particular point of significance. The disadvantages are the amount of time required for the interchange of information and the possibility of overlooking a significant area of inquiry for a given child.

Another way to obtain a comprehensive health history is through use of a printed form designed specifically to gather health information that will be most useful to the school nurse working with school-age children and youth. There are several advantages to using this type of data-gathering format. It is less time-consuming in the data-gathering phase of the interview and more detailed in scope. The questionnaires are easily answered with check marks in *yes* and *no* categories. The forms are sent home for the parents to complete prior to the interview. Additional depth can be achieved through the interviewing process when clarifying with the student or his parents those areas which they have indicated to be of concern. Sometimes the client fails to complete the form or partially fills it out. In these instances the form is used as an interview guideline.

Preschool screening clinics that used a series of printed forms for data gathering took place in Minnesota in the spring of 1978. Fig. 12-1 shows a child screening form. In addition to the usual biographical information found on this type of a form, there are areas for recording the child's primary care and dental providers and their possible involvement with other health care and social service agencies. This readily available information assists the school nurse when communicating information with other health care professionals about the child's health status. Also provided is an area for re-

```
                                    Name _____
                                    Record number _____
                                    Date_____
                                    Birth date _____

                          CHILD SCREENING
                  FAMILY AND PERINATAL HISTORY

Address _____ Telephone number _____
Directions to home _____
```

Medical	Physician's name _____
	Address _____
	_____
	Date of last visit _____
	Reason for visit _____
	_____

Dental	Dentist's name _____
	Address _____
	_____
	Date of last visit _____
	Reason for visit _____
	_____
	Was dental treatment completed? _____No _____Yes _____Not needed
	If no, why not? _____
	Is another dental appointment scheduled?_____
	If yes, when? _____

```
Other     Have you received services from:            No       Yes
          1.  County public health nurse             _____    _____
          2.  County Welfare--Financial Aid or Social
              Services                               _____    _____
          3.  Mental Health Center                   _____    _____
          4.  Other specialists                      _____    _____
              If so, state name, address, and reason
              for service.
              _____
              _____
              _____
```

```
Father

     Place of employment _____
     Telephone number _____
```

```
Mother

     Place of employment _____
     Telephone number _____
```

```
Brothers and     1.
sisters
                 2.

                 3.

                 4.
```

Fig. 12-1. Child screening: family and perinatal history. (Reprinted with permission of the Minnesota Department of Health.)

Continued.

		No	Yes
Brothers and sisters--cont'd	5. 6. 7. 8.		
General information	1. Have there been any major changes in the family situation in the last year, such as a family moving, loss of someone close, or a serious illness of either parent?	___	___
	2. Do you have any concerns about your home or family situation that might be affecting your child's growth or development?	___	___
Perinatal history	1. Was there anything unusual about this pregnancy, labor, or delivery?	___	___
	2. Did the child have any difficulty at birth or shortly after birth?	___	___
	3. Was the child premature?	___	___
Referral information given (to be filled in by screener)			

Fig. 12-1, cont'd. Child screening: family and perinatal history.

cording names of siblings. Using this area to record the siblings' birthday/age, general health status, and school of enrollment assists the school nurse to assess the child's placement in the family constellation and provides identify-

ing information for contacting other siblings while in school, if necessary.

A child health history form is shown in Fig. 12-2. It gathers pertinent past and present medical information, growth and development mile-

---

Name _____
Record number _____
Date _____
Informant _____

CHILD HEALTH HISTORY
(0 to 6 Years)

I. Past medical history			No	Yes

Hospitalizations
1. Has your child ever been hospitalized? ____ ____
2. If yes, list dates, hospital, and reason. ____ ____

Childhood illnesses
Has your child had any of the following:
1. "Red" or "hard" measles (rubeola)
2. German or 3-day measles (rubella) ____ ____
3. Meningitis ____ ____
4. Chicken pox ____ ____
5. Scarlet fever ____ ____
6. Rheumatic fever ____ ____
7. Mumps ____ ____
8. Pneumonia ____ ____
9. Diabetes ____ ____
10. Streptococcal infections ____ ____
11. High fever (104° F for longer than 2 days) ____ ____

Other illnesses
1. Has your child ever had any important illnesses for which he/she was not hospitalized? ____ ____
2. If yes, list dates, type of illness, and treatment given. ____ ____

Allergies
Has your child ever had problems with any of the following:
1. Asthma or hay fever ____ ____
2. Food allergy ____ ____
3. Eczema ____ ____
4. Drug or medication allergy ____ ____
5. Nose or eye allergy ____ ____
6. Severe reaction to insect stings ____ ____

Accidents
1. Has your child ever had any serious accidents or injuries? ____ ____
2. Has your child ever become poisoned? ____ ____
3. Has your child ever had any broken bones? ____ ____
4. Does your child have frequent accidents? ____ ____

Special health care
1. Has your child ever undergone any special tests for health problems? ____ ____
2. Has your child ever been seen by a specialist? ____ ____
3. Is he/she under the care of a specialist now? ____ ____

Fig. 12-2. Child health history. (Reprinted with permission of the Minnesota Department of Health.)

Continued.

		No	Yes
Growth and development	When did your child do the following? 1. Sit alone _____ 2. Walk alone _____ 3. Say single words _____ 4. Use two-word sentences _____ 5. Become toilet trained _____ 6. Do you think your child should be doing more than he/she is doing for his/her age?	____	____

II. Present medical history		No	Yes
General	1. Does your child have a poor appetite?	____	____
	2. Does your child eat too much?	____	____
	3. Does your child have an excessive thirst?	____	____
	4. Does your child have sleep problems?	____	____
	5. Does your child have too much or too little energy?	____	____
	6. Does your child have any physical restrictions?	____	____
	7. Does your child take any medications regularly?	____	____
Skin	1. Does your child have problems with rashes?	____	____
	2. Does your child bruise easily?	____	____
	3. Does your child have any unexplained lumps or spots?	____	____
	4. Does your child get hives or eczema?	____	____
Eyes	1. Does your child have any problems with his/her eyes?	____	____
	2. Do your child's eyes turn in or turn out when tired?	____	____
Ears, nose, and throat	1. Has your child had two to three episodes of ear problems in a year?	____	____
	2. Does your child have any trouble hearing?	____	____
	3. Has your child had two or more throat infections in a year?	____	____
	4. Does your child have frequent nosebleeds?	____	____
	5. Does your child get swollen glands frequently?	____	____
Respiratory	1. Has your child had four to six colds in a year?	____	____
	2. Does your child get a severe cough with colds?	____	____
	3. Does your child have trouble getting rid of a severe cough?	____	____
	4. Does your child have shortness of breath at times?	____	____
	5. Does your child have asthma or wheezing problems?	____	____
Cardiovascular	1. Do your child's hands and fingers turn blue when he/she plays hard?	____	____
	2. Does your child have heart trouble?	____	____

Fig. 12-2, cont'd. Child health history.

			No	Yes
Gastrointestinal	1.	Does your child have stomachaches?	____	____
	2.	Does your child have a problem with foods disagreeing with him/her?	____	____
	3.	Does your child have diarrhea frequently?	____	____
	4.	Does your child have trouble with constipation?	____	____
	5.	Does your child vomit frequently?	____	____
Urinary	1.	Does your child have an interrupted, dribbling, or weak urinary stream?	____	____
	2.	Does your child complain of pain upon urination?	____	____
	3.	Does your child have a strong or unusual odor of urine?	____	____
	4.	Is your child toilet trained? Answer if child is 2 years or more.	____	____
Skeletal	1.	Does your child complain of pains in his/her legs, arms, back, or joints?	____	____
	2.	Has your child had any broken bones?	____	____
	3.	Does your child toe in, toe out, limp, or walk funny?	____	____
Neuromuscular	1.	Does your child lose his/her balance in unusual ways?	____	____
	2.	Does your child have any unexplained movements or jerks?	____	____
	3.	Has your child ever had convulsions or seizures?	____	____
	4.	Does your child have any weakness in his/her body?	____	____
	5.	Does your child have unusual staring spells?	____	____
	6.	Does your child fall down more than most children?	____	____
Lead	1.	Does your child chew any unusual things such as woodwork, pencils, crib, paint chips, plaster?	____	____
	2.	Do you live in a house built before 1950 that has peeling paint on the walls, woodwork, ceiling, doors, or outside of the house?	____	____
	3.	Does your child seem tired, fussy, or cranky for more than 4 to 6 hours every day?	____	____

III. Psychosocial history

		No	Yes
Behavior problems	Are you concerned about your child in any of the following areas?		
	1. Bedwetting	____	____
	2. Wetting during the day	____	____
	3. Bad dreams	____	____
	4. Biting nails	____	____
	5. Thumbsucking	____	____
	6. Stammering or stuttering	____	____
	7. Nervous habits of any kind	____	____
	8. Irritability, easily upset	____	____
	9. Restlessness	____	____
	10. Day dreaming, preoccupied	____	____

Fig. 12-2, cont'd. Child health history.

Continued.

			No	Yes
Behavior problems--cont'd	11.	Glum, sulky, moody	___	___
	12.	Wanting too much attention, comfort, or support	___	___
	13.	Feelings hurt easily	___	___
	14.	Breath holding	___	___
	15.	Contrary, stubborn, uncooperative	___	___
	16.	Selfishness, inability to share	___	___
	17.	Jealousy	___	___
	18.	Bad temper	___	___
	19.	Anger	___	___
	20.	Destroying things on purpose	___	___
	21.	Lying	___	___
	22.	Disobedient	___	___
	23.	Clumsiness, awkwardness	___	___
	24.	Bowels	___	___
	25.	Speech	___	___
	26.	Does your child require more work than you expected?	___	___
	27.	Has your child failed to live up to your expectations?	___	___

Nurse's comments _____

_____

_____

_____

_____

_____

_____

_____

_____

_____

_____

_____

_____

_____

_____

_____

Fig. 12-2, cont'd. Child health history.

stones, and psychosocial history. Depth in problem identification and preliminary psycho-educational planning is achieved through the interview in which the school nurse reviews the form with the child's parent(s). The behavioral history area is of particular significance for the child entering school. With additional clarify-ing comments by the parent(s) about the child's characteristics, the school nurse can begin problem solving with them and making specific recommendations to the kindergarten teacher that will assist the child in adjusting optimally to school.

The form shown in Fig. 12-3 depicts clearly

Name _____

Record number _____

Date _____

Informant _____

EPS IMMUNIZATION RECORD

Where does child usually receive immunizations? _____

Give month and year of each immunization.

	No. 1	No. 2	No. 3	No. 4	No. 5
DPT (diphtheria, pertussis, tetanus, or 3 in one)	☐	☐	☐	☐	☐
Td (after age 6) (tetanus, diphtheria)	☐	☐	☐	☐	
Oral polio	☐	☐	☐	☐	
Rubella (German measles)	☐				
Mumps	☐	or MMR	☐		
Rubeola (red measles)	☐	or other	☐		
Tetanus (lockjaw) (booster, e.g., emergencies)	☐	☐	☐	☐	

Tuberculin skin test   Date   Result

_____   _____

_____   _____

_____   _____

_____   _____

Has this child ever reacted to an immunization?   No ____ Yes _____

If so, what and how? _____

Comments: _____

_____

_____

_____

_____

Fig. 12-3. Early Periodic Screening (EPS) immunization record. (Reprinted with permission of the Minnesota Department of Health.)

Minnesota Departments of Health and Education

IMMUNIZATION REQUIREMENTS FOR ADMISSION TO MINNESOTA SCHOOLS

Minnesota Statutes 1978, Section 123.70, requires that all children entering a Minnesota public, private or parochial elementary school, day care center or nursery school for the first time be immunized against diphtheria, tetanus, pertussis, polio, measles, mumps and rubella. These requirements can be waived only if a properly signed medical or conscientious exemption is filed with the school. IN ORDER FOR YOUR CHILD TO ENTER SCHOOL, THIS FORM MUST BE COMPLETED, SIGNED, AND ON FILE PRIOR TO ADMISSION AT THE SCHOOL YOUR CHILD WILL ATTEND. The information you provide on this form will be available to the local public health agency and the Minnesota Department of Health to determine if your child has received the minimum recommended immunizations.

Step 1

Name	Birthdate	School	Grade

Parent or Guardian	Address	Telephone

Step 2

IMMUNIZATION HISTORY/MINIMUM RECOMMENDATIONS

Enter the MONTH AND YEAR the child received each dose of the following vaccines. One measles, mumps, and rubella, three polio, and four DTP are the minimum recommended doses for admission to school. This section, when completed, must be signed by a physician or public immunization clinic.

DO NOT USE (✓) OR (X).

TYPE OF VACCINE	1st Dose Month-Year	2nd Dose Month-Year	3rd Dose Month-Year	4th Dose Month-Year	5th Dose Month-Year
DTP Diphtheria-Tetanus-Pertussis					
POLIO					
MEASLES		I certify that the recommended number of immunizations have been received for school admission.			
RUBELLA					
MUMPS		Signature of Physician or Public Immunization Clinic Date			

Step 3

IF THE CHILD HAS NOT RECEIVED THE MINIMUM RECOMMENDED DOSES, YOU MUST CHOOSE AT LEAST ONE OF THE FOLLOWING THREE ALTERNATIVES BY PLACING AN "X" IN THE APPROPRIATE BOX AND OBTAINING THE REQUIRED SIGNATURE(S):

1. [ ] In addition to having received measles, mumps, and rubella vaccine, the above named child has commenced a schedule to receive adequate doses of DTP/Td and/or polio vaccine:

   _____
   Signature of Physician or Public Immunization Clinic   Date

   Note to Parents: I understand that if this step is chosen, I intend to submit an amended certificate within 10 months to the school verifying completion of the DTP and/or polio vaccine schedule. I understand that my child may be excluded from school if the vaccine is not received within a 10 month period.

   _____
   Signature of Parent or Legal Guardian   Date

2. [ ] I hereby certify that the physical condition of this child is such that immunization would endanger the life or health of the child. Indicate vaccine(s) _____

   _____
   Signature of Physician   Date

3. [ ] I hereby certify by notarization that immunization for my child is contrary to my conscientiously held beliefs. Indicate vaccine(s) _____

   _____
   Signature of Parent or Legal Guardian   Date

   Subscribed and sworn to before me this _____ day of _____ 19 _____

   _____
   Signature of notary

Fig. 12-4. Immunization requirements for admission to Minnesota schools. (Reprinted with permission of the Minnesota Department of Health.)

the child's immunization status. This form has the advantage of showing precisely which immunizations the child has received. They must be recorded by month and year to maintain complete accuracy of administration. It also indicates the primary source of immunizations and any reactions that might have occurred with their administration.

Many states have mandatory immunization requirements for children prior to school entrance. Immunization against all preventable childhood communicable diseases, such as by use of diphtheria and tetanus toxoids and pertussis vaccine (DTP) (five doses), poliovirus vaccine (four doses) and measles, mumps, rubella (MMR) vaccines for children entering school in Minnesota became mandatory in April, 1978. The form for compliance with that law is shown in Fig. 12-4. Although this form does not gather information about reactions to previous immunizations, that data can be made a part of the past medical history. A community's level of protection against these childhood communicable diseases can be assessed by computing the percentage of compliance with the law within each school district's entering kindergarten class. Furthermore, immunization booster programs can be planned from this baseline data.

Periodic updating of the initial comprehensive health history is achieved at three intervals during the years a student is enrolled in school. The intervals used in some districts are at grades four, seven, and ten. This update of information can be achieved through further parental completion of questionnaires, teacher notation of health defects, and student response to self-administered questionnaires.

Using teacher's observations of student health and behavior as an adjunct to the initial health history data base is most helpful for viewing the "total child." Teachers are in a unique position to observe a child's daily classroom functioning and peer relationships. Ritter (1976) found that a simple checklist for teacher observations of body symptoms, behavioral traits, and adjustment factors was superior to a *yes/no* category designation for recording teachers' health observations. Fig. 12-5 shows the form used by school nurse practitioners (SNPs) in the elementary schools of the Penn Manor School District in Pennsylvania. These observations can be the basis for subsequent in-depth conferences with teachers about a child's health condition. Systematic input by teachers, capi-

talizing on their close and continual interaction with children, assists the school nurse in evaluating the health status of children.

Another mechanism for obtaining interval health history data is the student self-administered questionnaire. As young people mature, it is of utmost importance that they be given responsibility for their own health care. They should be given that amount of responsibility commensurate with their level of maturity. Giving secondary students the opportunity to personally respond to a health questionnaire involves them in decision making about personal health concerns. This tends to increase their sense of responsibility toward themselves.

Research indicates that the yes/no category type of questionnaire is reliable for collecting health information from adolescents. In a recent study, a health questionnaire designed to collect data on body systems, emotional-social areas, and the student's academic adjustment was administered to seventh- and tenth-grade young people. The results indicated that a significantly high correlation existed between the historical data gathered and the physician's findings (Beitz, 1976).

Administering the health history form to adolescents can be done by the school nurse within the educational setting or in cooperation with regularly scheduled early and periodic screening (EPS) clinics sponsored by the local county community health service. The form currently being used by Minnesota's Ramsey County Public Health Nursing Service in their EPS clinics is shown in Fig. 12-6. The instrument is designed to collect past health information and data specific to problems that commonly occur during adolescence. The student is directed to check either the no or yes column opposite each question. In this manner problem areas are identified, and further information about the student's health concerns is achieved in the interview between the student and nurse. Health educational programs can be developed to meet the adolescent group needs when statistics suggest a high incidence of specific health problems. Thus a more thorough understanding of each student and the health status of the class as a whole is obtained.

Systematic interviewing as it relates to acute complaints

As in any service providing health care, the school health service receives numerous acute episodic complaints. These complaints are usu-

Text continued on p. 265.

```
                    TEACHER'S HEALTH OBSERVATIONS

     Name of child_____Date_____

     Grade_____Class_____

     Name of teacher_____

     Please check items as directed.  Add comments next to the item or at

     the end of the form.

     A.  Observations of child's body

         Check any of the following you have noticed:

         Eyes
            1.  Eyes crossed in or out
            2.  Red, runny, or itchy eyes
            3.  Deformity of eyes

         Ears
            4.  Discharge or running from ears
            5.  Deformity of ears

         Skin and hair
            6.  Skin rash
            7.  Lack of cleanliness of skin or hair
            8.  Sores on skin
            9.  Nits in hair
           10.  Pale or sallow skin, or other color
           11.  Evidence of physical abuse or harsh punishment
           12.  Unusual scars

         Nose
           13.  Continuous runny nose
           14.  Deformity of nose

         Chest
           15.  Wheezing sounds in chest

         Bones and muscles
           16.  Deformity of spine
           17.  Deformity of hands, arms
           18.  Deformity of legs, feet
           19.  Deformity of head

         Appearance
           20.  General neglected appearance
           21.  Appears too thin
           22.  Appears too fat
```

Fig. 12-5. Teacher's health observations. (From Ritter, A. M.: 1976. J. School Health **46**(4):235-237.)

B. Observations of child's body functions and symptoms

Check any of the following that the child complains of or demonstrates
more severely or more frequently than most classmates of same age:

Movements
23. Clumsiness
24. Limp or abnormal gait
25. Poor coordination
26. Poor writing or drawing
27. Convulsions, fits, or spells
28. Spells of inattention or staring into space

Speech
29. Unclear speech
30. Delayed speech
31. Stammering or stuttering

Vision
32. Poor vision

Hearing
33. Poor hearing

Nose
34. Frequent nose picking

Head
35. Headaches

Mouth
36. Drooling

Skin and head
37. Frequent scratching

Chest
38. Cough
39. Short of breath with exercises

Gastrointestinal
40. Poor eater
41. Recurrent stomachaches
42. Soils self with bowel movements

Urinary
43. Frequent urination
44. Wets pants

C. What is your general opinion of this child's health?

Check one of the following:

45. Perfect health
46. Specific problem(s) as noted, but generally healthy
47. Not in good health

Fig. 12-5, cont'd. Teacher's health observations.

Continued.

D. Observations of child's behavior

Check any of the following that the child demonstrates more severely or more frequently than most classmates of the same age:

48. Temper tantrums
49. Impulsive behavior
50. Explosive behavior
51. Hyperactivity or restlessness
52. Extremely quiet or withdrawn
53. Sleepy or lethargic
54. Tics or grimacing
55. Wanting too much attention
56. Contrary or stubborn
57. Selfish in sharing
58. Fighting with other children
59. Purposely destroys things
60. Masturbates
61. Nail biting
62. Thumb sucking
63. Frequent or prolonged absence from classroom
64. Cannot follow directions
65. Tasks incomplete
66. Uncooperative
67. Poor attention span
68. Poor verbal behavior
69. Lacks self-confidence
70. Child is not progressing in emotional development
71. Child is not progressing in intellectual development

E. What is your general opinion of this child's behavior?

Check one of the following:

72. Behavior is appropriate for age range
73. Behavior is relatively inappropriate for age range
74. Behavior is definitely limiting learning abilities

F. Observations of child's social adjustment

Check if you have noticed any problems in the following areas:

Home
75. Problem in child's relationships at home
76. Problem in parents' attitude to child
77. Poor parental attitude to child's problem
78. Evidence of neglect of the child
79. Evidence of physical abuse or severe punishment of the child

School
80. Problem in child's adjustment to school
81. Problem in child's attitude to school
82. The child's absenteeism is a problem
83. Performance is not at grade level or is a problem
84. The child is not developing satisfactorily in school

Further observations and explanations of items checked:

Fig. 12-5, cont'd. Teacher's health observations.

HEALTH HISTORY (14 to 21 years)

ALL INFORMATION ON THIS HISTORY FORM WILL BE KEPT CONFIDENTIAL

Name _____

Date _____

I. Past medical history

			No	Yes
Hospitalizations	1.	Have you ever been hospitalized?	____	____
Other illnesses	1.	Have you ever had mononucleosis, rheumatic fever, hepatitis, poliomyelitis, or other?	____	____
Allergies	1.	Do you have any allergies?	____	____
Accidents	1.	Have you ever had any serious accidents?	____	____
	2.	Have you ever been knocked unconscious?	____	____
Special health care	1.	Have you ever undergone any special test for health problems?	____	____
	2.	Have you ever been seen by a medical specialist?	____	____
	3.	Are you under the care of a specialist now?	____	____

II. Present medical history

			No	Yes
General	1.	Do you have a poor appetite?	____	____
	2.	Do you have an excessive appetite?	____	____
	3.	Do you have an excessive thirst?	____	____
	4.	Are you overweight?	____	____
	5.	Are you underweight?	____	____
	6.	Have you had a sudden weight loss or gain?	____	____
	7.	Do you have difficulty sleeping?	____	____
	8.	Do you have too much or too little energy?	____	____
	9.	Do you feel you are being abused by your parents, teachers, or peers?	____	____
Skin	1.	Do you have problems with rashes?	____	____
	2.	Do you have acne?	____	____
	3.	Do you have any unexplained lumps or spots?	____	____
	4.	Do you bruise easily?	____	____
Eyes	1.	Do you wear glasses or contact lenses?	____	____
Ear-nose-throat	1.	Have you had earaches or discharge in the past 6 months?	____	____
	2.	Do you have trouble hearing?	____	____
	3.	Do you have frequent nosebleeds?	____	____
	4.	Do you have trouble swallowing?	____	____

Fig. 12-6. Adolescent health history. (Modified from the Minnesota Department of Health form MCH/EPS 147; reprinted with permission from the Ramsey County Public Health Nursing Service and the Minnesota Department of Health.)

Continued.

			No	Yes
Respiratory	1.	Do you have any hoarseness?	____	____
	2.	Do you cough a lot?	____	____
	3.	Do you wheeze?	____	____
	4.	Do you have trouble breathing at times?	____	____
	5.	Do you smoke cigarettes?	____	____
	6.	Do you have frequent colds?	____	____
Cardiovascular	1.	Do you have chest pains?	____	____
	2.	Do you have high blood pressure?	____	____
	3.	Do you have coldness, numbness, or discoloration of hands or feet?	____	____
	4.	Do you have attacks when your heart beats very fast?	____	____
Gastrointestinal	1.	Do you have abdominal pains or discomfort?	____	____
	2.	Do you become nauseated?	____	____
	3.	Do you have indigestion?	____	____
	4.	Do you have diarrhea or constipation?	____	____
	5.	Do you ever have blood in your stool?	____	____
Urinary	1.	Do you have trouble urinating?	____	____
	2.	Do you have painful or burning urination?	____	____
	3.	Do you urinate more frequently than every 3 hours?	____	____
	4.	Do you have any blood in your urine?	____	____
	5.	Do you have bed-wetting problems?	____	____
Skeletal	1.	Do you have pains in your legs, arms, back, or joints?	____	____
	2.	Do you limp?	____	____
	3.	Have you had broken bones?	____	____
	4.	Do you have swollen joints?	____	____
Neuromuscular	1.	Do you have headaches?	____	____
	2.	Do you have any paralysis?	____	____
	3.	Do you have any numbness?	____	____
	4.	Are you clumsy?	____	____
	5.	Do you lose your balance?	____	____
	6.	Do you have dizziness?	____	____
	7.	Do you have unexplained movements or jerks?	____	____
	8.	Do you have seizures or convulsions?	____	____
	9.	Do you have staring spells?	____	____
	10.	Have you ever fainted?	____	____
	11.	Do you have unexplained "attacks" of any kind?	____	____

Fig. 12-6, cont'd. Adolescent health history.

			No	Yes
Sexual	1.	Do you have questions about menstruation, masturbation, venereal disease, wet dreams, discharges, petting, intercourse, homosexuality, birth control, sexual development, or pregnancy that you would like to discuss with someone? Please underline.	____	____
	2.	Would you like to know where to get help or learn about venereal disease, pregnancy, birth control, or information about sex?	____	____
	3.	Have you ever had intercourse?	____	____
	4.	Are you sexually active now?	____	____
	5.	Is intercourse painful?	____	____
	6.	Do you have concerns about your sexual activity?	____	____
Female	1.	When did you begin menstruating? Month_____ Year_____		
	2.	Do you have painful periods?	____	____
	3.	Do you have an irregular cycle?	____	____
	4.	How long does your period last?	____	____
	5.	Do you have excessive bleeding with your periods?	____	____
	6.	Do you have problems or questions about menstruation?	____	____
	7.	Do you have any unusual odor or discharge from your vagina?	____	____
Male	1.	Do you have any concerns about wet dreams?	____	____
	2.	Do you have a discharge from your penis?	____	____
	3.	Do you have any pain or lumps in your groin?	____	____
Medications and drugs	1.	Are you taking any prescribed medications?	____	____
	2.	Do you use nonprescription drugs other than aspirin, vitamins, or laxatives?	____	____
	3.	Do you drink or use drugs?	____	____
	4.	If yes, does drinking or using drugs		
		a. make you feel better with yourself or others?	____	____
		b. cause you to lose control, become aggressive, get drunk, or have a memory loss?	____	____
		c. make you feel badly afterwards?	____	____
		d. affect your reputation, your relationship with your family or friends?	____	____
		e. cause you to have problems with the law?	____	____
		f. decrease your ambition or drive, affect your personality?	____	____
	5.	Is anyone in your family having problems with alcohol or drugs?	____	____

Fig. 12-6, cont'd. Adolescent health history.

Continued.

III. Psychosocial (If attending school, answer the following:)

			No	Yes
School	1.	Have you ever been in special classes?	___	___
	2.	Do you have difficulty with schoolwork?	___	___
	3.	Do you dislike school?	___	___
	4.	Do you consider dropping out of school?	___	___
	5.	How many days have you missed school?	___	___
Peers	1.	Do you have trouble making friends?	___	___
	2.	Do you have trouble keeping friends?	___	___
	3.	Do you fight a lot with kids your age?	___	___
	4.	Do you prefer to be alone?	___	___
	5.	Are you without a close friend?	___	___
	6.	Do you spend most of your time with your family?	___	___
	7.	Are you afraid or uncomfortable with the opposite sex?	___	___
Mood	1.	Are you a tense person?	___	___
	2.	Do you worry a lot?	___	___
	3.	Are you often unhappy?	___	___
	4.	Do you become angry often?	___	___
	5.	Do you find it difficult to talk to someone about things that bother you?	___	___
	6.	Do you have a lot of mood swings?	___	___
Identity	1.	Do you feel self-conscious?	___	___
	2.	Are you fearful of being rejected or sensitive to what others think of you?	___	___
	3.	Are you upset with your physical appearance?	___	___
Life values	1.	Does it bother you that your values and standards of behavior may be different from your parents?	___	___
	2.	Do you and your parents fight a lot?	___	___
	3.	Do you have trouble standing up to your own values?	___	___
	4.	Do you feel anyone is abusing you, physically, emotionally, and/or sexually?	___	___

Fig. 12-6, cont'd. Adolescent health history.

ally symptomatic in nature and need to be clearly described to define the problem involved. Systematic interviewing is most appropriately applied in the problem-centered interview; however, aspects of the process can be used in any type of interview. Symptom inquiry is the systematic mechanism of problem delineation (Malasanos et al., 1977). While school nurses have learned to assist students with elaboration of concerns, they have not always been systematic in this process. By using the following seven variables of symptom inquiry, the school nurse can assist the student with clear and complete problem description and lay the foundation for problem identification:

body location The anatomical place where the symptom is located.

quality or characteristics What the symptom is like, its comparison or analogy to some other type of discomfort.

quantity Number, size, extent, and intensity of the symptom.

chronology The time sequence or pattern of the symptom. When did the symptom start and how long did it last?

setting or environmental factors The circumstances in which the symptom occurred.

aggravating and alleviating factors Actions taken by the client that make the symptom worse or better.

associated manifestations Those things which occur along with the symptom; pertinent negatives or those things usually expected with the complaint, but absent in this instance should be noted.

Table 12-1 shows two examples that clarify and delineate a student/client's concern with use of the seven variables of symptom inquiry.

The student's answers to inquiries within each variable will stimulate further questioning. This will clarify and more completely describe his complaint and lead the nurse to an assessment. The accuracy with which the concern is delineated depends on complete exploration of the ramifications of the seven areas during the data collection and systematic interview (Malasanos et al., 1977).

Table 12-1. Suggested questions to elicit symptom description

Variable	Example one: "My stomach hurts."	Example two: "I've got these funny spots."
Location	"Show me where it hurts."	"Point to where you see the spots."
Quality	"What is the pain like?"	"Are these spots like any you've had before?"
Quantity	"How badly does it hurt?" "How much does the hurt keep you from doing things?"	"How many spots do you have?" "Where else do you have these spots?"
Chronology	"When did you first notice the stomach-ache?" "How long have you had it?"	"When did you first notice the spots?" "How long have you had these spots?"
Setting	"Where were you when the stomachache started?" "What class are you coming from? . . . going to?"	"Are you eating any different foods than usual at your house?" "Does anyone else in your house or class have these spots?" "Are you taking any medicine?" "Is your mom washing clothes with a different soap?"
Aggravating and alleviating factors	"What seems to cause the pain?" "Does anything you do make it worse? . . . better?" "Have you taken anything for the hurt?" "Did it help?"	"Does anything you do make it worse? . . . better? "Have you put anything on it?" "Did that help?"
Associated manifestations	"Have you noticed any other hurt besides in the stomach?" "Are there any other changes?" "What is your bowel movement like today?"	"Have you noticed anything else, any other changes besides the spots?"

Review of systems (ROS)

The ROS portion of the health history is designed to elicit any additional information about the student's body systems that was not revealed previously in the history. A series of questions is asked that relate to symptoms commonly present in functional problems of each body system. The questions are asked about symptoms that may have been encountered in the immediate past or current illness. The ROS can be completed as a separate part of the health history, or, as some examiners prefer, it can be performed concurrently with the physical assessment as the practitioner examines each body region.

It is important that "pertinent negatives" are noted in the physical systems review. This means that where one might expect a symptom such as "fever" to occur and the client indicates "none," it should be so noted. For example, fever usually accompanies a complaint or concern of "earache." If this is denied by the student, a pertinent negative statement, such as "no fever" or "denies temperature elevation" should be recorded. Often negative information can be as significant as the positive when analyzing and identifying health problems.

The ROS inquiry is associated with the comprehensive health history and the history of the current acute complaint. It is considered the final check for eliciting significant data prior to the physical assessment. For further information on specific questions related to ROS, see the Suggested Readings on assessment listed at the end of the chapter.

PHYSICAL ASSESSMENT

As changes in the health care delivery system evolve and more emphasis is placed on preventive care, a variety of ambulatory child health care sites are developing. One of these developing health care delivery sites is the community school. As evidence of this trend, Colorado, New York, North Dakota, and Utah received a total of $4.8 million in grants to educate school nurses in the practitioner role and to improve delivery of health services in the schools.* It is logical that as the school nurse's role is expanded to that of school nurse practitioner, health maintenance of the school-age child will be delivered from the community school base. This means that comprehensive health assessments as well as those delineating acute com-

plaints are being performed more frequently, and school nurse practitioners are expanding their role in this direction (Nader et al., 1978). Therefore it is imperative that school nurses develop expertise in the use of physical assessment skills.

Physical examination is the second portion of the health assessment. After gathering a thorough health history, physical assessment involves examination of the student/client's body systems as well as special attention concentrated in those areas of concern revealed by the history. For example, if the student voices a current concern of "dizziness," the school nurse should increase her efforts in the neurological portion of the examination.

Tools of assessment

Four major modalities of examination are used as tools in assessing the client's physical health status: inspection, palpation, percussion, and auscultation. Each basic technique of examination is applied equally with varying emphasis on the different regions of the body, depending on the client's age and the significance it has for revealing abnormalities within a particular system. For example, inspection is the most important examining technique in assessing the skin of an infant, whereas palpation is of greatest use when examining the abdomen in all age groups. Percussion, inspection, and auscultation are equally important techniques for examining the chest of adults, and auscultation is of greatest significance when assessing the cardiac status in all age groups. Effective use of these examination methods is based on practice and validation by clinical preceptors of the nurse's accuracy.

Inspection

Inspection means the observation or thorough visualization of each part of the body. It also includes listening for unusual audible sounds and paying particular attention to odors that may be emanating from the student. Inspection can be enhanced by the use of instruments, such as the otoscope and ophthalmoscope, for greater visualization of structures.

Palpation

The technique of palpation requires training the fingers to be sensitive to specific sensations, since it involves feeling and touching. The most sensitive parts of the hand are used for discriminating different sensations. For example, the

---

*News release from the Robert Wood Johnson Foundation: 1978. Princeton, N.J., Aug. 2.

pads of the fingers are used to augment the examination of maculopapular rashes that are revealed through inspection. Gross skin temperature can be assessed with the dorsum of the hand. Vibration is best determined by using the palmar surfaces of the hands, while position and consistency of a structure is examined by using one's grasping fingers. Tenderness of the abdomen, tremors in the extremities, moisture and texture of structures such as the hair, as well as masses and abnormal accumulations of fluid are assessed through the use of touch. Individual structures can be assessed as to position, shape, size, and consistency by using the hands and fingers (Malasanos et al., 1977).

Percussion

Percussion involves a cause-and-effect relationship of tapping the fingers over a surface, such as the chest or abdomen, and listening for the resulting sound. The sound produced is classified as to its intensity or loudness, pitch or frequency, and quality. This enables the examiner to detect whether the tissue beneath the skin is filled with air, such as the lungs, or is solid, like the heart.

Auscultation

Auscultation is the process of listening, which is direct or immediate when done with the unaided ear. Mediate auscultation is accomplished with the aid of a sound augmentation device such as a stethoscope. Auscultation as an examining modality is most useful in assessing lung or breath and heart sounds in the chest (Malasanos et al., 1977).

• • •

Experience and practice will promote skillful use of these modalities of examination. Because we see only what we know, concentration and meticulous attention to detail are critical to effective physical assessment. Repetition in the use of these skills is essential for defining both normal and abnormal structures. Thus developing skills in the major modalities of physical examination is essential for the expansion of the school nurse's role in health assessment.

General assessment

The general survey or assessment is the formation of an impression by the school nurse after briefly observing the total child/student. This general inspection of the whole child reveals an overall status of health, any outstanding characteristics, and sets the stage for details the nurse pursues in the physical assessment. Generally, observations are made as to age, sex, race, body symmetry, posture, nutrition, development, emotional status, skin condition, and apparent signs of stress and distress (Malasanos et al., 1977).

An example of the record of the general survey of a child attending the preschool comprehensive screening clinic might read:

Cooperative, inquisitive, 5-year-old black male, somewhat overweight, with slight limp favoring the right side, is well hydrated and in no acute distress.

This observation cues the practitioner to the child's readiness for school by virtue of his cooperative and curious nature as opposed to being clinging and shy.

The practitioner will also thoroughly inquire regarding the child's nutritional habits, eating patterns, and relationships with family members during either the history taking or exit interview. She will pay particular attention to the abdomen, gastrointestinal system and habits of elimination, and the extremities and neurological system when performing the physical assessment.

Clinical measurements, such as height, weight, blood pressure, temperature, pulse, and respiration are usually considered routine. They are extremely important measurements for assessing body functions and developing disease states. Of particular interest to the school nurse are the results of screening tests such as for vision and hearing. The screening results plus laboratory tests such as urinalysis and hemoglobin levels are included here as usual routine measurements because they are a part of regular health maintenance of the school-age child and directly affect the child's ability to function in normal school routines. These measurements are performed in any physical assessment, whether completed by the nurse or an assistant. The nurse is responsible for determining whether the results fall outside normal parameters and require subsequent health counseling and/or referral.

A similar survey is also made when the school nurse observes students as a group. Each child is a member of a classroom group and is therefore viewed both as an individual and a group member. Meaningful psychosocial, behavioral, and sociodynamic data is collected when the nurse communicates with teachers about the health status of her class members. It

Table 12-2. A systematic method for order of performing the assessment versus its order of recording

Order of performance	Order of recording
General observations and vital signs	Vital signs
Head, including cranial nerves	General observations
Neck	Head, eyes, ears, nose, and
Posterior thorax	throat (HEENT)
Anterior thorax and lung examination	Neck
Breasts and axillary areas	Lymphatic system
Heart	Breasts
Abdomen	Thorax and lungs
Extremities, including basic neurological system	Heart
Male external genitalia	Abdomen and external genitalia
Rectal examination	Back
Pelvic examination	Rectal area
Fundus (if eyedrops are required)	Extremities
	Neurological system
	Skin
	Pelvic examination

is also helpful to observe children in their usual classroom milieu or routine to validate this information. Sometimes the group takes on specific character traits, such as being "excessively verbal" or "hostile in response." This has implications for the nurse in her own interactions with individual children from that classroom as well as in her work with that faculty person.

Systems assessment

As with systematic interviewing, physical assessment of the body systems demands an organized, detailed approach. Generally, the examination proceeds cephalocaudal (head to toe) unless the client is sufficiently upset to disallow this sequence of progression. In these instances, the examiner must vary her approach, assisting the client to feel at ease and lessening his anxiety by being assertive and providing comfort measures. Those areas of examination which demand explicit cooperation from the client, such as auscultation of the heart and palpation of the abdomen, may need to be performed at times when the client is quiet, even though they may be out of sequence.

Furthermore, the assessment proceeds from general to specific. A general survey of each region precedes the detailed examination within each region of the body. For example, the arms and hands are inspected before zeroing in on the child's nails and nailbeds.

Performance of the physical assessment will differ from the way in which it is recorded, since the examination is performed by regions. It is then recorded by organ systems (Murphy and Brown, 1977.) Table 12-2 is a brief outline suggesting a systematic method for the order of performing the assessment versus its order of recording. For a detailed explanation of what the nurse looks for in the physical assessment of each body region, see the Suggested Readings at the end of the chapter.

Physical assessment with acute complaints

Clients appear at the school health service each day with numerous acute complaints or concerns, ranging from minor to significant health concerns. Regardless of the seriousness of the complaint, it is of considerable importance to the student. With increasing skill in physical assessment, school nurses and school nurse specialists/practitioners are able to deal with the concern quite effectively.

After the seven variables of symptom inquiry are used to delineate and clarify the concern, physical assessment is performed. Consideration is given to the nature of the complaint and symptoms. Those structures in the systems located both immediately above and below the location of the symptoms are examined. For example, when the student complains of his "ear hurting," the practitioner will examine the eyes, ears, nose, pharynx, neck, heart, and lungs. In doing so she will use the four modalities of examination employing such aids to assessment as the otoscope, ophthalmoscope, and stethoscope as necessary. In this manner, she is able to clearly identify the nature of the concern and employ problem-solving techniques to appropriately resolve it.

COMPLETE HEALTH ASSESSMENT AT PERIODIC INTERVALS

To achieve the goals of health promotion, high-level wellness, and prevention of disease, complete health assessment, including both the health history and physical assessment, is necessary at periodic intervals. Changes occur along with peak times for onset of disease as children grow and develop. This necessitates entry into the health care system in which maintenance and promotion of healthful living can benefit children. Complete health assessment for the school-age child has a wellness focus and occurs at specific predetermined intervals.

Focus on wellness

Wellness is basic to learning. Although Chinn's (1973) study documented a relationship between health or some degree of illness and classroom problems, the specific relationship is unclear. Nonetheless, nursing has been beneficial in helping schoolchildren achieve educational goals. The current emphasis on health assessment is gaining acceptance as a mechanism for identifying and resolving health problems that interfere with learning.

The complete health assessment that occurs at periodic intervals throughout a student's school career has a wellness focus. This is imperative, since a student must be in as high a state of wellness as possible to avail himself of the learning situation. High-level wellness has been defined by Dunn (1977:9) as ''. . . an integrated method of functioning which is oriented toward maximizing the potential of which the individual is capable, within the environment where he is functioning.'' This definition has specific implications for complete health assessment of the school-age child. It implies that high-level wellness is directional, indicating the child's functioning is forward and upward. Second, it encompasses the total child, his physical, emotional, cognitive, and social development and functioning. Since the child cannot be subdivided, the wellness concept as it relates to health assessment allows the whole child as a personality in his own uniqueness to be observed. Third, the definition implies a changing environment that demands

adaptation on the part of the child as he grows.

By using a wellness focus in the health assessment of children and youth during their school years, the school nurse can assist them in reaching their highest potential of functioning and adapting positively within their family, school, and community milieus.

Health assessment intervals

In the school-age child, health assessment usually occurs at preschool (age 3 or 4), kindergarten (age 5), grade four (age 9), grade seven (age 12), and grade ten (age 15). Using these intervals for complete health assessment allows the school nurse to maximize anticipatory guidance opportunities, emphasize prevention of disease, and effectively manage developmental crises.

In addition to the comprehensive health history and physical assessment, the complete health assessment also includes detailed information about the student/client's development, psychosocial status, dental health, nutrition, and specific habits. These components are updated from the initial health history data base at the interval health assessment. There are many opportunities for health teaching and counseling. The health information discussed is based on the individual needs determined in the assessment visit.

The purpose of health assessment of the preschool child is to gather a thorough initial data base. Preschool clinics offer an excellent opportunity for assessing development and readiness for learning. Speech and language are other important assessments that should be done at this time. Early identification of developing language lags during the preschool clinic increases the potential for alleviation. Subsequent problems of peer relationships due to speech difficulties can also be avoided. During the preschool years nutritional patterns and habits are forming. These clinics can be organized to collect thorough diet histories, followed by nutritional counseling and dental hygiene teaching. The preschool clinic is a very important time for providing parents with concrete information that will help them further prepare their child for school entry.

The first interval health assessment is completed on entering kindergarten. Essential developmental and other information that may have been missing from the preschool assessment is added to the data base. Stresses a child encounters in developing new relationships on entry into school can be identified. Data collected about the entering kindergarten class is the basis for preliminary educational planning to meet the needs of individual kindergartners and the class as a whole.

Health assessment of fourth graders reveals considerable growth in stature, development, and social relationships. Physical growth takes on new dimensions with the child's increase in height and weight. It is significant at this assessment to determine the degree to which the child is integrating the psychosocial tasks of "industry versus inferiority" (Erikson, 1963). By fourth grade the child's permanent dentition is nearing completion. Also, dental caries are documented to be the number one health problem of the school-age child (Nader, 1974). Thus the child should be considered a partner in his own dental health practices. Teaching correct toothbrushing techniques and dental health habits is one mechanism for beginning to emphasize the student's responsibility for his own body and health status. Since children of this age will soon experience prepubertal changes, another important aspect of this assessment is the anticipatory guidance discussions with the child and his parents about the onset of puberty and the accompanying physical and psychosocial changes.

Health assessments of seventh- and tenth-grade students can be organized so that the students themselves take the major role and responsibility. With seventh-grade students, the health assessment focuses on assisting the student with preparation for an increase in activity level, adjustments to new routines found in secondary school, physical and emotional changes, and developing heterosexual relationships.

The tenth-grade assessment emphasizes students' responsibility for themselves with preparation for entry into the wider health care system. Participation through provision of health history information and contracting as a part of the decision making regarding health problems is the beginning of this preparation. Highlighted during assessment at adolescence is the students' use of tobacco, alcohol, and other drugs. During this interval health assessment, high priority is placed on assisting adolescents with health problems, roles and interpersonal relationships with family and friends, and the psychosocial tasks of "identity versus role confusion" (Erikson, 1963).

Performing health assessments with children and youth at these intervals assists the nurse in systematically providing necessary health services through effective problem identification and individual student needs assessment.

PROBLEM-ORIENTED HEALTH RECORD (POHR)

The value of the cumulative school health record lies in the information it contains and the manner in which it is used. A record that is mandated by law to be kept, but which has little concrete data, is useless to the health professionals in the school setting. The impact of problem-oriented recording on nursing practice, delivery of health care, and revolutionizing of record keeping in all aspects of the health care industry is well documented (Yarnell and Atwood, 1974). In keeping with the trend in other health delivery sectors, school health is beginning to implement a problem-oriented approach to improve health care. More and more school districts are revising their record system in favor of the POHR. Following are several criteria that a good school health record system should meet (Boone, 1974):

1. Cumulative—easily depicts essential health history, screening, and assessment data through the years.
2. Accurate—contains data useful in promoting the student's health.
3. Accessible—data easily retrieved.
4. Uniform format—record easily portrays essential health information about the student, yet a uniform record is used for all.
5. Confidentiality—mechanism for protecting the information contained within the record.

The 1974 Family Education Rights and Privacy Act is an added impetus for implementing the POHR. Since this legislation gives parents or guardians the right to view their child's school records and prevents disclosure of information without written permission to anyone outside the school system, school health personnel are concerned about developing a record system that organizes health information for objectivity, clarity, uniformity, and factual accuracy (Oda and Quick, 1977).

Rationale for application of the POHR to the school setting

The POHR can and should be adapted to the school setting. There is no single approach to the POHR, so it must be individualized to fit specific situations. Yet the components and mechanism of use remain the same, making this approach valuable as an aid for greater understanding in interdisciplinary and interinstitutional use.

The POHR approach emphasizes the client and his problems. Care of the whole student/client is facilitated through concise, yet thorough assessment, problem identification, and plans. It becomes an interdisciplinary record focusing on the client's needs, as opposed to the traditional "source-oriented" record, in which the health care professional entered comments in the appropriate section of the chart. The POHR implemented in the school setting should focus on the student's ongoing health status during the years he is in school and should be shared by the members of the educational health team.

The new accessibility law presents school districts with a dilemma in record keeping, since up to the present some comments contained in school health records might be considered libelous. The POHR approach, in part, is an answer to this dilemma because an entry must be analyzed and justified. All conclusions reached in the assessment statement are based on recorded supporting data. The format of recording forces the recorder to enter only information that is pertinent to the identified problem and prevents the record from being cluttered with irrelevant information.

Implementation of the POHR in the school setting can take several forms. If the school system is quite small, all health records for students in grades kindergarten to twelve can be changed simultaneously with transfer of information to the new format. In a large school district, this approach might prove to be an overwhelming task. When large numbers of records must be changed, health service personnel can change to the new system with a phased-in approach, using the new record with entering kindergartners, new students to the district, and groups of students or classes that are scheduled for interval health assessments. The POHR (Fig. 12-7) is being implemented by the Minneapolis Public Schools, using a phased-in approach. This record is 8½ × 11 inches and designed as a folder, which provides a place to file reports, correspondence, flow sheets, and other notes pertinent to the student's health status. As a folder it serves as a section containing health data, which then is easily filed in the student's educational cumulative file.

In summary, while the POHR approach has many advantages, its implementation and use are often confounded by resistance. The POHR concept is a logical means of organizing client health care that results in effective problem solving. Using this approach challenges traditional ways of functioning. The POHR is interdisciplinary, increasing communication and cooperation among health care providers. It is more than a record-keeping system, since its use affects the practice of all health care professionals. It increases the responsibility and accountability of the recorder. It is a mechanism for all nurses to expand their roles. For school nurses, the POHR is an opportunity to include the educational health team in the care of the school-age child and to increase the effectiveness of the nurse's link with other health care providers.

Components of the POHR

There are three structural components of the POHR: the data base, the problem list, and the narrative notes (Woolley et al., 1974). Each of these major structural areas contains subsets that will be briefly explained.

First, the *subjective data base* includes student identification information and all health history data. The *objective data base* comprises the physical assessment, measurements, laboratory findings, general survey, and screening results. Physical assessment results, measurements, laboratory findings, and general survey should be included in the POHR folder as inserts. Cumulative screening results are easily recorded in a sequential order from year to year as they are performed (Fig. 12-7).

The growth chart is an important device for monitoring height and weight parameters over time. It is essential that these measurements be graphed for adequate interpretation of the child's physical growth status. A place is provided for this, since male and female growth grids have been printed directly on the back side of the POHR folder (Fig. 12-7), making growth data by percentile readily accessible.

Student identification information can easily be placed by means of a computer sticker onto the record when it is opened. Significant immunization, developmental, and past medical history data are permanently transferred to the outer portion of the POHR. The remaining comprehensive health history information is maintained within the folder as a part of the initial data as it is acquired on entering students.

The second structural component of the POHR is the problem list. The mechanism for

Text continued on p. 276.

PUPIL HEALTH RECORD

PROBLEM LIST

		DATE ONSET	DATE RESOLVED
HEALTH MAINT. YEAR:			
1	HEALTH EXAM. (date)		
	IMMUNIZATIONS		
	DENTAL COMPL. (date)		
	HEALTH CLASSIF.		
2			
3			
4			
5			
6			
7			
8			
9			
10			

IMMUNIZATION HISTORY

IMMUNIZATION	ORIGINAL SERIES COMPLETED	BOOSTER DATES
DIPHTHERIA		
TETANUS		
PERTUSSIS (Whooping Cough)		
POLIO (Oral)		
MUMPS		
RUBELLA (German Measles)		
RUBEOLA (Red Measles)		

TUBERCULIN TEST	DISEASE OR VACCINE		
	DATE		
	TYPE		
	RESULT		

DEVELOPMENTAL HISTORY

	AGE
Sit Alone	
Walk Alone	
Talk Words	
Talk Sentences	
Bladder Train	
Bowel Train	

PAST HISTORY

CHECK (✓) if child has had —

Strep Throat	
Scarlet fever	
Rheumatic fever	
Chickenpox	
Red Measles	
German Measles	
Epilepsy	
Mumps	
Asthma	
Heart Disease	
Diabetes	
Serious Accident (Specify)	
Surgery (Specify)	
Allergies (Specify)	
Other (Specify)	

Fig. 12-7. Pupil health record. (Reprinted with permission of the Minneapolis Public Schools.)

SCHOOL HEALTH SCREENING AND FOLLOW-UP RECORD

GRADE	YEAR	VISION										HEARING			DENTAL	SCOLIOSIS			OTHER
		ACUITY		M/B*		+LENS*		COLOR		COMMENTS	R	L	COMMENTS		P	R	COMMENTS	
		R	L	P	R	P	R	P	R										

* M/B — MUSCLE BALANCE (e.g., Worth 4-Dot test)

+ LENS — PLUS LENS TEST FOR HYPEROPIA

25-6210 (12E) Graphic Services — Print Shop 1979 8 7

MINNEAPOLIS PUBLIC SCHOOLS

Student No. _____   Sex _____   Birthdate _____

Name (last, first, middle) _____

Parents Name _____

Address _____   Phone _____

Continued.

Fig. 12-7, cont'd. Pupil health record.

NARRATIVE NOTES

DATE	PROBLEM NUMBER AND TITLE	FINDINGS (Subjective & Objective)	ASSESSMENT & PLAN	SIGN EACH ENTRY

Fig. 12-7, cont'd. Pupil health record.

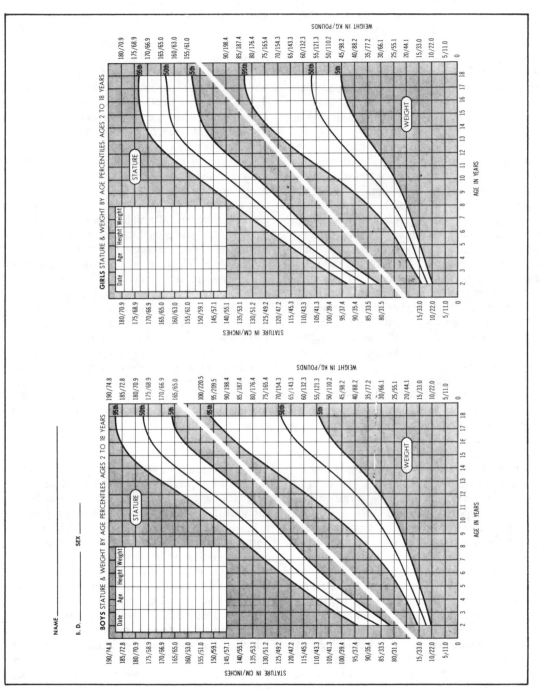

Fig. 12-7, cont'd. Pupil health record.

developing the problem list is analysis of the subjective and objective data. Through the nursing process, problems are identified and sequentially placed in the problem list. Thus the problem list becomes the index to the POHR, where the nature and interrelatedness of a student's problems can be quickly observed (such as No. 2, "language lag," and No. 3, "recurrent or chronic ear infections"). The problem list is continuously updated. Changes and dates of such occurrences should be entered as problems are clarified and modified and diagnoses are confirmed and/or resolved.

An active problem can be defined as a concern, need, or "some aspect of the client which requires further attention for observation, diagnosis, management or education" (Yarnell and Atwood, 1974:219). The problems may be expressed as symptoms, physical findings, abnormal laboratory findings, emotional or psychosocial maladaptations, medical diagnoses, or nursing assessments. The problem should be stated at the highest perceived level of refinement. For example, an adolescent who is exhibiting signs of depression should have the problem identified as "manifestations of depression," rather than the individual symptoms of loss of appetite, crying without control, and sleep disturbances.

Temporary problems are generally considered to be acute and self-limited episodes that are not significant to the student's present or future health status. Examples of temporary problems might be "minor cuts" or "poison ivy." If, in the judgment of the school nurse or her designated assistant, the problem is considered to be acute and self-limiting, it should be so noted at the beginning of the narrative note entry as a temporary problem (TP).

All problems require a plan, since problems represent student health needs. Following are three basic components to the plan:

1. Reference to additional data and diagnostic information that must be collected before validated conclusions can be drawn.
2. Specific interventions, including present and planned future interventions such as symptomatic treatments, counseling, advice given, consultation, and referral.
3. Client health education provided or planned.

The plan is recorded by problem and sequentially after each encounter with the student. Plans are written thoroughly, yet concisely, in the narrative notes using the subjective, objective, assessment, and plan (SOAP) format.

The last structural component of the POHR is the narrative notes, which contain ongoing, chronological, and sequential written commentary about referenced problems, flow sheets, and the discharge summary. With the exception of brief telephone calls, which are simply entered as they occur, narrative notes are written using the SOAP format.

The SOAP method is helpful in organizing information for purposes of charting the student's progress objectively and accurately. *Subjective data* is historical information and refers to the student's reactions or feelings about the problem. *Objective data* includes the physical assessment, relevant laboratory and diagnostic findings, and astute observations made by the health professional. *Assessment* is a statement that explains the significance of the subjective and objective data after it has been analyzed and synthesized. The *plan* includes written specific courses of action that are being taken to resolve the problem. The plan is based on the information contained in the data base from which the problem is defined (Berni and Readey, 1978).

Flow sheets are used whenever recurrent observations are required or when nursing care activities need to be recorded repetitively. Some examples of situations in the school setting to be recorded on flow sheets might be the newly diagnosed diabetic's daily urine testing, the hyperkinetic child's medication routine, the hypertensive faculty member's weekly blood pressure readings, and the obese adolescent's biweekly weigh-in. The chronic disease flow sheet is an excellent mechanism for coordinating and tracking the various therapies, consultations, and referrals that are a part of ongoing care for a child with a chronic condition (Schmitt, 1973). The flow sheets are a rapid and efficient means of gathering data and become a permanent part of the record as an insert into the folder (Woolley et al., 1974).

The final portion of the narrative notes is the discharge summary. This is written at the time of graduation from high school or when the record is transferred to another school district. The summary statement reflects the degree to which goals have been met in the resolution of the student's health problems. The discharge summary is significant because it describes the student's health status for the next health professional.

A tool for communication

Communication itself is an age-old problem. Strategies for alleviating or at least reducing communication problems encountered in delivering health care deserve consideration. The POHR is a mechanism to improve communication with the student/client, members of the educational team, and other health care providers.

The POHR is a valuable tool for objective and forthright sharing of information with the student/client, since the school nurse contracts with him about his health concerns. The problem list and mutually developed plans can be reviewed together with the student. Using the record in this manner can increase the trust level between the nurse and students because the written communication is completely open, well documented, and easily understood. Review of the record also helps the student take responsibility for and participate actively in his health care as he is developmentally able.

Effective implementation and use of the POHR improves communication among educational team members. Teachers, school counselors, educational specialists, psychologists, social workers and administrators are also members of the educational team that the school nurse must reach on behalf of students. As a part of the student's cumulative record, information contained in the POHR is readily accessible to all professionals in the school setting. Although there may be problems getting a POHR system started, as these difficulties are overcome, the systematic POHR can become the vehicle for communication and student advocacy within the school district. Thus written communication is becoming more and more important as the school nurse interacts with an increasing number of persons.

The POHR should also be used as a basis for teacher-nurse conferences. Since the conference setting is a means of establishing rapport between health and teaching personnel, the POHR should serve as a vehicle for exchange of health information about students. Eisner and Oglesby (1972:349) suggest that the primary purpose of the teacher-nurse conference is "to bring the teacher's health observations about each child to someone who can initiate further action." These conferences provide a systematic mechanism for input regarding student health, and the observations become a part of the POHR.

As educational team members use the POHR, both verbal and written communication are stimulated. In the end, communication and service are of greater benefit to the student, and

duplication of effort among personnel is decreased.

Another way in which the POHR can be used as a tool for communication is in the referral process. Professional communication is becoming increasingly important in the school nurse's roles as student advocate and liaison between the educational facility and other health care providers. School nurses have valuable input in contributing to the total health care of the child. Referrals are more clear when the SOAP format is used and goals with expected outcomes are stated. Written referrals and information interchanges are major mechanisms through which collaboration with physicians and other institutions is achieved.

According to Atwood et al. (1974:232), communication benefits occur between nurses and physicians:

. . . Physicians become better acquainted with what nurses can and should do. In so doing they become more involved in teaching and assisting nurses to practice more effectively. Nurses also have more opportunity to understand physicians' practice styles and to share some of their specialized knowledge with physicians.

If professionals in the educational setting use a recording method similar to that of increasing numbers of health care providers and agencies, interagency communication will improve and health care services to children will be enhanced.

A tool for planning nursing care

The nursing process is a problem-solving approach to delivering nursing care. The problem-oriented record concept, like the nursing process, involves deliberative thinking and becomes a mechanism of thought. Thus the problem-oriented method of recording complements nursing practice and facilitates its documentation.

Because the record is interdisciplinary, development of care plans becomes a collaborative action. With use of this systematic communication among health professionals, each learns from the other (Niland and Bentz, 1974). For example, a psychologist might use the SOAP format to record her interactions with an adolescent exhibiting concerns consistent with depression, including results of the Minnesota Multiphasic Personality Inventory. This information alerts the school nurse to specific psychological data and preliminary plans the psychologist has developed. The school nurse adds her observations of fatigue, lassitude, and anorexia. Together they can develop and support each other's plans of intervention from each discipline's unique vantage point. Subsequent observations are according to collaboratively developed plans. The teacher-nurse conference and educational team conference are verbal mechanisms for multidisciplinary input into the student's health care plan.

Systematic thinking promotes systematic planning and acting. Since the nursing process involves the cycle of data collection, assessment, planning intervention, and evaluation of interventions, updating the record is facilitated by using the problem-solving approach of POHR. Updating the record provides an opportunity to review and modify nursing care plans based on outcomes of previous interventions. An example might be that of a ninth-grade student returning to school after a 10-day absence and a diagnosis of mononucleosis, with a note from her physician indicating that she may have activity as tolerated. A problem-oriented update note after the student's readmission might read as follows:

No. 2 Mononucleosis: diagnosed 1/10/79 by Dr. Jones.
January 20, 1979. Informant: Jane.
S Attended school half days for the past week as arranged; feels "very tired"; expressed feeling "more tired Monday and Tuesday than later in the week"; on arrival home in afternoon needs to nap for 2 to 3 hours; some throat soreness on swallowing; appetite continues to be decreased; homework "piling up."
O Temperature: 99° F, P = 64, R = 18
Blood pressure: 110/72
Weight: 100 pounds
General characteristics: Pale and drawn face; alert, but sluggish in verbal response.

Physical examination

Head, eyes, ears, nose, and throat (HEENT): Normocephalic; pupils equal, round, react to light (PERRL), red reflex, conjugate gaze; TMs translucent, landmarks present, and sharp cone of light bilaterally; no nasal discharge; R pharyngeal erythema with no secretions.
Neck: R occipital node slightly enlarged, 1 cm; no tenderness.
Chest: Heart, S_1 S_2, rate regular, no murmur. Lungs, clear anteriorly and posteriorly to auscultation.
Abdomen: Normal bowel sound, liver and spleen not palpable.
A Slowly recuperating from mononucleosis, with throat irritation, poor appetite, and 5-pound weight loss from predisease level; concerned about amount of makeup work, especially in view of low energy and high fatigue level.
P 1. Maintain attendance at half days, monitor activity tolerance midweek.
2. Arrange fruit juice break and ½-hour rest midmorning.
3. Repeat throat culture.
4. Contact teachers regarding extension of time limits for assignments and possible revision of expectations based on previous performance.
5. Discuss with Jane reasonable physical limitations that must continue during this phase of convalescence, rest regimen, and diet. Encourage diet of high carbohydrate and protein foods.
6. Telephone call to mother, Mrs. Johnson, regarding progress and change in routine.
7. Send progress information interchange to Dr. Jones.

This example integrates the nursing process with the SOAP format of recording, employs expanded role assessment skills, and applies the problem-oriented record system to the educational setting.

A tool for client education

The basis for assumption of responsibility for one's own health is knowledge. The POHR becomes a practical teaching tool for imparting this health knowledge. As young people grow and mature they are able to take on increasing responsibility for their own health care. In the educational setting this can only happen if the school nurse has the expectation and confidence that, depending on their age and developmental status, students can be responsible and should be included in the decision making regarding their own health.

In using the POHR as a tool for client education, it is important to involve the student in the recording process. For example, after teaching the diabetic student to test his own urine, the school nurse could show him the diabetic flow sheet and explain how to record the urine test results, interpret their meaning, and discuss his role in maintaining the flow sheet as a part of his permanent POHR. In so doing, she is actively teaching about diabetes as it relates to him as an individual and is helping him take responsibility for accurate testing, interpretation, and recording of results. In this case she is also teaching the student the basis for communication with his physician and subsequent decision making regarding management of his disease.

A tool for accountability, responsibility, and audit

Nurses are becoming more áccountable to the health care consumer and responsible for the quality of nursing care they deliver. Among the reasons for this increased accountability are the change in nurse practice acts and the greater autonomy occurring in our country today. Along with increasing accountability, the nurse is also liable and needs to clearly document the care provided in order to be protected from unfair legal entanglements. Nurse practice acts apply to all settings in which nurses find employment. Thus the school nurse must also provide a means for documenting the care she is providing and be accountable and responsible for its quality (Berni and Readey, 1978).

As previously mentioned, the nursing process and the POHR concept are both problem-solving approaches and are therefore complementary. Using the POHR approach is a mechanism for written documentation of the nursing care given. Thus the POHR in the educational setting is the vehicle through which client care audit and documented evidence of nursing accountability is conducted.

The specific auditing method varies from one institution to another. In school health, record audit is in the beginning stages. Generally, record audit should have the following characteristics:

1. *Thoroughness.* An analysis of the health care professional's ability to complete the assigned tasks. Is the collected data complete?
2. *Reliability.* An analysis of the health care professional's ability to correctly, repeatedly, and routinely complete tasks. Is the collected data correct and complete on all clients seen?
3. *Analytic sense.* Does the record reflect disciplined and logical thinking? Are problems identified at the highest level of refinement and based on the health care professional's perception and understanding? Is opinion avoided?
4. *Efficiency.* Were appropriate steps taken quickly to resolve problems?

These elements make up the basis of an effective record audit (Neelon and Ellis, 1974). The documented record is then compared against a preexisting standard of what should be contained in the record, using these elements of analysis. The procedure should be considered a learning experience, an opportunity to grow as new ideas for effective nursing care are generated.

SUMMARY

Systematic assessment of the school-age child as a part of school nursing practice in the educational setting is in its infancy. As the practitioner movement evolves and the school nurse's role expands, use of systematic assessment as an integral part of health maintenance and promotion will increase. Using the systematic interviewing process is a means for developing an effective data base both in comprehensive health assessment and acute complaint situations. Physical assessment is a systematic way of looking at children and youth. Combining the health history with physical assessment produces the complete health assessment for the purpose of identifying and resolving health problems of schoolchildren.

The POHR is an effective way to document nursing care. It can be used as a tool for communication, client health education, and for the health care professional's accountability and responsibility of providing quality care. Adapting the problem-oriented concept to the school health record provides advantages and client outcomes well worth the efforts involved.

REFERENCES

Atwood, J., Mitchell, P. H., and Yarnall, S.: 1974. The POR: a system for communication, Nurs. Clin. North Am. **9**(2):229-234.

Beitz, D.: 1976. Health appraisal in secondary schools, J. School Health **46**(6):322-324.

Berni, R., and Readey, H.: 1978. Problem-oriented medical record implementation: allied health peer review, 2nd ed., The C. V. Mosby Co., St. Louis.

Boone, S. F.: 1974. A new approach to school health records, J. School Health **44**(3):156-158.

Brown, M. A., and Murphy, M. A.: 1975. Ambulatory pediatrics for nurses, McGraw-Hill, Inc., New York.

Chinn, P.: 1973. A relationship between health and school problems: a nursing assessment, J. School Health **43**(2):85-91.

Dunn, H. L.: 1977. What high-level wellness means, Health Values: Achieving High-Level Wellness, **1**(1):9-16.

Eisner, V., and Oglesby, A.: 1972. Health assessment of children. VIII, The unexpected health defect, J. School Health **42**(6):348-350.

Erikson, E. H.: 1963. Childhood and society, W. W. Norton & Co., Inc., New York.

Hogue, C. C.: 1977. Epidemiology for distributive nursing practice. In Hall, J. E., and Weaver, B. R.: Distributive nursing practice: a systems approach to community health, J. B. Lippincott Co., Philadelphia.

Lynch, A.: 1975. Use of health history and problem-oriented medical record to upgrade school health care and staff roles, Pennsylvania Department of Health, Harrisburg, Pa. (Unpublished manuscript.)

Malasanos, L., Barkauskas, V., Moss, M., and Stoltenberg-Allen, K.: 1977. Health assessment, The C. V. Mosby Co., St. Louis.

Minnesota Department of Health: 1976. EPSDT 1976 Minnesota guidelines, MCH-V-H, Oct., Minneapolis.

Murphy, M. A., and Brown, M. S.: 1977. Health maintenance for children. In Reinhardt, A. M., and Quinn, M. D., editors: Current practice in family-centered community nursing, vol. 1, St. Louis, The C. V. Mosby Co., pp. 191-211.

Nader, P. R.: 1974. The school health service: making primary care effective, Pediatr. Clin. North Am. **21**(1):57-73.

Nader, P. R., Conrad, J., Williamson, M., McKevitt, R., and Berrey, R.: 1978. The high school nurse practitioner, J. School Health **48**(1):649-653.

Neelon, F. A., and Ellis, G. J.: 1974. A syllabus of problem-oriented patient care, Little, Brown & Co., Boston.

Niland, M. B., and Bentz, P. M.: 1974. A problem-oriented approach to planning nursing care, Nurs. Clin. North Am. **9**(2):235-245.

Oda, D. S., and Quick, M. J.: 1977. School health records and the new accessibility law, J. School Health **47**(4):212-216.

Ritter, A. M.: 1976. Using a teacher's health observation form to evaluate school child health, J. School Health **46**(4):235-237.

Schmitt, B.: 1973. The chronic disease flow sheet in ambulatory pediatrics, Pediatrics **51**(4):722-730.

Sills, G. M., and Hall, J. E.: 1977. A general systems perspective for nursing. In Hall, J. E., and Weaver, B. R.: Distributive nursing practice: a systems approach to community nursing, J. B. Lippincott Co., Philadelphia.

Woolley, F. R., Warnick, M. W., Kane, R. L., and Dyer, E. D.: 1974. Problem-oriented nursing, Springer Publishing Co., Inc., New York.

Yarnell, S. R., and Atwood, J.: 1974. Problem-oriented practice for nurses and physicians, Nurs. Clin. North Am. **9**(2):215-228.

FORMAL SCHOOL NURSE PRACTITIONER PROGRAMS

University of California, Los Angeles (UCLA)
UCLA Extension
Division of Nursing
10995 LeConte Avenue
Los Angeles, California 90024
Phone: 213/825-3115

University of Colorado—Contact persons:
Henry K. Silver, M.D.
Professor of Pediatrics
Department of Pediatrics
University of Colorado
Medical Center
4200 East Ninth Avenue
Denver, Colorado 80262

Ms. Judith B. Igoe
Associate Professor
University of Colorado
School of Nursing
4200 East Ninth Avenue, C287
Denver, Colorado 80262
Phone: 303/394-8581

Louisiana State University (LSU)
LSU School of Nursing
420 South Prieur Street
New Orleans, Louisiana 70112
Phone: 504/943-2431

Northeastern University
College of Nursing
11 Leon Street
Boston, Massachusetts 02115
Phone: 617/437-3136

Pennsylvania State University
Codirector: Grace Laubach
Assistant Professor
Hershey Medical Center
Hershey, Pennsylvania 17033

Rutgers University
College of Nursing
Box 101
Piscataway, New Jersey 08854
Phone: 201/564-4343

San Diego State University
School of Nursing
5402 College Avenue
San Diego, California 92182
Phone: 714/286-5356

SUGGESTED READINGS

Alexander, M. M., and Brown, M. S.: 1974. Pediatric physical diagnosis for nurses, McGraw-Hill, Inc., New York.

American Academy of Pediatrics: 1972. Standards of child health care, American Academy of Pediatrics, Evanston, Ill.

Brown, M. S., and Murphy, M. A.: 1975. Ambulatory pediatrics for nurses, McGraw-Hill, Inc., New York.

Chinn, P. L.: 1979. Child health maintenance: concepts in family-centered care, 2nd ed., The C. V. Mosby Co., St. Louis.

Chinn, P. L., and Leitch, C. J.: 1979. Child health maintenance: a guide to clinical assessment, 2nd ed., The C. V. Mosby Co., St. Louis.

Christie, R. W.: 1976. Periodic comprehensive health assessment and a problem-oriented medical record for public school students, J. School Health **46**(5):256-262.

DeAngelis, C.: 1975. Basic pediatrics for the primary health care provider, Little, Brown & Co., Boston.

Joint statement of the American Nurses' Association: 1978. Guidelines on educational preparation and competencies of the school nurse practitioner, J. School Health **48**(5):265-268.

CHAPTER 13

Screening programs as tools in school health

SUSAN J. WOLD

As noted in Chapter 1, the value of school health activities has been increasingly challenged in recent years, resulting in cutbacks in some school health services and the elimination of others. If school health is to remain a viable concept, then school health activities must be well planned and their outcomes adequately documented. Fenske (1975) believes that this can be best accomplished through development of *programs* rather than proliferation of *services*. In distinguishing between programs and services, Fenske states that a *program* is based on *documented* needs; this ensures the program's relevance for the population served. In addition, a program has specific goals and objectives; this allows both determination of a program-specific budget and evaluation of the program as a whole based on the projected goals or outcomes. In other words, because a program is *outcome oriented*, its accountability is built in. In contrast, Fenske describes *services* as "open ended." Thus large amounts of money may be spent without demonstration of accountability for results, other than tabulation of services rendered or numbers of individuals served; hence, services tend to be *process oriented*, measuring "wing flaps" rather than outcomes. The conclusion to be drawn is obvious: demonstration of the accountability and merits of school health requires that *delivery of school health services occur only within a defined school health program*.

For the same reasons, *screening* should also occur *only as part of a screening program* (Lessler, 1972; North, 1974). In addition, it is important to remember that "screening is not and cannot be a substitute for other elements of health care" (North, 1974:639). Screening is only one way to alert people to the possible need for health care; it is *not* a system for health care delivery (North, 1974). According to Less-

ler (1972, 1974), the distinction between *screening* and a *screening program* is clear: *screening* is a means of acquiring significant data about a population, whereas a *screening program* uses the data to remediate the problems or defects that were identified. The distinguishing characteristic, then, is *intervention*, which is an essential component of a screening program.

As discussed in Chapter 2, one of the functions of the school health program is to protect students' health through disability limitation; this is accomplished through early diagnosis and prompt treatment (Chapter 5). As a means of promoting early diagnosis and prompt treatment, a carefully planned and implemented screening program is therefore an appropriate component of school health. Indeed, because it reveals important data about the population (students) screened, a screening program can be a very effective *tool* in planning, implementing, and evaluating outcomes of portions of the overall school health program.

To enable the nurse and other school health team members to effectively employ a screening program as a school health tool, the remainder of this chapter will discuss the following:

1. Planning, implementation, and evaluation of an effective screening program within the context of a school health program
2. Conditions or problems for which screening of school populations is recommended and appropriate screening procedures or tests to be used

PLANNING, IMPLEMENTATION, AND EVALUATION OF A SCHOOL HEALTH SCREENING PROGRAM
Planning the screening program

In any programming effort, careful planning is essential. Failure to weigh all pertinent variables and to use sound problem-solving skills will result in a program that is inefficient and ineffective; hence the need for careful and comprehensive planning cannot be overstated. Although planning an effective school screening program may seem to be a relatively simple, yet time-consuming task, in reality, planning a screening program requires some complex decision making.

In planning a school screening program it is essential that the planners recognize that *all* of the decisions they will make will depend on their value system. This is true for two reasons. First, there is no universally "right" screening program for planners to simply select and implement, because health problems and needs vary by such factors as geographic location and age. Thus determination of a population to screen and conditions for which to screen them will depend on the health needs and problems *perceived by the program planners*. Second, because the screening program is only one component of the overall school health program, it must "fit" within the particular objectives of that total program. Therefore the determination of whom to screen and for what will be based on the thrust of the total school health program in that school district at that point in time. Since health needs and problems vary among and within population groups, obviously the thrust and scope of overall school health programs will vary as well. In other words, school screen-ing program planners need to begin by clearly articulating their *philosophy* regarding school health and screening as a component of school health *before* determining the scope and nature of the screening program.

The process of planning, implementing, and evaluating a school screening program is illustrated in Fig. 13-1. Although the various considerations and aspects of the program are listed sequentially, it is possible and often desirable to consider some aspects simultaneously. For example, in identifying the objectives and evaluative outcome criteria (EOCs) during the "planning" phase of the screening program, it is also logical to simultaneously consider certain aspects of the "evaluation" phase to determine how, when, and by whom the objectives and EOCs will be evaluated.

It should also be noted that the model depicted in Fig. 13-1 is *cybernetic* in that it relies on feedback to control or modify behavior (Bailey and Claus, 1975). In this model, the "feedback loop" is the means by which the outcomes of the evaluation are fed back into the system as planning inputs. This ensures that the results of the program evaluation are actually used to improve the efficiency and effectiveness of the screening program.

Scope of the screening program

One of the primary considerations in planning a screening program is determining its

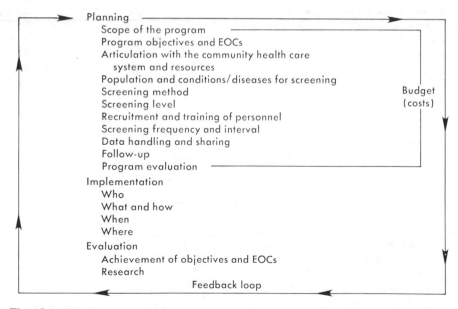

Fig. 13-1. Planning, implementation, and evaluation of a school health screening program.

scope, which Webster defines as "extent of treatment, activity, or influence . . . range of operation." In other words, the planners must decide how comprehensive the program will be in terms of the population to be screened and the number and range of conditions for which they will be screened. Establishing the scope of a screening program thus entails choosing between *selective screening* and *multiphasic screening* (Chapter 5). If the currently vogue multiphasic screening is chosen, then Lessler (1972) cautions that the tests selected should have high reliability and be simple, accurate, minimally inconvenient for the individual being screened, and quickly administered and interpreted. Also, a screening program should be established only after careful review of the accepted principles and criteria for screening. This means that in planning a multiphasic screening program, the planners must resist the temptation to "throw in" other superfluous tests and procedures just because they have access to some nifty new gadget or equipment and to a captive population. The program planned must be based on the needs of the population screened and on the availability of follow-up resources.

If, in contrast, the program is to include selective screening, then the planners must clearly identify how and why the specific group(s) within the population and the specific conditions for which they are to be screened were selected. These selections obviously depend on and (should) flow from the philosophy of the planning group concerning school health and the role of screening within it.

Program objectives and EOCs

Once the scope of the screening program has been established, a logical next step is to identify the specific objectives and EOCs. These should be stated as outcomes not as steps in a process. That is, the program's objectives should be *behaviorally* stated and focused on the *results* of the program. The EOCs represent the breakdown of individual objectives into their specific, finite, and *measurable* behaviors. The specificity or measurability of the EOCs is the key to their usefulness in any program. The more specifically they are stated, for example, through inclusion of the *number of times* a behavior will occur or the *date* by which the behavior(s) will occur, the more readily their attainment or lack of attainment can be determined. In other words, the measurability of

EOCs is directly proportional to the specificity with which they are stated. Because the EOCs represent division of the objectives into smaller behaviors, the sum of which should equal attainment of the entire objective, it follows logically that the list of EOCs should be sufficiently exhaustive to include all behaviors, which, when collectively achieved, indicate that the entire objective has been met. That is, the sum of the behaviors specified in the EOCs equals achievement of the particular objective.

Articulation with the community health care system and resources

As discussed in Chapter 5, successful outcome of a screening program requires collaboration between the school health team and other community health care professionals and resources in (1) determining and communicating the criteria to be used for referral of those being screened for further evaluation and (2) determining what, how, and by whom follow-up will be done. To prevent later sabotage of the program, such collaboration should be initiated *early* in the planning phase and maintained throughout the implementation and evaluation phases as well.

Population and conditions/diseases for screening

Decisions concerning whom to screen and for what need to be made concurrently, since decisions about one will affect the other. That is, determination of the specific population to be screened for a particular condition, disease, or defect depends on who is at risk of having or developing that particular health problem. For example, if plumbism (lead poisoning) is one of the conditions sought in a screening program, incidence and prevalence data suggest that the high-risk population includes 15- to 36-month-old children living in old, substandard housing in the eastern, southern, and midwestern United States (Chisholm, 1975); hence the focal population for plumbism screening would include 1- to 3-year-olds residing in such housing.

Again, as noted in Chapter 5, the school nurse is uniquely qualified to assess the particular health needs of the school population through such methods as epidemiological surveys; such survey data can be invaluable in planning selective screening programs. The school nurse's expertise is also essential in then determining for which diseases or conditions the overall school population or its subgroups are to be screened. The criteria to be used in selecting diseases or health needs for screening include the importance of the condition as a health problem, availability of accepted treatment for identified patients, availability of diagnostic and treatment resources, existence of a recognizable latent or early symptomatic stage of the disease or condition, adequate understanding of the disease's natural history, and economic balance between the cost of case finding and the cost of medical care for the condition.

Screening method

Selection of the particular test or procedure to be used in screening for a given disease or condition is based in part on value judgments made by the planners. These judgments are based on the relative importance assigned to the sensitivity, specificity, predictive value of a positive result, or efficiency of the test by the program planners. Acceptability of the test is likewise important. Frankenburg (1975b) notes further that the *appropriateness* of a screening test must also be considered, especially if the child's cooperation is required. He suggests that the appropriateness of a test be weighed in terms of the child's age, communicative skills, and sociocultural experiences. He believes that consideration of the child's communicative skills and cultural experiences are especially important for psychological or language screening and for other tests or procedures that rely on learned behavior.

Another important consideration in choosing a test for inclusion in a screening program is the cost. The direct costs of a screening test include the costs of the equipment and supplies (durable and disposable) needed to administer the test, training personnel to perform the test, personnel time to conduct the test (including labeling and transporting any specimens), and recording test results and interpreting them to the persons being screened (children) and their families (Frankenburg, 1974). Thus, when there is more than one suitable test available, cost-effectiveness becomes an important factor in test selection.

Screening level

After selecting a screening test or procedure, the planners must next determine the screening level (the value or score at which the test is considered "positive"). This is an important decision because the numbers of false positives and false negatives contribute to the indirect costs of the overall screening program, both monetary and psychological. The screening level selected will vary from one program and locale to another, based on consideration of these factors: the outlook for a person with the disease, existence of treatment facilities, mental status accompanying knowledge or suspicion of the disease, by whom diagnostic follow-up will be done, likelihood of repeat screening, and whether or not healthy individuals are sought.

Budget (costs)

An unavoidable reality that must be dealt with in planning a screening program is the budget. The amount of funding available will directly affect the scope of the program, the population to be screened (numbers), the screening level (tolerable numbers of false negatives and false positives), and selection of the specific screening test or procedure (cost-effectiveness).

The literature (Eisner and Oglesby, 1972a; Scriver, 1974; Frankenburg, 1974, 1975a) is replete with admonitions to would-be planners of screening programs to consider *all* the costs, direct and indirect, of a screening program and to weigh them against the potential benefits of the program. As these authorities point out, the total costs of the screening program include costs related to follow-up activities such as counseling and interpretation of results, personnel time for relocating individuals needing to be rescreened before any referral is made, and costs (personnel time, postage, secretarial services, etc.) of notifying those being screened of arrangements made for diagnostic examination and of making the actual referral.

Eisner and Oglesby (1972a) point out that other frequently overlooked screening costs are the costs of diagnosis and treatment. The cost of diagnosis varies, depending on the cost of the diagnostic procedure itself and on the cost of diagnosis of false positives or overreferrals. Thus a screening test that is inexpensive to administer may actually be very expensive if there are many overreferrals requiring expensive and elaborate diagnostic follow-up (Frankenburg, 1975b). As an example of the costs of overreferral, Eisner and Oglesby (1972a) cite a study in which children were screened for vision defects using the Snellen test; although the test was calculated to cost less than $.50 per student screened, the actual costs per correct referral came to nearly $63.00 per student when the costs of professional examination for the false positives were added in! In addition to the costs of diagnosis, the screening program must also include anticipated costs of treatment for those who need it. These costs must be added on to the total projected costs of the overall program in deciding if indeed the overall benefits of the screening program outweigh the costs. Failure to consider *all* costs related to screening (direct and indirect) results in a misleading economic evaluation of the program and may in the long run jeopardize acceptance of legitimate and well-planned programs.

The size of the screening program budget reflects the conscious or unconscious importance and priority of the screening program within the school health program as a whole. If the budget is too small, the scope and quality of the program may suffer. In her role as manager of health care, the school nurse must gather and present to those individuals who control the purse strings appropriate data documenting the need for the screening program and the expected outcomes, relative costs, and anticipated benefits. This requires assertiveness, persistence, and leadership on the nurse's part.

Recruitment and training of personnel

Another important consideration in planning a screening program is recruitment and training of personnel. Cost-effectiveness is important here. There must be sufficient personnel to reduce the per capita screening time to an acceptable and safe level; this means that the number of persons recruited to conduct and follow up the screening must be adequate to handle the expected volume of clients or individuals being screened. In addition, the personnel must be properly trained so that they can administer the test(s) accurately and score them appropriately. Generally, it is advisable to periodically reevaluate the skills of personnel and retrain them if necessary to ensure the continued quality and continuity of the program. It is also important to carefully match the skills and abilities of personnel with the tasks assigned to them. If a professional person, such as the school nurse, is assigned to administer screening tests that could be just as reliably administered by a trained technician or volunteer, then the costs of the screening are needlessly increased, and at the same time, the nurse is prevented from more effectively using her skills for other aspects of the screening program.

Screening frequency and interval

In planning the school's screening program, it is also important to consider the timing of the screening: how often it will be done and at what intervals or age groups. This decision is obviously related to the selection of the population to be screened. For example, in screening for vision and hearing defects among schoolchildren, it may be advantageous to conduct the screening early in the year before defects have interefered unduly with students' learning; this also allows maximal time for follow-up for students who need corrective lenses or hearing aids. The interval selected for screening might be alternate grade levels, such as one, three, five, seven, and nine; this provides for periodic rescreening of all students as they advance through the grade levels. Decisions about screening frequency and intervals are related to the philosophy and values of the program planners and may be influenced by budgetary limitations as well.

Data handling and sharing

According to Lessler (1972, 1974), careful planning regarding data handling and sharing is very important. The data gathered must obviously be relevant and accurate if it is to be useful. Lessler believes that screening data is important not only as a means of evaluating program effectiveness but is also important for follow-up for individual students. He states that screening results should be shared with all of the child's caregivers, including parents, teachers, physicians, and others, to prevent duplication or gaps in service. Due to prevailing privacy laws, such plans for data handling obviously require "informed consent" and preferably written permission when findings are to be communicated from one system or agency to another. Plans for data handling also have implications for recruitment and orientation of personnel for the program; those recruited must be able to maintain appropriate confidentiality without confounding legitimate and authorized requests for data sharing.

Finally, it is important that the data be collected, recorded, and stored in appropriate ways to afford maximum retrievability and usefulness. If the data is to be used for research purposes, planners must be sure that the format for recording is consistent with the research design. If research or program evaluation plans call for periodic data collection and comparisons, then the data must consistently be collected and recorded using similar or identical categories; this avoids comparisons of "apples" with "oranges."

Follow-up

Although it often receives far too little attention, follow-up is the most important aspect of screening. Again, failure to provide adequate follow-up for screenees is unethical and even immoral (Chapter 5)! Follow-up activities provide the best measure of the screening program's outcomes and benefits—mere lists of numbers of persons screened and the categorization of the findings are only "wing flaps." In other words, early detection of health problems or needs is only a beginning step toward improved health; the ultimate outcome depends on what happens *after* the actual screening.

In planning follow-up activities for a screening program, one of the first concerns should be interpretation of scores or test findings. That is, when is a test considered "positive" and who will interpret the scores? As noted earlier, this is another aspect of screening that requires careful ongoing collaboration with health care professionals and resources in the community. Those professionals who will be receiving referrals requesting diagnostic study for persons with a positive test result must understand and accept the standards and criteria used in making the referral; otherwise, the program may be discredited and sabotaged.

Other aspects of follow-up requiring close collaboration with area health care professionals include deciding what to do about borderline or questionable scores; how, when, by whom, and to whom referrals will be made for diagnostic workup and possible treatment; to whom screening results (negative and positive) will be communicated and by whom; in what instances rescreening will be done; and who will assume responsibility for counseling individuals and families to accept and follow through with the referral. Indeed, this latter aspect of counseling has been shown to have significant impact on the outcome of referrals: a study of Philadelphia schoolchildren revealed that intensive counseling of parents by school nurses significantly improved the rate of defect correction (Campbell et al., 1970).

Mayshark et al. (1977:201) cite the following six specific functions or purposes of good follow-up:

1. Provision of useful personal health status data to students for their use

2. Interpretation of health data and conditions to parents to encourage procurement of needed care for children
3. Motivation of students and parents to seek necessary treatment
4. Promotion of students' self-responsibility for their health within developmental limits
5. Contributing to the health education of students and parents
6. Obtaining educational programs geared to the individual needs and abilities of exceptional or handicapped students

These functions all relate to health education for those students being screened and their families. As discussed in Chapter 4, health education is a primary prevention strategy and a means of promoting high-level wellness. The long-range importance of health education and other primary prevention strategies cannot be overstated: if such efforts succeed, then screening and other early detection efforts for some health problems can be decreased or eliminated. Surely, this is a worthwhile goal. Thus the long-range follow-up for screening programs *must* include attention to primary prevention efforts to reduce the at-risk population.

However, primary prevention does not always work and, as previously noted, primary prevention strategies may not always exist. Thus, in some instances, there will be a continuing, long-term need for case finding. This need for continued case finding is also an important aspect of follow-up. In setting the screening level (the point at which the test is considered positive) future case finding plans are important; if rescreening is planned within a reasonable time, then the tolerable level of false negatives may be increased, since repeat screening increases the probability of detection. In any event, the hazards of "one-shot" screening efforts have already been thoroughly discussed, and the salient point is clear: long-range plans must be made for continued case finding.

Program evaluation

A final aspect of the program to be considered during the planning phase is program evaluation. The essence of program evaluation will be discussed later in this chapter, but it is important to note at this point that the kind of program evaluation planned has some effects on other aspects of the screening program. For example, if the program evaluation depends on collection and analysis of certain pieces of data, then plans for implementation of the screening program must detail how, when, and by whom that data will be collected. Obviously, these plans for program evaluation relate back to the objectives and EOCs developed in the early planning stages and must therefore be congruent.

Implementation of the screening program

During this phase of the screening program, the main task is to enact the plans that have been made; that is, the objectives and EOCs must be translated into *means* or activities for achieving the desired outcomes. These means must be spelled out in sufficient detail so that all personnel involved know what they are responsible for and to whom they are accountable.

Implementation is another challenge to the management skills of the school nurse and others involved with the screening program. Logical application of management process suggests that the first step in program implementation is to formulate policies (guides to decision making) and procedures (series of steps taken to implement objectives) (Chapter 18). Basically, the issues in implementation are who, what and how, when, and where.

Who

One of the first "who" questions is: Who specifically is included in the population to be screened? For example, if plans are made to screen all first-graders in a particular school district for vision problems, all the first-graders need to be located and identified before the screening procedure can be carried out; this includes arranging for informed consent to participate, such as through written parental permission, and arranging for any needed transportation to the screening site. Another "who" concern is: Who are the personnel who will participate in all phases of the screening program? This includes plans for recruitment and training as well as decisions concerning lines of authority and accountability.

What and how

This category includes all the activities necessary to carry out the entire program and to whom they are assigned. Thus details of the screening procedure itself, such as ordering supplies, arranging for facilities, arranging the clinic or screening room for efficient traffic flow, establishing the screening rate (numbers screened per hour), and who will conduct the actual screening are included. Other relevant details involve follow-up activities, including plans and methods for rescreening, counseling students and parents about screening findings, referral of students for diagnosis and treatment, plans for assessment of defect correction, establishment of primary prevention programs, and modification of individual educational experiences or programs as needed. The details of program evaluation also must be addressed. What exactly needs to be done to assess achievement of the program's EOCs?

When

Timing of various elements of the program is also important. When (time of year, dates, hours) will the screening procedure be carried out? When will the various follow-up activities be started or scheduled? When will the program evaluation be completed?

Where

One of the last implementation questions is "where." Where will the screening take place? Where (location of health professionals and other community resources) will students needing further evaluation or testing be referred? Where will screening data ultimately be stored after the program is completed? Where can interested parents, students, or other community residents obtain additional information about the program before, during, and after its implementation?

Evaluation of the screening program

Although evaluation of the screening program as a whole occurs after the fact, a great deal of formal or informal evaluation goes on throughout all phases of the program. For example, if the routing pattern established for the screening clinic proves to be inefficient, the pattern can be altered to correct the problem without waiting for the formal program evaluation to point out the problem. In other words, evaluation must be done as part of the day-to-day activities of the program so necessary corrections can be made promptly. Obviously, lines of authority must be respected in initiating change, but generally there should be no other reason for delay. The one notable exception would be in situations where research is part of the screening program. Depending on the nature of the research (process oriented versus outcome oriented), changes in procedure to improve efficiency may or may not be possible without jeopardizing the study's validity and outcome.

Formal summative program evaluation is generally based on two major components: achievement of the stated objectives and EOCs and outcomes of formal research. These areas merit careful review and assessment, because the results of the evaluation provide the feedback loop back to the planning phase (Fig. 13-1). If the program is to improve, evaluation results must be fed back into the planning process as data.

Achievement of objectives and EOCs

Since EOCs represent the subdivision of objectives into their specific and measurable behaviors, they are therefore the means for assessing attainment of objectives as well. If the EOCs were carefully written during the planning phase and are indeed *measurable* as stated, then evaluation of the program in terms of its EOCs requires only that the actual data and behaviors collected and recorded during the program be compared against the standards that were set (EOCs). That is, one need only reread each EOC and decide "yes" or "no" that the EOC has been met. No other inference or interpretation is needed; the EOC was either achieved or it was not—there are no "gray" areas here. If any EOC was not achieved, then inference and analysis may be useful in determining the cause. It might be that the EOC was not stated clearly or specifically enough, or perhaps the EOC was not appropriate as a measurement of achievement of the objective for which it was used. Analysis of the nonachievement can provide useful insights into the structural weaknesses of the program and should be carefully considered when the program is revised or redone.

Research

Another important and all too often overlooked means of program evaluation is research. North (1974) and Lessler (1972) have emphasized the importance of periodic monitoring or evaluation of screening programs to determine whether or not they are achieving the intended results. Research is a means of such evaluation. Frankenburg (1975a) cautions that the prevailing view of screening as a "panacea" for many health problems may result in proliferation of screening programs that are unnecessary and ill advised. The obvious risk of that approach is "overkill," which Frankenburg fears may result in complete abandonment

of screening before it has been fully evaluated as a health tool. Thoughtfully designed and carefully executed research studies can provide sound evaluative data about screening. The net result can then be appropriate rather than indiscriminate use of screening.

A number of suggested research emphases have been described in the literature (Commission on Chronic Illness, 1957; Lessler, 1972; Frankenburg, 1975a). First, there is a recognized need to determine the prevalence (total number of current cases), incidence (number of new cases per year per 100,000 population), and distribution within the population by age and population group of various diseases and health problems. This type of research is important in determining if a disease or condition is an important health problem, which is one of the criteria or principles for screening (Chapter 5). This kind of study can also be helpful in pinpointing the at-risk groups within the general population, which allows better focusing of screening efforts.

A second research priority suggested in the literature is to study the natural history of diseases or health problems to improve our understanding. These kinds of studies can help determine the earliest possible detection time (compared with the usual time of detection) and the optimal time for treatment. In addition, such studies could assess the impact of early detection (by screening) on the outcome or course of the disease or defect. Such data is essential in deciding whether or not screening is worthwhile for a given disease or health problem; if earlier detection does not provide any benefit for the individual in terms of improved prognosis, then screening for that problem may not be warranted.

Another category of needed research in screening includes studies to evaluate the effectiveness of existing early detection methods and to refine them as required. This includes studies to establish the validity (sensitivity and specificity), reliability (efficiency), and yield of current screening and other early detection methods. This category also includes experimental studies on such factors as screening level to *improve* the validity, reliability, and yield. Research to establish optimal screening conditions (such as age and sex of the person being screened, facilities and equipment needed, time of year or day) and to determine the preparation and qualifications needed by the screeners is also necessary.

A fourth goal of screening research would be

to evaluate the appropriateness and effectiveness of follow-up activities. This could include studies of the way screening findings are interpreted to those being screened, timing of follow-up actions, and research documenting the outcomes of referrals, including studies on the availability and adequacy of community resources to handle the referrals. Virtually all aspects of follow-up merit further study; if follow-up is acknowledged as the most important aspect of the screening program, then it logically deserves careful study to improve results.

The final research area identified in the literature is perhaps the most difficult to tackle: evaluation of the screening program's overall effectiveness. Such studies are involved and challenging because of the sheer complexity of the program. Among the specific aspects to be studied within the context of total program evaluation is the adequacy of the program in terms of its focus; that is, are the diseases or health concerns on which the program is based really important and valid for this population? Are there other health needs that might be alleviated by screening which are not part of the current program? Likewise it is important to study the structure and administration of the program; if the purposes and foci are found to be appropriate, but the structure and administration are cumbersome and ineffective, then the program requires modification to ensure its success. Research can point out these deficiencies and can also be designed to evaluate the modifications made after previous evaluations. Ultimately, though, the most important measure of a screening program's effectiveness will be the net improvement of the population's health status that occurred once the program was initiated. Obviously, studies that can be designed to demonstrate a cause-effect relationship will greatly enhance the likelihood that the program will continue to receive funding. In these times of tight budgets, nothing speaks louder to administrators who control purse strings than *documented results*. For that reason, research will continue to be an essential feature of screening programs.

In summary, screening activities must be provided *only* within the context of a carefully planned and executed screening program. The planners must ensure a good "fit" between the screening program and the philosophy and objectives of the overall school health program and should expect to provide relevant data for evaluation of the program's effectiveness and efficiency. Finally, planners must be prepared to make conscious value judgments in planning the program and to be held accountable for those judgments. They must recognize and accept the fact that there is no one "right" school screening program that can be universally applied. In short, the buck stops here.

SUGGESTED SCREENING FOCI AND METHODS

Again it must be stated that the details of a screening program, specifically, selection of the population groups to be screened, methods to use, frequency of screening, and personnel requirements, *must* be decided by the particular group or agency offering the program. The material included in this discussion is intended *only* to guide decision making, not to supplant it. The suggestions included have been compiled and extracted from current literature, but even as this book goes to press, many of these ideas may have become outdated as a result of recent research.

The discussion of suggested screening foci and methods in the remainder of this chapter will be presented within these organizational categories: periodic health assessment, growth and development, learning disabilities and behavior problems, sensory processes, orthopedics, and illnesses and health problems. These groupings have been arbitrarily made; the order of presentation is based on personal preference and does not necessarily denote priority.

Periodic health assessment

Periodic health assessment includes four specific topics: the health history, physical examination, "open-ended" procedures, and early and periodic screening, diagnosis, and treatment (EPSDT). Because they *can* be excellent sources of early detection of health problems, these activities are good sources of baseline data about a population. Baseline data can then be used to help plan a screening program that is relevant to the population.

Health history

Authorities (North, 1974; American Academy of Pediatrics, 1977) generally agree that the health history is perhaps the most important part of any health assessment. Indeed, North (1974) points out that 90% of all diagnosis is based on history. Unfortunately, history taking is often viewed as time consuming (which it is) and requiring less professional skill and judgment than a physical examination (which it does *not*). Although questionnaires filled out by the child, parent, or other informant may provide important historical data, the health professional's judgment and skills are needed to review and clarify the information and to evaluate its importance. The American Academy of Pediatrics (AAP), in their 1977 publication *School Health: A Guide for Health Professionals,* emphasized the importance of the examiner's review of the health history, regardless of the way (interview, questionnaire, etc.) it was obtained, *before* beginning a physical examination. Thus they view the medical history questionnaire as an adjunct to the examination and to the examiner's interview with the client; it is *not* a diagnostic or screening device in itself.

Techniques for eliciting a history were discussed in Chapter 12, and sample inventories were presented. Although the actual areas included will depend on the age of the child and the purpose of the history and subsequent physical examination, the AAP (1977) suggests that the health history include past health problems (physical and emotional) and their resolution, body systems review, past and current family problems involving some or all members, the child's academic progress and general school adjustment, immunization history, and health-related practices such as tobacco and drug use (including alcohol), and frequency, type, and duration of exercise. Jenne and Greene (1976) suggest inclusion of identifying personal data, such as name, birthdate, source of health care, general family information (living arrangements, age and sex of members, etc.), and additional data describing personal habits, such as usual bedtime on school nights, nutritional patterns, and any other relevant information.

Physical examination

No doubt the most hotly debated means for periodic health assessment of schoolchildren is the periodic physical examination. As noted in Chapter 1, medical examinations of children at school were begun in the 1920s as a means of discovering "defects." By the 1950s, the emphasis shifted away from physical examinations provided at school toward examinations by the student's private physician. However, requirements for periodic physical examination of children by a physician have persisted despite the shift in provider responsibility and despite research findings (Yankauer et al., 1955, 1956; Rogers and Reese, 1964; Iglehart et al., 1977) discounting the value of these examinations in detecting significant health defects.

Despite the conclusion by Iglehart et al. (1977:92) that the routine school physical examination is "a relatively ineffective casefinding procedure," and Eisner and Oglesby's (1971a) report that physicians generally regard school examinations as "unimportant bureaucratic requirements," periodic physical examinations for school-age children are required by law in some states and by school district policy in others. It is now generally accepted that these examinations *can* have merit in evaluating the total health status of the child and in providing appropriate education and other follow-up as needed *if* they are performed by a physician or nurse practitioner who is acquainted with the child's health history and who conducts the examination at an unhurried pace in an atmosphere conducive to cooperation and trust.

Since periodic physical examinations of schoolchildren are mandated by law or school policy throughout much of the country, the primary issue currently debated is the frequency and interval of these examinations. One of the considerations often voiced is cost; Eisner and Oglesby (1971a) unequivocally state that physicians' examinations are the most expensive procedure used for routine health assessment of children. Even when the examinations are offered without charge to the family through public or school-based clinics, the cost to taxpayers is significant, especially for a procedure whose value is questioned.

In areas where frequency of periodic medical examination of schoolchildren is not specified by law, the AAP (1977) recommends that guidelines be developed jointly by local school and medical officials, based on such factors as health needs of students, available community resources, and frequency, nature, and quality of other student health appraisal activities, such as screening programs, health inventories, and teacher observation. The intervals suggested by the AAP for these examinations and generally supported by others (Jenne and Greene, 1976; Mayshark et al., 1977; Anderson and Creswell, 1980) are as follows:

1. School entrance (first grade or kindergarten)
2. Middle school years (grade six or seven)
3. Before leaving school (grade eleven or twelve)
4. Children with identified health problems (initial referral and periodic monitoring of treatment)
5. Prior to participation in competitive or

rigorous athletics (may be an annual requirement)

6. Employment certification for minors (need determined by state law).

Anderson and Creswell (1980) also recommend that physical examinations be required for students referred by the nurse or teacher following observation and/or screening and for students new to the school system for whom there is no health record or whose health condition is questionable.

Despite continuing debate regarding the merits and recommended frequency for these examinations, the requirement stands. The important and nondebatable aspect of these examinations is the adequacy of follow-up for the findings and for those students who do not (and perhaps cannot financially) comply with the requirements. The school nurse or her designee must ensure that all problems uncovered through examination receive needed treatment and must assist students who cannot or have not arranged for their examinations to obtain necessary assistance.

Open-ended procedures

Eisner and Oglesby (1972c) point out that screening procedures and programs are limited in their ability to detect health problems by their very design; they only detect conditions for which the student is tested or examined and even then with varying validity and reliability. Thus adequate health assessment of schoolchildren requires use of *open-ended* procedures, or those which, according to Webster, are "adaptable to the developing needs of a situation."

Eisner and Oglesby (1972c) believe that schools should use "systematic observation of the child's activities" as a routine adjunct to school health examinations and screening procedures. They cite three basic open-ended methods of health assessment: physical examination, health inventories, and teacher-nurse conferences. The physical examination (Chapter 12) can be an open-ended assessment method *if* the examiner uses the medical history and symptoms to direct his examination; thus the examination proceeds as the history and findings direct it. If health examinations were routinely performed on schoolchildren following this approach, perhaps the findings would be more useful.

Health inventories, which are usually questionnaires filled out by the parent or child (adolescent) and returned to the school, generally include items about past illnesses, immunizations, and allergies. The information can thus be updated annually, which ensures that any modifications in the child's school program indicated by health status can be readily made and noted. However, as Eisner and Oglesby report, health inventories have not proved very useful in health assessment of students. One reason is that when they are scored like some screening tests, so that a "yes" answer regarding occurrence of a problem such as colds, vomiting, and fever is considered "positive," the net result is a high false positive rate. While these symptoms or problems *could* indicate serious disease, they are common occurrences and do not necessarily indicate a significant problem. Another problem with health inventories discussed by Eisner and Oglesby (1972c) is the language used in them. Sometimes, especially in areas where the population includes non-English-speaking persons, the questions on the inventory are incomprehensible. In addition, the items in an inventory obviously are based on the concepts of "health" and "disease" held by health care professionals; even if the language and intent of the questions are understood, the questions may seem meaningless and unimportant to the respondent. Also, such inventories may be viewed as close ended or "forced choice" questionnaires by the respondent; this may result in omission of important but unrequested clarifying information. Eisner and Oglesby conclude that an interview with the parent would in the long run be a more open ended and more reliable source of information concerning the child's health.

The last major method of open-ended health assessment discussed by Eisner and Oglesby (1972c) is the teacher-nurse conference. The purpose of the conference is to help the school nurse with her task of student health assessment and is based on the realization that the teacher is the best day-to-day observer of children other than their parents. The conference should be scheduled at least annually and on the nurse's initiative (Eisner and Oglesby, 1972c). In addition, the nurse should be available for interim conferences and consultation as needed. The conferences can be expedited by use of a checklist of typical observable signs of health, emotional, or behavioral problems of children. The checklist or tool can be distributed to teachers prior to the conference so they can take time to systematically observe their students. Orientation to the purposes and methods of teacher observation of students and teacher-nurse conferences should ideally be presented to the faculty each school year (in the fall) by the school nurse. This assists teachers to more effectively assess the health of their students and provides the nurse with an opportunity to become directly involved with the faculty and to clarify her role at the same time.

Early and periodic screening, diagnosis, and treatment (EPSDT)

Another type of periodic health assessment is the EPSDT program. During the 1960s, as noted in Chapter 1, the conservatism of the 1950s gave way to liberal ideas and proliferation of governmental programs; hence we had the "New Frontier" and the "Great Society." In 1965, in the midst of all this raised social consciousness, Title XIX of the Social Security Act was passed, creating the Medicaid federal medical assistance program to benefit the poor. Basically, within a few federal guidelines, Medicaid eligibility requirements are determined by the states; health care providers are then reimbursed for services rendered to eligible recipients, so that poverty is not a barrier to health care. Federal law stipulates that Medicaid programs *must* cover certain services, including inpatient and outpatient hospital services, physician, laboratory, and x-ray examination services, skilled nursing home services for those over 21 years old, family planning services, and EPSDT services for those under 21 years of age (Children's Defense Fund, 1977).

The EPSDT portion of the Medicaid program resulted from the 1967 "Early and Periodic Screening, Diagnosis, and Treatment" amendment to Title XIX of the Social Security Act (Children's Defense Fund, 1977). As amended, the law requires states operating Medicaid programs to *provide* EPSDT *services* to all children eligible for Medicaid. Thus, unlike the Medicaid program, which provides reimbursement only, EPSDT requires states to deliver services as well as provide reimbursement. Specifically, states are required to provide and pay for screening services for an eligible family within 60 days of their request. The services to be included are health and developmental history, physical growth measures (such as height and weight), developmental assessment, unclothed physical inspection, inspection of the ears, nose, mouth, and throat, including dental assessment, vision and hearing testing, tests for

sickle cell, anemia, tuberculosis, and lead poisoning, urine screening, other tests as indicated (such as blood pressure levels or chest x-ray examination), nutritional assessment, and assessment of immunization status (Children's Defense Fund, 1977). In addition, states must make available and pay for diagnostic services as needed and treatment services within the limits of the state Medicaid plan. States are also expected to develop some kind of outreach program to notify eligible families about services, develop contracts and agreements with existing health care resources to provide the services, and provide transportation to and from services (Children's Defense Fund, 1977).

The obvious intent of the EPSDT legislation was to provide preventive as well as curative services for high-risk children. However, as the Children's Defense Fund (CDF) (1977) points out in its comprehensive analysis *EPSDT Does It Spell Health Care for Poor Children?*, the answer to their title question is: "not necessarily." Compliance rates vary markedly throughout the country for a variety of reasons, such as lack of commitment to the program by states, inadequate outreach programs, and inadequate focus on diagnosis and treatment following the screening.

In their study of EPSDT, the CDF found that services were provided in a variety of ways from state to state. In some states, services are provided primarily by public health departments; in others, schools may participate in delivery of services. Because one of the major problems with EPSDT is that many eligible children do not get services, it is important for school nurses to be aware of this program and its services. In states where schools are directly involved in providing services, school nurses may participate in the actual screening; certainly, school nurses have a role in following up children from their schools who need further diagnostic study and/or treatment. Also, since one of the identified reasons for the failure of EPSDT to reach its goals was inadequate outreach, school nurses can do a great deal to publicize EPSDT services to eligible families in their schools and arrange whatever assistance they might need to take advantage of the services offered. In addition, if public health–oriented school nurses will provide EPSDT outreach services for *pre*schoolers in their school communities, then perhaps the number of *school-age* children with chronic health problems, poor nutrition, and incomplete immunizations from low-income families will decrease.

Growth and development

Among the time-honored practices in pediatrics and school nursing is assessment of growth and development of children. School nurses have long been interested in children's growth and development as compared with peers' growth and development and with standardized norms. As noted earlier, with the advent of EPSDT legislation, assessment of development and physical growth became required procedures for those children served in EPSDT clinics.

Physical growth

It is ironic to note (Eisner et al., 1972) that measurement of children's heights and weights has become a mindless routine, which is still performed "because we've always done it" or because "it just makes sense." The irony is that despite our vague assertions that these measurements are "important," there is a glaring absence of research data supporting the usefulness of height-weight data in identifying children with otherwise unsuspected health problems (North, 1974).

North (1974) suggests that because measurement of children's growth is generally reassuring to their parents, it may be justified on that basis alone. However, in school health programs where tight budgets necessitate careful priority setting, parental reassurance is not much of a justification for continuing a time-consuming procedure having dubious outcomes. Eisner et al., (1972) point out that despite routine recording of children's heights and weights as part of their health assessment, interpretation of the findings is often inadequate and is not integrated into the overall school health program. Thus the failure is not in collecting the data but results from misinterpretation and/or disuse.

Among the advantages of measuring children's heights and weights as cited by Eisner et al. (1972) is the fact that these measurements can be made by almost anyone—the skills of a nurse or physician are not required. These authors also believe that height and weight data can be useful in detecting nutritional and physical growth disorders when the raw data is converted to a standardized score or somehow compared against a standard, as in a growth chart. They believe that nutritional disorders can be estimated after a single observation, whereas physical growth disorders require serial observations for assessment.

Authorities (Eisner et al., 1972; North, 1974; McCammon, 1975) generally agree that growth charts, such as the Iowa Growth Charts, the Wetzel Grid, or the Stuart Grid, are useful in charting and comparing serial measurements of a child's height and weight with his own previous measurements and with accepted age-appropriate norms. However, as Eisner et al. (1972) caution, the use of heights and weights as a screening test for nutritional problems (such as obesity) or for growth disorders (such as dwarfism) is of limited value because (1) growth charts are relatively insensitive screening tests, (2) treatment of nutritional problems like obesity is relatively ineffective, and (3) growth disorders are rare. Also, as McCammon (1975) points out, there is a wide range of "normal" body sizes because individual growth is influenced by metabolism, which in turn is affected by other factors such as genetic makeup, nutrition, and illness.

Eisner et al., (1972) therefore believe that routine measurement of schoolchildren's heights and weights has not proven useful in school health programs. However, they believe that the following are legitimate uses for these measurements in school health:

1. As part of a health education program, such as a unit on growth or nutrition
2. As one kind of follow-up or evaluation of a nutrition program, such as a weight control group
3. As part of a nutrition survey *if* other corroborative measures, such as laboratory tests and skinfold measurements, are also used
4. As a screening test for detection of growth disorders *in locales where there is a common treatable condition,* such as hookworm or other chronic infections, resulting in growth failure

They rightfully conclude that if none of these situations applies, then measuring and recording children's heights and weights cannot be justified.

Development

Like physical growth measurements, developmental assessments have been a standard element in pediatrics, public health nursing, and school nursing for many years. Unlike physical growth measurements, though, developmental assessment has not aroused controversy about its merits. Authorities (Campbell and Camp, 1975; Erickson, 1976) generally acknowledge the importance of early and periodic screening of children's development in such areas as gross and fine motor skills, cognitive development, and personal-social behavior, including self-care activities and school readiness. Periodic developmental screening is recognized as *a* means of early detection for *some* handicapping conditions, such as cretinism and seizure disorders (North, 1974). Developmental screening also provides a means of documenting children's developmental achievements, thereby reassuring their parents. Thus for children who are found through repeated screenings to have a developmental lag or delay, screening results can be the impetus for early intervention; this can then prevent or minimize long-range complications for the child. For children whose performance is within normal limits on screening tests, developmental screening provides baseline data for additional health promotion.

The primary points of contention or controversy concerning developmental screening are centered on the validity and reliability of screening tools and procedures and on the way in which the data is interpreted and applied. North (1974) charges that (1) most available developmental screening tests do not have *documented* validity or reliability; (2) diagnostic criteria and effective treatments for many conditions leading to developmental delays have not yet been established; (3) research evidence showing how those classified as "abnormal" benefit from early detection and treatment is lacking; and (4) despite obvious negative consequences of mislabeling a child as "slow" or "retarded," the *benefits* of early identification through screening are not well documented. However, he concludes (1974:633) that "the importance of making *some* routine developmental observations seems to outweigh the uncertainties."

Most developmental tests or tools are designed to score or compare the behavior of a given child with accepted age-appropriate norms. Thus the child's behavior is compared with that of children of similar age and (preferably) socioeconomic and cultural background. The importance of serial or repeated testings before referring a child or before planning any intervention has been emphasized in the literature (North, 1974; Campbell and Camp, 1975; Erickson, 1976). In addition, Campbell and

Camp remind screeners that "abnormal" screening findings cause considerable anxiety for children and their parents; therefore children should *never* be labeled based only on screening results.

Selection of specific tests or tools for developmental assessment should follow consideration of such factors as age of children to be screened, the time frame (numbers of children screened and length of time available for each child's test), validity and reliability of the test (including similarities between the population used for standardization of the tool and the population to be screened), ease of administration (length of time to administer and qualifications and training needed by testers), and relative cost (Campbell and Camp, 1975). For increased time economy, North (1974) and Frankenburg et al. (1976) recommend use of streamlined, simplified tools such as the Denver Prescreening Developmental Questionnaire (PDQ) to identify those children needing a more thorough screening with a tool such as the Denver Developmental Screening Test (DDST). Children whose PDQ performance is questionable or deviant can thus be more thoroughly tested; likewise, children whose performance is clearly within normal limits need not be subject to lengthy and presumably unnecessary testing.

Although individual review and recommendation of specific screening tests is beyond the scope and intent of this chapter, there is a wealth of critical and analytical data concerning screening tests and procedures in the literature. (See the References and Suggested Readings at the end of the chapter.) There is an impressive array of tests and tools available for developmental assessment specifically. To facilitate the reader's awareness of developmental screening methods, Table 13-1 provides a list of some of the most commonly used methods by name and description (type); it also includes the age range for persons being screened and identifies suggested reference materials for further background and methodological information. This table is presented only as a basic reference for readers; it is not an endorsement or recommendation of any particular test. Selection of a particular test is the responsibility of the planners of the screening program.

In addition to the general developmental screening tests described in Table 13-1, four "school readiness" tests have been included. School readiness is related to overall development, since it is a function of the child's intel-

Table 13-1. Developmental screening tools

Test name	Type	Age range	References
Activities of Daily Living (ADLs) Assessment	Developmental (self-care)	Birth to adult	Coley, 1978
Denver Developmental Screening (DDST)	Developmental: personal-social, fine motor–adaptive, language, gross motor	Birth to 6 years	Campbell and Camp, 1975 Erickson, 1976 Frankenburg and Dodds, 1967 Frankenburg et al., 1970 Frankenburg et al., 1971a Frankenburg et al., 1971b Thorpe and Werner, 1974
Goodenough-Harris Drawing Test	Developmental (intellectual maturity)	3 to 15 years	Campbell and Camp, 1975 Harris, 1963a, 1963b
Maturity Level for School Entrance and Reading Readiness	School readiness	5 to 7 years	Banham, 1959 Goldstein, 1975
Preschool Attainment Record (PAR)	Developmental	6 months to 7 years	Campbell and Camp, 1975 Doll, 1966
Denver Prescreening Developmental Questionnaire (PDQ)	Developmental	3 months to 6 years	Frankenburg et al., 1976
Preschool Inventory (PI)	School readiness	3 to 6 years	Goldstein, 1975
Sprigle School Readiness	School readiness	4 years, 6 months to 6 years, 9 months	Goldstein, 1975
Vane Kindergarten Test (VKT)	Intelligence: school readiness, academic potential	4 years to 6 years, 6 months	Campbell and Camp, 1975 Vane, 1968
Vineland Social Maturity Scale	Development: social maturity	Birth to adult	Doll, 1965

lectual abilities, knowledge, prior experiences, and emotional maturity. All these factors collectively affect the child's ability or readiness to adapt to the school environment and the teaching-learning process. School readiness tests are designed to assess particular school-related skills such as those needed for reading and arithmetic (Goldstein, 1975); such tests may provide preliminary indications of children who may later be diagnosed as having learning disabilities. However, these tests are *not* diagnostic, and, as with other developmental tests, children should *not* be "labeled" on the basis of their performance on school readiness tests.

Learning disabilities and behavior problems

During the 1960s and 1970s, interest in "problem" or "difficult" schoolchildren increased. Children who were disruptive in class and "slow" to learn were now regarded in a new light; judgments like "lacks parental discipline" and "low IQ" gave way to increasing scientific evidence that these behaviors had identifiable physiological, environmental, and/or psychological origins. In addition, the advent of so-called special learning and behavior problems (SLBP) programs provided further evidence of the beneficial effects of early diagnosis and intervention on these children. For these reasons, in recent years school health programs and school nurses have been increasingly involved in developing and applying screening tests and procedures for early identification of high-risk children.

As Uyeda (1972) points out, there are more than thirty synonyms used by professionals to describe children with learning disabilities and behavior problems. For the purposes of this chapter, the following definitions will apply:

learning disability "Any condition which hampers a child from understanding, assimilating, and using the materials which are presented to him at school and at home" (Uyeda, 1972:214). Such disabilities are associated with central nervous system dysfunctions and appear (in various combinations) as impairments of "perception, conceptualization, language, and memory, and . . . control of attention, impulse, or motor function" (AAP, 1977:70). Mental retardation, sensory (visual or auditory) handicaps, severe emotional disturbance, and disadvantaged cultural background are not considered as learning disabilities (Kirk and Bateman, 1962; Uyeda, 1972).

dyslexia or reading disability A specific type of learning disability resulting in the child reading two or more levels below his grade (Bogle, 1973).

hyperactivity A syndrome characterized by four observable types of behavior: overactivity, distractibility, impulsiveness, and excitability; this syndrome is often associated with school failure and ultimately with a poor self-image (Woodard and Brodie, 1974).

It should be noted that some professionals use labels such as "brain-damaged," "brain-injured," "hyperkinesis" and "minimal brain dysfunction" to describe children with the learning disabilities syndrome or hyperactive syndrome just described. The AAP (1977) advises against the use of such labels because these terms incorrectly imply that the causes and process of pathogenesis are clearly understood. Indeed, as the AAP recommends, until adequate research data proving the causes and fully explaining the process of pathogenesis for these disorders is available, descriptive labels such as "learning disabilities syndrome" and "hyperactive syndrome" should continue to be used.

Because of difficulties in precise diagnosis of these syndromes and because there are overlapping symptoms, estimates of the prevalence of learning disabilities and behavior problems are imprecise. However, Uyeda (1972) believes that at least 15% of all schoolchildren have a learning problem, of which reading problems are the most common type. Woodard and Brodie (1974) suggest that 4% to 5% of all elementary schoolchildren are considered hyperactive; this is an average of one hyperactive child per American classroom. Furthermore, authorities (Woodard and Brodie, 1974; AAP, 1977) agree that boys are affected much more often than girls—perhaps even ten times as often. Children with learning disabilities and behavior problems not only experience frequent personal failure in regular classroom settings, but also interfere with the learning of other children. For all these reasons, learning disabilities and behavior problems affect significantly large school populations and are therefore important health problems. School health programming efforts directed toward early detection and early and appropriate intervention are important.

Although the available literature includes some interesting discussions of the etiology and populations at risk for learning disabilities and hyperactivity (behavior problems) (Kirk and Bateman, 1962; Ferinden, 1972; Woodard and Brodie, 1974; Mercer and Trifiletti, 1977), an in-depth review of current opinion is beyond the scope and intent of this chapter. Since Mercer and Trifiletti (1977) have completed and reported the findings from their comprehensive literature review, a brief summary of their findings is useful. After their review of research on learning disabilities, Mercer and Trifiletti (1977: 526-531) isolated the following five "possible predictors" of learning disabilities:

1. *Perinatal history,* documenting abnormalities such as prematurity, postmaturity, induced labor, prolonged labor, complications of delivery (including difficult, rapid, breech delivery, or cesarean section), cyanosis (natal or postnatal), incompatible maternal-infant blood types, and twinning; adoption was also implicated in some cases; *developmental history,* noting abnormalities such as late or abnormal creeping, late walking, prolonged tiptoe walking, late or abnormal speech, and ambidexterity after age 7 (that is, delayed establishment of laterality or handedness).

2. *Environmental factors,* including environmental deprivation (institutionalization), family size, the child's position within the family, and low socioeconomic status.

3. *Dental enamel defects,* specifically enamel hypoplasia (thinning or absence of enamel), hypocalcification (structural defect with resulting irregular texture), and hypomaturation (white or chalky areas; surface integrity unaltered). Enamel defects are more common in neurologically impaired children than in normal children.

4. *Physical anomalies* (minor), such as abnormal (± 1 to 1.5 standard deviations) head circumference, fine "electric" hair, ocular anomalies (epicanthus and hypertelorism), lowset, malformed, asymmetrical ears and/or adherent lobes, furrowed tongue, high palate, fifth finger of hand curved inward, and third toe of foot longer than second toe. (Dental enamel defects, already noted, are also physical anomalies.)

5. *Family history,* including history of par-

ental alcoholism, sociopathy, hysteria, and learning disabilities, history of alcoholism, hysteria, and sociopathy among male and/or female relatives (other than parents), number of siblings with learning disabilities, and current social or emotional stress in the family.

Based on their review of the literature, Mercer and Trifiletti (1977) concluded that no one particular anomaly occurring perinatally or during early childhood is in itself predictive of learning problems; rather, "constellations of anomalies" have been successful in predicting which children are high risk. Recognizing the importance of "pooling" these research findings into a workable whole, Mercer and Trifiletti designed a tool to be used within preschool screening programs to aid in early detection of children with learning disabilities.

Mercer and Trifiletti's tool, the Problem Learner Screening Procedures (PLSP), is intended to be an effective, rapidly administered and scored tool suitable for administration by (unspecified) school personnel. The validity is presumed by the authors, based on available research data and other literature they used in constructing specific items for the tool. Since no clinical trial of the PLSP had been done at the time of publication of their tool, the authors were unable to identify a specific "high-risk score." Hence, they encourage users of the PLSP to establish local normative guidelines. As shown in Tables 13-2 and 13-3, the PLSP consists of two parts: a parent questionnaire (which the authors suggest be mailed out during registration and returned by the first week of school) and a brief physical inspection (to be done by the school nurse) to detect minor physical anomalies.

As noted earlier, learning disabilities, including dyslexia, are often associated with hyperactivity or behavior problems (Haverkamp, 1970; Bogle, 1973; Woodard and Brodie, 1974). Indeed, often the first reported and most disturbing observation (to parents and school personnel) is that the child is hyperactive. That is, he is *consistently* overactive and on the move, easily distracted, impulsive, and excitable (Woodard and Brodie, 1974). The consistency and *persistence* of this behavior is what differentiates the truly hyperactive child from other children.

Fig. 13-2 provides a suggested checklist of behaviors that might be used to identify children needing further monitoring and evaluation

Table 13-2. Summary of PLSP parent questionnaire items and scoring weights

Item	Weight
Problems during pregnancy	1
Difficult delivery	2
Prolonged labor	1
Prematurity	1
Blood incompatibility	1
Low birth weight	1
Cyanosis	1
Adoption	1
Creeping late (after 9 months) or abnormal	2
Walking late (after 16 months)	2
Speech late (after 18 months) or abnormal	2
Problems with receptive language (30 to 36 months)	1
Ambidexterity (after 7 years)	2
Tiptoe walking prolonged (beyond 1 month)	1
Father history of alcoholism, sociopathy, hysteria	2
Father history of learning problems	1
Mother history of alcoholism, sociopathy, hysteria	1
Mother history of learning problems	1
Male relatives history of alcoholism, sociopathy, or hysteria	2
Female relatives history of alcoholism, sociopathy, or hysteria	1
One sibling with learning disabilities	1
More than one sibling with learning disabilities	2
Social or emotional stress in home at present	1
Institutionalization	2
Low socioeconomic status	2

*From Mercer, C. D., and Trifiletti, J. J.: 1977. The development of screening procedures for the early detection of children with learning problems, J. School Health **47**(9): 531.

of their behavior. The checklist might be completed by the parent, classroom teacher, and/or school nurse and could be the basis for a parent-nurse or teacher-nurse conference. The items included in the checklist are based on descriptive literature concerning hyperactivity (Haverkamp, 1970; Woodard and Brodie, 1974). This is not a standardized tool, nor have its validity and reliability been tested.

A simpler and quicker procedure than the PLSP for preliminary identification of children who are high risk for development of learning

Table 13-3. Summary of PLSP physical examination items and scoring weights

Anomaly	Weight
Head	
Circumference out of normal range for each age level	
>1.5 standard deviation	2
>1.0 standard deviation ≤ 1.5 standard deviation	1
Fine electric hair	1
Eyes	
Epicanthus: where upper and lower lids join with nose	
Point of union is deeply covered	2
Point of union is partly covered	1
Hypertelorism: approximate distance between tear ducts	
6 and 7 years = 3.2 cm	1
6 and 7 years ≥ 3.2 cm	2
Ears	
Adherent lobes: lower edges of ears extend	
Up and back toward crown of head	2
Straight back toward rear of neck	1
Asymmetrical	1
Mouth	
Dental enamel defects	
Enamel hypoplasia	2
Enamel hypocalcification	1
Enamel hypomaturation	1
High palate: roof of mouth is	
Definitely steepled	2
Flat and narrow at top	1
Hands	
Fifth finger markedly curved inward toward other finger	2
Fifth finger slightly curved inward toward other finger	1

*From Mercer, C. D., and Trifiletti, J. J.: 1977. The development of screening procedures for the early detection of children with learning problems, J. School Health **47**(9): 531.

disabilities is for the school nurse to follow up on all children who fail the reading readiness test usually given as part of the school readiness testing. The school nurse would take a thorough perinatal history on such children (Bogle, 1973) or could elect to use the PLSP to further assess their risk. Because this procedure only follows up children who have already experienced failure (on the reading readiness test), the yield from this type of case finding will probably be less than the yield from routine use of the PLSP for all preschoolers. However, in some school health programs, routine use of tools like the

PLSP may not be practical or advisable; in such cases, follow-up of children who have failed reading readiness and/or school readiness tests is an acceptable alternative.

As with all screening and early detection efforts, follow-up is the key to improved outcomes. Because children with learning disabilities and hyperactivity (behavior problems) have complex educational needs, interdisciplinary teamwork among the school health team or pupil personnel services team members is essential. Such teamwork must be maintained throughout the detection, diagnosis, and educational program planning processes (Haverkamp, 1970; Bogle, 1973; Woodard and Brodie, 1974; Logan, 1975).

Sensory processes

Because a child's ability to learn and to achieve academically depends to a great extent on the adequacy of his sensory processes, assessments of the child's vision, hearing, and speech and language skills become important baseline data in planning his educational program. The remainder of this discussion will focus briefly on considerations and recommendations for assessing children's vision, hearing, and speech/language.

Vision

Although there is general agreement that, ideally, every child should have a complete professional eye examination before starting school, the prohibitive costs and paucity of qualified professionals to perform the examinations has made this an unrealistic goal (Eisner and Oglesby, 1971b). Since most children entering school have *not* had a complete professional eye examination, and since visual problems, which increase significantly during the school years, must be detected promptly for optimal planning of children's educational experiences, it is likely that schools will continue to be involved in vision screening (Doster, 1971).

According to Eisner and Oglesby (1971b), most vision problems for which screening is done will be present at the time of school entrance and are not likely to develop later if they are not already present. Color vision and muscle balance are cited as examples; children with normal muscle balance (phoria or binocular coordination) and color vision at age 6 should continue having normal muscle balance and color vision throughout their school years. Therefore, Eisner and Oglesby (1971b) recom-

Behavior	Frequently	Seldom	Never
Overactivity			
Wears out clothing quickly, before he outgrows them			
Has trouble getting to sleep			
Awakens early			
Breaks toys before he loses interest in them			
Moves about constantly			
Cannot sit quietly for long			
Rocks back and forth, fidgets			
Talkative			
Perseverates (continuously repeats one behavior)			
Distractibility			
Is easily sidetracked (has a short attention span)			
Does not finish activities (such as homework)			
Frequently loses personal possessions (toys, coat, books)			
Cannot concentrate on an interesting task when multiple stimuli are present			

Behavior	Frequently	Seldom	Never
Impulsiveness			
Tends to be accident prone			
Is clumsy			
Laughs or cries easily			
Talks out of turn in class			
Is fearless			
Is uninhibited			
Viewed as a "pest" by others			
Excitability			
Has frequent temper tantrums			
Is aggressive: fights with peers and siblings			
Low frustration tolerance			
Is a clown or show-off			
"Overreacts" to unanticipated changes in routine			

Fig. 13-2. Checklist of behaviors associated with hyperactivity. (Modified from Woodard, P. B., and Brodie, B.: 1974. Nurs. Clin. North Am. **9**(4):728-729; and Haverkamp, L. J.: 1970. J. School Health **40**(5):229-230.)

mend that vision screening procedures be divided into two types: initial screening and subsequent screening.

Eisner and Oglesby point out that lack of agreement concerning the recommended nature and scope of initial vision screening procedures has resulted in controversy. They believe the root of the disagreement concerns philosophies of treatment—that is, at what degree of abnormality should a child's visual defect(s) be treated? This controversy unfortunately sometimes degenerates into a power struggle between groups of professional eye care specialists in the community, with optometrists and ophthalmologists "locking horns" in the debate. Because of the divisive and self-defeating consequences (for achievement of screening program objectives) of such conflict, Eisner and Oglesby strongly endorse establishment of an advisory planning committee represented by various eye care specialists as well as by parents, school officials, and others.

Authorities (Eisner and Oglesby, 1971b; Spollen and Davidson, 1978) agree that the next best thing to a complete eye examination by a qualified specialist is the Modified Clinical Technique (MCT) developed at the University of California during the 1950s. The MCT includes tests of visual acuity, binocular coordination (muscle balance), refractive error, and observation for ocular pathological conditions; its prime advantages are its moderate cost and low rate of underreferrals (false negatives). However, the usefulness of the MCT is limited by the necessity of having optometrists or ophthalmologists administer it; it cannot be given by nurses or teachers (Eisner and Oglesby, 1971b).

In contemplating inclusion of vision screening as part of the school health program, planners may be interested in prevalence rates of various visual problems among children. One of the important vision problems identified by Barker and Barmatz (1975) and Jenne and Greene (1976) is *amblyopia ex anopsia,* or "lazy eye" blindness, which is a dimness of vision that may result from unrecognized and untreated strabismus (muscle imbalance); the prevalence of amblyopia varies from 0.4% for children between ages 3 and 4 to 2% to 3% among school-age children. The prevalence of strabismus, also called "crossed eyes" or squint, is estimated to be between 1% and 4%, depending on the age group studied (Barker and Barmatz, 1975). Color vision deficiencies are

sex-linked hereditary traits affecting males more often than females; national estimates are that 7% to 7.5% of boys are affected, whereas less than 1% of girls are involved (Jenne and Greene, 1976). The most common vision problems are refractive errors, including hyperopia (farsightedness), myopia (nearsightedness), and astigmatism (inability to clearly see vertical and horizontal lines simultaneously). Refractive errors vary in prevalence from 6% to 7% among 6-year-olds to 15% among 15-year-olds (Barker and Barmatz, 1975). As Barker and Barmatz further note, the prevalence of these visual problems tends to increase with age, with the optimum time for treatment occurring between ages 4 and 6. Because symptoms of visual problems often do not appear until age 8 or 10, routine screening of asymptomatic children is advisable (1975). In fact, since the optimal time for treatment is between ages 4 and 6, comprehensive vision screening of *preschoolers* (Spollen and Davidson, 1978) is recommended.

Recommendations regarding age groups and frequency for vision screening vary (Doster, 1971; Jenne and Greene, 1976; AAP, 1977; Anderson and Creswell, 1980). Generally, authorities agree that vision screening should be done on entering school (including kindergarten or first grade as well as students who transfer into the school district). The National Society for the Prevention of Blindness (NSPB) (1969) advises full screening of acuity, hyperopia, and muscle balance at least every 2 or 3 years, with acuity-only testing done in the intervening years. Exact grade levels for screening can be locally determined. Based on the findings of their study of vision defects among preschoolers, Spollen and Davidson (1978) recommend that if financial or manpower resources are limited, priority should be given to elementary schools with large enrollments of children from low-income families. This recommendation resulted from data indicating that children from low-income families had three times as many referrable vision problems as children from high-income families.

In addition to the foregoing recommendations for deciding which children to screen and when, Jenne and Greene (1976) and Anderson and Creswell (1980) encourage individual follow-up, including any indicated vision testing, for children observed by teachers, parents, or the nurse to do the following: hold books too close or too far away when reading, have difficulty seeing the blackboard or other distant ob-

Table 13-4. Vision screening procedures for preschool and school-age children

Test	Purpose/description	Age group	Referral criteria	References
Cover test	Muscle balance or binocular coordination: observes errors in eye alignment with gaze fixed at distant and then near point to estimate deviation from parallel; detects heterophoria (latent strabismus) and heterotropia (manifest or frank strabismus)	Preschool and older	Given in prism diopters (D) for deviations: >1 D vertically >6 D inward >4 D outward at 20 feet >8 D outward at near distances	AAP, 1977 Eisner and Oglesby, 1971b NSPB, 1969 Spollen and Davidson, 1978
Direct observation (by nurse or teacher)	Observe (with or without ophthalmoscope) for obvious ocular pathological conditions	All ages	Nonallergic inflammations Frank strabismus Corneal or lenticular opacities Any detectable disease process	AAP, 1977 North, 1974
Hardy-Rand-Ritter (HRR) test	Color vision	Same as Ishihara test	Not applicable (see Ishihara test)	Doster, 1971 Jenne and Greene, 1976
Ishihara test	Color vision: uses pseudoisochromatic plates for color discrimination (red-green, blue-yellow)	Flexible, sixth or seventh grade	None; color blindness is not treatable; failure on test indicates need for vocational and predriver's training counseling	AAP, 1977 Doster, 1971 Jenne and Greene, 1976
Maddox Rod test	Muscle balance: uses stereoscopic machines	Preschool and older	Same as Cover test	Doster, 1971 Eisner and Oglesby, 1971b NSPB, 1969
Massachusetts vision test	Combination test using Snellen chart, plus lens and Maddox Rod test	Preschool and older	See individual tests	Eisner and Oglesby, 1971b
Miscellaneous machines: Bausch and Lomb School Vision Test Keystone School Telebinocular Test Titmus School Vision tester	Multiple use	Consult test manuals	Consult test manuals	Barker and Barmatz, 1975 Doster, 1971 Individual test manuals
Plus lens	Hyperopia (farsightedness): child attempts to read Snellen chart while wearing convex lenses of +2.25 D (preschool to fourth grade) or +1.75 D (fourth grade and older)	Preschool and older	Refer all children *who can* read 20/20 line	AAP, 1977 Doster, 1971 Eisner and Oglesby, 1971b NSPB, 1969

Continued.

Table 13-4. Vision screening procedures for preschool and school-age children—cont'd

Test	Purpose/description	Age group	Referral criteria	References
Snellen illiterate E chart	Visual acuity: child points out which direction E is facing	Preschool and grades one, two, and three	3 years: 20/50 or less 4 to 9 years: 20/40 or less Two-line acuity difference between R and L (anisometropia)	AAP, 1977 Anderson and Creswell, 1980 Barker and Barmatz, 1975 Doster, 1971 Eisner and Oglesby, 1971b Jenne and Greene, 1976 NSPB, 1969
Snellen mixed letter chart	Visual acuity: correctly reads letters	Fourth grade and older	10 years and older: 20/30 or less anisometropia	Spollen and Davidson, 1978 Same as above

jects clearly, cross their eyes, squint or frown when trying to see, rub their eyes excessively, shut or cover one eye while reading, blink excessively while doing close work, tilt their heads to see better, or complain of blurred or double vision, headaches, eye fatigue, or an inability to see well.

Table 13-4 presents an abbreviated list of available vision screening tests and procedures that may be incorporated into a school screening program. Further description and explanation of these and other tests may be found in the references cited in the table. Selection of specific tests should be made locally. Regardless of the test(s) selected, rescreening before referral is recommended as a means of minimizing costly overreferrals.

Barker and Barmatz (1975) also caution that vision screening outcomes are affected by procedural and situational factors, including the child's previous exposure to the test, how he feels (absence of fatigue, hunger, and anxiety), age and maturity, the test area lighting (too bright light may interfere with detection of refractive errors), presence of distractions, and personality and skills of the screener.

Hearing

In comparison with the issues surrounding vision testing, auditory screening is relatively noncontroversial. Although estimates of the prevalence of hearing loss vary (Northern, 1975; Jenne and Greene, 1976; AAP, 1977), approximately 3% to 6% of all children are affected. Authorities generally agree that early detection of medically remediable hearing loss helps prevent related problems in speech, social, and educational development.

Because early intervention for hearing impairment is advised (Eisner and Oglesby, 1971c; Northern, 1975), early and periodic screening of pediatric populations is suggested. Specifically, screening of high-risk neonates (risk is established from perinatal and family history) (Northern, 1975) and acoustic impedance testing of middle ear conduction for 2- to 4-year-olds with chronic or recurrent otitis media is encouraged (Northern, 1975). The AAP (1977) urges hearing tests for all preschoolers by age 4. Annual testing for children in kindergarten and grades one through three is suggested (Eisner and Oglesby, 1971c), with follow-up testing every 2 to 3 years thereafter; students should be tested at least once during junior and senior high school (AAP, 1977).

In addition to periodic screening for asymptomatic populations, auditory testing for children with known chronic and/or recurrent hearing problems should be provided as needed and at least annually (AAP, 1977). Jenne and Greene (1976) further recommend testing for any child exhibiting observable indications of possible hearing loss, including inattentiveness, asking to have questions or directions repeated, close watching of others' faces when speaking (attempts to lip-read), turning one ear toward a speaker, difficulty copying dictation, irrelevant responses to verbal questions or statements, mispronunciation of words, inappropriate speech volume (too loud or too soft), lack of response to sounds located next to or behind the student, failure to achieve up to his ability scholastically.

The two most common types of hearing loss in children are sensorineural and conductive (Woodford, 1973; Northern, 1975). *Sensorineural* losses vary in severity from mild to profound and are often frequency specific (especially affecting higher range frequencies); such losses are generally irreversible (Woodford, 1973). Sensorineural losses result from inner ear defects, auditory nerve damage, or damage to the auditory center in the temporal lobe of the brain (Northern, 1975; Jenne and Greene, 1976). Known causes of sensorineural losses include viral (especially measles and mumps) and bacterial infections; prolonged exposure to loud noises such as rock bands, gunfire, motorcycles, and power mowers; ototoxicity; congenital abnormality; and head trauma (Woodford, 1973; Northern, 1975; Jenne and Greene, 1976). Treatment for these losses includes auditory training with amplification devices (hearing aids), special education including lipreading, and speech therapy (Northern, 1975; Jenne and Greene, 1976).

Conductive hearing loss, which is the most common loss in children, results from a problem in the external ear canal, tympanic membrane, or middle ear cavity that interferes with transmission of sound (Northern, 1975). Causes include impacted earwax, foreign objects (beans, erasers, etc.) in the ear canal, otitis media, congenital abnormalities, and ruptured or scarred eardrums secondary to trauma or infection (Woodford, 1973; Northern, 1975; Jenne and Greene, 1976). Conductive losses can be mild or more severe and are considered "significant" when they interfere with the child's ability to communicate effectively

(Northern, 1975). Many cases of conductive loss respond to medical or surgical treatment (Jenne and Greene, 1976). However, Woodford (1973) points out the frustration involved in diagnosing and treating conductive losses; these losses fluctuate over time, so that a child who is referred to a physician for follow-up may not be experiencing the loss at the time of medical evaluation. This is another strong argument for the necessity of rescreening before referring a child (although children with a true and chronic conductive loss may experience these frustrating fluctuations over time).

Auditory screening is accomplished using pure tone audiometry. The two methods available are *threshold testing*, to establish the lowest volume (intensity) level at which the child can hear tones of a given frequency, and *sweep check testing*, to establish which frequencies can be heard when the volume remains fixed (Eisner and Oglesby, 1971c; AAP, 1977). The primary unresolved issue in hearing screening concerns which frequencies should be tested (Eisner and Oglesby, 1971c). It is suggested that program planners form an advisory committee represented by experts in audiology to help establish local testing plans and criteria, as well as plans for referral and follow-up.

Following studies (Harrelson et al., 1969) demonstrating the relative superiority of individual audiometry over group testing, group tests have become infrequent. Suggested individual auditory screening tests are listed in Table 13-5. These tests can be rapidly administered by a trained technician (or a school nurse).

Regardless of the test or screening procedure chosen, certain factors affecting the outcome of the test must be considered: suitability of the testing environment (avoidance of extraneous environmental noise and other distractions that may increase the number of false positives); calibration of the audiometer to ensure accuracy; and personal characteristics of the child at that time, such as illness, lethargy, boredom, anxiety, inattentiveness, and lack of cooperation (Northern, 1975).

Speech and language

For a child to grow and develop normally and benefit from school experiences, he must be able to communicate effectively with others. In assessing a child's communication, Weiss and Lillywhite (1976) appraise five areas: hearing, speech, voice, rhythm, and language. According to their definition, any "disorder of hearing,

Table 13-5. Auditory screening tests

Name	Description	Age group	References
Impedance audiometry	Uses acoustic impedance bridge instrument to assess middle ear	3 to 16 years	Northern, 1975
Preschool screening audiometry	Individually administered pure tone sweep check; cooperation of child gained through use of toys that child drops into box when he hears tone	3 to 5 years	Katz, 1972 Northern, 1975 Rose, 1971
School screening audiometry	Individually administered pure tone sweep check; may be followed by threshold testing	5 to 16 years	Eisner and Oglesby, 1971c Jenne and Greene, 1976 Katz, 1972 Northern, 1975 Rose, 1971
Verbal auditory screening of children (VASC)	Individually administered, or two children may be tested simultaneously; child's task is to listen to recorded word lists of gradually decreasing loudness and point to corresponding picture of named object	3 to 5 years	Northern, 1975

speech, voice, rhythm, or language, singly or in combination, that prevents an individual from adequately receiving communication from another person or communicating messages to another person, or both'' constitutes a *communication disorder* (1976:243).

Because good communication is important in the child's social and academic growth, early detection of communication disorders, before irreparable harm is done, is essential. Drumwright (1975) estimates that 12% to 15% of preschoolers and early school-age children have speech disorders that are serious enough to require treatment. She advocates speech and language screening for preschoolers (using the youngest age groups appropriate for each test) so that early intervention can be initiated. She believes that intervention is most successful with very young children, whose verbal skills are not firmly established. Since hearing problems and their detection have already been discussed, the remainder of this discussion will focus on the areas specifically included as ''speech'' and ''language.''

Before further describing methods for detecting children with speech or language problems, terms used in this chapter should be clarified as follows (Weiss and Lillywhite, 1976):

speech Refers ''primarily to articulation—the clarity, intelligibility, and accuracy of the phonemes used alone and combined in words'' (1976:100).
phoneme ''A unit of speech sound that may be a

single sound . . . or a combination of two sounds that makes one unit . . .'' (1976:250).
language ''Connected speech, words, phrases, sentences, paragraphs. The organized, connected structure of verbal communication as differentiated from speech'' (1976:246).

In determining which children need further assessment of their speech and language skills, lists of problematic behaviors that are associated with (but not necessarily indicative of) communication disorders, such as the one presented in Table 13-6, may be helpful. In addition, Gardner (1974) advises school nurses to review students' health records and to assess the speech and language abilities of children who have or have had speech and language therapy, hearing problems, poor motor coordination or other neurological handicaps, reconstructive oral surgery, severe dental malocclusion, chronic illness, cerebral palsy, or a special education classification.

In deciding which children need further study and/or intervention following review of checklists like Table 13-6, Weiss and Lillywhite (1976:124) suggest consideration of these questions:

Is there a deviation from normal?
Is communication interfered with?
Is attention called to it?
Is communication difficult to understand?
Do others tease or reject the child?
Are emotional or psychological problems resulting?

Table 13-6. Behaviors associated with speech/language disorders*

Assessment area	Problem behaviors
Articulation	Speech not readily intelligible unless listener knows subject matter Speech not 100% understandable by age 48 months Omits, substitutes, or distorts any phonemes after age 7 Most initial consonants omitted after age 3 Tongue is visible between upper and lower teeth when producing /s/ sound Speech sounds generally "slushy" Child is concerned or teased about speech (at any age)
Voice	Sounds chronically hoarse or breathy Complains of frequent hoarseness Coughs or clears throat frequently Voice frequently sounds nasal, monotonic, dysphonic, or whiny Pitch sounds abnormally high or low Abnormal volume (too loud or too soft)
Rhythm	"Struggles" to get words out; hesitates, stops and starts over Struggle accompanied by facial mannerisms such as blinking or tics Seems to have more trouble with sounds and syllables than with whole words Frequently repeats or prolongs individual sounds (stutters) Unable to produce any sounds at times Talks too fast or too slow
Linguistic development	Uses inappropriate grammar, such as pronoun usage, verb tense, pluralization, and direct objects at age 60 months Sentence word sequences incorrect (telegraphic, reversed, or confused) by age 48 months Has not begun asking questions by age 36 months Has trouble formulating thoughts, which leads to inappropriate verbal response Is concerned and/or teased about language used Illogical relationship between sentences Limited expressive vocabulary (fewer than 200 to 300 simple words) by age 60 months Does not use auxiliary verbs by age 48 months
Inner language concept development	Has difficulty with spatial concepts, quantitative concepts, and time concepts Has difficulty describing object's size, shape, color, or texture

*Modified from Weiss, C. E., and Lillywhite, H. S.: 1976. Communicative disorders: a handbook for prevention and early intervention, The C. V. Mosby Co., St. Louis; and Gardner, J. O.: 1974. Identification of children for speech and language referral, J. School Health **44**(5):255-256.

Table 13-7. Speech and language tests

Test name	Type	Age range	References
Denver Articulation Screening Examination (DASE)	Articulation	2½ to 6 years	Drumwright, 1975 Drumwright et al., 1973
Houston Test for Language Development	Language	Part I: 6 months to 3 years Part II: 3 to 6 years	Drumwright, 1975
Riley Articulation and Language Test	Articulation and language	Kindergarten, grades one and two	Drumwright, 1975
Templin-Darley Screening Test of Articulation	Articulation	3 to 8 years	Drumwright, 1975 Templin and Darley, 1969
Verbal Language Development Scale (VLDS)	Language	0 to 15 years	Drumwright, 1975

If the answer to most of these questions is "yes", referral is advisable.

Formal screening of selected children can be accomplished through tests such as those included in Table 13-7. Drumwright (1975) recommends referral of any children who achieve "abnormal" scores on formal tests.

Orthopedic screening

Following the success of pioneering programs conducted in the early 1960s (Cronis and Gleeson, 1974), orthopedic screening of school populations increased in popularity and credibility. Some authors (Banta, 1974; Cronis and Gleeson, 1974) encourage thorough assessments and inspections of children to detect a variety of orthopedic problems, including hip dysplasia, lordosis (swayback), kyphosis (humpback), genu valgum (knock-knees), genu varum (bowlegs), miscellaneous foot problems, and poor posture. However, this discussion will be confined to screening specifically for scoliosis because it is the most important and most serious of the pediatric orthopedic problems for which screening is available.

Scoliosis

The term *scoliosis* is used to describe a lateral, S-shaped curvature of the spine that may occur in the cervicothoracic, thoracic, or thoracolumbar regions (Banta, 1974). Etiologically, scoliosis is classified into two main types: nonstructural, or functional, scoliosis and structural scoliosis. *Nonstructural,* or *functional, scoliosis* involves no vertebral changes—such curves are postural or compensatory (such as for a leg length discrepancy) and disappear during forward or lateral bending; correcting the exogenous cause (such as poor posture) will correct the scoliosis; medical treatment is usually not indicated (Wynne-Davies, 1973; Hill and Romm, 1977). *Structural scoliosis* (Fig. 13-3) refers to a lateral curvature in which the vertebrae are rotated, producing visible changes such as the characteristic "rib hump" that is visible with the patient in Adams (forward-bending) position; early detection and treatment of structural scoliosis is vital in preventing or minimizing progressive disability (Lezberg, 1974; Weiler, 1974; Hill and Romm, 1977).

Structural scoliosis is etiologically classified as idiopathic, congenital, neuropathic, myopathic, osteopathic, thoracogenic, and miscellaneous (Shifrin, 1971). By far the most common type of scoliosis, with estimates of prevalence ranging from 70% (Hill and Romm, 1977) to 80% (Sells and May, 1974), is *structural idiopathic scoliosis,* the causes of which are poorly understood as the label implies. However, recent studies have demonstrated a genetic basis (probably transmitted by an autosomal dominant gene) for idiopathic scoliosis (Wynne-Davies, 1973; Banta, 1974; Hill and Romm, 1977). This genetic basis for scoliosis has led to broadened screening efforts to include siblings of affected children as well (Shifrin, 1971; Wynne-Davies, 1973; Wallace, 1977).

Precise prevalence figures for scoliosis are lacking, but estimates suggest that approximately 4.5% to 5% of children are affected (Sells and May, 1974; Hill and Romm, 1977; Wallace, 1977), with girls affected nearly eight times as often as boys (Banta, 1974). Idiopathic scoliosis is further classified as *infantile,* which affects children ages 0 to 3 years (usually boys), showing a left thoracic curve; *juvenile,* a right thoracic curve with onset between ages 4 to 10 years; and *adolescent,* which affects children age 10 years to skeletal maturity (primarily girls) usually showing a right thoracic or right thoracolumbar curve (Banta, 1974). According to Sells and May (1974), 80% to 90% of all cases of idiopathic scoliosis occur in preadolescent or adolescent girls.

Detection of idiopathic scoliosis in its early presymptomatic stage is difficult for a number of reasons. Children age 10 and older tend to be generally healthy and therefore do not necessarily have regular physical examinations. For those who do have periodic physicals, assessment of the back may not be included or may not be properly done. In addition, postural changes due to spinal curvature develop insidiously, so that the child and his parents may not notice them. This is further complicated by the fact that parents of older children and adolescents generally do not see their children undressed and therefore have no opportunity to observe the change. Adolescents who are aware of the change are not likely to report it, since the abnormality threatens the body image and identity they are trying to establish (Sells and May, 1974; Hill and Romm, 1977). Indeed, in some cases the first observation that something is wrong is the result of ill-fitting clothes (due to one shoulder being higher than the other, for example) or an uneven hemline (Shifrin, 1971; Barrett, 1977).

Because (for reasons just given) scoliosis is

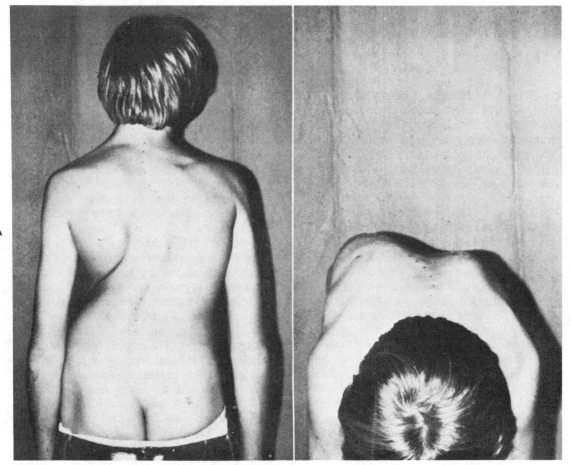

Fig. 13-3. Structural scoliosis. **A,** Structural scoliosis: the classic s-shaped curve. **B,** The characteristic "rib hump" as viewed in Adams position. (From Hill, P. M., and Romm, L. S.: 1977, MCN 2(3):157.)

not likely to be detected early by parents, family physicians, or children themselves, and because early treatment of scoliosis minimizes the severity of this incurable condition, screening of at-risk groups is an important case-finding tool. Early detection of scoliosis allows use of non-surgical treatment such as the Milwaukee brace; if treatment is delayed, spinal fusion may be necessary and yet not totally safe or satisfactory (Shifrin, 1971; Lezberg, 1974). The severity of the scoliotic curve increases rapidly during the adolescent growth spurt (Shifrin, 1971; Banta, 1974; Hill and Romm, 1977), adding to the urgency of early detection and treatment for adolescents. As Shifrin (1971) warns, untreated scoliosis can have serious complications in adulthood, including cardiopulmonary failure, chronic back pain, psychological problems re-

sulting from the changed body image, and employment problems due to employers' reluctance to hire persons with known back deformities.

Thus the school can make an important contribution to students' immediate and long-range health by providing scoliosis screening. The high-risk population, for whom annual (Wallace, 1977) or semiannual (Lezberg, 1974) screening is suggested, includes students age 10 and older, especially those in grades five through nine, plus the younger siblings (of any age) of students who are known to have scoliosis (Lezberg, 1974; Hill and Romm, 1977; Wallace, 1977).

Although detailed explanations of the screening examination procedure are available (Shifrin, 1971; Banta, 1974; Cronis and Gleeson,

1974; Lezberg, 1974; Weiler, 1974), the description included here will be brief. Most of these authors suggest that school nurses and physical education teachers be trained to perform the screening examinations. The actual screening can be done during physical education classes or at another scheduled time. The students should be dressed in a manner that does not conceal the back and chest; bathing trunks or shorts for boys and bathing suits or halter tops and shorts for girls are suggested (Hill and Romm, 1977). Students should be examined in the Adams forward-bending position from both front and rear to detect any rib hump (prominence or projection of rib cage) or lateral spinal curvature. The students should also stand erect with the feet together so the back may be inspected for any asymmetry, such as differences in shoulder and hip heights, an observable spinal curve, prominence of either scapula or hip, and any difference in size of the spaces between the arms and trunk (Hill and Romm, 1977).

Rescreening for those who fail the initial test is recommended (Sells and May, 1974). Since *any* spinal curvature is abnormal, students found with even the slightest spinal abnormality should be referred for further evaluation (Shifrin, 1971). Again, because of the rapid progression of scoliosis during adolescence, the immediacy of follow-up should be emphasized.

Other health problems and illnesses

In addition to the kinds of screening discussed previously in this chapter, planners of school screening programs may wish to consider the relative merits of screening for some other health problems or illnesses as well. To assist with such decision making, this discussion will briefly highlight additional health problems or defects for which screening of school populations may be contemplated. Due to limitations of space and scope, much of the relevant data concerning these screening tests is summarized and presented in Table 13-8. The reader is encouraged to consult the references cited with each test and others listed at the end of the chapter for more detailed discussion of these procedures and factors affecting their proper use.

Dental disease

Dental screening has been a traditional part of school health programs in the past. Children's needs for ongoing dental care have been well documented, and quality dental services are now widely available. Because dental screening for the purposes listed in Table 13-8 must be done by a dentist or dental hygienist, it is very costly. In fact, some authors (Eisner and Oglesby, 1972a) believe that the costs of dental screening often outweigh the benefits. Their recommendation, which makes good sense, is that in schools where most children receive good dental care, a screening program can be useful in identifying the few who need treatment. However, preventive dental health is important for all children, and even in schools where dental screening is uneconomical, good dental health education should be provided.

Cardiovascular disease

Another assessment category for which screening of school populations is sometimes suggested is cardiovascular disease. As shown in Table 13-8, cardiovascular screening is usually undertaken to detect congenital heart disease (CHD), rheumatic heart disease (RHD), and hypertension. These screening procedures can be useful in identifying those few children who have serious cardiac or vascular problems. However, some of the test procedures, such as the PhonoCardioScan, involve expensive equipment and skilled personnel to give and interpret the test. Thus the tests can be very expensive, especially if small numbers of children are being screened. Another factor in deciding whether to include cardiac screening in a program is the effect of the findings on the child's life. Some children have been erroneously "labeled" as cardiac patients through such screening, resulting (for some) in severe curtailment of their activity level and life-style. Again, if such screening is undertaken, careful interpretation of results and referral to a cardiologist for evaluation should be planned to avoid the psychological damage that results from labeling.

Communicable disease (tuberculosis)

Another traditional focus of the school health program has been communicable disease control. Of those diseases, tuberculosis (TB) received perhaps the most attention and has been the basis for mass screening efforts. However, the incidence and prevalence of TB have now dropped; Edwards (1974) reports that the number of new positive reactors to tuberculin skin tests among children entering school has been less than three children per 10,000 per year, a rate of 0.2%. Approximately 80% of new TB

Table 13-8. Screening for miscellaneous health problems

Assessment category/ health problem or defect	Screening method(s)	Screening population/ age group	Criteria for referral	References
Dental				
Dental caries	Use of tongue blade and flashlight to examine teeth for visible decay	Ages 3 years and older periodically Under age 3 years if any problems are noted	Penetrable soft discolored lesions on tooth crown	Bruck, 1975
Periodontal disease	Observation of color, texture, and shape of gums; check presence of subgingival calculus	Same as above	Overt inflammation and hemorrhage (eruptive gingivitis around loose primary and newly erupted secondary teeth is common and *not* in itself cause for referral)	Bruck, 1975 North, 1974
Malocclusion	Observation of bite, spacing, crowding, and overlapping of teeth; note missing teeth	Same as above	Any lower teeth outside upper teeth when biting together; presence of two teeth in space for one; overlapping teeth	Bruck, 1975
Cardiovascular				
Heart disease (HD) Rheumatic (RHD) Congenital (CHD)	Physician or nurse practitioner examination	All ages; only effective method for infants	Examiner's judgment; positive history for HD	Eisner and Oglesby, 1972b Thompson, 1975
	PhonoCardioScan computerized recording of heart sounds; best technique for large-scale screening of schoolchildren; can help "delabel" children; based on questionable cost-effectiveness and sensitivity, low RHD prevalence, and yield; blanket use is *not* recommended; use in geographic areas with high incidence of acute rheumatic fever and low socioeconomic status (SES) may be helpful	RHD: early teenage years, after junior high entrance, and after senior high entrance CHD: at birth and during first few months of life; it is *not* epidemiologically valid to screen schoolchildren for CHD General use: ages 4 years and older	Children whose test results are "outside normal limits" or "technically unsatisfactory" after second screening	Eisner and Oglesby, 1972b Matanoski et al., 1977 Thompson, 1975

Continued.

Table 13-8. Screening for miscellaneous health problems—cont'd

Assessment category/ health problem or defect	Screening method(s)	Screening population/ age group	Criteria for referral	References
Hypertension	Blood pressure: moderate elevations occur in 2% to 3% of children screened; medical significance of these elevations is unknown; suggest blood pressure measurement during routine health appraisals but not as screening initiative	School-age children	Persistent systolic blood pressure of 130 mm Hg or above and/or diastolic blood pressure of 90 mm Hg or above in children under 10 years; persistent systolic blood pressure of 140 mm Hg or above and/or diastolic blood pressure of 95 mm Hg or above in children over 10 years	AAP, 1977
Communicable disease				
Tuberculosis	Tuberculin skin tests			
	Mono-vacc (liquid concentrated old tuberculin)	All close (household or classroom) contacts of known TB patients: test initially and repeat 3 months after contact ends	Mono-vacc: *any* induration; confirm with Mantoux test	AAP, 1977 Edwards, 1974; 1975
	Tine test (dried concentrated old tuberculin)		Tine test: 2 mm induration; confirm with Mantoux test	AAP, 1977 Edwards, 1974; 1975
	Mantoux test (PPD-T 5TU) (intradermal administration)	All school personnel annually by Mantoux test; routine testing also recommended for children in families with history of TB, in neighborhoods or housing projects with TB prevalence higher than general community, with TB signs and symptoms, with increased risk due to special medical conditions (diabetes, neoplastic or immunological disease, and those on steroids or immunosuppressive drugs) *if* their TB skin test is positive	Doubtful reaction: 5 to 9 mm induration; positive reaction (basis for further diagnostic study) is 10 mm induration or more	AAP, 1977 Edwards, 1974; 1975

Special conditions

Condition	Test	Target population	Criteria	References
Plumbism	Free erythrocyte protoporphyrin (FEP)	High-risk children (those residing in old, substandard housing in eastern, southern, and midwestern United States); risk increases during summer months; target age group is 1 to 3 years	FEP ≥ ten times normal level and all with abnormal findings	Chisholm, 1975; Moriarty, 1974
	Blood lead concentration	Same as above	≥ 50 μg Pb/100 ml	Chisholm, 1975; Moriarty, 1974; AAP, 1977; North, 1974
Anemia	Hemoglobin test requires blood sample; measured in grams per 100 ml (g/100 ml)	Neonates and 1-year-olds; screen at school entry if no previous hemoglobin test was done; adolescents	Hemoglobin levels *less than**: 11 g/100 ml, ages 6 months to 10 years; 12 g/100 ml, ages 10 to 14 years; 13 g/100 ml, ages 14 years and older for males; 12 g/100 ml, ages 14 years and older for females	AAP, 1977; North, 1974
	Hematocrit test requires blood sample; expressed as percent (%)	Same as above	Hematocrit levels *less than**: 34% ages 6 months to 10 years; 37% ages 10 to 14 years; 41% ages 14 and older for males; 37% ages 14 and older for females	AAP, 1977; Eisner and Oglesby, 1972a; North, 1974
Asymptomatic urinary tract infection	Microculture technique (Testuria, Quantikit, or Uricult); midstream specimen preferred	Preschool girls (as soon as they can void on request); adolescent girls	Colony counts of 100,000/ml	Dodge, 1974; Eisner and Oglesby, 1972a; Kunin, 1974; North, 1974
	Microscopic examination	Same as above	Same as above	

*From American Academy of Pediatrics: 1977. School health: a guide for health professionals, Appendix G, American Academy of Pediatrics, Evanston, Ill. Copyright American Academy of Pediatrics.

cases are now found through follow-up of contacts of known cases or by examination of symptomatic persons seeking medical care. Therefore it is now recommended that routine periodic tuberculin testing of school-age children (using the methods and criteria presented in Table 13-8) be undertaken *only* if and when the prevalence of tuberculin sensitivity (known positive reactors) exceeds 1% or 10 per 1000 children (Edwards, 1974).

Plumbism

In 1970, the Surgeon General released a report advising periodic screening of blood lead levels for "all young children who live in or visit old dilapidated buildings" (Moriarty, 1974) and recommended stringent guidelines for follow-up and treatment of those with excessive levels of lead in the blood. This report was and is controversial, as is much of the debate concerning the true risks of plumbism. One of the previously discussed criteria for selecting conditions or diseases to include in a screening program is the adequacy of understanding of the natural history of the disease. The importance of having an agreed on policy regarding whom to treat as patients has also been discussed. In the case of plumbism, both of these criteria are unresolved and subject to much debate. Therefore screening efforts to detect plumbism should ideally by restricted to the population identified by age and location of residence in Table 13-8.

Anemia

Probably the most important age group to screen for anemia is infants, both neonates and 12-month-old infants (North, 1974). North believes that infants whose hemoglobin or hematocrit levels are normal at age 12 months probably are not at risk of anemia again until they begin their adolescent "growth spurt." Therefore screening of school-age children as a routine procedure is not necessary (except for those children entering school with no prior testing of hemoglobin or hematocrit levels) and is not always accepted by children (because it hurts) or their parents (because the test "breaks" the skin). Specific recommendations are included in Table 13-8.

Asymptomatic urinary tract infections

Screening for urinary tract infections is another controversial procedure. The most reasonable conclusion seems to be that it can be valid and useful *if* the population screened is limited to those most at risk—preschool age and adolescent girls. Specific tests and referral criteria are given in Table 13-8.

Other miscellaneous conditions

Among the screening procedures purposely omitted from Table 13-8 are those for *bacteriuria, glucosuria,* and *albuminuria*. Based on available references, screening for these conditions among school-age populations cannot be justified (Eisner and Oglesby, 1972a; Kunin, 1974; North, 1974; Dodge, 1975; AAP, 1977).

CONCLUSION

Although the information presented in this chapter is hardly more than a cursory overview of the careful planning needed to initiate and implement a screening program, it does provide data for basic decision making. The most important point to be retained from this chapter is that successful screening efforts are those contained within carefully planned and thoughtfully executed screening *programs*. Because well-planned screening programs have a holistic child health focus, they are important tools for achieving the objectives of the school health program.

REFERENCES

American Academy of Pediatrics: 1977. School health: a guide for health professionals, American Academy of Pediatrics, Evanston, Ill.

Anderson, C. L., and Creswell, W. H.: 1980. School health practice, 7th ed., The C. V. Mosby Co., St. Louis.

Bailey, J. T., and Claus, K. E.: 1975. Decision making in nursing, The C. V. Mosby Co., St. Louis.

Banham, K.: 1959. Maturity level for school entrance and reading readiness manual, American Guidance Service, Inc., Circle Pines, Minn.

Banta, J. V.: 1974. Early recognition of orthopedic problems in childhood, J. School Health **44**(1):38-40.

Barker, J., and Barmatz, H.: 1975. Eye function, Chapter 12. In Frankenburg, W. K., and Camp, B. W., editors: Pediatric screening tests, Charles C Thomas, Publisher, Springfield, Ill.

Barrett, M. J.: 1977. Surviving adolescence in a back brace, MCN **2**(3):160-163.

Bogle, M. W.: 1973. Relationship between deviant behavior and reading disability: a retrospective study of the role of the nurse, J. School Health **43**(5):312-315.

Bruck, T. L.: 1975. Dental screening, Chapter 11. In Frankenburg, W. K., and Camp, B. W., editors: Pediatric screening tests, Charles C Thomas, Publisher, Springfield, Ill.

Campbell, M. T., Garside, A. H., and Frey, M. E. C.: 1970. Community needs and how they relate to the school health program: S.H.A.R.P.—the needed ingredient, Am. J. Public Health **60**(3):507-514.

Campbell, W. D., and Camp, B. W.: 1975. Developmental screening, Chapter 14. In Frankenburg, W. K., and

Camp, B. W., editors: Pediatric screening tests, Charles C Thomas, Publisher, Springfield, Ill.

Children's Defense Fund: 1977. EPSDT, does it spell health care for poor children?, Children's Defense Fund, Washington D.C.

Chisholm, J.: 1975. Plumbism, Chapter 10. In Frankenburg, W. K., and Camp, B. W., editors: Pediatric screening tests, Charles C Thomas, Publisher, Springfield, Ill.

Coley, I. C.: 1978. Pediatric assessment of self-care activities, The C. V. Mosby Co., St. Louis.

Commission on Chronic Illness: 1957. Chronic illness in the United States, Vol. I: Prevention of chronic disease, Harvard University Press, Cambridge, Mass.

Cronis, S., and Gleeson, A. W.: 1974. Orthopedic screening of school children in Delaware, Phys. Ther. 54(10): 1080-1083.

Dodge, W. F.: 1975. Bacteriuria, Chapter 6. In Frankenburg, W. K., and Camp, B. W., editors: Pediatric screening tests, Charles C Thomas, Publisher, Springfield, Ill.

Doll, E. A.: 1965. Vineland social maturity scale condensed manual of directions, 4th ed., American Guidance Service, Inc., Circle Pines, Minn.

Doll, E. A.: 1966. Preschool attainment record: manual, American Guidance Service, Inc., Circle Pines, Minn.

Doster, M. E.: 1971. Vision screening in schools—why, what, how, and when? Clin. Pediatr. 10(11):662-665.

Drumwright, A. F.: 1975. Speech and language, Chapter 15. In Frankenburg, W. K., and Camp, B. W., editors: Pediatric screening tests, Charles C Thomas, Publisher, Springfield, Ill.

Drumwright, A. F., Van Natta, P. A., Camp, B. W., Frankenburg, W. K., and Drexler, H. G.: 1973. The Denver articulation screening exam, J. Speech Hear. Disord. 38(1):13-14.

Edwards, P. Q.: 1974. Tuberculin testing of children, Pediatrics 54(5):628-630.

Edwards, P. Q.: 1975. Tuberculosis, Chapter 7. In Frankenburg, W. K., and Camp, B. W., editors: Pediatric screening tests, Charles C Thomas, Publisher, Springfield, Ill.

Eisner, V., and Oglesby, A.: 1971a. Health assessment of school children. I. Physical examinations, J. School Health 41(5):239-242.

Eisner, V., and Oglesby, A.: 1971b. Health assessment of school children. III. Vision, J. School Health 41(8): 408-411.

Eisner, V., and Oglesby, A.: 1971c. Health assessment of school children. IV. Hearing, J. School Health 41(9): 495-496.

Eisner, V., and Oglesby, A.: 1972a. Health assessment of school children. V. Selecting screening tests, J. School Health 42(1):21-24.

Eisner, V., and Oglesby, A.: 1972b. Health assessment of school children. VII. Heart sound screening, J. School Health, 42(5):270-271.

Eisner, V., and Oglesby, A.: 1972c. Health assessment of school children. VIII. The unexpected health defect, J. School Health 42(6):348-350.

Eisner, V., Oglesby, A., and Peck, E. B.: 1972. Health assessment of school children. VI. Height and weight, J. School Health 42(3):164-166.

Erickson, M. L.: 1976. Assessment and management of developmental changes in children, The C. V. Mosby Co., St. Louis.

Fenske, J. M.: 1975. A new rationale for school health programming, J. School Health 45(10):569-576.

Ferinden, W. E.: 1972. The role of the school nurse in the early identification of potential learning disabilities, J. School Health 42(2):86-87.

Frankenburg, W. K.: 1974. Selection of diseases and tests in pediatric screening, Pediatrics 54(5):612-616.

Frankenburg, W. K.: 1975a. Principles in selecting diseases for screening, Chapter 1. In Frankenburg, W. K., and Camp, B. W., editors: Pediatric screening tests, Charles C Thomas, Publisher, Springfield, Ill.

Frankenburg, W. K.: 1975b. Criteria in screening test selection, Chapter 2. In Frankenburg, W. K., and Camp, B. W., editors: Pediatric screening tests, Charles C Thomas, Publisher, Springfield, Ill.

Frankenburg, W. K., and Dodds, J. B.: 1967. The Denver developmental screening test, J. Pediatr. 71(8):181-191.

Frankenburg, W. K., Dodds, J. B., and Fandal, A. W.: 1970. Denver developmental screening test manual, rev. ed., University of Colorado Medical Center, Denver.

Frankenburg, W. K., Camp, B. W., and Van Natta, P. A.: 1971a. Validity of the Denver developmental screening test, Child Dev. 42:475-485.

Frankenburg, W. K., Camp, B. W., Van Natta, P. A., and Demersseman, J. A.: 1971b. Reliability and stability of the Denver developmental screening test, Child Dev. 42: 1315-1325.

Frankenburg, W. K., van Doorninck, W. J., Liddell, T. N., and Dick, N. P.: 1976. The Denver prescreening developmental questionnaire (PDQ), Pediatrics 57(5): 744-753.

Gardner, J. O.: 1974. Identification of children for speech and language referral, J. School Health 44(5):255-256.

Goldstein, A. D.: 1975. School readiness and achievement, Chapter 16. In Frankenburg, W. K., and Camp, B. W., editors: Pediatric screening tests, Charles C Thomas, Publisher, Springfield, Ill.

Harrelson, O. A., Ferguson, D. G., Killian, G. P., and Zimmer, I.: 1969. Comparison of hearing screening methods, J. School Health 39(3):161-164.

Harris, D. B.: 1963a. Children's drawings as measures of intellectual maturity: a revision and extension of the Goodenough draw-a-man test, Harcourt Brace Jovanovich, Inc., New York.

Harris, D. B.: 1963b. Goodenough-Harris drawing test manual, Harcourt Brace Jovanovich, Inc., New York.

Haverkamp, L. J.: 1970. Brain-injured children and the school nurse, J. School Health 40(5):228-235.

Hill, P. M., and Romm, L. S.: 1977. Screening for scoliosis in adolescents, MCN 2(3):156-159.

Iglehart, V. R., Conner, D., and Sinnette, C. H.: 1977. A comprehensive school health program in Harlem: a retrospective view, J. School Health 47(2):88-93.

Jenne, F. H., and Greene, W. H.: 1976. Turner's school health and health education, 7th ed., The C. V. Mosby Co., St. Louis.

Katz, J.: 1972. Handbook of clinical audiology, The Williams & Wilkins Co., Baltimore.

Kirk, S. A., and Bateman, B. D.: 1962. Diagnosis and remediation of learning disabilities, Exceptional Child 29:73-78.

Kunin, C. M.: 1974. Current status of screening children for urinary tract infections, Pediatrics 54(5):619-621.

Lessler, K.: 1972. Health and educational screening of school-age children—definition and objectives, Am. J. Public Health 62(2):191-198.

Lessler, K.: 1974. Screening, screening programs and the pediatrician, Pediatrics **54**(5):608-611.

Lezberg, S. F.: 1974. Screening for scoliosis: preventive medicine in a public school, Phys. Ther. **54**(4):371-372.

Logan, B. A.: 1975. Kindergarten screening program for learning disabilities, J. School Health **45**(7):413-414.

Matanoski, G. M., Henderson, M. M., Stine, O. C., Courpas, C., Hepner, R., and Walker, S.: 1977. Evaluation of a screening program for heart disease, Am. J. Public Health **67**(7):609-611.

Mayshark, C., Shaw, D. D., and Best, W. H.: 1977. Administration of school health programs: its theory and practice, 2nd ed., The C. V. Mosby Co., St. Louis.

McCammon, R. W.: 1975. Postnatal growth, Chapter 3, Growth measurements. In Frankenburg, W. K., and Camp, B. W., editors: Pediatric screening tests, Charles C Thomas, Publisher, Springfield, Ill.

Mercer, C. D., and Trifiletti, J. J.: 1977. The development of screening procedures for the early detection of children with learning problems, J. School Health **47**(9): 526-532.

Moriarty, R. W.: 1974. Screening to prevent lead poisoning, Pediatrics **54**(5):626-628.

National Society for the Prevention of Blindness: 1969. Vision screening of children, National Society for the Prevention of Blindness, New York.

North, A. F.: 1974. Screening in child health care: where are we now and where are we going? Pediatrics **54**(5): 631-640.

Northern, J.: 1975. Auditory Screening, Chapter 13. In Frankenburg, W. K., and Camp, B. W., editors: Pediatric screening tests, Charles C Thomas, Publisher, Springfield, Ill.

Rogers, K. D., and Reese, G.: 1964. Health studies: presumably normal high school students, Am. J. Dis. Child. **108**(12):572-600.

Rose, D. E.: 1971. Audiological assessment, Prentice-Hall, Inc., Englewood Cliffs, N.J.

Scriver, C. R.: 1974. PKU and beyond: when do costs exceed benefits? Pediatrics **54**(5):616-618.

Sells, C. J., and May, E. A.: 1974. Scoliosis screening in public schools, Am. J. Nurs. **74**(1):60-62.

Shifrin, L. Z.: 1971. Recognizing scoliosis early, Am. Fam. Physician **4**(6):76-82.

Spollen, J. J., and Davidson, D. W.: 1978. An analysis of vision defects in high and low income preschool children, J. School Health **48**(3):177-180.

Templin, M. C., and Darley, F. L.: 1969. The Templin-Darley tests of articulation, 2nd ed., Bureau of Educational Research, University of Iowa, Iowa City, Iowa.

Thompson, R. S.: 1975. Cardiac Screening, Chapter 8. In Frankenburg, W. K., and Camp, B. W., editors: Pediatric screening tests, Charles C Thomas, Publisher, Springfield, Ill.

Thorpe, H. S., and Werner, E. E.: 1974. Developmental screening of preschool children: a critical review of inventories used in health and educational programs, Pediatrics **53**(3):362-370.

Uyeda, F. F.: 1972. The detection of learning disabilities in the early school age child, specifically the kindergarten child, J. School Health **42**(4):214-217.

Vane, J. R.: 1968. The Vane kindergarten test, J. Clin. Psychol. (Supplement) **24**(2):121.

Wallace, A.: 1977. A scoliosis screening program, J. School Health **47**(10):619-620.

Weiler, D. R.: 1974. Scoliosis screening, J. School Health **44**(10):563-565.

Weiss, C. E., and Lillywhite, H. S.: 1976. Communicative disorders: a handbook for prevention and early intervention, The C. V. Mosby Co., St. Louis.

Woodard, P. B., and Brodie, B.: 1974. The hyperactive child: who is he? Nurs. Clin. North Am. **9**(4):727-745.

Woodford, C.: 1973. A perspective on hearing loss and hearing assessment in school children, J. School Health **43**(9):572-576.

Wynne-Davies, R.: 1973. Genetic aspects of idiopathic scoliosis, Dev. Med. Child Neurol. **15**(6):809-821.

Yankauer, A., and Lawrence, R. A.: 1955. A study of periodic school medical examinations. I. Methodology and initial findings, Am. J. Public Health **45**(1):71-78.

Yankauer, A. et al.: 1956. A study of periodic school medical examinations. II. The annual increment of new defects, Am. J. Public Health **46**(6):1553-1562.

SUGGESTED READINGS

Eisner, V., and Oglesby, A.: 1971. Health assessment of school children. II. Screening tests, J. School Health **41**(7):344-346.

Frankenburg, W. K., and Camp, B. W., editors: 1975. Pediatric screening tests, Charles C Thomas, Publisher, Springfield, Ill.

Hodgson, W. R.: 1968. Audiometric screening and threshold norms, J. School Health **38**(6):373-376.

Hollien, H., Wepman, J. M., and Thompson, C. L.: 1969. A group screening test of auditory acuity, J. School Health **39**(8):583-588.

Kaluger, G., and Kaluger, M. F.: 1979. Human development: the span of life, 2nd ed., The C. V. Mosby Co., St. Louis.

Meskin, L. H., Kenney, J. B., Martens, L., and Meskin, E. R.: 1977. A preventive dental program for "high risk" children, J. School Health **47**(5):293-295.

Murray, R., and Zentner, J.: 1979. Nursing assessment and health promotion through the life span, 2nd ed., Prentice-Hall, Inc., Englewood Cliffs, N.J.

Parker, P. W.: 1974. The nurse's role in the early periodic screening, diagnosis, and treatment program, ANA Clin. Sess., American Nurses' Association, San Francisco.

Schoenwetter, C. D.: 1974. Primary care's responsibility to early success in school, J. School Health **44**(6):307-309.

PART VI

Systematic processes in school nursing

CHAPTER 14

The nursing process and the nurse-client contract

SUSAN J. WOLD

Nursing's quest for full recognition as a profession in its own right has been stymied by a number of factors. One of the most obviously limiting factors has been the fact that nursing has been the "stepchild" of medicine, to whom nursing historically looked for education and training, supervision, and employment. When responsibility for providing nursing education was finally assumed by nurses, medicine's hold over the profession loosened, and the drive toward professionalism was launched. However, as nursing leaders and educators soon realized, nursing did not have a body of knowledge that was uniquely its own; hence, of necessity nurses borrowed concepts and theories from other professions and disciplines to guide their practice.

A related problem is the fact that without a clearly defined, scientifically tested body of knowledge that is universally accepted as "nursing," nurses have not consistently provided sound, comprehensive, and well-thought-out client/patient care. The varying educational preparation levels (associate degree, diploma, and baccalaureate degree) for entry into nursing have further complicated the problem of providing consistently high-quality and scientifically based client/patient care. Indeed, the lack of agreement about what nursing is, how it should be practiced, and by whom has all too often resulted in nursing by intuition instead of nursing by systematic process.

The ability of nursing to achieve full stature and recognition as a profession will depend in large part on nurses' ability to define, articulate, and defend their practice and on their ability to *document* the process and outcomes of practice. Application of the nursing research process (Chapter 17) will help articulate nursing theory, standards of practice, and nursing care approaches. However, the responsibility for providing high-quality, scientifically based nursing care and for documenting and evaluating outcomes rests with the individual professional nursing practitioner. To carry out that responsibility, the nurse must use another systematic process: the nursing process.

In the remainder of this chapter, two systematic processes will be described: the nursing process and the process of contract setting. Both processes are essential for provision of high-quality nursing care to clients in all settings. These processes are discussed together because they are interdependent; that is, successful application of the nursing process requires involvement of the client in his own care (through a nurse-client contract), and successful application of the contract-setting process depends on the use of the nursing process. These processes will be *discussed* consecutively to avoid confusion. However, in actual practice, these processes may *occur* simultaneously and may therefore overlap to some degree.

THE NURSING PROCESS

According to Yura and Walsh (1973), the nursing process was first mentioned in the literature during the 1950s but was not widely discussed until the 1960s. They report that the initial reaction of many nurses to introduction of the term "nursing process" was: "Oh, we've been doing that all along." Yura and Walsh agree that nurses have generally used the nursing process in assessing clients' needs and planning nursing care to meet them; however, they believe that deliberative evaluation of outcomes, which is an integral step in the nursing process, has not always been carried out. In addition, as noted earlier, logical nursing care planning based on careful assessment of needs, as well as thoughtful implementation of nursing care and thorough evaluation of process and

317

outcomes are necessary components of nursing practice if nursing is to be a full-fledged profession.

Definition and purpose

The nursing process has been described (Yura and Walsh, 1973:1) as "central to all nursing actions" and as the "very essence of nursing." One might logically expect that a process so fundamentally important to a profession would be clearly understood and uniformly defined by all practitioners. However, that is not the case with the nursing process. It is ironic and somewhat amusing to note that members of the nursing profession, who are frequently challenged by other health care professionals to articulate and account for their practice, cannot even agree among themselves as to the number and labeling of the steps in this process, which has been described as the "essence of nursing"! Indeed, estimates of the number of steps in the nursing process vary from three (Carlson, 1972; Boland et al., 1975) to four (Yura and Walsh, 1973; Marriner, 1979) to five (Bloch, 1974; Stuart and Sundeen, 1976).

However, review of the literature indicates that despite disagreements about the number of steps in the process or their labels, these differences are primarily semantic; the actual process described is the same. For the purposes of this chapter, the following definition of the *nursing process* proposed by Yura and Walsh (1973:23) will be used:

The nursing process is an orderly, systematic manner of determining the client's problems, making plans to solve them, initiating the plan or assigning others to implement it, and evaluating the extent to which the plan was effective in resolving the problems identified.

As described in this definition, then, the steps in the nursing process are assessment (which includes data collection and nursing diagnosis or problem definition), planning, implementation, and evaluation. It should be noted, however, that identification of specific steps in the nursing process does not mean that nursing practice consists of discrete, strictly sequential steps beginning with assessment and ending with evaluation. Rather, the "steps" in the process may be used concurrently and recurrently; thus reassessment of the client's needs may continue throughout the process, and evaluation may result in reassessment and possible revision of the plan and its implementation (ANA, 1973).

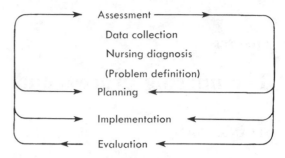

Fig. 14-1. The nursing process.

Thus the nursing process is a continuous cycle (Marriner, 1979) (Fig. 14-1).

The overriding purpose of any nursing practice actions of course is to promote high-level wellness for the client within his capabilities, whether that client is an individual, family or group, or community (Stuart and Sundeen, 1976). As Carlson (1972) more specifically explains, the basic purpose of the nursing process is to encourage the nurse to use a problem-solving approach as she assists the client to achieve his optimal level of wellness. In other words, the nursing process discourages nursing by intuition and encourages nursing by systematic process.

Assessment

As illustrated in Fig. 14-1 and as defined by Bloch (1974:692), *assessment* includes "both the process of data collection and the interpretation of such data." Together, these two actions make up the first step of the nursing process, since without assessment there can be no systematic development of a nursing care plan.

Data collection

According to Bloch (1974:692), *data collection* is "the gathering of more or less objective facts without an interpretive component." For the nursing diagnoses or defined problems to accurately reflect the client's health status, the data collection on which they are based must be thorough. Thoroughness can be ensured by use of a systematic approach to data collection and by continuous efforts to update it. In fact, this type of comprehensive data collection is an expectation for which all nurses are held accountable, as indicated in Standard I of the ANA (1973):

The collection of data about the health status of the client/patient is systematic and continuous. The data are accessible, communicated, and recorded.

This standard further specifies that the kinds of data to be collected include biophysical and emotional status; growth and development; cultural, religious, and socioeconomic background; performance of activities of daily living (ADLs); coping and interaction patterns; environmental factors; availability and accessibility of resources (human and material); client's perception of and satisfaction with his health status; and client's health goals (ANA, 1973).

The assessment factors just identified are common to all persons. However, depending on the unique characteristics of the client and his situation, the data collection procedure must be adjusted and adapted to ensure that all data relevant to this particular client at this point in time are collected and recorded. The setting in which the nurse practices may also influence the data collection procedure to some extent (Yura and Walsh, 1973). For example, the school nurse, whose clients are primarily school-age children and youth, would most likely focus on those factors which her knowledge, experience, and school health program goals indicate are most important in meeting the needs of that population. Thus the school nurse might focus on growth and development, emotional status, and coping patterns for her school-age population in general and might focus more specifically on management of ADLs, biophysical status, emotional status, availability of resources, and coping patterns (plus any other pertinent areas of concern) for the handicapped child who is adjusting to the school environment. These latter suggestions are merely examples and not exhaustive or comprehensive lists of assessment factors especially relevant for the school nurse within her setting. The nurse must always rely on her judgment and knowledge base in deciding which assessment areas to pursue in depth.

There are usually a number of data sources regarding the client's health status. One obvious source of data is the client himself. The nurse, using her systematic assessment skills (Chapter 12) and helping relationship skills (Chapters 10 and 11) collects data from the client through physical assessment procedures (inspection, auscultation, palpation, and percussion); history taking; and other nurse-client communication opportunities, such as the interview (structured, using an interview guide, nursing history form, data base, or checklist; semistructured; or unstructured).

Other sources of data include the client's family and "significant others." For the schoolchild, the significant others may include peers, teachers, school counselors, ministers, coaches, and other health care professionals to name just a few. The nurse may collect data from these persons through interviews, case conferences, or sharing of records (which, incidentally, must be done within the legal and ethical limits imposed by privacy or confidentiality laws, policies, and guidelines).

In addition, the client's current health record as maintained within the nurse's practice setting, whether that is a school, hospital, clinic, or other facility, is a ready source of important data concerning the client's health status and history *if* that record contains complete documentation of health history and prior health problems, including any interventions and their outcomes, and *if* that data is recorded in an intelligible and retrievable format, such as the POHR. For the schoolchild, another potential source of relevant data may be the student's cumulative record, which contains data concerning all aspects of his school experience, including psychological and achievement test data, grade and course transcripts, and other descriptions of the child's behavior and school participation.

As specified in the ANA standard concerning data collection (p. 318) the data collection procedure should be systematic and continuous, and the collected data should be recorded in an accessible or retrievable format. The POHR, as described in Chapter 12 and further elaborated on by Vaughan-Wrobel and Henderson (1976) and Berni and Readey (1978), is one format that more than adequately meets those criteria. Because the steps of the POHR format (generation of a data base, development of a problem list, formulation of a nursing care plan, implementation of the plan, and monitoring and evaluation of outcomes through ongoing SOAP and evaluation of EOC achievement) closely approximate the steps in the nursing process, the POHR format can be initiated in most settings with little or no adjustment of the nurse's approach to problem identification and problem solving. The format of the POHR enhances retrievability of data because there is a "right" place to record all kinds of data as well as the interpretation of that data. Furthermore, the POHR system is readily understood by other health care professionals, which improves the communication between those professionals; this is an especially important feature for school health records, which follow a child from one institution and/or district to another. Thus, although the POHR is not "the" only format for school health records, it is an ideal format.

Nursing diagnosis or problem definition

Once the data collection has been completed, the nurse is ready to conclude the assessment by interpretation of that data through formulation of a nursing diagnosis or definition of problems. Because nurses have been successfully socialized to believe that diagnosis is the sole province of the physician, they have been generally reluctant to state their assessments with any strong conviction and have scrupulously and timorously avoided use of the word "diagnosis" to describe their conclusions; in fact, in those situations where nurses have risked diagnosing, they have too often qualified their diagnoses with modifiers like "seems to have . . ." and "appears to be. . . ."

Because of the strong medical connotation of the word "diagnosis" and because of the general reluctance of nurses to apply it to the assessments they make, Bloch (1974) suggests use of the term "problem definition" as a substitute for "nursing diagnosis." However, Bloch's (1974:692) description of *problem definition* as the process "where judgment is brought to bear on the data by critical analysis and interpretation," applies (by her own admission) to the process of *nursing diagnosis* as well. Indeed, the definitions of nursing diagnosis proposed by others (Chambers, 1962; Komorita, 1963; Durand and Prince, 1966; Rothberg, 1967) are so similar to the description of *problem definition* just given that the differences are largely semantic. The importance of universal adoption of the term *nursing diagnosis* to describe the outcomes of nurses' assessments has been clearly articulated by Gordon (1978:264), who warns that:

. . . Until nurses can name the health problems they treat, nursing will remain a vague entity to legislators, third-party payers, administrators, professional colleagues, and sometimes to other nurses.

Therefore, because of the importance of nursing diagnosis to the economic and professional survival of nursing and because the term is becoming increasingly acceptable to nurses, in the remainder of this chapter the term *nursing diagnosis* will be used to describe the outcomes of the nursing assessment process. The specific definition used for nursing diagnosis will be the one advanced by Gebbie and Lavin (1975:114); according to their definition, *nursing diagnosis* denotes "the judgment or conclusion that occurs as a result of nursing assessment."

The mandate for formulation of nursing diagnoses is clearly presented in the second standard of nursing practice established by the ANA (1973):

Nursing diagnoses are derived from health status data.

Although there is no universally accepted format for statement of nursing diagnoses, there is widespread agreement concerning the purpose of nursing diagnoses and their basic content. As a result of this predominant spirit of agreement, the recent literature concerning nursing diagnoses has focused primarily on refinement of the diagnostic process and taxonomic classification of nursing diagnoses in current use (Gebbie and Lavin, 1975).

The ANA's rationale for inclusion of a standard mandating formulation of nursing diagnoses is that data analysis to determine the client's health status is a necessary precursor to identification of nursing care needs and subsequent development of a nursing care plan. In diagnosing the client's health status, the ANA suggests that the client's health data be compared with existing norms to detect any deviation from them. These norms could include standardized accepted ranges of "normal" as in laboratory test data or could entail comparison of the client's present status with his former "normal" or baseline data. Once deviations from the norm are detected, the diagnostic process requires that the degree and direction of the deviation (that is, above or below normal) be noted (ANA, 1973).

The nursing diagnosis process also involves identification of the client's capabilities and limitations. Examples of data to be assessed for this purpose include the client's management of ADLs and overall coping patterns. In addition, it is important that the nursing diagnoses formulated for the client are related to and congruent with the diagnoses developed by the other professionals who are also caring for the client in some capacity (ANA, 1973). If their diagnoses are *not* congruent, their care plans are also likely to be incongruent; the unfortunate result of these inconsistent care plans is likely to be conflicting goals for the client, possibly indicating that the nurse is actually working *against* other health care team members. The net outcome of all this confusion and conflict among the caregivers is likely to be the client's conclusion that (1) they do not know what they are doing (resulting in the client's total lack of faith in their ability to manage his care), (2) these caregivers therefore cannot be trusted to safely care for him, and (3) since they all seem to contradict one another, ignoring all of them is the safest option. Unfortunately, this latter conclusion may well be "hazardous to his health," since by ignoring *all* advice and assistance, the client may unwittingly be "throwing the baby out with the bath water."

Suggestions as to the content of nursing diagnoses have been offered by a number of authorities, including Gebbie and Lavin (1975) and Yura and Walsh (1973). In addition to their suggestions, Gordon (1978:265-266) proposes that nursing diagnoses be developed with the following three components:

1. *State-of-the-patient* (client) or *health problem*. Qualifying or quantifying adjectives or other means are used to indicate stages, phases, or levels of the problem.
2. *Etiology of the problem*. Identification of the cause is important because the kind of treatment or other nursing action to be carried out will depend on the cause of the problem.
3. *Signs and symptoms*. These are the patient behaviors used to make the diagnosis.

Gordon refers to these components collectively as the problem-etiology-signs/symptoms (PES) format for nursing diagnoses and points out that this format can be readily adapted to most charting or record-keeping systems, including the POHR.

Nurses across the country are working to develop and refine the classification systems for nursing diagnoses that were proposed at the First National Conference on the Classification of Nursing Diagnoses held in St. Louis in 1975. The detailed proceedings of that conference have been scrupulously reported by Gebbie and Lavin (1975) so that all nurses can review and critique them. There are many divergent opinions concerning the precise content, wording, format, and classification of nursing diagnoses. It is therefore important that *all* nurses review and react to these proposals and that *all* nurses become involved in the process of refinement in some way, since the decisions that will be made will affect standards of practice for *all* nurses. The goal of this process is to assist nurses in defining and articulating the health problems they treat; nurses cannot and do not wish to make *medical* diagnoses, which are distinctly different from nursing diagnoses (Soares, 1978). However, nurses can and must articulate their assessments, and nursing diagnoses are the means for doing so.

Planning

The purpose of the planning phase is to identify solutions for the client's diagnosed problems. During the planning process, then, goals are formulated, priorities are established, persons responsible for implementing the plan are designated, and a written nursing care plan or "blueprint for action" is formulated as the end product of the planning process (Yura and Walsh, 1973).

While health care professionals, including nurses, are too often accustomed to "taking over" and making parental yet well-intentioned decisions on behalf of the client, it is important to remember that the client is responsible for his own health and well-being. Therefore, although the nurse and other health care professionals certainly have a knowledge base and clinical expertise to apply on the client's behalf, the client should be included in the problem-solving and decision-making processes. The problem, after all, belongs to the client and usurping his right to participate in the process of planning its solution can not only interfere with his ability and motivation to assume responsibility for his health, but can also jeopardize the success of the plan. Therefore, to ensure that the plan for solution of his health problems is appropriate and realistic and to increase the likelihood of his compliance with it, the client must participate in the planning process.

Planned outcomes: goals and EOCs

Once nursing diagnoses have been formulated (or problems defined), solutions or treatments must be planned. However, nursing actions cannot be planned until the desired outcome is known. Thus the nursing care plan must identify *goals* or desired outcomes. Indeed, the nursing standards published by the ANA (1973:Standard III) further emphasize the importance of goal setting:

The plan of nursing care includes goals derived from the nursing diagnoses.

The assessment factors published with the standard as means of evaluating compliance with it, emphasize the importance of *mutual* goal setting, which should include the client/

patient and others involved in his care. In addition, the assessment factors specify that the goals should be stated in *realistic* and *measurable* terms, with a *designated time period* for their achievement (ANA, 1973).

Although this expectation that goals be stated realistically in measurable terms (behaviorally) and with a specified time frame seems reasonable, it is not always easily achieved. For students and other uninitiated persons, writing behavioral goals is an acknowledged problem (Marriner, 1979). First of all, it is often difficult for students, because of their lack of experience, to know what goals are realistic for a given client; for that reason, and because of their idealism and enthusiasm, students may unrealistically expect a client to completely and immediately change a lifelong behavior pattern as a result of their nursing actions. To avoid unrealistic expectations that jeopardize success, the nursing care plan must be based on a realistic assessment of the client's ability and willingness to change his behavior.

Another problem confronting students and others in writing behavioral goals and objectives for the nursing care plan involves stating those goals and objectives in *measurable* terms. So-called behavioral objectives that are written with verbs such as "knows" or "understands" or "appreciates" are *not* measurable as stated. The nurse must therefore decide what *behaviors* she expects to occur that will indicate the client does indeed "know," "understand," or "appreciate"; examples of appropriate behavioral verbs would include "verbalizes," "demonstrates," "applies," and "describes." The inability of many students and graduate nurses to write behavioral, measurable goals and objectives is partially the result of inexperience in writing goals and objectives and partially due to gaps and omissions in nursing curricula. For those reasons, many baccalaureate nursing students and graduate nurses educated in years past simply have not had the opportunity to learn to write measurable goals. However, while lack of experience and educational preparation are valid explanations of the problem, they must *not* be used as excuses for continued ignorance. Skill in writing behavioral goals and objectives is essential for all nurses, and individual practitioners must assume responsibility for developing such skills, whether through use of self-directed, programmed learning methods (Mager, 1962) or through more formal means such as enrollment in continuing education courses and workshops.

The ANA's (1973) assessment factors for nursing Standard III also specify that the nursing goals established "maximize functional capabilities" of the client; in other words, the client should be assisted to achieve his optimal level of functioning within whatever limitations or handicaps he may have. Furthermore, the stated goals must be consistent with the client's growth and development, biophysical status, behavioral patterns, and the available and accessible human and material resources.

As discussed in Chapter 13, the measurability of the nursing goals or objectives is enhanced by the use of EOCs, which represent the subdivision of a particular goal or objective into its specific, finite component behaviors, the sum of which equals achievement of the entire objective. Therefore the list of EOCs for a given goal should be sufficiently exhaustive to include *all* behaviors, which, when collectively achieved, indicate that the overall goal or objective has been met. In addition, the usefulness of EOCs is directly proportional to their specificity; their specificity can be enhanced by stating the *number of times* a behavior will occur, the *frequency* with which it will occur, the *conditions* in which it will occur (if appropriate), the *time period* allowed for achievement, as well as a *precise description* of the behavior itself.

Priority setting

Because it is not feasible or humanly possible to focus equally on all the client's health problems or nursing diagnoses simultaneously, priorities must be established. As defined by Marriner (1979:89), *"priority setting is the process of establishing a preferential order in the delivery of nursing care."* Those problems or nursing diagnoses assigned "high" priority would be dealt with first, problems of "medium" priority would be considered next, and problems considered to be of "low" priority would be solved last.

The process of priority setting requires the input and judgment of both the nurse and client. As Yura and Walsh (1973) point out, life-threatening problems or diagnoses are obviously "high" priority, from the perspective of both the nurse and client; examples of such problems include hemorrhage, airway obstructions, and poison ingestion.

Maslow's (1954) hierarchy of needs can also be used to prioritize client problems. According to his hierarchy, man's most basic needs, which must be satisfied first, are *physiological* needs for food, water, sex, clothing, and shelter. At the next step in the hierarchy are *safety* needs, which include both physical and economic security. The third rung in the hierarchy includes *belonging* needs, such as membership in a family and other groups, maintaining friendships, and feeling "accepted" by others. Above that level is man's need for *respect,* which includes self-esteem, status and prestige, and recognition for one's achievements. At the top of Maslow's pyramidal hierarchy is man's need for achieving his fullest potential, which is called *self-actualization;* according to Maslow's theory, man cannot achieve his potential until all his lower level needs (physiological, safety, belonging, and respect) are satisfied, because his energy, both physical and psychic, is tied up with lower level and more urgent needs.

Theoretically, then, unless the client can be assisted to meet all his lower level needs, he may never be free to achieve high-level wellness and self-actualization. Therefore it is important for the nurse to help clients solve problems that are important to *them* and that perhaps indirectly contribute to their overall health. To achieve that, the nurse must obviously use helping relationship skills to learn the client's perception of his problems and their potential solutions; this will allow her to identify and more fully support his constructive coping efforts as well. If the nurse and client do not discuss and reach mutual agreement about the priority of the client's needs, they may find themselves working against each other. For example, a school nurse who is following up students referred for eye examinations, following a school vision screening program, may well expect to find some parents who do not follow through with the referral by seeking the needed eye examination for their child. If, instead of continuing to send written reminders or telephoning frequently for that purpose, the school nurse explores the problem more fully with the family, she may find that the child's need for eye care is of relatively low priority to the family, which is currently concerned about saving enough money to pay their heating bills for the winter. In such cases, the nurse must be prepared to help with problems (either through direct intervention or referral to another professional such as, in this case, a social worker) that are not necessarily handled by nurses routinely. The nurse must be willing to help with problems like the financial one just described *before* she can expect the family to comply with the specific "health" need that she identified.

However, it should also be noted that Maslow's hierarchy cannot be used as an "automatic" prioritizing device, whereby the nurse might assume that the lowest (most basic) level needs are always of the highest priority. The client's perceptions must *always* be determined to prevent such possibly fallacious assumptions. An example of the danger of such assumptions would be an adolescent who has developed a behavior pattern that includes spending Friday nights drinking beer and drag racing with his buddies. The school nurse or a counselor or any other adult might *expect,* based on Maslow's hierarchy, that the boy could be easily convinced to "mend his ways" by pointing out the safety hazards of that behavior: the risk of having an automobile accident due to both speeding and impaired functioning from alcohol usage. However, if in the adolescent's perception, the opinion of his peers is the most important need (which is likely, since adolescents are strongly influenced by their peers), then he is placing a higher priority on his belonging and respect needs than on his safety needs. Therefore, in working with this student, the school nurse would need to adjust her strategies accordingly, beginning by communicating with the student about the perceived discrepancies in problem solving and priority setting.

The priority assigned a given problem or need will also be influenced by other factors, including availability of resources, costs of needed services, and the amount of time required to solve the problem (Yura and Walsh, 1973). If, for example, the resources necessary to provide speech therapy for a child with multiple health problems are not available, then higher priority could be assigned to the child's other more immediately resolvable problems until speech therapy facilities can be located or provided. The school nurse could very appropriately concern herself with stimulating development of speech therapy facilities through lobbying and other approaches, while at the same time focusing her direct intervention toward the child's other health problems.

The time factor can also affect the priorities set; both the client and the nurse might assign comparatively high priority to a nonurgent problem simply because it is readily solved and can be quickly and immediately resolved. On the other hand, a problem that is viewed as chronic or long term and not readily solved might be assigned a lower priority even though it affects the quality of his day-to-day life. Thus priority setting involves complex decision making, which *must* include the perceptions of the client and relevant others who are involved in his care.

Planning intervention: what and by whom

Once the desired outcomes (goals and EOCs) are known and the priorities for achieving them have been set, the nurse's attention can be directed toward deciding *who* will carry out *which* interventions or planned actions (Yura and Walsh, 1973). This involves analyzing each desired outcome or goal and deciding *how* to achieve it. The proposed nursing actions and approaches may include a variety of means, such as health teaching, providing emotional support, and administering medical treatments and prescribed drugs. The nurse will need to rely on her knowledge and experience, critical thinking and decision-making skills, research findings (her own and those of others) concerning effective approaches and actions, and creativity in designing solutions to the client's problems.

Again, as noted previously, the client is an important source of input in planning intervention and should be consulted about previous intervention strategies and their acceptability to him as well as their success. If the nurse truly believes that the client is and should be responsible for his own health, then she will value his input into the process of planning nursing interventions.

Another important decision to be made in planning intervention for the client's health problems is determining *who* will assume responsibility for carrying out the designated actions (Yura and Walsh, 1973). In addition to consulting the client about the goals for his care and acceptable and known effective means to achieve them, the nurse will need to include him in deciding who will take the specified action. For some problems, the client himself may be the appropriate person to take action, with or without the assistance and support of the nurse and other members of the health care team. In other situations, the nurse may be the most appropriate person to intervene on his behalf, or she may delegate that responsibility to other nursing personnel or health care professionals. However, no matter who is chosen to carry out the problem-solving action, that decision must be made consciously and rationally, based on careful analysis of the level of skill and preparation needed to carry it out, qualifications (legal, experiential, and educational) of available human resources to take that action, and on principles and policies regarding delegation of nursing actions. This decision is far too important to be made haphazardly, since the competence and reliability of the person designated to carry out the plan(s) can critically affect the outcome.

The end product: the nursing care plan

The written nursing care plan is the end product of the planning process (Yura and Walsh, 1973), and its essential components are specified in the ANA (1973:Standard IV) standards for nursing practice:

The plan of nursing care includes priorities and the prescribed nursing approaches or measures to achieve the goals derived from the nursing diagnoses.

The rationale accompanying Standard IV specifies that nursing actions should be planned to promote the client's wellness (which is the basis for so-called health promotion strategies), as well as to maintain and restore his health.

The compliance assessment factors published with Standard IV (ANA, 1973) include the following criteria:

1. Specification of physiological measures to prevent or control specific problems (nursing diagnoses) and to achieve defined goals of care
2. Identification of psychosocial measures for dealing with specific diagnosed problems and for achieving specified client outcomes (goals)
3. Incorporation of relevant teaching-learning principles and inclusion of behaviorally stated learning objectives
4. Inclusion of approaches designed to provide a "therapeutic environment" for the client, including attention to physical, psychosocial, and interactional environmental factors
5. Specification of approaches to orient the client to new roles and relationships, appropriate health resources (human and material), modifications in the nursing care plan, and the relationship of changes in the nursing care plan to the overall health care plan
6. Utilization of appropriate and available resources to achieve the desired outcomes
7. Identification of an ordered sequence for nursing actions
8. Utilization of current scientific knowledge as a basis for planned nursing approaches

The precise format for the nursing care plan will vary from one agency or institution to another and may depend on the charting or record-keeping system used. Boland et al. (1975) point out the importance of using a format that is readily understood by all relevant nursing and health care personnel and easy to use. Marriner (1979) encourages writing care plans in pencil so that changes can be readily made without having to redo the entire plan. However, for nursing care plans that are written as part of a client's health record or chart, the use of pencil may not be advisable because such documents are considered legal, permanent records.

Another approach to nursing care plans described by Boland et al. (1975) is the "routine care" approach. In this approach, Kardex cards and/or health record forms may be preprinted with certain "usual" or "standard" problems that are expected to affect most clients. Other personalized problems can be added if indicated, but nursing care could be given on the basis of the standardized preprinted care plan alone. While this system has some advantages, including (1) reduction of planning and charting time and (2) improvement in overall quality of care in a given agency or setting by identifying approaches that are minimal expectations for the care of all clients/patients, there is a disadvantage as well. The potential disadvantage of such a system is that nursing care may be given by rote rather than by reason. If nursing care becomes so standardized, the individual needs and concerns of clients may be overlooked. Thus a decision to use standard or "routine" nursing care plans must be carefully made, including built-in controls to ensure that the plan is used appropriately and not in lieu of sound nursing planning.

Implementation

During the implementation phase, the nursing care plan is carried out or enacted. Thus this phase is action oriented toward achieving the desired outcomes specified in the plan. However, as Yura and Walsh (1973) caution, this phase should not be seen as a rote enactment of the care plan. Instead, the nurse must continually gather more data to refine her assessment and her plan, as well as to evaluate the accuracy and appropriateness of both. If the nurse discovers that portions of the care plan are ineffective, or if she finds that the client's needs have changed, then she must go back and revise her assessment (nursing diagnoses) and modify the care plan to incorporate the new data she collected.

If the nursing care plan includes participation by other health care professionals and personnel, the nurse must maintain good communication with them and review the plan with them periodically to ensure that the planned nursing approaches are consistently applied by all personnel. Failure to take such actions to ensure conformity with the plan may result in unintentional interference with the planned outcomes.

Evaluation

The last phase of the nursing process is evaluation. As defined by Gebbie and Lavin (1975: 115), *nursing evaluation* is "a systematic comparison of patient [client] responses obtained as a result of nursing interventions with the response expected." In other words, evaluation compares "what is" with "what should be."

Boland et al. (1975:87) describe the importance of evaluation in terms of its contribution to the nurse's accountability. As they define it, *accountability* is "the state of being responsible for one's acts and being able to explain, define, or measure in some way the results of decision making." As noted repeatedly throughout this book, school nurses must be accountable for their actions and must document their effectiveness if they are to survive in the political and fiscal jungle of the public school system.

The nursing care standards developed by the ANA (1973) provide one means of increasing the accountability of the nurse by specifying for what quality of care she is accountable to her peers. The ANA standards exemplify the *process-oriented* method of evaluation described by Bloch (1975). According to Bloch (1975), process-oriented evaluation focuses on the actions and competency of the *nurse* and can be measured from two perspectives: the care *given* (measured through direct observation and/or use of performance rating scales) or the care *received* (measured by patient/client-oriented scales and checklists and by retrospective audit of clients' charts or health records by methods such as the Phaneuf method).

Another method of evaluation of client/patient care discussed by Bloch (1975) is the *outcome-oriented* method, which uses EOCs or other similar methods to assess change in the client's behavior and/or health status. This method is very useful, but has one significant drawback: it does not indicate which, if any, of the planned (nursing) actions specified in the client's care plan were responsible for effecting the desired outcome. Therefore, in trying to determine which nursing approaches "work," the outcome-oriented evaluation method has definite limitations: this method only indicates that the desired change did or did not occur and provides no evaluation of the nursing approaches used.

As an alternative to the process-oriented evaluation method, which is limited by its exclusive focus on nurse actions, and to the outcome-oriented method, which is limited by its inattention to the nurse's actions, Bloch (1975) suggests use of the *process-outcome* method of evaluation. Bloch (1975:258) describes process-outcome evaluation as the ideal method of nursing care evaluation because "it allows examination of how the actions of providers relate to changes in the recipient of care."

As preparation for inauguration of process-outcome evaluation, the following tasks must be accomplished (Bloch, 1975:258):

1. Development of a set of measurable outcome criteria specific to nursing (if the purpose is to evaluate *nursing* care)
2. Development of reliable and valid methods for measuring these outcomes
3. Development of a set of measurable process criteria
4. Development of reliable and valid methods for measuring the process of nursing care in all various forms, including both the physical aspects of the process as well as the psychosocial and cognitive aspects
5. Testing of the various aspects of nursing practice in relation to patient outcomes, by applying process as well as outcome measurement

Bloch points out, however, that nursing is not yet ready to base its quality control efforts solely on process-outcome evaluation methods, since work on these tasks is still in progress and is nowhere near completion; however, she urges nursing to adopt as its goal steady and resolute progress toward completion of those tasks.

Regardless of the specific approach used, the ANA nursing care standards (1973, Standard VII) clearly convey the expectation that nursing care given should be evaluated:

The client's/patient's progress or lack of progress toward goal achievement is determined by the client/patient and the nurse.

Among the compliance factors accompanying this standard are the following expectations:

1. The client's progress toward goal achievement will be measured based on current data concerning his health status.
2. The effectiveness of nursing actions in accomplishing the client's goal attainment will be analyzed.
3. The client will participate in the evaluation of both goal achievement and nursing actions.
4. Long-term effects of nursing care for the client will be evaluated.

The value of the data from the evaluation process depends on how or if that data is used. If the data is simply recorded and then filed away for posterity, then the process has probably been a waste of time. Ideally, the evaluative data should become an input back into the nursing process. More specifically, as reflected in the last of the general nursing practice standards (ANA, 1973:Standard VIII):

The client's/patient's progress or lack of progress toward goal achievement directs reassessment, reordering of priorities, new goal setting and revision of the plan of nursing care.

Thus the results from the evaluation become a feedback loop and provide new data for reassessing the client's health status, reviewing the appropriateness of the nursing care plan, reviewing the actual implementation of the plan, and even reassessing the appropriateness of the evaluative strategies (Fig. 14-1). Again, as emphasized throughout this discussion of nursing process, the client's input should be solicited for this aspect of evaluation as well as for all other phases of the nursing process.

THE PROCESS OF CONTRACT SETTING

According to Sloan and Schommer (1975), the use of contracts in nursing and other helping professions has been a fairly recent development. Traditionally, contracts have been the sole province of business and law and have been formal, usually written, and legally binding agreements.

The incorporation of contracting into the day-to-day practice of mental health workers, counselors, social workers, nurses, and other health care personnel represents a dramatic shift in philosophy. Helping professionals have thus moved away from a benevolent, paternalistic orientation to helping and toward a philosophy of mutual respect, involvement, and cooperation. This shift in philosophy was undoubtedly difficult to make, since helping professionals (and health care professionals in particular) have traditionally been accorded a great deal of deference and respect, probably because of the tremendous power of life and death they wield over the client/patient. For some health care professionals, relinquishing any of their power (charismatic as well as helping) is uncomfortable and even threatening.

However, the benefits of sharing the "power" through mutual decision making with the client outweigh the misgivings that sometimes result. One of the benefits of nurse-client contracting is that the client thereby develops a relationship (with the nurse) in which he has respect and responsibilities. This feeling that his opinions are respected, coupled with successful completion of his responsibilities, can have a significantly positive effect on his self-esteem (Sloan and Schommer, 1975).

Another related benefit is that the contracting relationship provides the client with an opportunity to develop his problem-solving skills. For those clients (including children) whose life experiences leave them feeling "not OK" or "one down," the successful completion of a mutually negotiated contract can not only improve self-esteem, but can also help them to be responsible persons with improved chances for future successes, which, according to Glasser's Reality Therapy (Chapter 11), is the ultimate goal of "helping."

Another very important benefit of contracting is that it clarifies the nature of the nurse-client relationship by clearly articulating ownership of responsibilities for the client's care. This reduces the risk that the client will develop an unhealthy dependency on the nurse and averts the possibility that the client will manipulate the nurse into providing inappropriate services which allow him to avoid responsibility and independence (Brammer, 1973; Sloan and Schommer, 1975).

The contracting process has benefits for the nurse as well. As Sloan and Schommer (1975) point out, the contract encourages the nurse to maintain realistic expectations of both the client and herself. Since the contracting process involves *mutual* goal setting, the nurse should not find herself working toward one goal and the client focused on a different goal: the contract requires them to work together. For the nurse who may expect herself to somehow "save" everyone from the world and from themselves, the contract can reduce the frustration and fear of failure that result from a Messianic complex gone awry; the contract clearly establishes the client as responsible for his own improvement with the nurse acting as catalyst and helper.

The nurse-client contract
Definitions

In contrast to the traditional concepts of "contracting," in which the contractual agreement was formal and legally binding, such as marriage contracts, sales contracts, and employment contracts (Sloan and Schommer, 1975), the nurse-client contract is usually *not* legally binding and serves primarily as a working agreement or tool to accomplish mutual goals.

Among the definitions of contracts proposed in the literature is the following definition (Sloan and Schommer, 1975:222-223) of a community nursing contract:

. . . Any working agreement, continuously renegotiable, between nurse, patient [client] and family . . . [that may be] formal or informal, written or verbal, simple or detailed, signed or unsigned by patient [client] and nurse.

An important element of this definition is its description of nurse-client contracts as "continuously renegotiable." This proviso is necessary in helper-helpee contracts, especially those involving nurses and their clients/patients, because the health status of the client/patient may change rapidly and without warning. For that reason, the contract must have the inherent flexibility to be renegotiated as needed. Otherwise, the nurse and client may find themselves locked into a contract that is inappropriate and therefore not beneficial to the client's health and welfare.

Another important aspect of the nurse-client contract included in the Sloan and Schommer (1975) definition concerns the variability of format and structure. As they note, the contract can be "formal or informal, written or verbal, simple or detailed, signed or unsigned" (1975: 223). In deciding on the precise format for the contract with a given client, the nurse will need to use the nursing process *assessment* methods (data collection and nursing diagnosis) already discussed. Specifically, the nurse must consider the client's growth and developmental stage, biophysical status, emotional and mental health status, and usual coping patterns to decide if the client (1) can comprehend the nature and purpose of such a contract, (2) is capable of defining mutual goals and responsibilities, and (3) has the coping skills and resources to comply with the terms of the agreement. For example, a school nurse working with a severely retarded child might find a contract inappropriate because it is beyond the child's comprehension. However, a contract could be very effective in working with a child with behavior problems; in this instance, the contract might specify which disruptive behaviors the child would "give up" and what his rewards for doing so would be.

For the school nurse especially, the structure and complexity of any nurse-client contract must be carefully determined. The nurse's assessment of growth and development, particularly *cognitive* development, is very important in finding the most appropriate format and *wording* or language for the agreement. The kind of contract described in Fig. 10-1 may be very appropriate for young children from the time of school entrance through elementary school. For children who cannot read or write, a similar agreement could be reached, although it might be preferable to *verbally* negotiate the contract and to keep the terms *simple*. In addition, with young children time limits must be short, since small children (under the age of 7) lack a concept of time; to them, a week (and even an hour) often seems like an eternity. For older children and adolescents, the nurse-client contract may be written and more formal, include more sophisticated language, be more complex and detailed in its goals and responsibilities, and include a longer time span for completion.

In his discussion of *structuring* or defining "the nature, limits, and goals of the prospective helping relationship," Brammer (1973:60) makes a strong case for the importance of contracting. Brammer emphasizes the importance of specifying the kind of help offered, the qualifications and limitations of the helper, the time structure for the relationship, and any fees that may be involved (although the latter is not likely to be a part of a school nurse's contract with a student or other client within the school).

In accordance with this emphasis on the structure of the helping relationship, Brammer (1973:61) proposes the following definition, in which he describes a *contract* as:

. . . An agreement between the helper and helpee that they will work toward certain *goals,* that each will carry out specific *responsibilities* to achieve the goals, and that certain specific *outcomes* will be taken as evidence that the help was successful.

This definition, in contrast with that proposed by Sloan and Schommer (1975), provides a stronger emphasis on the *process* and essential elements for contracting and will therefore be the basis for further discussion of the contract-setting process in the remainder of this chapter.

Underlying philosophy

Although, as previously mentioned, the origin of contracting is firmly rooted in business and law, there is also a direct link between the importance and process of contracting within helping relationships and some of the theories and approaches to "helping" described in Chapter 11.

After spending 25 years trying to "treat, cure, or change" his clients, Rogers (1956), proponent of "client-centered therapy," discovered that the most appropriate and helpful strategy is to form a kind of *partnership* with the client, in which the client "discovers" his true feelings and problems and can "discover" (with the assistance of the therapist) the right solutions or course of action (Chapter 11). This assistance provided by the therapist is based on the "genuineness," "unconditional positive regard," and "accurate empathic understanding" that the therapist brings to the relationship, which create a climate in which the contract can be negotiated.

The tenets of Adlerian Psychology as modified by Dreikurs (Chapter 11) also provide a basis for use of contracts in helping relationships. Adlerians encourage participative decision making for their clients through use of the family council concept, in which the client family works together to make decisions about division of household labor, limit setting and discipline for the children, plus any other decisions affecting the family as a whole. This emphasis on participative decision making can be carried over into helping relationships as well; the decision-making skills of the client can be applied readily to negotiation of goals and responsibilities within the nurse-client contract.

Probably the most obvious link between helping relationship theories and approaches and the use of contracts is Glasser's Reality Therapy (Chapter 11). As noted in that discussion, Glasser believes mental health problems in our society are often due to irresponsibility on the client's part, perpetuated perhaps by feelings of failure. The goal of Glasser's Reality Therapy is to help the client become a responsible person, by first helping the client evaluate his behavior and admit that it has been irresponsible. The client is then asked to formulate a plan (goals and means for achieving them), make a commitment to carry it out, and evaluate his progress with the support of the helper or therapist. Although Glasser does not refer to this process as contract setting, the elements of planning, commitment, and evaluation are clearly congruent with the contracting process.

The contracting process

The importance of contracting in nursing practice has been recognized by the ANA and communicated in their code of ethics (ANA, 1976) and nursing practice standards (1973). Thus use of contracts is an accepted and *expected* component of nursing practice. In the very first paragraph of the "interpretive statements" that accompany the ANA's (1976:4) code of ethics is the following assertion:

Whenever possible, clients should be fully involved in the planning and implementation of their own health care.

The ANA's philosophical commitment to use of contracts in nursing is further evidenced by the wording of some of the nursing practice standards, including Standards V and VI (ANA, 1973):

Nursing actions *provide for client/patient participation* in health promotion, maintenance and restoration.

Nursing actions *assist the client/patient* to maximize his health capabilities.

Both these standards clearly mandate that the client should participate in his own nursing care and that the nurse's actions should facilitate his participation. In addition, Standard VI indirectly acknowledges that the client is responsible for his own health and that the role of the nurse is to *assist him* in achieving high-level wellness or optimal health. The ideal method for implementing both these standards is through the contract-setting process.

The contracting process as described by Sloan and Schommer (1975) has eight phases or steps, which are illustrated in Fig. 14-2 and will be individually discussed.

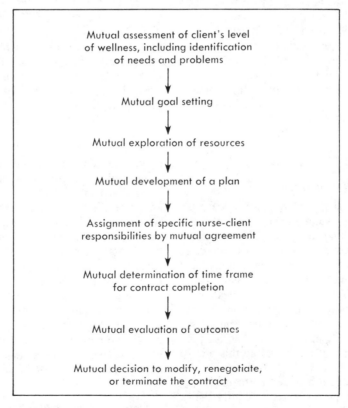

Fig. 14-2. The nurse-client contracting process. (Modified from Sloan, M. R., and Schommer, B. T.: 1975. The process of contracting in community nursing, Chapter 25. In Spradley, B. W., editor: Contemporary community nursing, Little, Brown & Co., Boston.)

Step 1: Mutual assessment of client's level of wellness, including identification of needs and problems

The key word in this first step of the contracting process and in the remaining steps is *mutual*. Through use of helping relationship skills in the data collection process, the nurse elicits the client's perception of his problems, needs, and concerns, after which the nurse shares her perceptions and observations with the client. By discussing and comparing their perceptions, the nurse and client reach agreement and understanding concerning the nature of the client's problem(s). This mutual assessment process helps ensure a positive outcome by getting the nurse and client "on the same wavelength," so that they can work together and not against one another.

Step 2: Mutual goal setting

As pointed out in discussion of the planning phase of the nursing process, the assessment factors published with ANA (1973) Standard III specify that the goal-setting process should include the client and others (family members and other professionals) involved in his care.

According to Sloan and Schommer (1975), during the mutual goal-setting phase the nurse and client need to consider collaborative strategies for solving the identified problems or meeting the needs of the client. In addition, they must decide where to begin: that is, from which vantage point to attack the problem. However, probably the most important decision to be made at this stage is determining what goals or outcomes are realistic and workable.

Step 3: Mutual exploration of resources

The third step in the contracting process is exploration of the available and accessible resources for achieving the goals. This not only includes assessment of material resources (such as equipment and clinics) and other human resources (such as significant others, health care professionals, and other official agencies), but it also entails assessment of the nurse and client as resources. Thus the nurse and client must now explore such questions as what unique qualities can each provide in solving this problem and what skills and energy is each willing to commit to this goal-centered partnership? It is also appropriate at this stage to clarify their expectations of one another to be sure that their respective working "styles" are compatible (Sloan and Schommer, 1975).

Step 4: Mutual development of a plan

The fourth step in the contracting process is development of their actual plan for achieving their mutual goals and resolving the problem(s) identified earlier. Their emphasis is now on actual strategies and actions to achieve the goals and may include delineation of both long-range and short-range plans, as well as prioritizing goals based on their relative importance and urgency.

Step 5: Assignment of specific nurse-client responsibilities by mutual agreement

During this fifth step in the contracting process, the strategies discussed during the previous stage are now translated into specifically assigned actions. Thus, from their earlier (step 3) generalized sharing of working styles and mutual expectations, the nurse and client now formalize their expectations by clearly assigning responsibility for completion of tasks and actions necessary for achievement of the goal(s).

Step 6: Mutual determination of time frame for contract completion

This sixth step is one of the most important, yet often overlooked, elements of the contracting process. Identification of the time frame, including time limits for completion, provides a kind of control over the working relationship between the nurse and client and avoids the risk of endless and aimless involvement for them. The time limits established provide a built-in evaluation mechanism, so that the effectiveness of the plan can be reviewed and further decisions made as to continuing as planned, modifying the plan, or terminating the relationship altogether (Sloan and Schommer, 1975). Again, as previously noted, the time frame must be reasonable to allow adequate testing of the plan's effectiveness and must also be reasonable in terms of the client's perception of time. This is especially important in working with young children whose conception of time is limited by their cognitive development; thus, for young children (under age 7, approximately), the time frame may need to be much shorter than that usually planned with adults, and, of course, the goals must be likewise limited in scope.

Step 7: Mutual evaluation of outcomes

In accordance with the time frame established and the responsibilities assigned to each,

Table 14-1. Congruence of the nursing process and contracting process

Nursing process	Contracting process
Step 1: Assessment	*Step 1:* Mutual assessment
Data collection	Client's level of wellness
Nursing diagnosis (problem definition)	Identification of needs and problems
Step 2: Planning	*Step 2:* Mutual goal setting
Planned outcomes: goals and EOCs	*Step 3:* Mutual exploration of resources
Planning intervention: what and by whom	*Step 4:* Mutual development of a plan
Development of nursing care plan	*Step 5:* Assignment of specific nurse-client responsibilities by mutual agreement
Step 3: Implementing	
Step 4: Evaluation	*Step 6:* Mutual determination of time frame
	Step 7: Mutual evaluation of outcomes
	Step 8: Mutual decision: modify, renegotiate, or terminate contract

the nurse and client must evaluate the success of the plan during the seventh phase of the contracting process. The importance of *mutual* evaluation has been emphasized by the ANA (and in this chapter's earlier discussion of evaluation within the nursing process). As cited earlier (ANA, 1973:Standard VII) mutual evaluation is one of the standards for nursing care regardless of practice setting:

The client's/patient's progress or lack of progress toward *goal achievement is determined by the client/patient and the nurse.*

Basically, this involves determining (1) whether or not the goals and planned outcomes were achieved; (2) if the goals were not achieved, why not (Were the goals realistic and were the strategies effective? Did both participants carry out their assigned tasks?); and (3) whether or not there are other problems (related or not related to the current contract emphasis) that need to be resolved through nurse-client contracting (Sloan and Schommer, 1975).

Step 8: Mutual decision: modify, renegotiate, or terminate the contract

Following careful evaluation during step 7, the nurse and client must decide during step 8 of the contracting process where to go from that point (Sloan and Schommer, 1975). If the problems identified were satisfactorily resolved and if no additional problems have surfaced, then the appropriate decision may be to terminate the relationship until and unless the client again needs help. If the evaluation revealed a flaw in precise identification of the problem(s), the strategies planned, or the division of labor to achieve the desired outcomes, then the nurse

and client may decide to modify and/or renegotiate the contract. This, too, (as noted in discussion of evaluation within the nursing process) is a process mandated by the ANA's nursing practice standards (1973:Standard VIII):

The client's/patient's progress or lack of progress toward goal achievement directs reassessment, reordering of priorities, new goal setting and revision of the plan of nursing care.

Thus, as with nursing process evaluation, the results of the evaluation process can become inputs to begin the contracting process again.

Congruence of nursing process and contracting process

As noted earlier in this chapter, contracting can be done in conjunction with the nursing process, despite the fact that they are considered to be (and have been presented in this chapter as) two distinct processes. There are many similarities between the two processes, and some overlapping of steps occurs. Thus, as illustrated in Table 14-1, these processes are quite congruent. The primary difference between them seems to be that the nursing process focuses on the *nurse's* actions and responsibilities, whereas contracting is a way of formally including the *client* in the nursing process, thereby acknowledging that the client is ultimately responsible for his own health and well-being and must therefore participate actively *with* health care professionals on his behalf.

CONCLUSION

Clients in all settings have come to expect (and rightfully so) that the nursing care they receive will be scientifically sound, safely and skillfully administered, and in accordance with their personal needs and preferences. For nurses to live up to these expectations in this era of knowledgeable and articulate health care consumers requires consistent application of systematic processes (in lieu of the former intuitive approach), including the nursing process and contracting. Although most of the literature describing these processes focuses on the nurse and patient in acute care settings (usually, hospitals), the nursing process and contracting are nonetheless readily applicable to clients and population groups (including schoolchildren) who are primarily well and in need of health promotion and primary prevention. These processes further provide means of articulating, documenting, and evaluating nursing skills and actions and therefore are important survival tools for today's school nurse.

REFERENCES

American Nurses' Association: 1973. Standards of nursing practice, American Nurses' Association, Kansas City, Mo.

American Nurses' Association: 1976. Code for nurses with interpretive statements, American Nurses' Association, Kansas City, Mo.

Berni, R., and Readey, H.: 1978. Problem-oriented medical record implementation: allied health peer review, 2nd ed., The C. V. Mosby Co., St. Louis.

Bloch, D.: 1974. Some crucial terms in nursing what do they really mean? Nurs. Outlook **22**(11):689-694.

Bloch, D.: 1975. Evaluation of nursing care in terms of process and outcome: issues in research and quality assurance, Nurs. Res. **24**(4):256-263.

Boland, M. H., Murray, R., Zentner, J., Nolan, N., and Lough, M. A.: 1975. The nursing process: a method to promote health, Chapter 4. In Murray, R., and Zentner, J.: Nursing concepts for health promotion, Prentice-Hall, Inc., Englewood Cliffs, N.J.

Brammer, L. M.: 1973. The helping relationship: process and skills, Prentice-Hall, Inc., Englewood Cliffs, N.J.

Carlson, S.: 1972. A practical approach to the nursing process, Am. J. Nurs. **72**(9):1589-1591.

Chambers, W.: 1962. Nursing diagnosis, Am. J. Nurs. **62**(11):102-104.

Durand, M., and Prince, R.: 1966. Nursing diagnosis: process and decision, Nurs. Forum **5**(4):50-64.

Gebbie, K. M., and Lavin, M. A.: 1975. Classification of nursing diagnoses, Proceedings of the First National Conference on the Classification of Nursing Diagnoses, October 1-5, 1973, The C. V. Mosby Co., St. Louis.

Gordon, M.: 1978. Nursing diagnoses and the diagnostic process, Chapter 25. In Chaska, N. L., editor, The nursing profession: views through the mist, McGraw-Hill Book Co., New York.

Komorita, N. I.: 1963. Nursing diagnosis, Am. J. Nurs. **63**(12):83-86.

Mager, R. F.: 1962. Preparing instructional objectives, Fearon • Pitman Publishers, Inc., Belmont, Calif.

Marriner, A.: 1979. The nursing process: a scientific approach to nursing care, 2nd ed., The C. V. Mosby Co., St. Louis.

Maslow, A. H.: 1954. Motivation and personality, Harper & Row, Publishers, Inc., New York.

Rogers, C. R.: 1956. A counseling approach to human problems, Am. J. Nurs. **56**(8):994-997.

Rothberg, J. S.: 1967. Why nursing diagnoses? Am. J. Nurs. **67**(5):1040-1042.

Sloan, M. R., and Schommer, B. T.: 1975. The process of contracting in community nursing, Chapter 25. In Spradley, B. W., editor: Contemporary community nursing, Little, Brown & Co., Boston.

Soares, C. A.: 1978. Nursing and medical diagnoses: a comparison of variant and essential features, Chapter 26. In Chaska, N. L., editor: The nursing profession: views through the mist, McGraw-Hill Book Co., New York.

Stuart, G. W., and Sundeen, S. J.: 1976. The nursing process, Chapter 1. In Sundeen, S. J., Stuart, G. W., Rankin, E. S., and Cohen, S. P.: Nurse-client interaction: implementing the nursing process, The C. V. Mosby Co., St. Louis.

Vaughan-Wrobel, B. C., and Henderson, B.: 1976. The problem-oriented system in nursing—a workbook, The C. V. Mosby Co., St. Louis.

Yura, H., and Walsh, M. B.: 1973. The nursing process: assessing, planning, implementing, evaluating, 2nd ed., Appleton-Century-Crofts, New York.

SUGGESTED READINGS

Brodt, D. E.: 1978. The nursing process, Chapter 24. In Chaska, N. L., editor: The nursing profession: views through the mist, McGraw-Hill Book Co., New York.

Murchison, I., Nichols, T. S., and Hanson, R.: 1978. Legal accountability in the nursing process, The C. V. Mosby Co., St. Louis.

Sundeen, S. J., Stuart, G. W., Rankin, E. S., and Cohen, S. P.: 1976. Nurse-client interaction: implementing the nursing process, The C. V. Mosby Co., St. Louis.

CHAPTER 15

Health education: a vital process for promoting and maintaining health in school community populations

SUSAN J. WOLD

As noted in Chapter 2, a major responsibility of the school health program is planning, implementation, and evaluation of a comprehensive health education curriculum to prepare students to assume responsibility for their own health. This responsibility resides within the school health *team,* which by definition includes administrators (including principals), teachers, social workers, psychologists, school nurses, and other health care professionals (such as physicians and dentists), nonprofessional assistants (including school health aides and volunteers), parents, and others deemed appropriate by the local school district or individual school. Thus design and implementation of an effective health education curriculum require the talents and cooperation of a number of people, including the school nurse. Indeed, for the school nurse, participation in the school's health education program is an opportunity to demonstrate her concern for health and wellness as opposed to disease and illness and to contribute to the emergence of "health-educated young adults" capable of making responsible decisions regarding health.

The thesis of this chapter, then, is that health education is a vital component of the school health program which contributes to health promotion and health maintenance among school community populations. To develop and defend this thesis, in the remainder of this chapter the following will be discussed:

1. The importance of health education in the school
2. Problems confronting school health education
3. Sources of health influence and education
4. Health education process and principles

5. Subject areas for inclusion in a school health education program
6. The role of the school nurse in school health education

THE IMPORTANCE OF HEALTH EDUCATION IN THE SCHOOL

Although health education has been an acknowledged component of the school health program since the late 1920s and early 1930s (Chapter 1), the importance and priority assigned to health education within school health programs varies widely across the country (Castile and Jerrick, 1976). Such variance in the quality and priority of school health education programs seems particularly ironic, since schools exist for the primary purpose of educating students to become responsible and self-sufficient adults, which should logically include educating them to be healthy, self-actualized adults. However, recognizing that such variance exists, it seems prudent to reaffirm the importance of health education in schools by briefly discussing what health education is, why it is an essential component of the school health program, and what it is intended to accomplish (purposes and goals).

Defining health education

The literature is replete with definitions of health education, health instruction, and school health education. As Bruess and Gay (1978) point out, because definitions of health education are logical extensions of one's definition and concept of "health," they are therefore based on conscious or unconscious value judgments concerning health. Thus persons or groups who view health as the absence of disease will conceptualize health education quite differently from those who view health as high-level wellness. For the purposes of this chapter, three definitions of health education will be briefly described.

The first definition of health education to be discussed is proposed by Bruess and Gay (1978: 424); according to their view, "school health education" may be defined as "the process of providing learning experiences for the purpose of influencing knowledge, attitudes, and conduct relating to individual and group health interests and needs. Health education will take place either through incidental or planned learning in separate courses or correlated courses." According to this definition, then, health education can be either formally planned as course content areas, or informal and unplanned, capitalizing on the incidental or so-called teachable moment. The purpose of health education based on this definition is to "influence" students' knowledge, attitudes, and behavior regarding their own and the community's health. Unfortunately, this definition does not describe the direction of that "influence" (although presumably it is intended to be *positive*) or the *outcome* of the process.

Another definition of health education proposed in the literature is Kaplan's (1972:9) definition, in which health education is viewed as "the provision of learning experiences which favorably influence knowledge, attitudes, and behavior in matters pertaining to individual and community health." Kaplan's definition, in contrast with that of Bruess and Gay, indicates that the intent of health education is to "favorably influence" students' knowledge, attitudes, and behavior. However, this definition likewise fails to indicate or even hint at the *outcomes* of such learning experiences and is therefore unacceptably incomplete.

In contrast with the perceived inadequacies of the two preceding definitions, the definition proposed by the Minneapolis Community Health Education Study Committee indicates clearly the projected outcomes for the learner. According to this definition, *health education* includes "the sum total of processes and experiences whereby people are helped to adopt and/or maintain positive health behaviors. These behaviors will make it possible for individuals to deal effectively with health-related disruptions, maintain present levels of functioning and move towards higher levels of well-being" (Kenney, 1977:32-33). Because this definition specifies desired outcomes for health education programs and is also consistent with my view of health as high-level wellness, the definition of health education proposed by Kenney (1977) will be adopted as the basis for this chapter.

Health education as an essential component of the school health program

Wellness behavior, defined as the "development of an individual's ability to actively seek to change his life situation so that he can function at his perceived maximum capacity and satisfaction" (Bruhn and Cordova, 1977:248), is *learned* behavior. While there are many sources of health influence for individuals, including the family, peers, and the media, the school also influences the wellness behavior of its students.

The interrelatedness of education and health has been described in the literature by a variety of authors, including Oberteuffer and Beyrer (1966), Neilson (1969), Haro (1974), Jacobsen and Siegel (1971), and Kaplan (1972). Specifically, Jacobsen and Siegel (1971:158) point out that the school "as the basic institution for formal education, *has a primary duty* to equip its pupils with those skills and tools of learning that will enable them to live productive, useful, happy and healthful lives." These authors go on to say that while the "basic subjects" such as English, science, social studies, and mathematics are very important "primary" concerns for the school, the following is also true:

. . . There *are many* highly important responsibilities and opportunities in health which are consistent with the school's primary functions. For example, the *quality* of a pupil's health and the *environment* in which he is taught, have a *direct bearing upon the quality of education a school can provide.* An essential component of education for future life is knowledge of health and healthy relationships.

In other words, Jacobsen and Siegel (1971:158) believe that for a school to successfully educate young people to live "productive, useful, happy and healthful lives," it must provide a school health program that includes the basic elements of healthful school environment, adequate health services, and comprehensive health education.

There are both health care professionals and lay persons (especially parents) who view health education as the purview and prerogative of the family. However, as a consequence of compulsory school attendance laws throughout the country, parents must delegate part of that responsibility for children's health education to the school, since children spend up to 6 hours per day, 5 days per week, 30 plus weeks per year under the care and supervision of the school (Oberteuffer and Beyrer, 1966). The school is thus morally and legally obligated to provide health education experiences to reinforce, clarify, expand, or correct (if necessary) the health education children receive at home. Such school health educational programs must be built around the following realization (Kaplan, 1972:8):

. . . There is a mutually interdependent relationship between education and health: one needs health to become educated; one needs education to maintain health; and, one needs health to make use of one's education.

Purposes and goals of school health education programs

Health education programs have generally been viewed as primary prevention and health promotion measures, designed to prevent disease and disability and to promote "health" as it is perceived by the program's planners. Based on the definition of health education adopted for this chapter, the purpose of school health education may be perceived as the provision of learning experiences that result in development of self-actualized health-educated adults, capable of making and carrying out responsible decisions concerning their own health and that of the community (whether local, regional, national, international, or global) in which they live.

The purpose and importance of health education within the school health program have been more eloquently described by Califano (1977) and Jacobsen and Siegel (1971). In reporting how his experiences as a parent convinced him that children develop behaviors early in life which will affect their health, Califano (1977: 334) acknowledged the following:

Perhaps the single most important contribution school health programs can make to promote health is to emphasize the importance of lifestyles, and the environment, and to teach children how to use the health system.

Califano (1977:335) further points out that today's children are tomorrow's health consumers; for that reason, it is imperative that schools teach them to be "discriminating consumers of health care" so that as adults they will be "capable of using the health care system more efficiently and effectively" [than many of today's adults].

A more specific and detailed description of the contribution and desired outcome of the school health education program is presented by Jacobsen and Siegel (1971:158) as follows:

The health education program must help the pupil obtain an understanding of the life processes and realize the extent of man's ability to correct or eliminate those elements which are a health hazard. The health program should enable the pupil to *acquire* and *maintain* a wholesome respect for the human body. The student should be taught how to develop patterns of healthful living and social relationships and how to accept a major responsibility for his own health and well-being and for the ecology of the community in which he lives. Finally, the school health education program should provide the pupil with knowledge of the communities [sic] health resources and how to use them.

The purposes and desired outcomes of school health education as described by these authorities (and others) are lofty and broad in scope. To successfully undertake such an educational program would obviously require careful planning and adequate resources (including skilled and qualified health educators). As mentioned in previous discussions concerning planning school health programs, the specific goals and objectives adopted for a particular school health program depend on the specific health needs that are present in the school community's population. Thus there can be no universally "right" school health education curriculum or program. Each school district (or individual school) will need to survey or otherwise determine the health needs of the population it plans to serve before designing and implementing its health education program.

While the precise details of a particular school health education program must be tailored to the health and educational needs of its "target" population, suggested goals, missions, and recommendations for health education programs are available in health and education literature. Some of these will be briefly highlighted in the remainder of this discussion.

According to Anderson and Creswell (1976: 222-223), school health education programs encompass the following three basic goals:

1. Development of *attitudes* and *ideals* to motivate individuals (students) to achieve

their optimal level of functioning or well-being

2. (Students') acquisition of *knowledge* appropriate and necessary for health promotion
3. Establishment of *practices* (behaviors) necessary for health

In their view, these three objectives are interdependent and reciprocal; thus, for example, health knowledge that is not coupled with appropriate health attitudes will not likely result in positive health habits or behaviors. Therefore the school health education program must address all three areas. To illustrate how general health education objectives can be written to incorporate these three areas, Anderson and Creswell (1976) list thirty-six school health education general program objectives, presented by category (health attitudes, health knowledge, and health practices or behaviors).

In an effort to determine more precisely the "missions" of health education, Shirreffs (1978) conducted a survey of college and university health educators, trying to establish the existence of a consensus regarding the goals or missions of health education. Although no consensus was reached, the "mission" that was most highly accepted was "to foster positive health attitudes and value development in individuals," followed by "to change behaviors and practices that detract from health to those which promote health in individuals" (1978: 332). Thus the importance of influencing health attitudes and behaviors as well as providing knowledge is valued by collegiate health educators, a position which supports that of Anderson and Creswell.

To clarify and declare their support for school health education programs, two professional organizations, the American Association for Health, Physical Education, and Recreation (AAHPER) and the American Academy of Pediatrics, have authored position statements detailing their recommendations concerning health education in the schools. According to the AAHPER position statement (1971:171), the following actions are recommended:

1. Development of a unified program of health instruction providing "scope and sequence" for grades kindergarten to twelve.
2. Emphasis on curriculum development including (a) delineation of specific courses (content, learning activities, and evaluation activities) and (b) coordination and integration of health courses with other academic subjects.

3. Involvement of school personnel, curriculum directors, lay members of the public, representatives of voluntary and official health agencies, plus available state and national consultants in health curriculum development.
4. Employment and provision of health teachers who are genuinely interested in health education and specifically prepared to teach health.

The position statement presented by the American Academy of Pediatrics (1978:503) supports the AAHPER position and recommendations as just described and adds the following recommendations:

1. Kindergarten to twelve comprehensive health education curriculum should be required for all students, and should be planned based on age and maturity of the children in each grade level; recommended subject areas include biology, physiology, genetics, accident prevention, venereal disease, sex education, alcoholism, drug abuse, mental health, parenting, environmental and consumer health, and preventive medicine.
2. The health education curriculum should help students apply facts and concepts in achieving "healthful living" and in making responsible, appropriate decisions to solve personal, family, and/or community health problems.
3. The collegiate preparation for *all* elementary and secondary teachers should include mandatory courses in health science.
4. Adequate financial support for health education programs should be obtained from local boards of education, state and federal governmental agencies involved with education, as well as from corporations, foundations, and special interest groups and organizations (such as the American Heart Association or the National Institute for Mental Health).
5. Health education programs for adults should be intensified as part of a "coordinated community health education effort."

Thus, while the specific programmatic objectives for school health education programs are determined by districts or individual schools, there are some generally accepted overall goals and outcomes recommended by professional organizations who have an interest in and commitment to school health and health education.

Having discussed (1) the meaning of the term "health education" as defined in this chapter, (2) why health education is an essential component of the school health program, and (3) basic goals, purposes, and other recommendations for planning and implementing a school health education program, it is both prudent and necessary to next discuss some of the problems confronting school health education.

PROBLEMS CONFRONTING SCHOOL HEALTH EDUCATION

In today's health-conscious society with its emphasis on "good" nutrition, physical fitness and weight control, mental health, environmental purity, and consumer participation in health care planning and delivery, it would seem logical to expect that health education would be an esteemed and prominent feature of the overall school educational program. However, as Aubrey (1972:285) points out in his description of health education as a "neglected child of the schools," this is not the case; indeed, quite the reverse is true:

With few exceptions, health education in the public schools of the United States has low status and esteem in the eyes of teachers, students, and administrators.

Furthermore, as Aubrey (1972:285) points out, this is not a new problem:

Health education has never been popular among either teachers or students. Teachers have seen health education as an imposition, another unit or lesson to be crammed into an already sardine-packed curriculum. Students too have reacted unenthusiastically to films and factual presentations loaded with admonitions and moralistic leanings unrelated to their everyday lives.

The regrettable result of this unpopularity plus the failure of the educational reform movement of the 1950s and 1960s to examine and revise health education curricula and strategies is as follows (Aubrey, 1972:285):

Today, health education retains its image as an amorphous area, somewhere between physical education and the nurse's office. . . . All too often the responsibility for health is placed in the hands of the physical education department or sundry members of the home economics staff. Rarely is it viewed as an integral or essential component in the total curricular experience of students.

In the preceding brief passages, Aubrey has identified a number of important problems confronting contemporary school health education programs:

1. Lack of prestige and esteem for health education on the part of administrators, faculty, and students.
2. As a result of this lack of prestige and esteem, faculty and students tend to be disinterested, and health education receives low or no priority.
3. Use of ineffective health education strategies, including a too heavy emphasis on "facts" and moralistic judgments.
4. Lack of integration of health education into the total school curriculum, resulting in fragmented, piecemeal health education offerings.
5. Lack of interested, motivated, and academically qualified teachers to carry out health education curricula, resulting in health "teaching" being done by unqualified, disinterested teachers who view health education as a burden and a chore.

These problems have also been recognized by other authors, including Sliepcevich (1964), Kaplan (1972), Means (1973), Newman and Mayshark (1973), and Haro (1974).

Not surprisingly, students themselves are very aware of the problems confronting school health education, as documented by a research study in which adolescents (high school students) were asked to identify their health needs (Wold, 1975). The student participants identified, as a primary concern, their need for information about immediate and cumulative effects of drug and tobacco usage, sex education, birth control/family planning, abortion, venereal disease, pollution, mental health, and existing health resources. However, the students were characteristically blunt and forthright in their expression of frustration and disappointment with the health education courses available to them at school. The students decried the policy of having health taught by physical education teachers, pointing out that this often results in use of the health class period to discuss what these teachers are presumably most comfortable with—sports. Another problem identified by the students was the use of outdated and thus irrelevant audiovisual aids, including films, pamphlets, books, and posters; they believed such materials contribute to student apathy. Finally, these students expressed concern about the "inflexibility" of the health course content, complaining that the curriculum is predetermined and not subject to "student-centered" revision in the classroom to make it more relevant to their needs and interests (Wold, 1975). Indeed, health education has become so routinized, in their opinion, that it is planned around calendar dates instead of student needs and interests. Thus, as one student wryly observed, "If this is December, it must be sex ed.!"

In addition to the school health education problems already addressed in this discussion, additional problems merit attention. Among these is the lack of comprehensive *mandated* health education programs throughout the United States. Castile and Jerrick (1976) report that only sixteen states have mandated comprehensive health education programs, although in some states such programs are optional and left to the discretion of individual school districts; in other states particular health subject areas may be mandated, such as drugs, tobacco, and alcohol or safety. Thus in states where comprehensive health education is required by law, quality health education programs might be presumed to exist.

However, Conley and Jackson (1978) point out that this conclusion may not be valid. Indeed, in their attempts to answer the question: "Is a mandated comprehensive health education program a guarantee of successful health education?" their inescapable conclusion was "not necessarily." Obviously, other factors, such as quality of the curriculum and instruction, and administrative and faculty interest and support, affect the outcome and success of school health education programs. However, as Aubrey (1972) notes, an additionally significant factor affecting the success of mandated health education programs is the extent of *enforcement* of existing laws and regulations. Thus failure of states to evaluate and monitor the quality of health education programs within their jurisdiction has only compounded the problem.

Another problem related to the lack of enforcement of existing health education standards and regulations concerns the lack of adequate funding to support both surveillance/evaluation activities (Aubrey, 1972) and program development and implementation activities (Sliepcevich, 1964; Means, 1973). Thus while federal and local governmental agencies may have paid lip service to the need for comprehensive and high-quality health education, financial backing has been limited; in fact, the national School Health Education Study by Sliepcevich (1964) relied heavily on private funding sources (Means, 1973) for support.

In addition to the lack of mandated comprehensive school health education programs nationwide, there has been a corresponding tendency toward continuation of ineffective "traditional" health education formats (Sinacore, 1978:216), which are readily perceived as such (ineffective) by students:

We can painfully recall the boring recitations of the names of bones and muscles, as if by some miracle,

this would lead to a healthier body. The bones and muscles approach is now referred to as the BM approach, and students have long since appropriately named courses of that type.

The need to develop effective teaching strategies is acute if successful health education outcomes are desired.

Yet another problem that plagues existing school health education programs and curricula is the fact that too often they are not based on careful assessment of the community's health needs (Jacobsen and Siegel, 1971; Newman and Mayshark, 1973; Kunstel, 1978). This may be due in part to the failure of school systems to view their school health programs as part of the overall community health program (Jacobsen and Siegel, 1971) and to integrate their school health program within the community's health system. As Kunstel (1978:220) points out, when schools fail to consider or assess the *community's* needs, the school health education program may have "critical gaps in its structure" and/or "neglect important opportunities to relate to the students' life experiences."

Finally, but certainly not of least importance or urgency, is the problem of inadequate research concerning all aspects of health education (Simonds, 1977), including curriculum design, age-appropriate presentation of particular content areas, age-appropriate teaching strategies and desired outcomes (objectives), long-range and short-range learning outcomes of health education strategies, and qualifications necessary for health educators. It seems that like school nursing, health education as a discipline has also operated largely on untested assumptions concerning such areas as health, health education, and health educators (Sechrist and Jones, 1979). For that reason, Sechrist and Jones (1979) propose that concerted efforts be expended on what they describe as "assumption analysis" in the hope that ultimately health education programs will be "based a little more on science and a little less on intuition."

In conclusion, health education, like school nursing, faces some important and weighty problems that affect its future. And, as in the case of school nursing, the solutions to many of these problems depend on two major strategies: (1) obtaining adequate funding for program development, implementation, and evaluation and (2) conducting research to document and justify outcomes and expenditures (cost-effectiveness). School health education programs are *generally* believed (at least by their proponents) to be important and effective primary prevention/health promotion strategies, but those beliefs must be proven.

SOURCES OF HEALTH INFLUENCE AND EDUCATION

In addition to recognizing that some very real and serious problems confront school health education programs, it is also important to realize that even well-designed and well-executed school health education programs are just *one* source of influence over children's health and health behavior. Indeed, children are influenced and "health educated" by a variety of sources, including their families, peers, other adults, institutions (school and church), and mass media, particularly television.

The family is an important, yet often overlooked, source of health education for children and youth. In fact, as Bruhn and Cordova (1977:249) point out, the family "is a primary factor in the learning of wellness behavior." However, the family may also be a primary factor in the learning of "illness-seeking" behavior, if its values and health knowledge and competence are such that wellness and health-promoting behaviors are not encouraged. During early childhood, until the child enters preschool, day care, or kindergarten, the family may be the primary influence over the child's health; that influence may be conscious and direct, as in the case of families who require children to be appropriately dressed for weather and climate conditions, bring children in for periodic health care, including immunizations, or are careful to provide a safe environment and safe toys. Or the influence may be subtle, unconscious, or indirect, as in the case of families in which sugary foods are used to reward acceptable behavior (thus setting up a potential pattern of emotional dependence on food, which may lead to later obesity), or families in which television is the primary source of stimulation for children (and at times may serve as babysitter), as well as families in which nutrition consists of "junk food," and smoking and drinking are the norm. Obviously, the family's direct and indirect influences over a child's health can be either positive *or* negative; however, regardless of whether the family attempts to consciously influence the child's health or does so without conscious effort or intention, the child is learning something about health and health values in his home.

Despite occasional parental protestations to the contrary, Bruhn and Cordova (1977:249) believe that families "have not done an adequate job of teaching children health practices or helping them to clarify conflicting values regarding health." As a result, they believe this responsibility has been relegated to others, including peers, schools, churches, and the media. From the time of their first venturing forth into the neighborhood or to the babysitter, day care center, or preschool, children begin to learn about health from persons other than their immediate families. The kinds of meals served by the babysitter or day care worker (sugar content, food group sources), the hygiene standards observed (handwashing, cleanliness of play areas), the emphasis (or lack of emphasis) on balanced rest and play, and the manner of discipline (verbal or physical, consistent or variable) are just a few of the physical, mental, or social health behaviors the child can observe. For those children whose parents are employed outside the home, adults other than their parents, such as babysitters, day care workers, or preschool teachers and aides, may become very powerful and consistent role models for health, exerting an influence that is potentially as strong as that of their parents.

As children mature, their peer group expands and becomes more important to them. School-age children, especially adolescents, begin to rely more heavily on the opinions and behaviors of their friends than on those of their parents. Thus children who may have been carefully taught at home that smoking is hazardous to health may begin to question that premise when they observe their friends smoking without any apparent observable ill effects. If the health behaviors of their peers are similar to those which they were taught at home, then familial health concepts and behaviors are reinforced; however, if their peers' health values and behaviors are different from those of their parents, the inevitable result is conflict and confusion.

Another likely source of influence on children's health attitudes and behaviors includes institutions and organizations like schools and churches. At school, children are exposed to and involved to varying degrees in a health education program designed to positively influence their health attitudes, values, and behaviors. However, while the school health education curriculum presumably has some effect on children's values and behaviors, it is not the only source of health influence in the school. Indeed, the conscious or unconscious role modeling of teachers, school nurses, and other school staff members must certainly be regarded as a powerful influence on children. Most preadolescents have high regard for their teachers' opinions and actively seek their approval. Teachers need to be aware of this "hold" they have over children and be sure that their verbal and nonverbal behaviors are congruent; that is, they must be sure they "practice what they preach." Teachers who give class lectures about the evils of smoking and then smoke in the presence of their students must realize the conflict this generates and recognize the possibly negative effect it may have on their credibility with students. Similarly, ministers and other respected adults encountered by the child through his church affiliation may also be contributing consciously or unconsciously to the child's health education; they too must realize the effect of their behavior and beliefs on children and exercise their influence wisely.

Finally, major though probably underestimated sources of influence over children's health attitudes and behaviors are the media, including magazines and books (especially comic books and other children's publications), newspapers, billboards, radio, and television. Even for preverbal children, the illustrations in magazines and newspapers of violence and sex must be regarded as potentially powerful messages about "OK" health behaviors and attitudes. Radio, television, and motion pictures are also known influences on children's behavior and values and are not necessarily *positive* influences. For example, children viewing programs like the popular "Incredible Hulk," in which the main character deals with his anger by turning into a raging monster, may conclude that it is "OK" to vent one's anger indiscriminately and without restraint. Likewise, some persons believe that violence on television can actually teach children how to commit crimes by imitation, as in the case of a teenager in Florida on trial for homocide whose legal defense was that the producers of "Kojak," a series about a New York City police lieutenant, were responsible for "teaching" him to commit murder and for glamorizing crime.

The ethics and effects of commercial advertising directed at children through such sources as comic books, magazines, radio, product packaging (including everything from the backs of cereal boxes to gum wrappers), and televi-

sion have also been hotly debated. Probably the most damning indictment has been made against television commercials that urge children to persuade their parents to buy sugar-coated cereals, candies, soft drinks, gooey, spongy, prepackaged bakery goods, or highly caloric and greasy "junk" food. While some people argue that parents ought to have enough stamina and sales resistance to say "no" to their children's requests for such foods, others argue that such advertising only increases the demands and pressures imposed on today's parents, who may, however reluctantly, "give in" to their children's demands to keep the peace; the result, then, may be temporarily relieved parental pressure, children who learn that mom and dad *can* be pressured successfully, increased sales and soaring profits for advertisers and manufacturers, and yet poorer nutrition for children, the ultimate "victims" in this game. In fact, according to a survey of 272 pediatricians reported and described by Bruyn (1978:475), television has failed abysmally to provide "useful information about nutrition, health, diseases, accident prevention, drug abuse, tobacco, and . . . how to make reasonable decisions." The respondents also believed that television programming failed to stimulate and encourage children to engage in "constructive activities" or creative play and offered less than ideal presentations of sex/gender roles and adult roles in general. While the long-range impact of extensive television viewing and exposure on children's development is as yet unknown, there is certainly cause for concern. One conclusion seems certain: whether positive or negative, television and other media sources are powerful influences on the health values and behaviors of our nation's children and must be regarded as sources of health education for them.

HEALTH EDUCATION PROCESS AND PRINCIPLES

Up to this point, this chapter has focused on the importance of health education in the school, some of the problems confronting school health education, and the likely sources of health influence and education for children and youth. With that discussion as background, the following areas pertaining to the actual process of health education will be discussed: observations on education of two theorists, the health education process, and principles relevant for health education.

Observations on education: two viewpoints

There seems to be a vast array of literature directed toward educators, in which numerous theories of teaching and learning are proposed and evaluated, and specific approaches and strategies for curriculum design and classroom or informal teaching are suggested. Because so much has been written on these topics, educators must read prolifically and discriminate carefully among the available ideas and suggestions if they are to stay abreast of new developments and avoid the pitfalls of faddism. Among the contributors to educational literature whose ideas of educational psychology and methods are widely respected are Carl Rogers and William Glasser.

The importance of freedom to learn: the views of Carl Rogers

Carl Rogers (1969:v) has been a respected and influential educator who, by his own admission, has been "experimenting and innovating" in his approach to students since the mid 1930s. Throughout that time, he has written and published extensively for and about educators. Because of that fact, it is difficult and hazardous to attempt to describe Rogers' philosophy and ideas about education in just a few paragraphs, since the result may be a dangerous oversimplification of his views. For that reason, this brief discussion of some of Rogers' ideas is prefaced by this disclaimer: this discussion is *not* intended as a comprehensive description of Rogers' work and beliefs and should not be construed as such; rather, the concepts and ideas included have been arbitrarily chosen for their particular relevance to health education.

Among his more unconventional and radical views on education and the teaching-learning process is Rogers' conviction (1969:103) that "teaching . . . is a vastly over-rated function." Rogers defends that seemingly heretical statement by pointing out that "to teach" is variously defined by Webster as "to instruct" or "to cause to know a subject." The problem with this, according to Rogers, is that such definitions assume that the "teacher" has a "superior vantage point" from which she can determine exactly what another person needs to know, which is a highly presumptuous view.

As an alternative to such traditional views of "teaching" as directing, guiding, and showing others (students) what and how to learn, Rogers proposes that the *aim* of education be reassessed. Instead of attempting to ensure that students *acquire knowledge,* Rogers urges that the goal of education be redefined to become *facilitation of learning.* In other words, he believes educators should assist students to "learn how to learn" and to learn how to adapt and change in our modern, nonstatic world. As he points out, the "facts" and knowledge that are accepted today as "truth," will be out-of-date tomorrow; therefore only those students who have truly learned how to think and adapt will be able to cope with life.

Thus as Rogers explains (1969:5), *in order for learning to be significant, it must be experiential;* experiential learning is characterized by these five attributes:

1. *Personal involvement*—the person (student/learner) is involved both affectively (feelings) and cognitively (intellectually) in the learning experience.
2. *Self-initiated*—even when the stimulus to learn is external or outside the person, the *sense of discovery* is intrapersonal or *internal.*
3. *Pervasiveness*—such learning affects the entire person of the learner, including his behavior, attitudes, and even his personality.
4. *Evaluated by the learner*—the *learner* bears primary responsibility for determining whether the learning experience meets his needs and expectations.
5. *Its essence is meaning*—"when such learning takes place, the element of meaning to the learner is built into the whole experience."

It is unfortunate that much of our formal educational system, including higher education, fails to incorporate these kinds of learning experiences.

To encourage experiential and significant learning, Rogers (1969) urges that the role of teacher be changed from "instructor" to *facilitator of learning.* Rogers goes on to identify three qualities or essential attitudes of the teacher/facilitator that facilitate learning. The first of these facilitator qualities is *realness* or *genuineness.* Rogers believes that when the facilitator presents herself to the learner as a "real" person without a facade to mask her genuine feelings, her effectiveness is enhanced. This kind of teacher, characteristically unafraid to be herself and to accept her own emotions, can feel comfortable expressing enthusiasm or boredom or anger or joy and will therefore be respected as a "real" person instead of a "faceless embodiment'' by her students. With this kind of respect from students, the teacher can generate greater interest and participation in classroom learning activities.

The second quality or attitude of the facilitator that Rogers (1969) emphasizes is *prizing, acceptance, and trust*. This attitude means that the teacher/facilitator ''prizes'' the learner or cares for him as a person, including his feelings and attitudes; the teacher views the learner/student as a separate, worthwhile, and trustworthy person. Another description of this attitude might be Rogers' term ''unconditional positive regard,'' which was discussed in Chapter 11 within the context of the helping or therapeutic relationship. Regardless of which term is used, the meaning is essentially the same: the facilitator accepts the person with all his imperfections and abilities, and trusts him to behave responsibly without anyone ''checking up'' on his performance.

Finally, the third facilitator quality or attitude that encourages self-directed, experiential learning is *empathic understanding*. This quality refers to the teacher's ability to see things through the student's eyes—that is, to understand the student's reactions and perceptions. The teacher who can display this kind of sensitive understanding increases the likelihood of significant student learning (Rogers, 1969).

The task for teachers or educators, then, according to Rogers (1969:131), is to create a climate in which students' intrinsic motivation is enhanced rather than dampened: ''to tap that motivation, to discover what challenges are real for the young person, and to provide the opportunity for him to meet those challenges.'' In short, the emphasis needs to be on providing the freedom to learn.

School-induced failure and some alternatives: the views of William Glasser

As noted in the discussion of Reality Therapy in Chapter 11, William Glasser is primarily a psychiatrist by background. However, Glasser believes his Reality Therapy principles can be applied not only to one-to-one therapeutic helping relationships, but also to our American educational system.

Both Glasser (1969) and Rogers (1969) seem to agree that ''traditional'' teaching-learning theories and approaches are less than optimally effective because, according to Glasser (1969: xiv), they are predicated on an ''educational philosophy . . . of noninvolvement, nonrele-vance, and limited emphasis on thinking.'' In other words, much of the ''school failure'' experienced by American children is due to the ineffectiveness of our educational system and philosophy and not to some personal defects of the children themselves.

More specifically, Glasser (1969) identifies two ''principles'' that contribute to lack of school achievement and, indeed, to school failure in this country. The first is what he calls the ''certainty principle,'' according to which there is a right and a wrong answer to every question; applying this principle, ''the function of education is then to ensure that each student knows the right answers to a series of questions that educators have decided are important'' (1969: 36). This kind of attitude obviously does not reward creativity or thinking ability; instead, the ''payoff,'' which may be anything from verbal recognition to a straight ''A'' report card, is awarded for giving the ''right'' answer.

The second principle that contributes to school failure is the ''measurement principle''; according to this principle, ''nothing is really worthwhile unless it can be measured and assigned a numerical value'' (1969:38). Thus the score of one student on a test is seen as educationally significant compared with the scores of other students. What students learn when these two principles are operationalized is that to be rewarded, they must ''learn'' the ''right'' answers and ''regurgitate'' them on request, as in testing situations. It seems highly unlikely that significant learning occurs within such an educational climate.

According to Glasser (1969), the solution to this growing problem of school-induced failure is to move toward an opposite educational philosophy—that is, a philosophy that emphasizes involvement, relevance, and thinking. Among the numerous methods he suggests for accomplishing this are (1) giving children a voice in determining both the curriculum and conduct ''rules'' for their school; (2) deemphasizing rote memorization of ''facts,'' encouraging instead problem solving, social responsibility, and thinking; (3) abolishing A, B, C, D, F grading and replacing it, perhaps, with a ''pass-superior'' system; and (4) frequent and regular use of what he calls ''classroom meetings'' of three types: social problem solving, open ended, or educational-diagnostic (1969).

Thus, while Glasser and Rogers have slightly different philosophies of education and teaching and learning, both are encouraging reforms

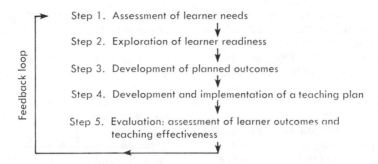

Fig. 15-1. Health education process.

within our educational system. Both wish to abolish educational styles and methods that encourage student passivity and uninvolvement, reward memorization at the expense of creativity and thinking, and, most of all, fail to respect and value students as persons in their own right. Only their semantics and labels are really different: Glasser dreams of schools without failure, while Rogers yearns for an educational system that provides students with the freedom to learn.

Health education process

While the philosophies of Rogers and Glasser address the educational system in general, their ideas are certainly relevant for persons charged with the responsibility of designing, implementing, and evaluating the school health education curriculum. Indeed, it should become apparent as the process of health education is described that incorporation of many of their ideas and beliefs could greatly improve the relevance, usefulness, and outcome of health education in our schools.

Although there are undoubtedly numerous conceptualizations or models of the teaching-learning process, each of which may be labeled and described as "unique," the process of education generally includes the same basic steps, regardless of any semantic differences in the labeling or sequencing of those steps. For the purposes of this chapter, the process of health education (Fig. 15-1) will be discussed using the following steps:

1. Assessment of learner needs
2. Exploration of learner readiness
3. Development of planned outcomes
4. Development and implementation of a teaching plan
5. Evaluation: assessment of learner outcomes and teaching effectiveness

The feedback loop (Fig. 15-1) indicates that the results of the evaluation process should be fed back to the first step (assessment of learner needs) and on through the process again to allow for meaningful revision.

Step 1: Assessment of learner needs

As Lussier (1972:618) points out, "Everything done by the educator is meaningless if it is not directed at the needs of the learner." This deceptively simple statement explains the often overlooked importance of ensuring that educational programs and curricula be designed with the learner in mind. Thus students' perceived needs and interests as well as their (statistically) probable risks of developing health problems and conditions should be assessed. For example, in a high school where the reported or estimated venereal disease rate is high, extra emphasis on sexuality and venereal disease prevention and treatment may need to be incorporated into the health education curriculum. Obviously, then, a survey of the school population's health needs should be done to ensure planning of a viable curriculum; such a survey or assessment might include analysis of vital statistics data (especially morbidity and mortality data), opinion surveys administered to students, teachers, administrators, parents, and other interested and involved parties, or analysis of data generated by review of students' school health records.

Such assessment of students' needs and interests is essential, since programs planned on the basis of "yesterday's" needs are likely to be received with yawns, outrage, or apathy and are unlikely to result in significant learning for students. Lussier (1972) describes several studies designed to counteract the problem of outdated curricula by assessing the health education needs and interests of school-age children and youth as well as college students. Studies done in the 1970s showed definite changes in student needs and interests as compared with studies from the 1950s and 1960s; for that reason, Lussier (1972) urges that health education curricula be continually updated to reflect these changes. Obviously, that also requires ongoing studies to assess students' needs and interests and incorporation of their findings into curricular revisions.

However, as Newman and Mayshark (1973) and Kunstel (1978) point out, assessment of *students'* health needs and interests alone is not adequate in planning a school health education curriculum. Rather, as they point out, the community at large is also part of the school's constituency; therefore in planning the health education curriculum, the needs of the local community must also be considered. As Kunstel (1978:220) warns, failure to do so results in a health education curriculum that is ''likely (1) to contain critical gaps in its structure and (2) to neglect important opportunities to relate to the students' life experiences.''

Thus, in assessing learner needs during this first step of the health education process, it is necessary and important to assess not only students' perceptions, but also statistical data, opinions of school personnel and parents, as well as the health needs of the local community. This kind of careful assessment and community focus helps ensure the timeliness and relevance of the school's health education curriculum, thus increasing the likelihood that significant learning will occur.

Step 2: Exploration of learner readiness

Once the learning needs of the target population are known, the next consideration is the learner's *readiness* and receptivity to the proposed teaching plan. It is generally not safe to assume that because a person has a ''need'' or a defined risk of developing or exacerbating some health condition or problem, he is psychologically ''ready'' to deal with the problem—and until he *is* ready, even the most articulate and creative teaching plan is likely to fall on deaf ears. For example, there are many smokers today who, despite their admittedly chronic coughs or other more serious sequelae such as emphysema, are stubbornly resistant to the well-intentioned efforts of their loved ones or other persons to induce them to quit smoking. Some of those smokers may even admit ''I know I *should* quit . . .'' but are simply not

''ready'' to deal with what they doubtless anticipate will be a painful process of changing their behavior. For such persons, health education campaigns (which appear to descend on them like a veritable blitzkrieg) directed at elimination of smoking behavior are not likely to succeed and may in fact increase their defensiveness and even cause them to smoke *more*.

Thus learner readiness and motivation are essential if health education efforts are to succeed. To some extent, student readiness undoubtedly depends on the approach of the teacher. If the style of presentation of the course content and material is dull and uninteresting, or, worse yet, irrelevant to students' lives, the interest level of students who were initially highly motivated and very receptive will wane.

Thus an important aspect of facilitating learner readiness is creating an optimal learning climate (Gross, 1977). Creating such a learning climate requires attention to both the physical environment and the psychological comfort of students. The physical environment should be sufficiently large, adequately lighted and ventilated, and comfortably furnished; furniture should be arranged in appropriate groupings to coincide with the planned teaching strategies. For example, if the planned teaching strategy is small group discussion, then a round table with chairs would be appropriate. Promoting students' psychological comfort can be partially achieved by attending to some of the physical environmental details just mentioned. However, the psychological climate depends more on the teacher's ''style'' than on physical environmental characteristics. Thus the approaches described by Rogers (1969) and Glasser (1969), such as genuineness, trust, unconditional positive regard, honesty, relevance, and involvement are likely to create a climate in which student interest and motivation are heightened rather than stifled, with the result that significant learning is both possible and likely.

Step 3: Development of planned outcomes

If the goal of education or the teaching process is for the learner to be changed as a result of the experience, whether that change be in his attitudes, values, or behaviors, then it is important to determine exactly what result or change is desired *before the actual ''teaching'' is begun*. That is, if an educational program or curriculum is to be effective, the desired terminal outcomes for the learner should be *planned* in advance of the actual teaching, since unless you know where you are going, you'll have trouble determining whether (and when) you have arrived. For this reason, an important next step in the health education process is determining behavioral objectives or planned terminal outcomes. In this chapter the terms *behavioral objective, planned terminal outcome,* and *terminal behavior* will be used interchangeably. To borrow Mager's (1962:2) definition, these terms refer "to the behavior you would like your learner to be able to demonstrate at the time your influence over him ends." That is, these objectives or outcomes reflect *learner behaviors* that are somehow *observable* or *measurable* at the conclusion of the health education process. Thus while the health educator (used here to refer to anyone who teaches or educates others about health) may also have objectives describing the intended *process* for teaching and learning, assessment of actual *learning* requires development and use of learner objectives and outcomes as well.

Specifically, the four benefits of behaviorally stated learner outcomes (behavioral objectives) are as follows (Gronlund, 1970):

1. They provide direction for the teacher/health educator as well as indicating to others her "instructional intent."
2. They facilitate and guide selection of course content, teaching strategies, and supplemental materials.
3. They facilitate the evaluation process, since tests are constructed to measure achievement of the course/student objectives.
4. When communicated directly to the student, behavioral objectives guide the student's learning activities by pointing out what he is expected to be able to do as a result of the course or program; in other words, the objectives can serve as a sort of study guide for students.

While stating behavioral objectives/terminal learner outcomes may seem like a relatively simple task, in practice it can be frustrating. While it is clearly beyond the scope or stated intent of this book to develop the reader's expertise in writing such objectives or outcomes, several helpful and intelligibly written references do address the issue of actually writing behavioral objectives (Mager, 1962; Gronlund, 1970; Dickinson, 1971.) However, following is a summary of some of the key points for writing behavioral objectives for health education (Mager, 1962; Gronlund, 1970):

1. Begin each objective with an *action verb,*

such as "discusses," "describes," "analyzes," "names," "predicts," "compares," and "contrasts." Verbs such as "knows," "understands," or "appreciates" are not appropriate because they are *not* observable or measurable.
2. Be sure the objective is stated as a learner performance outcome rather than as a teacher action or intent. For example, "Discusses effects of smoking on the cardiovascular system." (This is a learner behavior.) An example of a teacher intent (process-oriented) objective would be: "Describe for students current research findings concerning the physiological effects of smoking." While this is relevant for the teacher in planning her course or class session, it does *not* identify the expected change in student behavior (terminal outcome) and thus cannot be used to evaluate student learning.
3. Include only *one* desired outcome/behavior per objective; this facilitates choosing teaching strategies and evaluating outcomes. (If several behaviors are combined into one objective, the relative emphasis of each may be lost, and the measurement of achievement becomes more complex.)
4. Be sure that the stated objectives are appropriate to the learning needs, interests, and developmental/maturational level of the learner. For example, in planning a sex education curriculum for first-graders, it would not be appropriate to include a detailed clinical discussion of the anatomy and physiology of reproduction, since the students' cognitive development is not sufficiently advanced for them to be able to grasp such material.

It should also be noted that behavioral objectives are generally classified as occupying one of three "domains": cognitive (intellectual), affective (attitudinal or emotional), and psychomotor ("doing" or motor skills) (Bloom, 1956; Gronlund, 1970). All possible learning outcomes are believed to fit within one of these domains, and all three domains are relevant for health education. Within each domain, behaviors are further classified into levels based on complexity. Thus, for example, the levels within the cognitive domain, from lowest to highest, are knowledge, comprehension, application, analysis, synthesis, and evaluation (Bloom,

1956). In writing behavioral objectives, it is helpful to consult this taxonomy to be sure that the objectives are within the intellectual capabilities of the learners; for example, in working with first-graders, the most appropriate cognitive levels would include knowledge, comprehension, and application, whereas adolescents could benefit from the higher level objectives as well, including analysis, synthesis, and evaluation.

Thus, while stating behavioral terminal learner outcomes presents some difficulties especially for the novice, it is a vital step to be completed *before* attempting to actually "teach" a student or "change" his behavior and attitudes.

Step 4: Development and implementation of a teaching plan

Undoubtedly, many persons regard development and actual implementation of a teaching plan as the essence or "meat" of health education; sadly, some even regard this step as the *equivalent* of "teaching" or "education." While development and implementation of a teaching plan are unquestionably very important to the success of the health education program or curriculum, they cannot stand alone. That is, the teaching plan and its implementation must be based on steps 1 to 3 of the health education process: assessment of learner needs, exploration of learner readiness and development of measurable, planned outcomes that form the basis for the selection of specific subject matter and teaching strategies. Thus completion of the first three steps in the health education process provides the groundwork for development and implementation of the precise teaching plan during step 4.

Selection of an appropriate teaching strategy. Armed with the behavioral objectives (planned learning outcomes) developed during step 3 of the health education process, the major task during step 4 is to select the appropriate teaching strategy (or strategies) to help students achieve those planned outcomes. Selection of teaching strategies should be based on consideration and assessment of the following:

1. The nature of the subject matter
2. Students' preferred learning style(s)
3. Students' developmental and maturational levels
4. Cultural considerations and other individual differences

NATURE OF THE SUBJECT MATTER. In any teaching-learning situation, the nature of the subject matter or course content is an important determinant for selection of an appropriate teaching method or strategy. For subjects such as mathematics, in which certain facts must be learned (formulas, multiplication tables, equivalents, and theorems) as a basis for solving problems or manipulating numbers in some way, the appropriate teaching strategies would include some definite emphasis on memorization of "facts" and principles, followed by drills to test memory and skill in applying those facts and principles. In contrast, subjects like history or sociology, in which the meaning of events and population trends and characteristics depends on their interpretation by scholars and other persons, memorization and application of "facts" and principles are not enough. In such subjects, discussion of the meaning of events and their relative value and impact on society is very important. Thus the strategies for these courses might include lecture, discussion, and values clarification. In the case of health education (as will be discussed more fully later in this chapter), a combination of strategies, including factual presentations, discussion, demonstration, and values clarification, is appropriate and necessary. The point is that the nature of the subject matter itself helps determine how it can be most effectively taught and should therefore be a primary concern for educators in planning course and curricular content.

STUDENTS' PREFERRED LEARNING STYLE(S). In addition to the nature of the subject matter itself, selection of appropriate teaching strategies requires assessment of students' preferred learning styles. Some learners prefer and respond more positively to informal, unplanned, spontaneous health teaching that occurs at the "teachable moment." For example, a high school student who has the uncomfortable and frightening symptoms of gonorrhea may be more amenable to health teaching about venereal disease prevention, early diagnosis, and treatment than he was during his health class because he now feels the need for that information. That same student (like many adult learners as well) may usually be apathetic or even actively resistant to health education efforts that are formal, planned, and (in his view) not directly applicable or relevant. While health educators may find that attitude distressing and be tempted to go to any lengths to correct it, a better use of energy and creativity would be to recognize and capitalize on that student learning style, since attempts to "change" the students' learning style to a formal, planned classroom experience may only *increase* student apathy and resistance and alienate students from *all* health education efforts. In contrast with students who prefer the informal "teachable moment" approach to health education, some students respond more readily to planned, formal programs or classes and are readily able to see the applicability of the concepts to their lives. Therefore student preferences for formal versus informal teaching and learning should be considered and respected whenever possible.

Other aspects of student learning preference to be considered include (1) preferred degree of self-direction, (2) use of printed or audiovisual materials versus verbal lecture or discussion, (3) use of demonstration–return demonstration techniques for learning new skills versus the "trial-and error" approach, (4) use of group versus individual learning experiences, and (5) preferred pacing or rate of learning.

Regarding preferred level of self-direction, students who view themselves as independent may prefer to be given some basic materials and references plus minimal guidance and direction and then set free to carry out learning activities on their own. In contrast, students who feel a need for more structure and assistance will prefer less freedom and more directed activity.

Concerning use or nonuse of printed and other audiovisual materials, some students can learn more effectively if they can read pertinent materials and/or use other audiovisual materials like films or tapes to help them understand health concepts and content. However, for students who are poor readers due to language barriers, limited intelligence, dyslexia or other causes, or who dislike reading, printed materials such as books and pamphlets may be ineffective teaching aids; for such students, a verbal presentation is often preferable, perhaps accompanied by a film or other audiovisual resource that does not require reading skills.

Use of teacher demonstration followed by a student return demonstration is an effective strategy for some students as they attempt to master a new psychomotor skill, such as bathing a baby, taking a temperature, or splinting an arm. However, other students may prefer to have the teacher demonstrate the skill, yet do not find return demonstration helpful; these students may prefer a "trial-and-error" approach (with or without an initial demonstration of the skill) in which the skill is learned by independent experimentation.

Another student learning preference may involve the learning setting itself. Some students in certain courses may prefer and respond more readily to individual learning or "private" teaching; this may be true for skills such as playing musical instruments or learning health assessment techniques or for other subjects in which students may feel incompetent and in need of maximal assistance or for subjects that are embarrassing or highly personal, such as portions of sex education. In contrast, other students may prefer the interchange and stimulation of a group learning setting and find the feedback and ideas of their fellow students important to their own learning.

Finally, another factor to assess in determining students' preferred learning styles concerns the pacing of the course or program. The fact that students vary widely in their rate of learning and their willingness to progress rapidly creates problems for classroom teachers, who are thus confronted with a group of students who may have different pacing needs. However, while such differences among students may pose tactical problems for teachers, these differences must nonetheless be acknowledged and considered in planning teaching strategies. An example of the influence of student pacing differences on teaching strategies is the traditional practice among many primary grade reading teachers of assigning students to reading groups based on ability and performance; thus students who are poor readers are grouped together so that they can proceed at a pace that is comfortable for them, whereas students who are excellent readers will not have their progress halted because of "slow" group members. In teaching health, this technique of grouping students according to preferred pace or rate of learning or according to depth of interest in a topic or issue may also have merit.

The obvious conclusion to be drawn from this discussion is that individual preferences and differences among students concerning their learning style and pace must be recognized and considered in planning health education programs and activities. The list of factors to be assessed concerning learning style presented here is intended only as a guide and not as an exhaustive list of pertinent factors. Readers may wish to add to the list based on their own experience.

STUDENTS' DEVELOPMENTAL AND MATURATIONAL LEVELS. Another consideration in selecting an appropriate teaching strategy is students' developmental and maturational levels. This means that teaching strategies should be compatible with students' abilities to comprehend and participate in the teaching plan. Specifically, this refers to students' *cognitive* or intellectual developmental levels, which are closely related to age (chronological and biological maturity). Thus factors such as the following must be considered and/or modified in planning teaching strategies that are age appropriate and developmentally realistic:

1. *Vocabulary.* Students who have limited language and vocabulary skills must be addressed in simple language that they can comprehend; otherwise, the teaching-learning strategy is unlikely to succeed.

2. *Use of printed materials and other audiovisual resources.* As noted previously, students with poor reading skills or young children who have not yet learned to read are unlikely to benefit from pamphlets or other reading materials. Films, slides, audiotapes, and other audiovisual resources may be useful teaching tools with preliterate or illiterate students *if* their content and style of presentation are appropriate for the cognitive and maturational (age) developmental levels of the intended audience (students).

3. *Length and style of presentation.* Young children have relatively short attention spans and are therefore unable and unlikely to sustain interest in an activity or presentation for long period of time; for this reason, health teaching with these children should be planned as brief (10- to 15-minute) "lessons" and may need to be repeated more than once. Older children and adults can sustain interest in activities for longer periods (provided the activities are not viewed as boring or uninteresting). In addition, the style of presentation may need modification based on the development and maturity of the intended students. Young children, for example, may respond more positively to involvement activities, such as games and discussions and may be totally unresponsive to "lectures" or more formal didactic presentations. In contrast, adults may tolerate and even benefit from lectures about health concerns and should be able to sustain their interest and attention for at least ½ hour under normal circumstances.

Again, this list is not exhaustive, but serves to point out the importance of considering students' cognitive and maturational levels in selecting health education teaching strategies.

CULTURAL CONSIDERATIONS AND OTHER INDIVIDUAL DIFFERENCES. The final areas to be assessed prior to selection of appropriate teaching strategies is the cultural background and orientation and any other individual or group characteristics of the students. Cultural factors and other individual differences or characteristics are important because they affect individuals' perceptions and beliefs about health, illness, health-seeking behaviors, and other life areas. Thus a student's cultural beliefs about health may preclude his acceptance of health teaching or may generate conflict between his beliefs and those espoused by the health educator (Chapter 8). Health educators who are sensitive to the disparities between their own beliefs and those of their students' cultural and family groups can therefore address those differences and help students resolve or at least acknowledge whatever conflict exists. Furthermore, cultural and individual or familial differences among students may result in varied levels of interest in education and learning and may also affect students' specific learning needs. Thus students whose familial and cultural beliefs place positive value on education may be more motivated to learn than students whose families or cultural groups scorn or devalue education. In addition, students who may hold cultural beliefs about disease causation that are not accurate based on scientific evidence may need health education which is more intensively focused, at least initially, on *facts*. On the other hand, students who have an accurate understanding of disease causation that is supported by their family and cultural beliefs and practices will not need as intensive a focus on those basic facts. Thus, insofar as they affect students' perceptions and attitudes about health, health practices, and the importance of disease prevention and health promotion, cultural and other individual differences among students are important considerations in selecting an appropriate health teaching strategy.

Appropriate health teaching strategies. Following assessment of the nature of the subject matter, students' preferred learning styles and developmental/maturational levels, and cultural considerations and other individual differences, selection of a specific health teaching strategy can be accomplished. In the remainder of this discussion, a number of suggested health teaching strategies will be briefly highlighted. The reader is again cautioned that the strategies included in this discussion are only presented as a representative sample.

FACTS: ARE THEY ENOUGH? Health education has traditionally been a "fact-oriented" discipline, presumably based on the assumption that people respond to the kinds of empirical-rational approaches described in Chapter 19; that is, health educators have seemed to operate on the assumption that if people are presented with the facts, they will change their behavior and/or attitudes to reflect that new knowledge because they are "rational." Unfortunately, experience has not borne out this assumption, since despite repeated "factual presentations" (with a few scare tactics thrown in for good measure), many people have staunchly refused to change their life-styles by quitting smoking, using automobile seatbelts, decreasing the salt, cholesterol, and calories in their diets, or by adopting other suggested changes in life-style (Fors and Ulrich, 1977).

Obviously, then, facts are not enough. As Fors and Ulrich (1977) point out, one of the basic problems with "facts" is that they tend to be "other centered." That is, people tend to believe that health problems like cancer and heart disease will happen to someone else and not to them. A classic example of the misuse of "facts" in health education is alcohol and drug education. As Fors and Ulrich (1977:200) point out:

We have missed our schools and communities with our approach to alcohol education because we have emphasized alcoholism. Keep in mind that no one in the community feels that he or she will ever be an alcoholic—that happens to someone else.

Another example of the inadequacy of mere facts in health education is venereal disease education. As Snegroff (1975:37) points out, knowledge about venereal disease is not enough because it does not ensure that students will *behave* according to their knowledge:

In addition to imparting knowledge other attempts must be made to affect their attitudes and behavior so that more of them will take active measures to prevent contracting a venereal disease or will seek treatment if infected.

However, despite the failure of mere facts to motivate people to adopt healthy life-styles and health-seeking or "wellness" behaviors, facts *are* important components of health education programs *because they help individuals/students form attitudes about wellness* (Bruhn and Cordova, 1977); these wellness attitudes are the

precursors of health-seeking behaviors. In other words, facts have an important place in health education, but they must not be equated or confused with health education itself.

DEVELOPING AND CLARIFYING HEALTH VALUES. In their discussion of "a developmental approach to learning wellness behavior," Bruhn and Cordova (1977:252) point out that in addition to exposure to facts, students need to learn *skills* to enable them to *practice* the wellness behaviors they have been taught. However, the extent to which individuals actually adopt wellness behaviors will depend greatly on the degree to which they *value* wellness. For that reason, health educators need to focus more fully and directly on instilling health values in their students. Bruhn and Cordova (1977:252) believe that this is especially critical for early adolescents, who are beginning to make their lifelong plans:

Whether wellness ranks high in the personal value system of the individual or not, individuals need to be exposed to wellness as a value so that it can be considered along with future plans which the individual begins to make in early adolescence.

In contrast with facts, which are described as "other centered," *values,* defined as criteria used in making choices among alternatives, are personal or "me centered" (Fors and Ulrich, 1977:201). For that reason, values have "personal consequence" for individuals and are therefore more likely than facts to have an impact on an individual's health behavior. Thus it is important for students to have opportunities to develop and refine or clarify their health and wellness values. Values clarification includes many specific techniques or strategies, such as self-survey questionnaires; rank ordering of value statements; group discussions including self-disclosures of feelings, attitudes, and past or projected behaviors; and "games" or decision-making simulations (such as the "game" for adults in which a mythical committee is asked to decide which of a group of needy patients will be assigned the one vacancy on the hospital dialysis machine). For detailed discussion of values-clarification techniques and their impact on students, the reader is encouraged to consult references such as Raths et al. (1966), Simon et al. (1972), and Osman (1974).

INTERACTIONAL HEALTH TEACHING: GROUP DISCUSSION. A classroom technique that can be used for values clarification as well as for increasing student involvement in learning is group discussion. Since development of health and wellness values requires critical thinking and analysis, group discussion or interaction can provide students with helpful feedback and criticism to guide their thinking. In addition, when students have the opportunity to compare their experiences, values, behaviors, and beliefs with those of their peers, they are thus provided with another source of health values and behaviors against which their own perceptions can be tested; the result, of course, may be either reassuring (if students find their own values are consistent and compatible with their peers') or disquieting (if, for example, the students' views are challenged, debunked, ridiculed, or simply at great variance with those of their peers). Whether the outcome is reassuring or disquieting, discussion is a useful health education strategy.

SELF-DIRECTED STUDY. Another category of health education strategies is self-directed study, in which the learner proceeds at his own pace through a course of study that is either self-designed and self-structured or predetermined and/or prepackaged by others. This category therefore includes independent study, in which the student generally, with faculty input and guidance, determines his own learning objectives and plans learning activities and evaluation measures to implement and evaluate them, respectively. Self-directed study also includes programmed learning, in which students proceed at their own pace through written and/or audiovisual materials designed to help them achieve certain specified learning objectives; learning programs typically include the objectives or planned outcomes, the materials necessary for achievement of those objectives, and pretests and posttests to measure learning. Programmed learning seemed especially vogue during the late 1960s and early 1970s; while it is not quite so popular or common today, programmed learning and the so-called modular format described by Carpenter and Quiring (1978) are useful learning tools, especially for groups of students with varied abilities and interests or for students who need or prefer to learn at their own pace. Such "programs" or modules have reinforcement in the form of verbal encouragement and praise built into them, so students get immediate and continuing feedback concerning their progress.

ROLE MODELING. As noted earlier in this chapter, role modeling, whether conscious and purposeful or unconscious and unintentional, can be a powerful influence on health behavior and attitudes. For that reason, role modeling must be acknowledged as a health education strategy. Health educators, including school nurses, must ensure that their health behavior is consistent with their espoused beliefs and with generally accepted health standards. Thus, health educators and school nurses should avoid smoking and alcohol and other chemical abuse, eat nutritionally adequate and balanced meals, and attain and maintain reasonable physical conditioning both to safeguard their own health and to demonstrate or "model" healthy behavior for their students.

EXPERIENTIAL HEALTH EDUCATION. By now it should be obvious that health education needs to include more than mere presentation of "facts." Indeed, as Esty (1970:11) points out:

Health concepts cannot be taught only, they must be experienced, and must bring about a change of behavior and a responsibility for personal involvement through an understanding of the conditions necessary for the maintenance of physical and emotional well-being.

Furthermore, according to Bruhn and Cordova (1977:252), "the experiential application of wellness is essential if the concept is to have practical value." Thus, experts agree that health education needs to be experiential and needs to actively *involve* students if sustained behavioral change is an expected and desired outcome.

Some of Carl Rogers' basic ideas concerning definitions of experiential learning and creating a climate that fosters it have already been discussed in this chapter (pp. 341 to 342) and will not be repeated here. Instead, it seems more appropriate at this point to identify a few specific experiential learning strategies that may be useful for health educators. The reader is again cautioned that these are cited only as examples; experiential learning, by definition, includes an almost limitless variety of techniques and strategies, selection of which depends on the creativity, ingenuity, and preference of the health educators.

One example of an experiential learning strategy incorporates use of audiovisual materials, such as films, slides, records and audiotapes, pamphlets, books, television, newspapers, and other periodicals. These materials may be used as a passive form of information giving much like a lecture, or they may become the stimulus for active, learner-involved health education. For example, a provocative film about teenage sexuality and parenthood could become the basis for a lively discussion of those issues, followed by students' clarification of their own sexuality values, or conduction of a survey to assess their peers' values and behaviors and to determine the need for health education and other programs to deal with those problems. Another strategy might be to assign students particular television programs or commercials to watch and/or critique to discover how television influences health attitudes and behaviors. Since most students are likely to enjoy watching television, this kind of "homework" is likely to be completed and enjoyed. Still another possible strategy would be to encourage (older) students to make and film on videotape their own "commercials" and "public service messages" concerning health issues; this would allow students to increase their appreciation of the difficulties of making responsible public service messages, while at the same time would give them the experience of communicating positive health attitudes and behaviors.

A second example of experiential learning strategies is the use of demonstration and return demonstration as a technique in teaching skills or behaviors. An obvious illustration of this would be in first aid classes, where students could be shown how to splint or bandage a limb, followed by student return demonstration of the techniques to validate their learning. This kind of technique can be used for any observable behavior or skill, including first aid, cardiopulmonary resuscitation (CPR), physical fitness, health assessment techniques (temperature taking and assessment of blood pressure), and personal hygiene.

A third example of experiential learning strategies includes those especially appropriate for children, such as games, coloring books, puppets, dolls, and play (Zentner and Murray, 1975; Redman, 1980). While these strategies have been in use for quite some time as therapeutic measures and as mechanisms that allow children experiencing stress such as pending hospitalization and surgery to "act out" their fears, they are also useful as teaching aids with "well" children in settings such as schools. Especially for children who are preverbal or whose language skills are limited, nonverbal experiential methods, such as puppets and dolls, allow children to learn by actively participating in health education experiences.

Again, experiential learning strategies or techniques abound, and health educators, including all persons involved in health teaching, such as teachers, nurses, and other health care professionals, are limited only by their ingenuity and creativity as they select or devise experiential strategies to supplement whatever factual information may need to be given.

Step 5: Evaluation: assessment of learner outcomes and teaching effectiveness

Another critically important aspect of the health education process, and one too often overlooked or underemphasized, is evaluation of the *results* of the health education program or curriculum. Because the results of health education, in the form of changed knowledge, values, attitudes, and behaviors, measure the success of the health education program, they are important inputs to be fed back into the health education process at step 1 (Fig. 15-1). In evaluating the health education process, then, two basic dimensions should be assessed: (1) learner outcomes and (2) teaching effectiveness.

In assessing learner outcomes, the focus is on comparing students' *actual performance* following the health education program with the *planned terminal outcomes* developed during step 3. Based on the EOCs developed in conjunction with those behavioral objectives (planned terminal outcomes), following measurement of students' abilities to demonstrate the planned terminal outcome behaviors through whatever means are appropriate, such as testing or direct observation, some conclusion concerning the success of the health education program in helping students achieve program objectives can be reached. If the EOCs are completely satisfied, the program can be judged successful, assuming, of course, that the EOCs were valid, reliable, and appropriate measures of the program's projected outcomes. If any EOCs were not satisfied, then further assessment of *why* they were not achieved and *how* the program can be revised or improved to increase the likelihood of their achievement needs to be done. Such assessment of students' performance following completion of the health education program or curriculum helps measure *learning,* which is, of course, the purpose of the health education program.

However, in addition to focusing on students' *learning,* it is also prudent to assess the *effectiveness of the teaching strategy in facilitating learning.* The possibility always exists that the learning which occurred was coincidental and unrelated to the formal health education program or curriculum experienced by the students; perhaps the students would have discovered or "learned" the content *without* formal health education, or perhaps their learning occurred *despite* grossly inappropriate or ineffective health teaching. Therefore if health educators want to know how effective *they* are in facilitating and encouraging student attainment of health education objectives, they will need to gather data concerning perceived teaching effectiveness. Evaluation of teaching effectiveness usually entails consulting the consumers of the "service": the students themselves.

While some teachers may scoff at the importance and deny the validity of student ratings and opinions, student feedback is very important and useful. Children, especially preadolescents, tend to be too honest to be polite; that is, they share their honest, spontaneous perceptions without feeling that they need to "cushion" them to make them more acceptable. As a result, children can often provide very helpful opinions, both verbally and nonverbally (such as by yawning or fidgeting to indicate boredom or disinterest). Therefore careful attention to development of a teacher and course evaluation form or procedure can assist teachers in improving their teaching effectiveness in the long run. *However,* if teachers do not plan to use that student feedback, regarding it seriously in reviewing course objectives, format, and teaching style and strategies, then it is not appropriate to solicit students' opinions. Indeed, older students (adolescents, college students, and adults) candidly report in many instances that filling out course and instructor evaluation forms is "a waste of time" because "nobody ever uses them anyway—they never make the changes we suggest." If those pessimistic statements are true, they are a sad commentary on contemporary education. Students who have not become jaded as to the merit and usefulness of teacher evaluations can provide an important perspective on what does and does not work in education, and their opinions should be solicited and carefully considered.

In addition to solicitation of student opinions, teachers may wish to seek feedback from their peers regarding teaching effectiveness. This might be accomplished through peer review of course materials and lesson plans or through direct classroom observation of teaching style and effectiveness. However, another way of obtaining peer feedback without direct classroom observation (which may be disruptive or distracting) is through peer critique of videotaped or audiotaped classroom presentations. The teacher seeking feedback could tape her own performance and then ask her peers for feedback and suggestions. Videotape and audiotaping can of course also be used by the teacher herself as a means of reviewing her own performance and comparing her intentions at the time the "lesson" was planned with her perceptions of its success at the time it was presented and with her perceptions when viewing or hearing the actual tape after the class. Whatever methods are chosen for teacher evaluation, it is important for teachers to have some valued mechanism for obtaining useful feedback concerning their teaching effectiveness.

Thus, whether based on assessment of learner outcomes, teaching effectiveness, or some combination of the two, evaluation of the health education process is critically important. Although evaluation is often viewed as the *end* or final step in a process, it should be noted that evaluative data serves as an input for planning and program revision and is therefore a *beginning* of sorts (Fig. 15-1).

Principles relevant for health education

In applying the health education process, health educators may find their task easier if they adhere to certain teaching principles. A number of such principles for health teaching will be briefly discussed here.

The first principle of teaching is that *good teacher-learner (nurse-learner) rapport is important.* As Pohl (1968) points out, effective rapport between the teacher (nurse) and learner is important in (1) creating a climate that fosters learning; (2) allowing the teacher/nurse to become familiar with the student as a person and to therefore more readily assess learning needs and readiness; (3) increasing the student's comfort with the teacher/nurse, thus allowing him to ask questions and make mistakes; and (4) enhancing the teacher's credibility as a role model, thus increasing the likelihood that the student will value and imitate the teacher's behavior and example. This kind of rapport is established through application of the helping relationships skills and concepts discussed in Chapters 10 and 11.

A second teaching principle closely related to the first, is that *"teaching requires effective communication"* (Pohl, 1968:32). Basically, this means that the sender of a message (such as a teacher/nurse) needs to ensure that the receiver (student/learner) "gets the message," without distortion or misinterpretation. Clearly, this principle, like the first, requires application of helping relationship principles and skills. More specifically, this requires that the sender use language and vocabulary that are intelligible to the receiver, based on the receiver's maturity, development, experience, culture, and education. In addition, when the receivers are children, especially young children, the sender may need to use more nonverbal communication than verbal, since young children have limited language skills. With handicapped persons, such as the deaf or mute, communication by verbal discussion may not be possible; in these circumstances, other methods such as use of written notes or sign language may be helpful.

A third principle to facilitate health teaching is that *attention must be paid to the timing of and setting for health teaching* (Pohl, 1968). The timing must be appropriate in terms of duration and time of day planned for health teaching. That is, enough time should be allotted to cover the topic without exceeding the students' attention span; also, the class should be held if at all possible during a time when students are alert and not preoccupied with other thoughts and interests. The physical environment (setting) should also be conducive to student comfort, alertness, and physical and mental health; that is, the environment should be adequately large for the student group, well-lighted and ventilated, and comfortably furnished with the furniture arranged in groupings that facilitate comfort and involvement, such as chairs in a circle for discussion.

Among other health teaching principles *not* cited by Pohl, is the *importance of the health educator being well versed in the subject and able to present accurate information*. One of the major factors in student interest in learning is teacher credibility, which in turn depends to a great extent on the teacher's command of the subject area. If students detect uncertainty or inaccuracy on the part of the teacher, they are likely to be skeptical about the merits of her teaching. Therefore health educators should take time to prepare themselves fully for their classes or presentations; in addition, if, despite careful and thorough preparation by the health educator, students manage to ask a question that the teacher cannot answer (which seems to be a special, inborn talent of students!), she should be candid about her inability to answer that question, admitting that she simply does not know the answer but is willing to try to find it. Students generally respond very positively to this kind of candor—once they get over the shock of realizing that the teacher does not know everything!

In addition to being as well informed as possible, health educators must also be careful to avoid *"stimulus overload"* of their students. That is, the length of class sessions should, as previously suggested, be compatible with students' attention spans. In addition, the *volume* and scope of material covered during any one program or class session should be limited so that students have an opportunity to "absorb" and assimilate it. If too much material is covered at one time, or if too many different topics are discussed, students may feel overwhelmed or overstimulated, thus reducing their concentration and ability to learn.

Finally, another principle of effective teaching to apply to the process of health education is that when new skills or behaviors have been taught, it is important to *provide students' with opportunities to apply and practice them as soon as possible*. The longer the period of time between learning and practicing a skill, the less likely it is that the skill level will be maintained. Thus students who learn CPR techniques one day but do not have an opportunity to practice them for a week are not likely to remember how to accurately perform CPR.

The health teaching principles cited in this discussion are only a sample of the teaching principles that are described in the literature. For expanded discussion of the principles included here and for discussion of other principles not mentioned, the reader is referred to education literature sources such as Redman (1980).

SUBJECT AREAS FOR INCLUSION IN A SCHOOL HEALTH EDUCATION PROGRAM

Decisions concerning particular topics or issues to include in school health education curricula are complicated, emotional, and often troublesome. As noted elsewhere in this book concerning school health programs in general and school screening programs in particular, there is no one "right" program that is appropriate for all schools or all school districts. That is also true for health education curricula and for many of the same reasons. The most important reason is that because school and community populations have different composition and different health and educational needs, the kinds of school- and community-based health education curricula used in each school and locale need to be tailored to the unique needs and interests of their specific populations. In schools and communities where attention is *not* paid to unique programmatic needs, the likely result will be health education programs that contain gaps and yet also overlap other existing programs and services. For that reason, as noted earlier in this chapter, school health education curricula need to be *comprehensive in scope,* with content areas and relative emphases *based on assessment of needs and interests* and carefully *articulated and coordinated with existing community health education programs and services.*

Therefore readers who turned eagerly to this page, hoping to find a clearly delineated school health education curriculum identifying topics and issues, teaching strategies, and resource materials, all neatly organized by age/grade level, are bound to be disappointed. However, many of those kinds of suggestions, some based on research findings documenting validity and reliability, can be found among the many resources listed in the References at the end of this chapter or elsewhere in the abundant health education literature.

In lieu of providing a "standard" comprehensive, universally appropriate school health education curriculum, the goal of this discussion will be to identify some of the *general* health topics that are suggested in the literature by many authorities for inclusion in school health education programs. Again, the reader is cautioned that these suggestions are *not* all necessarily appropriate in all settings, and the relative emphasis placed on any particular health topic should be determined following careful assessment of local needs.

School health education curricula as outgrowths of health education philosophy

Willgoose (1973) reminds readers that the health education curriculum in any school or school system should reflect and be an outgrowth of an identifiable health education philosophy. That is, the health curriculum should not be a "thrown together" jumble of trendy or traditional topics, organized into isolated "mini courses" (which serve to isolate and fragment health education, instead of integrating it into the overall school curriculum). Rather, the health education curriculum should evolve from

careful articulation of beliefs about the purpose and role of school health education and particular health education needs and interests of the student population to be "educated." Faculty members, including school nurses and other involved health care professionals, therefore need to begin the process of planning their school health education curriculum by identifying their beliefs or philosophy about health education and its role and goals in the school. This philosophy then becomes a basis for determining which topics and issues to include as curricular content areas and may likewise suggest age or grade placement of particular subjects, as well as suggesting philosophically compatible teaching strategies.

Major health education curricular topics and priorities

The possible topics and priorities for school health education programs range from the "problem-oriented" list suggested by Sinacore (1978) to the expansive list of 370 diverse topics (organized into twenty larger categories) proposed by Hardt (1978). However, between those extremes is Hoyman's (1977:263-269) list of ten major health curricular areas:

1. *Health in ecologic perspective,* which focuses on man's interaction with and adaptation to his environment.
2. *The human life and death cycle,* beginning with conception and progressing through all life stages including death. This focus on the human life cycle includes the interrelationship between "self-awareness and death awareness" and the impact of both on life-style and mental health.
3. *Human population dynamics and health,* including how "population dynamics—population size, density, growth rate, doubling time, and so on—relate to human health, disease, longevity, and life style."
4. *Man and his diseases,* including "ecologic-epidemiologic balance and imbalance," and the principles of disease transmission, prevention, and control.
5. *Personality and life-style,* with an emphasis on promotion of mental and emotional health and "healthy self-fulfillment."
6. *Human sexuality,* including not only facts about reproduction, but also attention to attitudes, values, ethics, and behaviors, including controversial issues such as abortion, family planning/birth control, unwed pregnancy and parenthood, venereal disease, homosexuality, and sex roles and relationships.
7. *Bioethics,* which includes helping students develop an "ethical value system" by developing "their cognitive ability to make decisions about

moral problems," such as abortion, euthanasia, and genetic engineering.

8. *Consumer health education,* including how to be an informed and intelligent consumer of goods and services and thus less vulnerable to quackery and misleading advertising.

9. *Human genetics and health,* with an emphasis on developing "a basic understanding of the role of heredity and genetics in their [students'] lives." Suggested topics include human reproduction and sexual development, genetic factors in health, disease, and longevity, research issues, and "cloning" of humans.

10. *Global health and the "human prospect,"* including such topics as world distribution of food and energy resources, environmental pollution, demographics (including population "explosions" in underdeveloped countries), international public health and disease problems, and the impact of war.

Whether or how any or all of these areas is incorporated into a particular school health education curriculum will depend on the philosophy used to guide curriculum development. Likewise, the relative priority assigned to a topic or content area will be based on the philosophical orientation of the curriculum designers and should also reflect the unique health needs of that school's population.

THE ROLE OF THE SCHOOL NURSE IN SCHOOL HEALTH EDUCATION

As discussed in Chapter 2, the goal of the school nurse in her role as health educator is to "participate in health education program activities for children, youth, school personnel, and the community." The precise nature of that "participation" can be defined individually by school nurses, depending on their role perceptions, educational preparation, experience, and situational variables and constraints, such as workload and work volume, program priorities, and availability of health education specialists and consultants (both teachers and curriculum design planners).

However, it is hoped that all school nurses will view themselves as health educators and will participate to the fullest possible and practical extent in health education activities within the school health program, since health education is a key health promotion/primary prevention strategy. For the public health–oriented school nurse, for whom health promotion and disease prevention are major goals, health education thus becomes a critically important process.

As with some of the other systematic processes, such as research and management, which are used deplorably infrequently by school nurses and other nurses as well, health education is too often carried out nonsystematically and may also be anxiety producing for those nurses who do attempt it. Probably one of the reasons why nurses avoid use of the health education process and principles is the fact that many baccalaureate nursing curricula do not adequately prepare their graduates for their role as health educator; for students who have had no formal course work and/or field practice in education theory and methods, the source of their anxiety in health education situations is apparent.

However, another important reason why school nurses and other nurses do not make full use of health educational opportunities and methods may be their misguided perception of health education as some alien, mystical process, requiring "unique" talents and skills. Perhaps this mistaken view can be corrected by looking at the comparison in Table 15-1 of the health education process with the nursing pro-

Table 15-1. Comparison of the health education process with the nursing process

Health education process	Nursing process
Step 1: Assessment of learner needs ⟷	*Step 1:* Assessment A. Data collection B. Nursing diagnosis or problem definition
Step 2: Exploration of learner readiness ⟵	
Step 3: Development of planned outcomes ⟷	*Step 2:* Planning A. Goals and EOCs B. Priority setting C. Intervention: what and by whom
Step 4: Development and implementation of teaching plan ⟷	*Step 3:* Implementation/intervention
Step 5: Evaluation: assessment of learner outcomes and teaching effectiveness ⟷	*Step 4:* Evaluation

cess (Chapter 14). As Table 15-1 illustrates, both the nursing process and health education process are really adaptations of the basic problem-solving process to particular focal areas: client/patient care and education, respectively. Both involve assessment on which planning can be based, followed by development of a "plan" of action, followed by evaluation of results of that plan. Thus while the details of each process are somewhat unique, the two systematic processes are remarkably similar. It therefore seems reasonable to conclude that without need for a graduate degree in education, any nurse with competence in her use of the *nursing* process should be able to develop facility with the *health education* process as well. The biggest hurdle is likely to be helping nurses to view "health educator" as an appropriate role and an attainable goal.

While each school nurse must determine for herself the extent of her involvement in health education activities, she can participate in many ways. One obvious way, and one that has been used by many school nurses, is to capitalize on the "teachable moment" when a student expresses a need or interest in learning more about a health area, such as venereal disease, smoking, and interpersonal relationships. By providing informal health education at such times, the school nurse can truly make a difference in the lives of the young people, parents, faculty, or other persons with whom she comes in contact.

Another way for the school nurse to carry out her role as health educator is to participate in the planning of the school district's health education curriculum; through such participation, the nurse can influence the health content to which all students in the district will be exposed and can at the same time demonstrate her expertise and leadership at the district level. A possible and desired consequence, then, may be improved visibility and credibility for school nurses within that school system. However, for school nurses to be able to participate at this level requires that they have preparation in and knowledge of curriculum design, school administration and decision making, as well as having some political acumen, leadership ability, and assertiveness. In addition, school nurses participating in district-wide curricular decision making will also need health expertise (which they should already have) and knowledge of growth and developmental norms for children and youth, so that reasonable decisions can be made concerning age and grade level placement of various health topics and issues. Since school nurses should already have such background, they should be able to contribute meaningfully to the decision-making process.

Another health education activity appropriate for the school nurse is serving as a consultant to classroom teachers in preparation of their health "lessons." Because she is an expert on health, the nurse can assist teachers in planning specific content, selecting resource materials such as films, or devising activities appropriate for teaching or conveying particular content or ideas. Indeed, there are many lists of suggested materials (see references at the end of this chapter for examples) to be used for school health education. If the nurse keeps abreast of new ideas in her professional literature, she should be able to make many helpful suggestions. However, the school nurse needs to be assertive and take the initiative in offering herself as a consultant to teachers and others. Because many school nurses find themselves "swamped" with paperwork and first aid activities, health education consultation may often seem to be a low priority. However, the truly public health–oriented school nurse is philosophically committed to health education as a health promotion strategy and therefore extends herself and offers consultation to teachers and others, even though that may not be an activity included in her job description.

In addition to serving as a consultant to classroom teachers, the school nurse can serve as an in-service person for the faculty and school staff as a whole. For example, if the school receives handicapped students to be "mainstreamed" into regular classes, teachers and other school personnel, including food service workers, janitors, bus drivers, teacher's aides, and secretaries, may need some in-service education about the students' health problems and needs and ways school personnel can deal effectively with them. In schools where staff members are interested in learning about particular health topics for their own benefit, such as the effects of job stress on blood pressure, other physiological factors, and morale, the school nurse may, of course, suggest topics about which she feels comfortable speaking and offer to conduct sessions about them. If any health problem or disease begins to occur or suddenly increases in the school or community, the nurse may wish to discuss the problem and any preventive measures that can or should be taken.

Bowman (1977:119) makes a strong case for

direct involvement of school nurses in classroom teaching and points out that "nurses can give better examples of health problems than teachers, and students see the nurse as an expert." Classroom teaching also provides the nurse with an opportunity to meet students and be "checked out" by them in a nonclinical situation. If the nurse comes across as caring and approachable, students may be more inclined to seek her out for help with a problem or when they need a trusted adult in whom to confide. Classroom teaching also affords the nurse an opportunity to observe children in class and to note any children who may have problems that have gone thus far undetected; such children can be discussed with the teacher and perhaps followed up individually if necessary.

Still another activity for the school nurse in her role as health educator might be to act as a consultant or liaison with community persons and groups concerning their health education needs. It has already been noted that school health education programs should mesh with community programs, so that the needs of the community are met without unnecessary duplication or omissions; if the school nurse, as an involved community health care professional, can act as a liaison between the school and community, then a comprehensive, community-based health education program can become a reality.

In addition to citing many of the preceding suggestions for involving the school nurse in health education, an unsigned editorial in the *American Journal of Public Health* (The role of the school nurse in health education, 1971: 2155) encourages nurses to "promote legislation relevant to school health." This thread of increased legislative and political involvement is a recurrent theme in school health and school nursing (Chapter 19). By working for passage of legislation to improve funding for school health or to mandate comprehensive health education curricula in all public schools in the state, school nurses are contributing significantly toward the future of school health and health education and are helping ensure that schools achieve their goal of graduating health-educated young adults.

Finally, an important though vastly underrated means for the school nurse to carry out her role as health educator is role modeling (Gordon, 1974). As Glover (1978:175) points out, "Because much of what students learn is through observation, it is essential for health

educators to serve as *effective* models for their students." Glover (1978:176) goes on to warn:

Some students will value health in spite of us, but we can be much more effective by setting the proper example. The role of health educators as models is often overlooked, but it may be our most powerful change agent.

CONCLUSION

Most nurses are engaged in health teaching nearly every day of their professional lives, although they may not be aware of it. In fact, much of the health education done by nurses is done informally and without attention to "planned terminal outcomes" and "teaching plans." While that kind of loose, unstructured approach to health teaching at times may be appropriate, effective health education follows a systematic process as described in this chapter. Because of their focus on attaining and sustaining high-level wellness in school populations, school nurses need to expand their use of health education process, recognizing that it is vital for promoting and maintaining health in school community populations.

REFERENCES

AAHPER Position Statement: 1971. A unified approach to health teaching, J. School Health **41**(4):171.

American Academy of Pediatrics Committee on School Health: 1978. Health education, J. School Health **48**(8): 503.

Anderson, C. L., and Creswell, W. H.: 1976. School health practice, 6th ed., The C. V. Mosby Co., St. Louis.

Aubrey, R. F.: 1972. Health education: neglected child of the schools, J. School Health **42**(5):285-288.

Bloom, B. S., editor: 1956. Taxonomy of educational objectives: the classification of educational goals. Handbook I: Cognitive domain, David McKay Co., Inc., New York.

Bowman, M. R.: 1977. Nurses can and should teach health in the classroom, J. School Health **47**(2):118-119.

Bruess, C. E., and Gay, J. E.: 1978. Implementing comprehensive school health, Macmillan Publishing Co., Inc., New York.

Bruhn, J. G., and Cordova, F. D.: 1977. A developmental approach to learning wellness behavior. Part I: Infancy to adolescence, Health Values: Achieving High-Level Wellness **1**(6):246-254.

Bruyn, H. B.: 1978. TV's effect on children: an opinion survey of pediatricians, J. School Health **48**(8):474-476.

Califano, J. A.: 1977. School health message, J. School Health **47**(6):334-335.

Carpenter, M. Y., and Quiring, J. D.: 1978. Using modular format in teaching health concepts to primaries, J. School Health **48**(7):404-408.

Castile, A. S., and Jerrick, S. J.: 1976. School health in America, American School Health Association, Kent, Ohio.

Conley, J. A., and Jackson, C. G.: 1978. Is a mandated comprehensive health education program a guarantee of successful health education? J. School Health **48**(6):337-340.

Dickinson, D. J.: 1971. School nursing becomes accountable in education through behavioral objectives, J. School Health **41**(10):533-537.

Esty, G. W.: 1970. Health education in our schools and the health manpower shortage, J. School Health **40**(1):11-15.

Fors, S. W., and Ulrich, C. O.: 1977. Getting it together, Health Values: Achieving High-Level Wellness **1**(5):200-206.

Glasser, W.: 1969. Schools without failure, Harper & Row, Publishers, Inc., New York.

Glover, E. D.: 1978. Modeling—a powerful change agent,'' J. School Health **48**(3):175-176.

Gordon, S.: 1974. School nurse-teacher as health role model and health profession role model, J. N.Y. State Sch. Nurse Teach. Assoc. **5**:14-17, Spring.

Gronlund, N. E.: 1970. Stating behavioral objectives for classroom instruction, The Macmillan Publishing Co., Inc., New York.

Gross, E. A.: 1977. Hints for the health education student teacher, J. School Health **47**(9):546-549.

Hardt, D. V.: 1978. Health curriculum: 370 topics, J. School Health **48**(1):656-660.

Haro, M. S.: 1974. School health revisited, J. School Health **44**(7):363-368.

Hoyman, H. S.: 1977. Improving health curriculum scope in the modern world, Health Values: Achieving High-Level Wellness **1**(6):262-269.

Jacobsen, R. F., and Siegel, E.: 1971. Comprehensive health planning in the space age: the role of the school health program, J. School Health **41**(3):156-160.

Kaplan, R.: 1972. The school health division's position on health education, School Health Rev. **3**(4):4-10.

Kenney, J. B., chairperson: 1977. A study of community health education, United Way of Minneapolis Area, Community Planning and Research Division, Minneapolis.

Kunstel, F.: 1978. Assessing community needs: implications for curriculum and staff development in health education, J. School Health **48**(4):220-224.

Lussier, R. R.: 1972. Health education and student needs, J. School Health **42**(10):618-620.

Mager, R. F.: 1962. Preparing instructional objectives, Fearon • Pitman Publishers, Inc., Belmont, Calif.

Means, R. K.: 1973. Can the schools teach personal responsibility for health? J. School Health **43**(3):171-175.

Neilson, E. A.: 1969. The child—the school's most important concern, J. School Health **39**(1):1-7.

Newman, I. M., and Mayshark, C.: 1973. Health education planning and community perceptions of local health problems, J. School Health **43**(7):458-463.

Oberteuffer, D., and Beyrer, M. K.: 1966. School health education, 4th ed., Harper & Row, Publishers, Inc., New York.

Osman, J. D.: 1974. The use of selected value-clarifying strategies in health education, J. School Health **44**(1):21-25.

Pohl, M. L.: 1968. Teaching function of the nursing practitioner, Chapter 3, William C. Brown Co., Publishers, Dubuque, Iowa.

Raths, L., Harmill, M., and Simon, S. B.: 1966. Values and teaching, Charles E. Merrill Publishing Co., Columbus, Ohio.

Redman, B. K.: 1980. The process of patient teaching in nursing, 4th ed., The C. V. Mosby Co., St. Louis.

Rogers, C. R.: 1969. Freedom to learn, Charles E. Merrill Publishing Co., Columbus, Ohio.

The role of the school nurse in health education (editorial): 1971. Am. J. Public Health **61**(11):2155-2157.

Sechrist, W. C., and Jones, H.: 1979. Are basic assumptions we hold about health education defensible? J. School Health **49**(5):275-277.

Shirreffs, J. H.: 1978. A survey of the health science discipline—its relationship to other academic disciplines, J. School Health **48**(6):330-336.

Simon, S. B., Howe, L., and Kirschenbaum, H.: 1972. Values clarification: a handbook of practical strategies for teachers and students, Hart Publishing Co., New York.

Simonds, S. K.: 1977. Health education today: issues and challenges, J. School Health **47**(10):584-593.

Sinacore, J. S.: 1978. Priorities in health education, J. School Health **48**(4):213-217.

Sliepcevich, E. M.: 1964. School health education study: a summary report, School Health Education Study, Washington, D.C.

Snegroff, S.: 1975. Venereal disease education: facts are not enough, J. School Health **45**(1):37-39.

Willgoose, C. E.: 1973. Saving the curriculum in health education, J. School Health **43**(3):189-191.

Wold, S. J.: 1975. A descriptive survey of health needs perceived by inner city and suburban adolescents, unpublished master's study, University of Minnesota School of Public Health, Minneapolis.

Zentner, J., and Murray, R.: 1975. Health teaching: a basic nursing intervention, Chapter 5. In Murray, R., and Zentner, J.: Nursing concepts for health promotion, Prentice-Hall, Inc., Englewood Cliffs, N.J.

SUGGESTED READINGS

American School Health Association: 1967. Growth patterns and sex education: a suggested program kindergarten through grade twelve, American School Health Association, Kent, Ohio.

American School Health Association: 1968. Mental health in the classroom (booklet), J. School Health **38**(5a):1-44.

American School Health Association: 1972. Growth patterns and sex education: an updated bibliography, preschool to adulthood, American School Health Association, Kent, Ohio.

Atkins, N. P.: 1978. Principles of curriculum development applied to health education, J. School Health **48**(4):209-212.

Barrett, J. E.: 1979. Family life education—parental involvement, J. School Health **49**(1):15-19.

Breckton, D., and Sweeney, D.: 1978. Use of value clarification methods in venereal disease education, J. School Health **48**(3):181-183.

Bruess, C. E., editor: 1976. Professional preparation of the health educator, Report of the ASHA Committee on Professional Preparation and College Health Education Conference at Towson State University, January 29-30, 1976, J. School Health **46**(7):418-421.

Bruess, C. E.: 1979. School health education: general gains from specific tasks, J. School Health **49**(2):93-95.

Carveth, S. W.: 1979. Teaching cardiopulmonary resuscitation in the schools, J. School Health **49**(4):223-224.

Crase, D., and Hamrick, M. H.: 1977. Health education: a reexamination of purpose, J. School Health **47**(8):470-474.

Douse, M.: 1973. Health hints or health philosophy? J. School Health **43**(3):195-197.

Falck, V. T.: 1978. Involvement for learning in health programs, J. School Health **48**(3):168-170.

Finn, P.: 1977. Should alcohol education be taught with drug education, J. School Health **47**(8):466-469.

Friedman, L. A.: 1974. Impact of teacher-student dental health education, J. School Health **44**(3):140-143.

Gordon, S.: 1974. "What place does sex education have in the schools? J. School Health **44**(4):186-188.

Greenberg, J. S.: 1977. Stress, relaxation, and the health educator, J. School Health **47**(9):522-525.

Grollman, E. A.: 1977. Explaining death to children, J. School Health **47**(6):336-339.

Hagen, M.: 1978. Prenatal care training, J. School Health **48**(8):486-489.

Harris, W. H.: 1978. Some reflections concerning approaches to death education, J. School Health **48**(3):162-165.

Hart, E. J.: 1976. Death education and mental health, J. School Health **46**(7):407-412.

Hoyman, H. S.: 1970. Should we teach sexual ethics in our schools? J. School Health **40**(7):339-346.

Hoyman, H. S.: 1973. New frontiers in health education, J. School Health **43**(7):423-430.

Hoyman, H. S.: 1974. Sex education and our core values, J. School Health **44**(2):62-69.

Hunt, B. M.: 1978. Management of health problems and medical emergencies in the classroom, J. School Health **48**(8):469-470.

Jacobs, K.: 1973. The school nurse-teacher and health education, J. N.Y. State Sch. Nurse Teach. Assoc. **4**:11-14, June.

Jenne, F. H., and Greene, W. H.: 1976. Turner's school health and health education, 7th ed., The C. V. Mosby Co., St. Louis.

Kreuter, M. W., and Green, L. W.: 1978. Evaluation of school health education: identifying purpose, keeping perspective, J. School Health **48**(4):228-235.

Lockwood, J.: 1970. The effectiveness of health education programs for average and disadvantaged public school children, J. School Health **40**(1):15-16.

Mager, R. F.: 1968. Developing attitude toward learning, Fearon • Pitman Publishers, Inc., Belmont, Calif.

Mager, R. F.: 1973. Measuring instructional intent, Fearon • Pitman Publishers, Inc., Belmont, Calif.

Mayshark, C., Shaw, D. D., and Best, W. H.: 1977. Administration of school health programs: its theory and practice, 2nd ed., The C. V. Mosby Co., St. Louis.

Merkl, D. J.: 1973. Contributions of the school health nurse to the school drug program, J. Drug Ed. **3**(2):183-187.

Mills, G. C.: 1979. Books to help children understand death, Am. J. Nurs. **79**(2):291-295.

Moomaw, M. S.: 1978. Involving students in nutrition education, J. School Health **48**(2):121-123.

Mulholland, D. N.: 1978. A comprehensive dental health education program, J. School Health **48**(4):225-227.

National League for Nursing: 1976. Patient education, Publication No. 20-1633, National League for Nursing, New York.

Needle, R. H.: 1977. Factors affecting contraceptive practices of high school and college-age students, J. School Health **47**(6):340-345.

Neilson, E. A.: 1969. Health education and the school physician, J. School Health **39**(6):377-384.

Newman, I. M.: 1979. Teaching health in a natural history museum, J. School Health **49**(2):104-108.

Newman, I. M., and Mayshark, C.: 1973. Community health problems and the school's unrecognized mandate, J. School Health **43**(9):562-565.

Parcel, G. S., Luttman, D., and Meyers, M. P.: 1979. Formative evaluation of a sex education course for young adolescents, J. School Health **49**(6):335-339.

Parker, M. C.: 1979. Health education for the preadolescent: basic first aid, J. School Health **49**(5):266.

Podell, R. N., Keller, K., Mulvihill, M. N., Berger, G., and Kent, D. F.: 1978. Evaluation of the effectiveness of a high school course in cardiovascular nutrition, Am. J. Public Health **68**(6):573-576.

Price, J. H.: 1978. Dental health education for the mentally and physically handicapped, J. School Health **48**(3):171-173.

Redican, K. J., Olsen, L. K., and Mathis, R. M.: 1979. A comparison of the cognitive effects of two prototype health education curriculums on selected elementary school children, J. School Health **49**(6):340-342.

Riggs, R. S., and Evans, D. W.: 1979. Child abuse prevention—implementation within the curriculum, J. School Health **49**(5):255-259.

Sanzi, S. M., Jong, A., and Frankl, S.: 1975. A comprehensive approach to dental health in a school population, J. School Health **45**(4):228-230.

Schwartz, S.: 1977. Death education: suggested readings and audiovisuals, J. School Health **47**(10):607-609.

Shirreffs, J. H.: 1978. The relevance of health education to health activation and self-care, J. School Health **48**(7):419-422.

Shirreffs, J. H., and Degelsky, T. L.: 1979. Adolescent perceptions of sex education needs: 1972-1978, J. School Health **49**(6):343-346.

Stone, D. B.: 1979. School health education: some future challenges, J. School Health **49**(4):227-228.

Tevis, B. W.: 1978. Teaching ideas in cardiovascular health, J. School Health **48**(2):92-96.

Torrance, E. P.: 1963. Education and the creative potential, University of Minnesota Press, Minneapolis.

Walton, E. G., and Russell, R. D.: 1978. Affective mental health education with sight and sound experiences, J. School Health **48**(1):661-666.

Yarber, W. L.: 1979. Instructional emphasis in family life and sex education: viewpoints of students, parents, teachers and principals at four grade levels, J. School Health **49**(5):263-265.

CHAPTER 16

Epidemiology: a systematic approach to understanding and promoting the health of school populations

SUSAN J. WOLD

Historically, epidemiology, which is derived from the Greek words *epi,* meaning upon, and *demos,* meaning people, has been interpreted literally as the science that studies "what happens upon or befalls a population" (Anderson et al., 1962:14). Specifically, epidemiology focused on sudden dramatic increases in disease or *epidemics.* This focus on epidemics of such diseases as cholera, plague, smallpox, and yellow fever was easily justified, since these diseases constituted the most important threats to human health and life up to the twentieth century (Fox et al., 1970).

This early "doctrine of epidemics" thus defined the main function of epidemiology as investigation of epidemics to identify their sources, limit their spread, institute control measures, and prevent recurrence (Clark, 1965). Although this is still an important function, the scope of epidemiology has gradually broadened in recent years to ensure its continued viability as a health science. According to Clark (1965), the first expansion of epidemiology was from its original focus on epidemics to include the *endemic* (or usual occurrence) phases of *epidemic* diseases. The next expansion involved application of epidemiological concepts and approaches to the study of infectious diseases, those which result from infections (Benenson, 1975) and that do not only occur as epidemics; examples of such diseases include tuberculosis, malaria, leprosy, and rheumatic fever. The third expansion of epidemiology described by Clark (1965) resulted in its modern-day broad application, which will be discussed more fully in the remainder of this chapter.

The purpose of this chapter, then, is to pro-vide an overview of epidemiology. Although discussion of this important and fascinating science must be limited, one of the intended outcomes of this chapter is to whet the reader's appetite to learn more about epidemiology and its applications. In addition, and in accordance with the specific purpose of this book, another goal of this chapter is to encourage the reader to apply epidemiological concepts and methods within the school health program as a means of understanding and promoting the health of the school population. To accomplish these goals, in the remainder of this chapter the following will be discussed:

1. Definitions of epidemiology
2. Purposes of epidemiology
3. Functions of epidemiology
4. Epidemiological approaches
5. Principles underlying epidemiological practice
6. Disease development and control
7. Epidemiological investigative process
8. Applications of epidemiology
9. The role of the school nurse

DEFINITIONS OF EPIDEMIOLOGY

As described at the beginning of this chapter, epidemiology originated as an investigative science, charged with the responsibility to explain and reduce the incidence and prevalence of epidemic diseases. Despite the gradual broadening of focus, many authorities still view epidemiology as a disease-oriented specialty. Thus, most textbooks and other epidemiology references (Lester, 1957; Anderson et al., 1962; Smillie and Kilbourne, 1963; Fox et al., 1970; Schuman, 1973; Friedman, 1974; Mausner and

Bahn, 1974; Lilienfeld, 1976) propose definitions of epidemiology that are similar to the one offered by MacMahon et al. (1960:3), in which epidemiology is defined as "the study of the distribution and determinants of disease prevalence in man."

In contrast to this typically disease-oriented definition, however, some authorities (Clark, 1965; Roberts, 1967; Lough et al., 1975) now view epidemiology much more broadly. Roberts (1967) describes epidemiology as a particular method of studying "health conditions" and believes that it can be applied within *any* clinical practice area. Her specific definition of epidemiology (1967:55) emphasizes the importance of studying "health states and behaviors of populations in relation to their varied environments . . ." as a means of identifying and understanding the factors that influence morbidity (illness or disease occurrence) and mortality (numbers of deaths within a population).

Although Roberts' definition of epidemiology includes an emphasis on the study of health states and behaviors, her definition is also primarily disease oriented, since it views those factors as important in understanding illness, disability, and death. Thus, although her definition is broader than most, it fails to incorporate the preventive aspects of health. Because health promotion and disease prevention are (or ought to be) the primary concerns of the school nurse, the definition of epidemiology adopted as the basis for the discussion in the remainder of this chapter must reflect a health promotion/disease prevention focus. For that reason, the following definition will be applied (Clark, 1965:40):

. . . Epidemiology is a field of science which is concerned with the various factors and conditions that determine the occurrence and distribution of health, disease, defect, disability, and death among groups of individuals.*

Clark's definition not only includes an emphasis on *health,* but it also places that emphasis *first* chronologically. Thus, based on this definition, epidemiology is appropriately concerned not only with the study of disease and the factors influencing its distribution and spread, but also with individuals and groups who are apparently well, since by studying the healthy populations, factors that contribute to

*From Preventive medicine for the doctor in his community: an epidemiological approach by H. R. Leavell and E. G. Clark. Copyright © 1965 McGraw-Hill Book Company. Used with permission of McGraw-Hill Book Company.

high-level wellness can be identified. This should be especially important for school nurses and others who work within the school health program; if children and youth can be taught to adopt a healthy life-style, then the need for disease-oriented epidemiological studies will decrease.

It should also be noted that in contrast with the traditional health science focus on the *individual* and his health or disease, the units of study in epidemiology are *groups* (Friedman, 1974). Thus epidemiologists study populations and other groups of persons to learn what factors are associated with wellness and how disease occurs. The epidemiologist may also be concerned with individuals and their health or illness as a means of understanding a *pattern* or trend or to fill in the knowledge gaps concerning the natural history of a new or known disease; an example of this might be Legionnaire's disease, which is a respiratory, pneumonia-like disease first recognized in some individuals attending an American Legion convention in the 1970s. The individual illness experiences of each person with this disease were analyzed by epidemiologists in identifying the etiology and relevant preventive measures. Thus the new knowledge gained from studying individuals contributed to the understanding of the total group's experience; similarly, knowledge from group studies of well and/or diseased persons can be applied to the diagnosis, treatment, and disease prevention/health promotion strategies for individuals. In other words, while data about individuals is needed to effectively identify and study the group's experience, group data can likewise be applied to meeting health needs of individuals (Clark, 1965).

PURPOSES OF EPIDEMIOLOGY

The working definition of epidemiology adopted for this chapter emphasizes the study of both health and disease states within population groups. Although the definition describes what epidemiology *is,* some discussion of what epidemiology *does* and its purposes and functions is warranted.

According to Schuman (1973), there are two ultimate goals of epidemiology: (1) *control* of disease through eradication or reduction of incidence to the lowest possible level and (2) *prevention* of disease. As previously suggested, an appropriate third goal of epidemiology (and not necessarily in this order of priority), would be *promotion* of healthy life-styles and *high-level wellness* based on epidemiological analysis of factors that influence the occurrence and distribution of health within the population.

Obviously, these are lofty goals and are universal for *all* health care professionals. To appreciate the unique contribution of the field of epidemiology in meeting these goals, then, it is necessary to understand *how* the goals are approached. To clarify the contribution of epidemiology to health promotion, disease prevention, and disease control, Clark (1965) has identified six specific purposes* of epidemiology that will be briefly described; viewpoints of other writers and epidemiologists will be incorporated as appropriate.

The first purpose of epidemiology described by Clark (1965:45) is *analysis of the interrelationships of the agent-host-environment complex to discover "gaps" in knowledge of the natural history of disease(s) and to thereby contribute to prevention efforts.* Through careful analysis of the interplay of agent-host-environmental factors, the natural history and etiology of both infectious (such as mononucleosis or tuberculosis) and noninfectious (such as lung cancer or arteriosclerotic heart disease) diseases can be discovered. Once the natural history is well understood (based on careful documentation and analysis), then intelligent and appropriate interventions can be planned to treat those with the disease and to prevent disease development in others.

The second purpose or aim of epidemiology described by Clark (1965:45-46) is *description and analysis of disease occurrence and distribution based on variables such as age, sex, race, occupation, temporal frequency, periodic fluctuation, long-term or historical trends, and geographic distribution (and, according to Schuman [1973], ethnic groups, socioeconomic factors, culture, and genetic factors) in order to make community diagnoses and to estimate the risks of morbidity and mortality.* Thus the first task of the epidemiologist when confronted with a new disease or health problem or an outbreak of any disease is to document the number of cases and all other factors relevant to their occurrence. An example might be the sudden illness of thirty students at an elementary school. The epidemiological approach to identifying the students' illness and to estimating the risk of illness for other students requires prompt

and thorough data collection regarding the ill students' demographic characteristics (age, sex, race, etc.), as well as careful documentation of their individual illness experiences, including symptoms, time of onset, and duration of illness, plus any additional information about the students' activities prior to illness. In this example, the cause of disease might be traced to a contaminated food in the school cafeteria. If so, the precise community diagnosis and estimate of risk to others will depend on the nature of the contaminant and on the number of persons exposed to it. Certainly a food-borne illness such as hepatitis will have potentially more serious and widespread consequences (in terms of severity of illness and control of disease spread) than an outbreak of salmonellosis. For that reason, it is important to identify the exact cause of the illness as soon as possible.

A third purpose of epidemiology, according to Clark (1965:46), is to *help reduce knowledge gaps concerning the cause of disease processes through observation of the range, amplitude, and group behavior of clinical syndromes in populations.* Achievement of this aim would logically entail grouping of data about individual illness experiences to identify the commonalities. Thus persons with arteriosclerotic heart disease (ASHD) might be studied to find out how many of them are smokers, how much exercise they usually get, and how much saturated fat is included in their diets; such information helps compile a picture of the group's experience, which can then be used to identify and test hypotheses concerning the disease's etiology.

The fourth purpose of epidemiology described by Clark (1965:46) is to *study pressing and special health problems including new diseases, endemic diseases, epidemics, and administration problems or operations research.* Thus, in addition to the study of individuals' clinical illness experiences and behaviors associated with the "clinical syndromes" included in the third purpose of epidemiology, the fourth purpose involves study of *all* aspects of a disease or health problem and is concerned with *immediate* problems and new diseases such as Legionnaire's disease or toxic shock syndrome (TSS). This purpose also includes study of endemic (widely prevalent within a given geographic area) and epidemic (occurring in excess of the usually expected numbers) diseases. An example of a disease that could be considered both endemic and epidemic is gonorrhea. Gon-

---

*Copyright © 1965 McGraw-Hill Book Company. Used with permission of McGraw-Hill Book Company.

orrhea can be cited as an example of a health problem that also results in administrative problems. Because of the venereal transmission of gonorrhea and the social stigma associated with it, efforts to control its spread are only partially successful. Thus gonorrhea control presents some administrative problems, including the need to identify and treat more contacts of gonorrhea patients.

According to Clark (1965:46), the fifth purpose of epidemiology is to *measure the effectiveness of (evaluate) preventive and control programs*. Thus, based on the data collection and analysis described in the preceding purposes and after implementation of a planned program to prevent new cases and control spread of the disease, the appropriateness and effectiveness of the program are evaluated. Citing gonorrhea again as an example, a typical control and prevention program might include health education for high-risk populations (including adolescents and young adults), confidential clinics for diagnosis and treatment, and follow-up of known contacts of persons with the disease (which is probably the most difficult aspect of gonorrhea control). Evaluation of the effectiveness of this program would entail the following:

1. Analysis of the numbers of new cases discovered prior to, during, and after implementation of the program
2. Comparison of the gonorrhea rates among the target age groups of the health education campaign (adolescents and young adults) before and after the health education program
3. Analysis of client usage patterns at the program's gonorrhea treatment and testing clinics to determine what population is being served and if there is an increase in the numbers of persons (cases and contacts) tested and/or treated
4. Comparison of the numbers of contacts identified and followed up prior to and as a result of the gonorrhea prevention and control program

It is important to note that changes in any of these rates or numbers do not *prove* a causal relationship between the program and the outcome; program evaluation must be cautiously and conscientiously done, and any hypothesized cause-effect relationships carefully tested.

Indeed, MacMahon et al. (1960:7) believe that one of the purposes of epidemiology is to test "the validity of the rationale on which control programs are based by the use of epidemiologic data collected in conjunction with the programs." They further suggest that a control program can be considered an experimental design for testing hypothesized cause-effect relationships that were the basis for the program's development.

The sixth and last purpose of epidemiology identified by Clark (1965:46) is to *stimulate and encourage systematic scientific research to fill in knowledge gaps and to study other problems in the fields of public health, medicine, dentistry, preventive medicine, welfare, education, administration, and other important spheres (which should certainly include nursing)*. The importance of research in epidemiology and in all areas of the health sciences cannot be overstated; research is critically important in fully understanding the natural history of diseases and in determining which prevention and treatment measures are most effective.

However, in accordance with the definition of epidemiology adopted as the basis for this chapter, it seems appropriate to add a seventh purpose to Clark's list. Hence the following purpose of epidemiology is proposed: epidemiology should *contribute to knowledge about health and levels of wellness and how to promote them*. Clark's list of epidemiological purposes focuses on health problems, diseases, and evaluation of programs and measures designed to prevent and control health problems and diseases. Although important and relevant for epidemiology, these purposes seem somewhat shortsighted. Our knowledge of health and wellness and just what kinds of factors and lifestyles are important in achieving and maintaining those states is far from complete. Probably because of traditional widespread use of the medical model, great amounts of time, energy, and resources have been expended in studying specific diseases and health problems; as a result, many diseases that once were prevalent, crippling, or lethal, such as polio, tuberculosis, and smallpox, are now well controlled or (in the case of smallpox) considered to have been eradicated. However, relatively small amounts of time, energy, and other resources have been committed to the study of health and healthy persons. Certainly health care professionals (including school nurses and others responsible for planning and implementing school health programs) could more adequately "promote health" if they knew (based on sound scientific study) what factors—whether they be genetic, environmental, psychological and attitudinal, demographic, or behavioral—are associated with health, wellness, and longevity. Epidemiological studies that are prospective (forward looking) using cohorts (groups of persons believed to be disease-free) need to be undertaken to help increase our understanding of health and how to effectively promote it. For many health care professionals, this kind of approach will require a shift in philosophy and thinking patterns to move *away* from a consistently problem-oriented or disease-oriented approach and *toward* a health promotion stance.

FUNCTIONS OF EPIDEMIOLOGY

Achievement of the purposes and aims described here depends on how well epidemiologists carry out the functions identified by Clark (1965:41),* which are to "collect a variety of data from diverse sources, construct logical chains of inference to explain the multiple factors in disease causation, and thereby contribute to preventive medicine" (or public health). Thus epidemiologists are concerned with clinical data, statistical data and morbidity and mortality, interview data, and other kinds of data relevant to the question or area studied. The multiple factors involved in the health state or disease studied must be carefully examined so that logical, valid inferences can be formulated. In fact, the logical, systematic, and scientific investigative approach is the hallmark of epidemiology. Epidemiologists recognize that there are no shortcuts to problem solution; they also recognize the value and importance of careful data collection and descriptive studies, no matter how tedious they may be to complete. Indeed, the validity and reliability of the contributions of epidemiology to our understanding of disease prevention and control and health promotion depend on painstaking data collection and logical data analysis.

EPIDEMIOLOGICAL APPROACHES

Epidemiological approaches to solving problems and answering health-related questions are usually classified as one of three types: descriptive, analytic, or experimental (Schuman, 1973; Friedman, 1974; Lough et al., 1975). Although there are distinct differences among them, each of these three approaches is important in

---

*Copyright © 1965 McGraw-Hill Book Company. Used with permission of McGraw-Hill Book Company.

achieving the goals and purposes of epidemiology.

Descriptive epidemiology

The first type of epidemiological approach is *descriptive epidemiology,* which, according to Lough et al. (1975:151), describes "the occurrence and distribution of disease or health states." Descriptive studies document all facts relevant to disease (or health state) occurrence, such as the number of cases, when and where they occurred, and the age, sex, and other demographic characteristics of the persons affected (Schuman, 1973). In other words, descriptive epidemiology is primarily interested in *person, place,* and *time* aspects of health and disease states (Friedman, 1974).

Although the descriptive approach has been much maligned and dismissed as "trivial" and "worthless," it is an important first step in epidemiological investigations, especially when "new" diseases or health problems are encountered or when an outbreak of any disease occurs (Schuman, 1973; Friedman, 1974). Indeed, Friedman (1974) believes that the descriptive approach is fundamentally important and serves three basic purposes:

1. To alert health care professionals regarding the types of persons (according to age, sex, race, occupation, socioeconomic status, etc.) likely to be affected by or at risk of developing a disease, where (geographically) the disease will occur, and when (time of occurrence)
2. To facilitate rational regional health planning in communities regarding health facilities and resources needed to cope with existing health problems and needs
3. To provide clues about disease etiology and to generate questions and hypotheses for further study (using analytic or experimental approaches)

Analytic epidemiology

The second type of epidemiological approach is *analytic epidemiology.* Analytic epidemiological investigations begin with etiologic clues and the hypotheses generated through the descriptive approach and explore the possible associations or relationships (independent or unrelated, statistical association, or causal association) between various factors and disease occurrence (MacMahon et al., 1960; Lough et al., 1975). Analytic studies are further classified as (1) retrospective, or case-control, studies; (2)

prospective, or cohort, studies; and (3) cross-sectional studies (Schuman, 1973; Friedman, 1974).

Analytic retrospective, or case-control, studies

Analytic *retrospective,* or *case-control,* studies begin with a hypothesized relationship between occurrence of a disease (for example, lung cancer) and some factor (such as smoking). To test this suspected relationship, persons *(cases)* with the disease under investigation (in this instance, lung cancer) are compared with *controls* (persons selected by a suitable variable) based on the factor being studied (smoking habits). This approach is *retrospective* because it *looks backward* at the facts (occurrence of cases of lung cancer) and looks for significant differences in terms of the variable studied (smoking) between the two groups (cases and controls). The relationship between smoking and lung cancer could be investigated by determining the percentage of cases who smoke at all and who smoke "heavily" (as defined by the investigators) and the corresponding percentages of controls who smoke and smoke heavily. Any observed differences are then tested for statistical significance to rule out the possibility of "chance" occurrence (Schuman, 1973).

Not surprisingly, there are both advantages and disadvantages to the retrospective, or case-control, method (Table 16-1). As shown in the table, if cases and suitable controls are already available, case-control studies can be rapidly completed. In addition, another advantage is that only well defined cases, according to the criteria of the investigator, are selected, which avoids the problem of borderline cases. Likewise, controls can be rigidly defined and carefully matched. Finally, case-control studies are relatively inexpensive, which makes them an appropriate means for initially testing hypotheses (Friedman, 1974).

Despite these advantages, there are some notable disadvantages as well. One disadvantage of case-control studies is that using this method of study it is difficult to determine *relative risk,* defined as the risk of a person developing or contracting a disease or health problem if he has a certain attribute or characteristic, unless two conditions are met: (1) the cases are representative of the population and (2) the controls are representative of all noncases (Schuman, 1973).

Another disadvantage of using the case-control approach is the difficulty in verifying the accuracy of the diagnosis and other data. Especially in studies where the data is old or was collected by a number of different persons over a period of time, the validity and reliability are unknown; even in case-control studies where the cases were recently diagnosed, unless the investigator personally diagnosed all the cases or had access to comparable data about them that he knew was properly collected, the problems of interrater reliability are potentially great.

The third disadvantage is related to the second and concerns the difficulty of obtaining representative controls. According to Friedman (1974), selecting the control group is the most difficult decision to be made in carrying out a case-control study; problems arise from selection of a source (such as persons within a given health care facility or community) and from any additional matching of cases and controls.

Finally, accurate and unbiased data collection may also be a problem. Schuman (1973) believes this is especially difficult when data collection is done by interviewing. To avoid qualitative or quantitative differences in data collected from cases and controls, Friedman (1974) suggests that research assistants recording laboratory data not be told which persons are cases and which are controls; furthermore, he recommends that data collection interviews (if used) be structured so that any questions regarding disease status are not asked until *after* the questions concerning etiological variables have been asked.

Table 16-1. Retrospective, or case-control, studies

Advantages	Disadvantages
Quickly done	Cannot determine "relative risk"
Can accept only well-defined cases	Questionable data and diagnostic accuracy
Can define controls rigidly as needed	Difficulty of obtaining representative controls
Cheaper to carry out than prospective or cohort studies	Possible bias in data collection

Analytic prospective, or cohort, studies

The second group of analytic studies includes *prospective,* or *cohort,* studies. *Prospective* studies begin with a characteristic or factor believed to be associated with development of a disease (or health state) and follow up a *cohort*, or group of persons selected based on a common attribute, over time to determine whether the factor under study is associated with development of the disease or health state in question (Schuman, 1973; Friedman, 1974; Lough et al., 1975; Lilienfeld, 1976). In other words, prospective studies are forward looking and ongoing over a period of time. They begin with the independent variable or factor under study, such as smoking behavior, and follow up the cohort to determine the outcome or dependent variable (for example, development of lung cancer) resulting from exposure to the factor (Schuman, 1973).

As with other types of epidemiological studies, there are both advantages and disadvantages to the prospective approach (Table 16-2).

As illustrated in Table 16-2, an important advantage of the prospective approach is that relative risk, defined as "the ratio of the incidence rate of those exposed to a factor to the incidence rate of those not exposed," can be readily and reliably calculated based on the outcome (Mausner and Bahn, 1974:322). In other words, the calculation of relative risk is done directly, without worry about representativeness of cases; all cases are counted as part of the outcome (Schuman, 1973; Mausner and Bahn, 1974). For example, the prospective approach to studying the relationship between smoking and lung cancer is to compare the rate of lung cancer in smokers with the rate in nonsmokers. In this example, the cohort consists of smokers who are observed longitudinally (over time) to determine their rate or incidence of lung cancer compared with the lung cancer rate of a group

of nonsmokers. To calculate the relative risk of developing lung cancer for smokers, the incidence (number of new cases) of lung cancer in the smokers is divided by the lung cancer incidence (number of cases) in the group of nonsmokers. As a parenthetical note, relative risk for cigarette smokers of contracting and dying from lung cancer has been reported to be nine to ten times greater than the risk experienced by nonsmokers (Schuman, 1973; Lilienfeld, 1976).

A second advantage of the prospective approach is the lack of bias concerning the independent variable, which, in this example, is smoking behavior. Quite simply, when using the prospective approach, there can be no bias concerning the relationship of the independent variable (smoking) to the dependent variable or outcome (lung cancer) because the outcome is unknown (Schuman, 1973; Mausner and Bahn, 1974). As noted earlier in the discussion of retrospective studies, the possibility of bias is an important and potentially serious limitation of such studies; in that respect, the prospective approach is preferable.

A third advantage of the prospective approach is that diagnostic criteria for determining the presence of the disease or condition under study can be set in advance. This helps ensure diagnostic consistency and should enhance interrater reliability among diagnosticians. In addition, by predetermining diagnostic criteria, the investigators can exclude from their study persons whose clinical findings and test results are "borderline" or tentative. Likewise, by preselecting the diagnostic criteria to be used in their prospective study, investigators can choose diagnostic methods and tests that are highly sensitive and specific, while avoiding those tests and procedures which are subject to varied interpretations and, hence, have low interrater reliability.

The fourth advantage, and one that is unique to the prospective approach, is that it allows observation of multiple outcomes (Mausner and Bahn, 1974). By following a cohort longitudinally and evaluating the health status of its members periodically, investigators can observe the development of health problems, diseases, or other phenomena that may occur during the study. Thus there may be some serendipitous findings as well. For example, in prospective studies to observe the relationship between smoking and lung cancer, the findings have also revealed an association between

Table 16-2. Prospective, or cohort, studies

Advantages	Disadvantages
Relative risk can be readily and reliably calculated	Time consuming
No bias concerning independent variable	Expensive
Diagnostic criteria for study can be set in advance	Method is not at all useful when prevalence is low
Observation of multiple outcomes is possible	Maintenance of cohort is difficult

smoking and a variety of other diseases as well, including emphysema, coronary heart disease, peptic ulcer, and cancer of the larynx, mouth, esophagus, and urinary bladder (Mausner and Bahn, 1974). Although these findings were not anticipated or included in the study's design, they are nonetheless very useful and provide strong support for the potential epidemiological benefits of the prospective approach.

However, despite the benefits and advantages of the prospective approach, there are some significant disadvantages, which must be carefully weighed and considered before undertaking a prospective study. The first disadvantage is that the prospective approach is time consuming. For the investigators to observe the relationship over time between the characteristic or factor and the subsequent occurrence of disease, they must wait. Especially in studies where the long-term effects of exposure to some factor (such as asbestos fibers in a community's water supply) are being investigated, the cohort may need to be followed up over a period of 20 years or more—there are no shortcuts.

A second and potentially significant disadvantage of the prospective approach is economic; this type of study can be very expensive (Schuman, 1973; Mausner and Bahn, 1974). The increased costs of this approach are due to a number of factors. One factor is the length of time required to complete the study; maintaining the investigative team's supplies and salaries over time can be expensive, especially if the study continues for many years. Also, prospective studies use large cohorts, partly as a safeguard against attrition during the study; finding and maintaining contact with large cohorts over time can be very expensive.

A third disadvantage of the prospective approach is that for rare diseases, those which have low prevalence or incidence, this approach is too time consuming and costly to use. An example of a rare disease cited by Schuman (1973) is osteosarcoma, which occurs at a rate of about one case per 100,000 population and is believed by some investigators to be related to use of drinking water contaminated with radium. Because the prevalence rate is so low, a cohort of hundreds of thousands of persons would have to be studied to get significant results; the costs of obtaining and maintaining such a large cohort would be clearly prohibitive.

The fourth disadvantage is the difficulty inherent in maintaining the cohort for the duration of the study primarily because of attrition or loss of members to follow-up (Mausner and Bahn, 1974). Attrition can be due to lack of interest, population mobility or migration, or death. In addition, if cohort members experience any changes in their lives affecting their exposure to the variable(s) under investigation, error may be introduced into the findings. For example, in a study of the effects of smoking on subsequent development of lung cancer, any change in smoking habits (smoking more, less, or quitting altogether) may affect the findings of the study. Administrative problems of maintaining the cohort include possible loss of project staff members, funding cuts, and the logistics and costs of maintaining contact with cohort members (current mailing and telephone lists, postage). Because of these potential problems, careful planning is essential for successful completion of prospective studies (Mausner and Bahn, 1974).

Analytic cross-sectional, or prevalence, studies

The third type of analytic approach to epidemiology is the *cross-sectional* study. As defined by Friedman (1974:47),* a *cross-sectional* study examines "the relationships between diseases and other characteristics or variables of interest as they exist in a defined population at one particular time." The presence or absence of the disease (lung cancer, for example) and the presence or absence of the independent variable or characteristic under study (such as smoking habits), in each person in the study population or a sample drawn from that population, *are determined at one particular time.* Cross-sectional studies are also called *prevalence* studies, since they are concerned with the presence of a disease and an independent variable at a particular time in a particular population (Friedman, 1974; Lilienfeld, 1976).

The relationship between the disease or condition under investigation and the variable thought to be associated with it can be studied in two ways using the cross-sectional approach. The first method is to select two population subgroups based on their exposure to the independent variable to be studied; the prevalence of the disease or health state being investigated is then measured and compared for both groups (Friedman, 1974). In the example of the re-

---

lationship between smoking and lung cancer, the population (or sample) would be divided into two groups based on their use or nonuse of smoking tobacco; then the prevalence of lung cancer in each group at the time of the study would be determined, and the prevalence rates of the two groups would then be compared.

The second cross-sectional method divides the population into subgroups based on the presence or absence of the disease; the exposure of the groups to the independent variables is then observed and compared (Friedman, 1974). Again using the relationship between smoking habits and lung cancer, the population (or sample) under study is divided into groups according to the presence or absence of lung cancer; the percentage of smokers in each group is then determined. If there is a significantly higher percentage of diseased persons who are smokers, then the association between lung cancer and smoking merits further study.

Curiously, very little discussion of the cross-sectional approach is found in epidemiology reference books or textbooks. Indeed, among all the sources cited in this chapter's reference list, the cross-sectional approach is mentioned in only three (Schuman, 1973; Friedman, 1974; Lilienfeld, 1976) and even then is mentioned only in passing. In none of these references is there discussion of the advantages and disadvantages of this approach. However, Table 16-3 is an attempt to identify what seem to be the logical and obvious advantages and disadvantages of prevalence, or cross-sectional, studies.

The first advantage of cross-sectional studies

Table 16-3. Cross-sectional, or prevalence, studies

Advantages	Disadvantages
Strict diagnostic criteria for determining presence of disease can be set	Representativeness of cases can be a problem
Useful in defining and characterizing an at-risk population	Require larger number of subjects than retrospective, or case-control, studies
Lengthy time commitment not required	
Repeated studies useful in assessing time trends	
Less costly than prospective studies	

is the fact that the investigators can define the diagnostic criteria to be used in determining whether participants have the disease in question; this enables the investigators to strictly define the "cases" included in their study and eliminates problems of borderline cases or subjective and unsubstantiated data. The intended result of this strict definition of what constitutes disease is to improve the validity of the study's findings.

A second advantage of cross-sectional studies is their usefulness in defining and characterizing an at-risk population. As defined by Friedman (1974), a *population at risk* consists of those persons initially free of the disease under investigation. As he points out, identifying the population at risk is important as a first step in an incidence, or prospective, study; the population at risk can be used to form a cohort for studying disease development.

A third advantage of cross-sectional studies is that, in contrast to prospective studies, lengthy time commitment is not required for their completion. Although some time will be needed for careful selection of the study population and representative subgroups, cross-sectional studies focus on the association between an independent variable (smoking) and a dependent variable or outcome (lung cancer) *at one point in time*. Thus, although planning the study requires some time for population selection and for designation of strict diagnostic criteria, the data collection process is comparatively brief.

A fourth advantage of cross-sectional studies acknowledged by Friedman (1974) is their usefulness in assessing time trends. As noted in the discussion of disadvantages associated with prospective studies, maintenance of a cohort (population group under surveillance) is at best difficult. By repetition of prevalence, or cross-sectional, studies, some assessment of the time trends associated with other characteristics of a population can be made. This provides useful data without the necessity of maintaining a cohort over a long period of time.

The fifth advantage of cross-sectional studies is related to the third. Because these studies do not require the lengthy time commitments of prospective, or cohort, studies, they are therefore less expensive to conduct. In these days of elusive funding and inflationary spirals, cost is an important consideration.

From the limited discussion of cross-sectional studies in the available literature, two potential disadvantages can be discerned. The first disadvantage of these studies concerns the difficulty of ensuring that the cases included are representative of *all* cases of the disease under investigation (Friedman, 1974). Friedman points out that the prevalence of a disease (the total number of cases in the population at one point in time) is influenced by its *duration* (how long it lasts). Therefore persons whose disease is of short duration are likely to be *under*represented in a prevalence study at any one time, whereas persons whose disease is of long duration may be *over*represented. If, as Friedman points out, the characteristics of the long duration cases differ from the characteristics of *all* cases of the disease being studied, then the findings of the study may be skewed. Another factor that may result in nonrepresentativeness of the cases sampled for inclusion in a prevalence study is the removal of some cases from the community or population studied (Friedman, 1974). If some persons are institutionalized elsewhere or move away to a location offering special treatment facilities, they escape sampling procedures for inclusion in the community's prevalence study; this may adversely affect the representativeness of those who remain and thus may jeopardize the validity of the study's findings.

A second disadvantage of cross-sectional studies inferred by Friedman (1974) is that they tend to require larger numbers of participants (subjects) than do retrospective, or case-control, studies. Although Friedman offers no explanation regarding the need for a large number of subjects, the difficulties of securing a representative sample provide a plausible explanation. Despite these potential disadvantages, cross-sectional studies have some notable attributes as well. Although cross-sectional studies are *temporally* different from retrospective studies, in practice they are often conducted jointly because they are *methodologically* similar (Lilienfeld, 1976).

Experimental epidemiology

The third epidemiological approach is *experimental epidemiology*. This approach differs from descriptive and analytic epidemiology, which are *observational* in nature, because *experimental epidemiology* entails some *action, manipulation,* or *intervention* by the investigators of some variable affecting at least some (if not all) of the subjects of the study (Friedman, 1974). Usually, the subjects are divided into two groups: an *experimental group,* on whom the action is taken, and a *control group,* which is not acted on. This approach is often used to establish cause-effect relationships by adding, increasing, removing, or decreasing the experimental group's exposure to some factor and comparing the outcome in that group with the outcome in the control group.

Experimental epidemiological studies rely on two kinds of subjects: animals and humans (Schuman, 1973; Lilienfeld, 1976). Among the types of experimental epidemiological studies using animals as subjects are vaccine studies, attempts to produce epidemics of infectious diseases, experimental carcinogenesis, experimental induction of atherosclerosis, and virological studies of the pathogenesis of neurological diseases (Lilienfeld, 1976).

Experimental epidemiological studies using human subjects include the following (Lilienfeld, 1976):

1. Vaccine trials to determine the effectiveness of a vaccine against an infectious disease; the Salk polio vaccine studies of the 1950s (Francis et al., 1955) are an example.
2. Human volunteer studies in which infectious diseases are intentionally produced in the subjects; an example of this type of study is the Walter Reed Commission's 1900 to 1901 classic and unprecedented study of yellow fever (Reed, 1901).
3. Clinical trials of etiological agents; an example is the study by Kinsey et al. (1956) of the effects of varying concentrations of oxygen on development of retrolental fibroplasia (RLF), a leading cause of blindness among premature infants in the 1940s who were maintained in incubators.
4. Risk factor treatment studies in which the investigator intervenes in the usual pathogenesis of a disease by "treating" or ameliorating a risk factor associated with the disease; if the incidence of the disease is then reduced, a causal relationship between the risk factor and disease development may be more strongly suspected. An example of this type of study would be use of a drug to reduce elevated serum cholesterol levels as a means of preventing coronary heart disease; if the drug succeeds in lowering serum cholesterol and this results in lower incidence of coronary heart disease, then the causal link between hypercholesterolemia and coronary heart disease becomes stronger.
5. Cessation studies in which the effect on disease development of terminating some behavior or personal habit is investigated; thus to determine the causal relationship between cigarette smoking and lung cancer, a group of smokers would be selected and randomly assigned to two groups.

One group would continue to smoke and the second group would quit smoking. If the lung cancer mortality and/or morbidity are lower in the second group, the causal relationship is strengthened.

6. Studies of health care delivery methods; interest in continuity of health care resulted in development of studies like the one done by Becker et al. (1974) in which some clients of a federal Children and Youth (CY) clinic were assigned the same pediatrician for all clinic visits, whereas others were seen by the first available pediatrician on each clinic visit. The purpose was to determine the outcome of physician continuity in terms of client satisfaction, frequency of failed appointments, etc. Such studies of health care delivery represent a "new frontier" in epidemiology.

As with the epidemiological approaches already discussed, there are both advantages and disadvantages of the experimental approach as well (Table 16-4).

The first advantage of experimental studies is that they permit the investigator to influence the outcome by directly controlling the effects of extraneous factors on the phenomena under study (Lilienfeld, 1976). The experimenter controls these extraneous variables by assignment of subjects to different treatment or "exposure" groups. This ability to control the influence of extraneous factors is a distinct advantage compared with the descriptive and analytic observational studies discussed previously, in which the investigator can only wait and see what nature does.

The second advantage of experimental studies is their usefulness in demonstrating cause-effect relationships (Friedman, 1974). Cause-effect associations suggested by the findings of descriptive or analytic studies can be tested through controlled experimentation. If the action taken with the experimental group results in an outcome that does not also appear in the control group, the action is then presumed to be the cause of the outcome (Friedman, 1974). Thus cause and effect are demonstrated.

A third advantage of experimental studies is that the findings are directly applicable to prevention and health promotion efforts. If, for example, an experimental study or series of studies reveal that cigarette smoking causes lung cancer, then public health programs emphasizing the importance of quitting smoking as a preventive measure or, in the case of school-age populations, health promotional education campaigns to encourage young people never to begin smoking at all can be developed and implemented with sound scientific rationale and renewed credibility. Certainly public health educational campaigns are more likely to succeed when they are based on hard data rather than unsubstantiated, although well-intentioned, belief.

Some significant disadvantages to experimental studies also must be carefully weighed before any experimental project is undertaken. The first disadvantage is that experimental studies are complex and therefore difficult to carry out (Friedman, 1974; Lilienfeld, 1976). Investigators must therefore allow adequate time for careful planning and must be sure their studies are carefully controlled; failure to do so may invalidate the findings and perhaps discredit the experimental approach altogether.

The second disadvantage of experimental studies is related to the first and concerns the potential for bias on the part of the investigator. Bias may result primarily from the manner in which subjects are assigned to experimental and control groups and may occur consciously or, more likely, unconsciously. The remedy, according to Friedman (1974) and Lilienfeld (1976), is to use the *double-blind* study in which neither participants (subjects) nor investigators know to which group (experimental or control) the subjects have been assigned; this eliminates possible subtle and unintended alterations in approach to members of one group or the other. Thus in studies of the efficacy of a drug or vaccine in preventing an illness, placebos are given to members of the control group as a means of maintaining the "blindness" of the study.

A third disadvantage of experimental studies concerns the ethical problems posed by human experimentation (Friedman, 1974). Indeed, even animal experimentation causes some consternation among the general public, despite the

Table 16-4. Experimental epidemiological studies

Advantages	Disadvantages
Investigator can influence outcome	Complex and difficult to carry out
Useful in demonstrating cause-effect relationship	Potential for bias
	Human experimentation poses ethical problems
Findings applicable to prevention and health promotion efforts	Human experimentation presents methodological problems

documented importance of animal studies in clarifying the process of pathogenesis of many diseases and health problems (Lilienfeld, 1976). The ethical considerations of human experimentation are thoughtfully addressed by Friedman (1974). The potential for harm to the subject is the primary concern and is compounded by the uncertainty of the actual outcome. Therefore before deciding to use human subjects for epidemiological research, regardless of the specific type of study planned, the investigator must carefully calculate the potential risks to the subjects and compare them with the realistic projected benefits for those participants. The potential benefits for future groups and populations are important considerations as well, but the welfare and benefits of participation for the subjects of the study must be the first priority. Ethical abuses of human experimentation have resulted in the trend in universities and other research centers toward requirements for committee review and approval for all research studies using human subjects and for securing informed consent from all participants prior to beginning experimentation (Friedman, 1974). Obviously, for experiments involving pediatric populations such as schoolchildren, informed consent from the child's parent or guardian is necessary.

The fourth disadvantage of experimental epidemiological studies is related to the first disadvantage and concerns the methodological difficulties that arise in experiments with human subjects. In addition to ethical considerations regarding the appropriateness of using human subjects for a given study (which should be contemplated *only* after all possible and relevant animal studies have been done), these studies, like prospective, or cohort, studies, often encounter problems in maintaining the study group (Lilienfeld, 1976). Some studies lose participants through withdrawal after the study has begun, whereas in some studies, participants are somehow lost to follow-up through death, mobility, or other causes. In addition, bias may be more of a problem in human studies than in animal studies, especially when the study relies on use of volunteers; as Lilienfeld (1976) notes, volunteers have been shown to differ significantly from nonvolunteers in some studies, which may bias the findings of studies that rely heavily on volunteers. Thus, because of the risks of attrition in the subject pool or bias from subject selection, experimental studies present some very real methodological problems.

As noted at the beginning of this discussion, all three basic epidemiological approaches (descriptive, analytic, and experimental) contribute to the science of epidemiology in important ways. However, it must also be recognized, based on discussion of advantages and disadvantages of each method, that selection of a particular approach or combination of approaches depends on careful analysis and evaluation of the pros and cons of each in relation to the specific problem or health topic to be investigated.

PRINCIPLES UNDERLYING EPIDEMIOLOGICAL PRACTICE

According to Clark (1965), the principles governing epidemiological approaches to problem solving are related to the basic principles of all scientific inquiry. Specifically, Clark (1965) identifies four principles that underlie epidemiology: *exact observation, correct interpretation, rational explanation,* and *scientific construction.*

Exact observation

The principle of exact observation has been the hallmark of epidemiology over the years. Epidemiologists, whether they are using an observational (descriptive or analytic) or an experimental approach, recognize the importance of painstaking attention to details that may seem to others to be minutiae of little significance. Experience has demonstrated the importance of strict and precise attention to detailed observation in solving health problems and understanding the pathogenesis and mode of transmission of many diseases. Thus, as noted earlier, there can be no shortcuts within epidemiological investigations.

Correct interpretation

Following accurate and precise observation, epidemiologists must then carefully and honestly interpret the meaning of their observations. Error-free interpretation is critically important if the study's findings are to be applied in ways directly or indirectly affecting the health and welfare of the public. Perhaps the most likely hazard to correct interpretation of data is bias on the part of the investigator. An investigator hoping to find "the" answers to pathogenesis and treatment of some new or perplexing disease might knowingly or unknowingly introduce subjective bias into her interpretation to support a hypothesis. Review of epidemiological data and methodology by qualified peers can help avert unintended misinterpretation of findings. However, the problem of deliberate misinterpretation of findings, which is hoped to be a rare occurrence, is more difficult to detect and solve. This is actually an ethical question that seems to be perpetuated and even encouraged to some extent by current funding procedures; when research grants are awarded by organizations or corporations who have a vested interest in obtaining findings and other documentation that supports their practices or lauds the apparent safety and merits of their products, then the risk of bias in data interpretation is increased.

For example, during the 1960s, research findings documenting the apparent hazards of consumption of cyclamates (artificial sweeteners used primarily by diabetics and other weight-conscious persons) were revealed and subsequently presented to the federal Food and Drug Administration, who then banned the sale of cyclamates in this country despite the protests of the manufacturers. Some time later the public learned that the research data on which the cyclamate ban was based had been funded by the sugar industry. The potential for conflict of interest is obvious and should serve as a warning about the need for unbiased study of health-related issues. Indeed, the same potential problem would exist if the only studies of the association between smoking and the risk of developing lung cancer were funded by the tobacco industry.

Without belaboring the importance of correct and unbiased interpretation of epidemiological study findings, it should be noted that because of the trust in health care professionals by the general public, great care must be taken to conduct and interpret the findings of epidemiological and all other kinds of health studies with the greatest care and integrity. Failure to do so may not only result in breach of trust and loss of public confidence in all aspects of health care, but may also prove hazardous to the public's health if inaccurate or biased findings are used to plan or modify programs and policies affecting health, safety, and welfare.

Rational explanation

This principle is inextricably tied to the preceding principle of correct interpretation. Not only must bias be avoided in interpreting the data, but "intelligent, sensible, [and] reasonable" explanations of the occurrence of the results must be given (Clark, 1965). Thus drawing on data and theories from other disciplines, such as microbiology, anthropology, biostatistics, and demography, epidemiologists must present reasonable explanations for the observed phenomena.

Scientific construction

As indicated by Clark (1965:42), this principle involves application of "expert knowledge and technical skill" in gaining new knowledge about health and disease states. Thus the development of the science of epidemiology requires careful building of its theoretical bases through studies of all three basic types (descriptive, analytic, and experimental) and integration of their findings with those of all other relevant disciplines, which include, according to Clark (1965): clinical medicine, biological sciences (zoology, parasitology, entomology, etc.), chemistry, physics, nutrition, demography, anthropology, sociology, genetics, psychology, meteorology, and statistics.

Although nursing is conspicuously absent from Clark's list of "relevant disciplines" with which epidemiological findings should be integrated, integration of epidemiological findings into nursing is important and necessary in strengthening nursing's theory building efforts. In addition, epidemiological studies can be used to document the effectiveness of nursing services by demonstrating changes in the health status of client populations following nursing intervention (Chapter 17). In other words, despite Clark's omission of nursing from his list of disciplines that are "relevant" to epidemiology, nursing can and should incorporate epidemiological findings into theory building, plans for nursing services and interventions, and for evaluation of intervention and program effectiveness.

These four scientific principles are the basis for epidemiological process and must be rigorously applied to all epidemiological studies regardless of the nature of the problem or health state under investigation or the setting in which the study takes place. In this way, the contributions and credibility of epidemiological studies will be enhanced.

DISEASE DEVELOPMENT AND CONTROL

Earlier in this chapter, the gradual expansion of epidemiology from a disease orientation to a health orientation was described, and a definition reflecting that shift in emphasis was adopted. No doubt, the future role of epidemiology as a health science will depend on its attention to health and health states and identification of health behaviors and habits that promote high-level wellness. However, there will always need to be some focus on disease causation and control as well because even as some diseases are well controlled or even eradicated (smallpox, for example) others (such as Legionnaire's disease and toxic shock syndrome) are emerging. Indeed, as technology becomes increasingly sophisticated, the kinds of diseases and traumas to which humans are exposed likewise become increasingly complex.

Like most other health care professionals, school nurses are frequently confronted with various illnesses among their school-age populations. It may therefore be helpful to review selected theories and concepts of disease development and control from an epidemiological frame of reference. However, because of the tremendous volume of data and material available concerning disease development, modes of transmission, and control, it is not feasible or appropriate to present a comprehensive discussion of these lengthy and involved topics. Therefore this discussion will be abbreviated and selective. For more detailed discussion of these topics the reader is referred to MacMahon et al., 1960; Smillie and Kilbourne, 1963;

Clark, 1965; Fox et al., 1970; Friedman, 1974; Mausner and Bahn, 1974; and Lilienfeld, 1976.

Definition of "disease"

According to Fox et al. (1970:45), *disease* is a "state of dysfunction, subjectively or objectively *apparent*." Thus disease is characterized as dysfunctional and as being *apparent* in some way; according to this definition, an infection or some other pathological process that has not progressed to the point of overt recognizable signs and symptoms would not necessarily be considered a disease.

Lilienfeld (1976:46) illustrates the complexity of the concept of disease in his discussion of the *spectrum of disease,* which he defines as "the sequence of events that occurs in the human organism from the time of exposure to the etiological agent to death." As illustrated in Fig. 16-1, this spectrum of disease includes two major subdivisions: subclinical manifestations and clinical disease.

In the case of infectious diseases, the spectrum of disease is renamed the *gradient of infection,* defined (Lilienfeld, 1976:46) as "the sequence of manifestations of illness in the host reflecting his response to the infectious agent . . . [extending] from death at one extreme to 'inapparent infection' at the other" (Fig. 16-2). As Lilienfeld further explains, the frequency

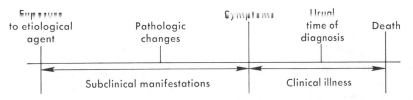

Fig. 16-1. The spectrum of disease. (From Lilienfeld, A. M.: 1976. Foundations of epidemiology, Oxford University Press, New York.)

Inapparent infection	Mild disease	Severe disease	Death
No signs or symptoms (also termed subclinical infections)	Clinical illness with signs and symptoms		

Fig. 16-2. The gradient of infection. (From Lilienfeld, A. M.: 1976. Foundations of epidemiology, Oxford University Press, New York.)

with which these various gradations occur varies with each infectious disease; for example, more than 90% of persons infected with measles develop clinical illness, whereas approximately 66%, or two-thirds, of those infected with mumps develop clinically recognizable illness (Lilienfeld, 1976).

Endemic versus epidemic disease

In discussing the concept of disease it is also important to distinguish between *endemic* and *epidemic* disease occurrence. As defined by Lester (1957:1434), an *epidemic* is "a sudden increase in the prevalence of a disease above the endemic level." *Endemic* level is then defined as "the incidence which is commonly present in a community" (Lester, 1957:1434). Thus the definition of epidemic focuses on a *sudden* and *unusual* or *unexpected increase* in the number of cases of the disease *in a given community*. In other words, occurrence of an epidemic is not determined by any absolute number of cases; instead, the history of the particular disease over time within a specified population is the basis for deciding whether the number of cases occurring in that population at any one time is a sudden and unusual increase and hence is an epidemic (Schuman, 1973). Whereas in many Third World countries the endemic level of a disease such as typhoid fever might be hundreds or thousands of cases, in most parts of the United States the occurrence of even one or two cases of typhoid fever might constitute an epidemic.

Measurement of disease: rates

To distinguish between endemic and epidemic occurrence of a disease within any population and geographic area, some way of measuring the disease experience is necessary. Calculation of *rates* provides a means for expressing the number of events (such as illnesses, births, deaths, etc.) within a given population. The general composition of epidemiological rates is shown in the following formula (Schuman, 1973):

$$\text{Rate} = \frac{\begin{array}{c}\text{Number of occurrences of events in a}\\\text{population of a given geographic area}\\\text{during a specified time}\end{array}}{\begin{array}{c}\text{Total number of individuals of the same}\\\text{geographic area exposed to the risk of the}\\\text{event during the same time interval}\end{array}}$$

Rates that describe disease occurrence are called *morbidity,* and rates describing deaths are called *mortality* (Mausner and Bahn, 1974).

Probably the two most widely used and applied morbidity rates, and ones that are especially relevant for school nurses working with school-age populations, are *prevalence* and *incidence*. Although those two terms were clarified and discussed in Chapter 5, it is appropriate to summarize that discussion here. The *prevalence* of a disease is the total number of cases of the disease at a specified time divided by the total population at that time (Friedman, 1974; W. S. Morris, 1975). The formula for its calculation is as follows (W. S. Morris, 1975:126):

$$\text{Prevalence} = \frac{\begin{array}{c}\text{All cases of the disease}\\\text{at a given time} \times 1000\end{array}}{\text{Population at given time}}$$

Thus prevalence expresses the total number of cases of the disease at any one point in time, regardless of when they developed. In contrast, the *incidence* of a disease measures the number of cases of the disease that develop within a specified time period (usually per year) per total population (Friedman, 1974; W. S. Morris, 1975). The formula for calculation of incidence is as follows (W. S. Morris, 1975):

$$\text{Incidence} = \frac{\begin{array}{c}\text{Number of new cases of}\\\text{specific disease in year} \times 1000\end{array}}{\text{Population on July 1}}$$

Thus the prevalence includes *all* cases in the population, whereas the incidence measures the rate of occurrence of *new* cases per specified time period. Calculation of these morbidity rates helps determine the endemic or usual rate of occurrence of various diseases in a population; once the endemic level is known, identification of epidemic occurrences is possible.

Multifactorial models of disease causation and development

Despite pressures from the general public to find "the" cause of cancer or "the" cause of heart disease, epidemiologists realize that there is never any one cause of a particular disease. Rather, the etiology of any disease is *multifactorial* or attributable to multiple causes (Schuman, 1973; Mausner and Bahn, 1974). This multiple causation helps explain why not everyone who is exposed to a communicable disease such as tuberculosis, influenza, or the common cold actually gets sick.

Mausner and Bahn (1974) emphasize the importance of an *ecological approach* to the explanation of disease occurrence. As defined by Webster, *ecology* is "the totality or pattern of relations between organisms and their environment.'' Because humans (as organisms) share their world (environment) with other organisms, together they make up the same ecological *system*. A *system,* according to Webster, is made up of *interdependent* and *interacting* parts or *elements* that are *in equilibrium;* therefore any change in one part of the system affects the other parts or elements by altering the balance or equilibrium among them. To use an ecological approach in explaining the occurrence of disease in humans the *relationships* between humans, other organisms, and their collective environment must be studied, because they are all elements of the same ecological system and are therefore interdependent and interacting with one another. In other words, an *ecological approach* to explanation of disease occurrence *analyzes the interaction among the various elements of the ecological system, recognizing that no single element acting alone is responsible for disease causation.*

Although the importance of an ecological approach to studying disease occurrence is widely accepted, no one ecological model or approach has been universally adopted. In fact, a number of ecological models have been proposed and are described in the literature (Mausner and Bahn, 1974). Two of the more commonly encountered ecological models are the *web of causation* and the *agent-host-environment* complex.

Web of causation

MacMahon et al. (1960) have generally been credited with development of the *web of causation* model (Friedman, 1974; Mausner and Bahn, 1974). Basically, the web of causation model conceptualizes disease causation as a complex network or *web* of contributing factors (MacMahon et al., 1960). According to this model, all kinds of factors are considered, and their complex interactions with each other and with the disease itself are analyzed (Friedman, 1974). These interrelationships are generally diagrammed so that the overall web can be visualized. From the visualization of the network

of relationships, strategies can be planned for disrupting some of those relationships and thus reducing the occurrence of the disease.

Agent-host-environment complex

Another ecological model for explaining disease occurrence is the *agent-host-environment complex,* which has been the classic epidemiological model of disease causation over the years and is still widely respected and applied today. As indicated by its name and illustrated in Fig. 16-3, the agent-host-environment complex focuses on the interactions among three groups or classes of factors: agent, host, and environmental factors (Fox et al., 1970).

Agent. According to Lough et al. (1975: 148),* an *agent* is ''an element, a substance, or a force, either animate or inanimate, that initiates or perpetuates a disease under proper environmental conditions or following contact with a susceptible host.'' As characterized by Fox et al. (1970:34), the agent is the ''primary or true cause without which a specific disease cannot occur.'' Thus, although the agent is not ''the'' only cause of a specific disease, it is a crucial element, since without it, the disease could not occur. As an example, the agent for tuberculosis is the tubercle bacillus *(Mycobacterium tuberculosis);* without it, tuberculosis cannot occur. However, not all persons exposed to or infected with *Mycobacterium tuberculosis* develop tuberculosis as a clinical disease; therefore although the tubercle bacillus is an essential element for development of tuberculosis, it is not the only causative element involved in occurrence of the disease.

The role of the agent in disease development is influenced by a number of variables, which, in the case of infectious diseases, include (1) the *numbers* or ''dose'' of the agent; (2) the ability of the agent to enter the host (victim), which is known as its *infectivity;* (3) the agent's

*From Lough, M. A., Murray, R., and Zentner, J.: 1975. Concepts of epidemiology, Chapter 6. In Murray, R., and Zentner, J.: Nursing concepts for health promotion, Prentice-Hall, Inc., Englewood Cliffs, N.J. By permission.

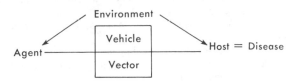

Fig. 16-3. The agent-host-environment complex. (Modified from Schuman, L. M.: 1973. Course materials and lecture notes, Public Health 5-330 Epidemiology I, University of Minnesota, Minneapolis.)

ability to produce disease, or its *pathogenicity;* and (4) the *transmissibility* of the agent from host to host (Schuman, 1973).

Transmissibility of the agent from host to host sometimes involves transportation of the agent by some other animate or inanimate object. As shown in Fig. 16-3, the agent may be carried to the host by an *inanimate intermediary* or *vehicle,* such as food, water, milk, serum, or plasma, or it may be transported by an *animate* or *living creature* (which may or may not be altered or damaged itself) referred to as a *vector,* examples of which include mosquitoes, ticks, or lice (Schuman, 1973).

As shown in Table 16-5, agents are generally classified into four groups: nutritional elements

Table 16-5. A classification of agent, host, and environmental factors which determine the distribution of diseases in human populations*

Classification	Examples
Agents of disease—*necessary etiologic factors*	
Nutritive elements	
Excesses	Cholesterol
Deficiencies	Vitamins, proteins
Chemical agents	
Poisons	Carbon monoxide, carbon tetrachloride, drugs
Allergens	Ragweed, poison ivy, medications
Physical agents	Ionizing radiation, mechanical
Infectious agents	
Metazoa	Hookworm, schistosomiasis, onchocerciasis
Protozoa	Amoebae, malaria
Bacteria	Rheumatic fever, lobar pneumonia, typhoid, tuberculosis, syphilis
Fungi	Histoplasmosis, athlete's foot
Rickettsia	Rocky Mountain spotted fever, typhus
Viruses	Measles, mumps, chickenpox, smallpox, poliomyelitis, rabies, yellow fever
Host factors *(intrinsic factors)*—*influence exposure, susceptibility, or response to agents*	
Genetic	Sickle cell disease
Age	
Sex	
Ethnic group	
Physiologic state	Fatigue, pregnancy, puberty, stress, nutritional state
Prior immunologic experience	Hypersensitivity, protection
Active	Prior infection, immunization
Passive	Maternal antibodies, gamma globulin prophylaxis
Intercurrent or preexisting disease	
Human behavior	Personal hygiene, food handling, diet, interpersonal contact, occupation, recreation, utilization of health resources
Environmental factors *(extrinsic factors)*—*influence existence of the agent, exposure, or susceptibility to agents*	
Physical environment	Geology, climate
Biologic environment	
Human populations	Density
Flora	Sources of food, influence on vertebrates and arthropods, as a source of agents
Fauna	Food sources, vertebrate hosts, arthropod vectors
Socioeconomic environment	
Occupation	Exposure to chemical agents
Urbanization and economic development	Urban crowding, tensions and pressures, cooperative efforts in health and education
Disruption	Wars, floods

*From Lilienfeld, A. M.: 1976. Foundations of epidemiology, Oxford University Press, New York.

(both excesses and deficiencies), chemical agents (including poisons and allergens), physical agents, and infectious agents (Lilienfeld, 1976). It is important to note, however, that as a result of our increasingly complex and sophisticated technology and life-styles, the list of possible agents of disease is growing. In some cases, nutritive materials such as eggs and multiple vitamins that were once regarded as "good for you" are now recognized as potentially hazardous to health, especially when used to excess. In other cases, the list of agents is expanded due to discovery or manufacture of materials that are ultimately proven to be more harmful than helpful; an example of this type of material is DDT, an insecticide originally hailed as an effective, safe, and vital tool for agriculture but later found to be carcinogenic in humans. As man's capabilities for exploring extraterrestrial territories improve, he will no doubt encounter new forms of infectious and other types of agents.

Host. The *host* is a "person or organism capable of being infected or affected by an agent."* Thus the host is the one who actually becomes ill—the "victim" of a disease.

The likelihood that a host will contract a disease depends in part on *intrinsic* host factors or variables that influence the host's *exposure, susceptibility,* and *response* to an agent. As shown in Table 16-5, these host factors include genetic endowment, age, sex, ethnic or cultural group background, physiological state, prior immunological experience, presence of other preexisting disease conditions, and behaviors such as diet, occupation, hygiene, and use of health care resources (Schuman, 1973; Lilienfeld, 1976).

Environment. The *environment* includes "all that is external to the agent and the human host(s) immediately in question including fellow men" (Fox et al., 1970:35). With such a global definition of environment, obviously the potential array of environmental, or *extrinsic,* factors available is practically limitless. These environmental factors influence the existence of the agent, exposure potential of the host, and the host's susceptibility to the agent (Lilienfeld, 1976). Environmental factors are generally classified into three groups: physical, biological, and socioeconomic (Fox et al., 1970; Lilienfeld, 1976).

Interaction of agent-host-environment factors. The interaction of these agent-host-environment factors is analogous to the balance of a lever, weighted on one end by the agent and on the other by the host, over a fulcrum (the environment) as illustrated in Fig. 16-4. The agent-host-environment complex as depicted in Fig. 16-4 is a concept based on the following three biologically derived premises (Clark, 1965:50):

1. Disease is the result of an imbalance between disease agent and host (man).
2. The type and extent of this imbalance depends on the specific nature and characteristics (intrinsic factors) of both host and agent.
3. The characteristics of agent and host and their interactions are directly related to and largely influenced by aspects of the physical, biological, and socioeconomic environment; the environment acts by bringing agent and host into contact with each other and by influencing their characteristics and interactions.

When all three factors are in balance, then health exists. If changes occur in the agent, host, or environment, then the balance is disturbed and disease may occur (Fox et al., 1970). In other words, the interaction among agent, host, and environmental forces is dynamic and the balance somewhat precarious, with the result that even seemingly minor and subtle changes in any one of them can sufficiently alter the equilibrium to produce disease.

For example, the dramatic drop in the incidence of measles during the 1970s can be traced to altered host susceptibility, resulting from widespread immunization of the susceptible at-risk (pediatric) population. Indeed, laws passed in many states requiring proof of immunization against measles, rubella, mumps, polio, and other serious communicable diseases prior to school enrollment have dramatically reduced the overall incidence of these formerly prevalent threats to pediatric populations by reducing the numbers of susceptible hosts. This, then, is an example of interfering with the disease-producing interaction among the agent, host, and environment to prevent disease and lower its incidence. However, in communities where parents have been complacent about immunizing their children, sporadic outbreaks of diseases like measles and diphtheria have been reported. Such outbreaks illustrate an imbalance

---

*From Lough, M. A., Murray, R., and Zentner, J.: 1975. Concepts of epidemiology, Chapter 6. In Murray, R., and Zentner, J.: Nursing concepts for health promotion, Prentice-Hall, Inc., Englewood Cliffs, N.J. By permission.

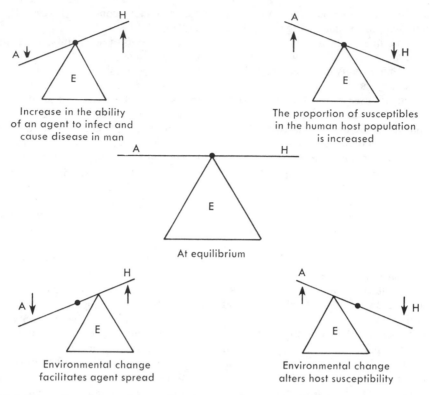

Fig. 16-4. Interaction of agent, host, and environment factors. *A,* Agent; *H,* host; *E,* environment. (From Fox, J. P., Hall, C. E., and Elveback, L. R.: 1970. Epidemiology: man and disease, The Macmillan, Co., New York.)

between agent and host and are further evidence of the tenuous and dynamic balance among the agent, host, and environmental factors.

Classification of diseases

Based on a variety of systems, diseases can be classified as acute or chronic, infectious or noninfectious, and functional or therapeutic. Regardless of the particular system adopted, classification of diseases is epidemiologically important as a means of procuring homogeneous groupings for epidemiological study (Mausner and Bahn, 1974). In fact, as noted in the discussion of epidemiological approaches (descriptive, analytic, and experimental), deciding which persons or subjects are to be considered diseased or ''sick'' is often a critically important aspect of the methodology of epidemiological study; studies of a particular condition or disease in which classification of persons is based solely on reported symptoms are likely to yield different findings from those using more precise diagnostic decision-making criteria such as laboratory tests or other ''hard'' data.

Mausner and Bahn (1974) also emphasize the importance of subdividing groups of diseased persons into clinical groups of the greatest possible precision as a further means of enhancing the feasibility of epidemiological study. Thus, for example, infectious diseases could be subdivided or subclassified based on the mode of transmission of agent to host; an example of this type of subclassification is presented in Table 16-6.

In addition to careful classification of diseases to facilitate epidemiological study, Lester (1957) points out the importance of disease classification as a means of facilitating diagnosis and treatment. Thus diseases may be classified according to anatomical location, such as gastrointestinal or musculoskeletal diseases, or according to disease agent, such as viral or bacterial diseases.

According to Lester (1957), diseases are epidemiologically classified by mode of transmission (Table 16-6) as direct or indirect or active or passive. Lilienfeld (1976:36) proposes a system of disease classification for infectious

Table 16-6. Classification of communicable diseases by mode of agent-host transmission

Modes of transmission	Examples of diseases
Direct transmission	
Direct contact	
Skin to skin	
Skin to mucus membrane	Syphilis, gonorrhea, other venereal diseases
Mucus membrane to skin	
Droplets (from nose and throat of infected person)	Chickenpox, influenza, measles, mumps
Fecal-oral	Infectious hepatitis, shigellosis (or bacillary dysentery)
Indirect transmission	
Vehicle borne	
Food	Infectious hepatitis, salmonellosis
Water	Typhoid fever, cholera, leptospirosis
Milk	Brucellosis, infectious hepatitis, bovine tuberculosis
Biological products (such as blood and plasma)	Infectious and serum hepatitis, and malaria
Fomites (contaminated articles such as toys, clothes, bedding, dressings, surgical instruments)	Pediculosis, acute bacterial conjunctivitis, and enterobiasis
Vector borne	
Simple mechanical transfer	Trypanosomiasis (African sleeping sickness), tularemia, anthrax
Harborage in gastrointestinal tract of vector	Louse-borne typhus fever
Biological	Malaria, yellow fever
Airborne	Tuberculosis
Droplet nuclei	Psittacosis
Dust	Q fever

conditions based on what he calls "selected epidemiologic features," including dynamics of spread through human populations, portal of entry into the host, principal reservoir (usual or natural habitat of an infectious agent) or source of infection, and cycles of the agent in nature. Such systems of epidemiological classification of diseases facilitate diagnosis and treatment and are very useful in devising methods to control the spread of disease as well, which is, of course, a primary purpose of epidemiology.

Disease control: manipulation of agent-host-environment
Infectious or communicable diseases

Control of infectious or communicable diseases can be accomplished in a variety of ways. Obviously, the greater the understanding of the natural history of a disease, the more opportunities and methods there are for interrupting the chain of infection and thus halting or preventing spread of the disease. Lester (1957) advocates identifying and focusing on the "weakest link" in the chain of infection or taking action against the factor that is most amenable to disruption through known control methods. Following are possible methods for interfering in transmission of infectious diseases: (1) attacking the agent

directly, (2) increasing host resistance, (3) reducing the available reservoir of infection, (4) reducing vehicular spread, (5) attacking the vectors, and (6) treating known cases (Lester, 1957; Lombard, 1975).

Attacking the agent. The emphasis here is on eradication of the agent by such measures as chemical disinfection and use of heat, steam, and ultraviolet rays to destroy the agent directly wherever it is found. Thus environmental sanitation as well as use of antibiotics are effective measures for attacking the agent.

Increasing host resistance. Improving the host's resistance can be accomplished by immunization against the particular disease, provided an effective and safe vaccine exists. When immunization is not feasible, the host's resistance can be improved to a limited extent by improving his overall health and lowering his susceptibility through provision of adequate nutrition, rest, and hygiene, and any other health behaviors or practices that contribute to wellness.

Reducing the reservoir. The *reservoir* of an infection (defined as the place or habitat where the organism usually grows and multiplies) can include other persons with frank clinical cases of the disease, persons with subclinical infections, and *carriers* (infected persons who harbor the agent/organism without obvious clinical disease and who are potential sources of infection for others). The reservoir can also include animals, particularly domestic animals and rodents, or it can be a plant, such as a mold or fungus (Anderson et al., 1962).

Reduction of the reservoir can be accomplished by destruction of animal reservoirs by slaughter, a method used for control of bovine tuberculosis (Anderson et al., 1962), or by regulation of importation and transportation of animal reservoirs, as in the control of psittacosis by regulation of the importation of parrots, parakeets, and similar birds (Lombard, 1975). In the case of human reservoirs, treatment with antibiotics and other chemotherapeutic agents is helpful. In some cases, the carrier state can be terminated through surgery (as in use of tonsillectomies for diphtheria carriers) or by administration of antibiotics (Anderson et al., 1962).

Reducing vehicular spread. The most important or usual vehicles for spread of disease are milk, water, food, and biological products such as blood and plasma; *fomites* (all inanimate vehicles except the foregoing) are relatively unimportant vehicles for the spread of most diseases (Anderson et al., 1962). Methods of reducing vehicular spread include environmental sanitation measures such as use of chemical disinfectants, use of heat (dry and steam), plus specific procedures like pasteurization to kill organisms or retard their growth. In the case of diseases spread through contaminated food supplies, improved hygiene of food handlers is an important control measure; for water-borne infections such as typhoid fever, chemical disinfection (chlorination) of water supplies may be useful.

Attacking the vectors. For some diseases like malaria or yellow fever that are transmitted by vectors (mosquitoes, to be specific), control of the vectors may be an important means of preventing spread of the disease. This may be accomplished through altering their usual environment, such as by eliminating wet, swampy breeding areas, or by efforts to kill the vectors directly through spraying of insecticides.

Treating known cases. Finally, the spread of infection can be halted or prevented by treatment of known cases, such as by administration of antibiotics plus other palliative measures. This, obviously, is also a means of reducing the reservoir of infection, a goal which can be more readily achieved for some diseases if the known cases are isolated as well until they are beyond the time of communicability of the disease (Lester, 1957).

Noninfectious diseases

Control of noninfectious diseases parallels control of communicable diseases in that the emphasis is on discovering and intervening at the most amenable point in the natural history of the disease. Thus by analyzing what is known about the agent-host-environment complex for a particular disease, appropriate control measures can be initiated.

Using levels of prevention as a conceptual frame of reference, an important control measure for cancer would be secondary prevention or early diagnosis and prompt treatment. If cancers can be detected and treated before metastasis occurs, then the prognosis for the patient is much more positive than it would be following metastasis.

At the tertiary prevention level, rehabilitation of patients is the intent; for a postmastectomy patient this would include assistance with psychological adjustment to change in body image following loss of a breast and physical retraining of muscle groups to regain arm functioning. An additional aspect of rehabilitation for this cancer patient might appropriately include psychological adjustment to the possibility of death and loss of self-esteem and employment.

At the primary prevention level, health education of the public concerning signs and symptoms of cancer, known or suspected risk factors, and recommended life-style alterations to reduce these risks is an important, although perhaps overwhelming, approach to control. In addition, strict enforcement of existing environmental safety codes, like those intended to reduce air and water pollution, plus enactment of new strict measures as indicated can improve the environment by reducing or eliminating some agents of noninfectious disease.

The important point to remember concerning control of disease (both infectious and noninfectious), is that it is *not* necessary to understand the complete etiology of a disease or health problem to initiate effective preventive measures—even knowing or understanding one small aspect can allow for implementation of some type of prevention and control (MacMahon, et al., 1960). Obviously, however, disease control through manipulation of agent-host-environment factors will be more effective if the natural history of the disease, including the roles and interactions among the agent, host, and environment, is well understood. For that reason, every possible effort should be made to understand the natural history of the disease through descriptive, analytic, or experimental study.

EPIDEMIOLOGICAL INVESTIGATIVE PROCESS

The ultimate test of any body of knowledge is in its usefulness and applicability. This is also true for scientific disciplines such as epidemiology. For that reason, it seems prudent to now discuss the applicability of epidemiological concepts and principles within the epidemiological investigative process.

According to Clark (1965:48),* the *epidemiological* method or *process* refers to the "application of scientific principles to investigations of conditions affecting groups in the population by the collection of information for analysis and by scientific research." The epidemiological method or process as defined by Clark and others (Lester, 1957; MacMahon et al., 1960; Friedman, 1974) is an orderly, systematic approach to solving epidemiological problems concerning health and disease. Although this approach has been primarily applied to infectious disease problems, it is a basic investigative approach that can be used to study noninfectious diseases or other health concerns and problems as well (Clark, 1965).

As described by Clark (1965) and illustrated above, epidemiological investigative process has five steps: (1) definition of the problem, (2) appraisal of existing data, (3) formulation of hypotheses, (4) testing of hypotheses, and (5) conclusions and applications. Clark points out that although these steps are usually followed in the sequence listed, it is not always necessary to do so. As Clark (1965) states, the precise starting point chosen by the investigator will depend on the investigator's experience and interest, the overall objectives of the investigation, and the nature and extent of the problem. However, to avoid thoroughly confusing the reader, the steps of the epidemiological investigative process will be discussed in the order listed.

Step 1: Definition of the problem

This step involves comparing the current incidence of the disease or health condition with

---

*Copyright © 1965 McGraw-Hill Book Company. Used with permission of McGraw-Hill Book Company.

> **EPIDEMIOLOGIC INVESTIGATIVE PROCESS***
>
> *Step 1* Definition of the problem
> ↓
> *Step 2* Appraisal of existing data
> ↓
> *Step 3* Formulation of hypotheses
> ↓
> *Step 4* Testing hypotheses
> ↓
> *Step 5* Conclusions and applications
>
> *Modified from Preventive medicine for the doctor in his community: an epidemiologic approach by H. R. Leavell and E. G. Clark. Copyright © 1965 McGraw-Hill Book Company. Used with permission of McGraw-Hill Book Company.

the previous and/or usual occurrence. The investigator needs to decide whether the current number of cases (incidence) is greater than would be expected at this particular time under these circumstances. If the incidence is significantly higher than usual, the investigator may conclude (regardless of the absolute *number* of cases) that an epidemic exists (Clark, 1965).

Step 2: Appraisal of existing data

During this step, the epidemiologist's observations are focused on *time, place,* and *person* (Lester, 1957; Clark, 1965). The emphasis on *time* includes questions regarding seasonal trends and cyclic occurrence, secular (long-term) patterns, incubation period (for infectious diseases), and chronological dates of onset for the current outbreak or group of cases. *Place* is studied in terms of geographic location of cases, geophysical characteristics (such as mountainous versus flat terrain), climate and weather, population concentrations (urban versus rural), biological environment (vector and pest harborage), and other environmental characteristics such as industrial facilities (and their environmental impact), and political, social, and economic structure and climate, which affect health policies, health care delivery strategies, quality of available health care and resources, and health values and philosophies (Mausner and Bahn, 1974). Observations of *person* emphasize age, sex, race, socioeconomic status, health history, disease experience, occupation, cultural and religious background, marital status, and other family-related variables such as family size, birth order, maternal age, and parental deprivation due to loss, separation, or divorce (Lester, 1957; Clark, 1965; Mausner and Bahn, 1974). The investigator's appraisal of this data plus any other information germane to the study provides the basis for step 3.

Step 3: Formulation of hypotheses

Based on all the data collected and assessed during step 2, tentative or "working" hypotheses are formulated (Lester, 1957; Clark, 1965). The purpose of these working hypotheses is to provide a tentative explanation of the cause of the disease or condition under investigation. The importance of providing at least a tentative hypothesis is, according to Clark (1965), that it allows something to be done to halt the disease's progression; the working hypothesis may also suggest measures to prevent spread of the (infectious or communicable) disease to others including control measures such as immunizations, environmental sanitation, or treatment measures for known cases. In addition, the working hypotheses may provide a basis for further investigation or study, including experimental studies.

Step 4: Testing hypotheses

During step 4 the hypotheses formulated during the previous step are actually tested by systematically and comprehensively searching for additional cases. These new cases are then analyzed and compared with the data gathered and appraised during step 2; in this way the new data is compared with previous data regarding such aspects as disease characteristics, natural history of the disease, and mode of transmission. Thus through analysis of these additional cases and the investigation of them, efforts are made to validate the hypotheses formulated during step 3 (Clark, 1965).

Step 5: Conclusions and applications

During this step, data analysis is done, including computation of morbidity (such as attack rates, incidence, and prevalence) and mortality (including fatality rate and age-specific and other specific rates). Using *all* available evidence and data, the facts are evaluated and the findings compared with the expectations stated in the hypotheses. The findings can then be applied to controlling the disease problem and preventing occurrence of additional cases. The findings of epidemiological investigations may have far-reaching consequences on peo-

ple's everyday lives, such as the adjustments required if the local water supply is found to be a source of disease and is temporarily shut off or the impact on a community's economy if an industry is shut down because of alleged environmental pollution. Therefore it is important that applications of investigative findings be based on sound scientific reasoning and on review and analysis of *all* relevant data; Clark (1965:68) warns that incomplete studies may result in inaccurate conclusions and may generate what he calls "false leads for future prevention." If the facts seem to fit more than one hypothesis, Clark urges that additional data be gathered and analyzed until a consistent and coherent picture can be formed.

Not surprisingly, the steps of the epidemiological investigative process bear a striking resemblance to the steps of the research process as outlined in Chapter 17. Both processes provide a systematic approach to problem solving, and both processes, if properly conducted, identify conclusions and outcomes that can be applied to improve and enhance the health and wellness of populations. As noted previously, the epidemiological investigative process has been most widely applied to the investigation of epidemics and other communicable disease problems; however, the process is a basic problem-solving method that can be used for other health concerns as well, including noninfectious chronic and/or acute diseases and other health states and concerns.

APPLICATIONS OF EPIDEMIOLOGY

It should now be apparent, after this discussion of epidemiology as an investigative science, that epidemiological concepts, principles, and methods are widely applicable to the study and amelioration of a variety of diseases and health problems and to health promotion efforts as well. In this discussion, applications of epidemiology will be highlighted and summarized.

Examples of the application of epidemiological concepts, principles, and methods have been incorporated throughout this chapter. However, it seems appropriate at this point to highlight and summarize the general applications of epidemiology as a means of assisting the reader to synthesize these ideas.

As Lough et al. (1975) point out, many nurses and other health care professionals apply epidemiological findings and principles within the context of their daily practice without recognizing these ideas as epidemiological in origin. Indeed, it is likely that many health care professionals (including nurses) have had no formal exposure to epidemiological concepts through course work or field experience and thus may have a limited or inaccurate perception of the scope and usefulness of epidemiology, despite the fact that many accepted disease detection and control measures in use today originated from epidemiological studies.

The following primary applications of epidemiology are described and illustrated at length by J. N. Morris (1975:262-263):

1. To *study the history of the health of populations,* including fluctuations in the incidence of disease occurrence and changes in the nature and appearance of diseases; such data may be useful in projecting future occurrences.
2. To *diagnose a community's health* and the health of its residents through the following means:
   a. Measurement of incidence, prevalence, distribution, and severity of disease and disability and other health problems and assessment of their impact on mortality experience (ages, causes, etc.) in the population
   b. Determination of the relative importance of specific health problems as a basis for priority setting
   c. Identification of groups requiring special attention for health-related problems and concerns
   d. Monitoring community life-styles and changes and their effects on the community's health
3. To *study the operation of health services and recommend improvements;* this includes assessment of the effectiveness of existing services and resources in meeting community health needs (and should include assessment of efficiency of services as well). Operational research also includes analysis of the adaptability of health resources in meeting the changing needs of the community and demands for new services and resources to cope with changing needs. Operational research data can be used for local, regional, state, federal, and international health planning.
4. To *estimate individual risks* of disease, accident, defect, and disability and the *chances of avoiding them* based on group and population experiences and rates.
5. To *identify syndromes* through description and study of signs, symptoms, and other disease characteristics (such as agent, host, and environment factors) that occur with a disease to distinguish between it and similar illnesses.
6. To *complete the clinical picture* of chronic diseases and *describe their natural history.* This entails studying and following up not only symptomatic patients who seek medical care but also

cohorts of persons who may experience subclinical disease. It also involves following remission, relapse, adjustment, and disability experiences in defined populations.
7. To *search for causes of both health and disease* through the study and comparison of groups' experiences with disease, defect, disability, and mortality. The search for causes of health and disease is based on groups defined by their composition, inheritance, experience, behavior, and environment. Suspected etiological factors may be tested through naturally occurring "experiments of opportunity" or planned experiments. Exposure to risk factors as well as the impact of "healthy" behaviors (such as moderate exercise, low saturated fat diet, nonsmoking, etc.) can be studied as they affect health and morbidity.

A reasonable addendum to Morris' list of applications as just presented would be *recommending specific courses of action for preventing and controlling disease, defect, and disability* based on the kinds of studies described in Morris' list of applications plus other epidemiological approaches described earlier in this chapter, such as cohort studies and experimentation. Epidemiologists collect data concerning disease occurrence and causation and should be able to suggest control and prevention measures for diseases whose natural history is well understood; in that sense, epidemiologists can provide direction and leadership in preventive medicine and public health. In addition, epidemiologists can also study the effectiveness of preventive and control measures and recommend changes in strategy based on the effects of existing programs and efforts on morbidity and mortality. In other words, in addition to studying and describing morbidity and mortality experiences as suggested by Morris, epidemiologists can assume leadership in implementing and evaluating the effectiveness of prevention and control programs.

Another area for application of epidemiological concepts and approaches is *health promotion.* As noted earlier, from its earliest roots in investigating and controlling outbreaks of communicable diseases, epidemiology has gradually evolved to a discipline interested in other kinds of diseases and health problems. However, epidemiology remains largely focused on diseases and health problems, with little emphasis on health and its promotion and maintenance. It is encouraging to note that in the postscript to his book J. N. Morris (1975) suggests that the "next leap forward" in epidemiological studies will be a shift in emphasis away from morbidity and mortality and to ". . . healthy processes, to the social, cultural, and economic conditions and sources of the people's good health." J. N. Morris (1975) believes this shift in emphasis will assist health care professionals to more effectively promote "normal" functioning, improve the disease resistance and defenses of populations, and assist populations to achieve their potential for growth and development.

THE ROLE OF THE SCHOOL NURSE

As Lough et al. (1975) point out, epidemiological concepts and approaches are applicable in all practice settings and can be used by all health care professionals, including nurses. However, as Roberts (1967) notes, nurses have tended to look to physicians for completion of epidemiological studies of diagnostic syndromes and development of corresponding plans of care. Although Roberts offers no explanation for the reticence of nurses to initiate epidemiological studies, the probable reasons include nurses' lack of knowledge of epidemiology generally, their traditional and well-socialized subservience to physicians, lack of adequate preparation in research methods, and often limited role perceptions. In addition, for those nurses who do have background in epidemiology, are skilled and motivated researchers, view themselves as colleagues with physicians instead of as handmaidens, and have broad conceptions of their role and functions, involvement in epidemiological studies may nonetheless be impossible due to demands and limitations placed on them by others.

This is certainly a problem for many school nurses, who are assigned to "cover" a number of schools with total populations of perhaps thousands of students. For such nurses, no matter how great their motivations may be, involvement with epidemiological or other kinds of studies may seem impossible. However, despite the difficulties involved, epidemiological studies and application of epidemiological concepts on a less formal basis can contribute to understanding and promoting the health of school populations and should therefore be used whenever and wherever feasible.

School nurses can independently or collaboratively plan and implement epidemiological studies of diseases or health problems observed within their school populations. For example, studies describing the occurrence of accidents among schoolchildren, including assessment of agent, host, and environmental factors, could be done using the suggestions of Parrish et al. (1967) as a guide. Since accidents are recognized as a major threat to the health and well-being of children, such studies to identify the most prominent and correctable causes could provide baseline data for design of a health education component on accident prevention.

Epidemiological studies can contribute to understanding and control of outbreaks of communicable diseases among school populations as well. For example, as described by W. S. Morris (1975), the school nurse might use the epidemiological investigative process to determine the nature of an influenza-like illness in a school population. Based on the outcome of this investigation, recommendations concerning control of the disease and treatment for known cases could be collaboratively planned by the nurse and other school health team members such as the physician and school principal or administrator. If the cause of the disease is found to be related to poor hygiene and food-handling techniques, then some health education for students and/or staff may be indicated.

Epidemiological studies of chronic diseases affecting school-age children are also appropriate concerns for the school nurse. Safyer and Miller (1977) report that cancer is the second most frequent cause of death among children under 15 years of age (accidents are number one) and indicate that approximately 7500 children per year are affected. Certainly school nurses should be interested in learning more about the cause of cancer in children. Safyer and Miller (1977) believe that school health professionals can provide important etiologic clues based on their observations of schoolchildren; they also emphasize the importance of epidemiological follow-up of children with cancer to assess factors such as the family's medical history and any "peculiarities" of environmental exposures experienced by the child and his family. They urge that any unusual findings be forwarded to an appropriate research center for evaluation.

An example of a health problem that can be studied epidemiologically is the dramatic increase in teenage pregnancies, a problem that has been investigated by Hansen et al. (1978). The study by Hansen et al. illustrates the use of vital statistics and rates as a means of assessing health experience of some population group. The avowed intent of their study, and one that is appropriate for other school-based epidemiological studies, was to attempt to identify groups within the (school) population needing special preventive programs.

School nurses can also (collaboratively or independently) plan and implement longitudinal epidemiological studies, such as the three-phase study described by Roberts et al. (1969) and Basco et al. (1972). This study looked at illness-absence patterns and attempted to identify child and family characteristics associated with them. The investigators plan to use that data to develop an experimental school nursing practice program to meet the needs of the "vulnerable" population—those children with health problems resulting in frequent and consistent absences. Longitudinal and cohort studies of school-age populations may prove very useful in school health, although they are costly and time consuming to carry out.

For school health professionals unable to conduct or participate in longitudinal studies, retrospective, or cross-sectional, studies may be viable alternatives. Certainly school health records, if they are up-to-date and complete, can provide a wealth of data concerning the health of school populations. Categorization and analysis of such group data may provide important insights into the health and health trends of school populations—information not usually revealed through review of individual health records.

Application of epidemiological approaches and principles may also provide means of evaluating the effectiveness of school nursing services. As emphasized throughout this book, school nurses must take the initiative in compiling and documenting data supporting the benefits of their services for the population served (schoolchildren). If a school nurse has provided special services for students with particular needs—such as the frequently absent students described in the Basco (1972) study—then epidemiological data documenting her success in reducing the number of absences by these students can help demonstrate the outcomes of her service. Studies documenting the effectiveness of school nursing services *must* be done if school nurses expect to justify their continued employment.

In short, epidemiology is a fascinating and important investigative discipline, the principles and concepts of which are readily applied in all practice settings. For the school nurse in particular, application of epidemiological concepts and approaches may provide important in-formation concerning the health of the school-age populations with whom she works and may also provide the means for the nurse to demonstrate the benefits and outcomes of her services in maintaining and promoting health.

REFERENCES

Anderson, G. W., Arnstein, M. G., and Lester, M. R.: 1962. Communicable disease control, 4th ed., The Macmillan Co., New York.

Basco, D., Eyres, S., Glasser, J. H., and Roberts, D. E.: 1972. Epidemiologic analysis in school populations as a basis for change in school nursing practice—report of the second phase of a longitudinal study, Am. J. Public Health 62(1):491-496.

Becker, M. H., Drachman, R. H., and Kirscht, J. P.: 1974. A field experiment to evaluate various outcomes of continuity of physician care, Am. J. Public Health 64(11): 1062-1070.

Benenson, A. S., editor: 1975. Control of communicable diseases in man, 12th ed., American Public Health Association, Washington, D.C.

Clark, E. G.: 1965. The epidemiologic approach and contributions to preventive medicine, Chapter 3. In Leavell, H. R., and Clark, E. G.: Preventive medicine for the doctor in his community: an epidemiologic approach, 3rd ed., McGraw-Hill Book Co., New York.

Fox, J. P., Hall, C. E., and Elveback, L. R.: 1970. Epidemiology: man and disease, The Macmillan Co., New York.

Francis, T., Korns, R. F., Voight, R. B., Boisen, M., Hemphill, F. M., Napier, J. A., and Tolchinsky, E.: 1955. An evaluation of the 1954 poliomyelitis vaccine trials: summary report, Am. J. Public Health 45(5):1-63.

Friedman, G. D.: 1974. Primer of epidemiology, McGraw-Hill Book Co., New York.

Hansen, H., Strom, G., and Whitaker, K.: 1978. School achievement: risk factor in teenage pregnancies? Am. J. Public Health 68(8):753-759.

Kinsey, V. E., Jacobus, J. T., and Hemphill, F. M.: 1956. Cooperative study of retrolental fibroplasia and the use of oxygen, Arch. Ophthalmol. 56:481-543.

Lester, M. R.: 1957. Every nurse an epidemiologist, Am. J. Nurs. 57(11):1434-1435.

Lilienfeld, A. M.: 1976. Foundations of epidemiology, Oxford University Press, Inc., New York.

Lombard, O. M.: 1975. Biostatistics for the health professional, Appleton-Century-Crofts, New York.

Lough, M. A., Murray, R., and Zentner, J.: 1975. Concepts of epidemiology, Chapter 6. In Murray, R., and Zentner, J.: Nursing concepts for health promotion, Prentice-Hall, Inc., Englewood Cliffs, N.J.

MacMahon, B., Pugh, T. F., and Ipsen, J.: 1960. Epidemiologic methods, Little, Brown & Co., Boston.

Mausner, J. S., and Bahn, A. K.: 1974. Epidemiology: an introductory text, W. B. Saunders Co., Philadelphia.

Morris, J. N.: 1975. Uses of epidemiology, 3rd ed., Churchill Livingstone, Edinburgh.

Morris, W. S.: 1975. Epidemiology: the community nurse's whodunit. In Archer, S. E., and Fleshman, R.: Community health nursing: patterns and practice, Duxbury Press, North Scituate, Mass.

Parrish, H. M., Wiechmann, G. H., Weil, J. W., and Carr, C. A.: 1967. Epidemiological approach to preventing school accidents, J. School Health 37(5):236-240.

Reed, W.: 1901. The propagation of yellow fever: observations based on recent researches, Med. Record **60**(6): 201-209.

Roberts, D. E.: 1967. Strengthening nursing practice through epidemiology. In American Nurses' Association, ANA Regional Clinical Conferences, Appleton-Century-Crofts, New York.

Roberts, D. E., Basco, D., Slome, C., Glasser, J. H., and Handy, G.: 1969. Epidemiologic analysis in school populations as a basis for change in school nursing practice, Am. J. Public Health **59**(12):2157-2167.

Safyer, A. W., and Miller, R. W.: 1977. Childhood cancer: etiologic clues from epidemiology, J. School Health **47** (3):158-164.

Schuman, L. M.: 1973. Course materials and lecture notes, Public Health 5-330 Epidemiology I, University of Minnesota, Minneapolis, unpublished material.

Smillie, W. G., and Kilbourne, E. D.: 1963. Preventive medicine and public health, 3rd ed., The Macmillan Co., New York.

SUGGESTED READINGS

Archer, S. E., and Fleshman, R.: 1975. Community health nursing: patterns and practice, Duxbury Press, North Scituate, Mass.

Kane, R. L.: 1974. Disease control: what is really preventable? Chapter 6. In Kane, R. L., editor: The challenges of community medicine, Springer Publishing Co., Inc., New York.

Kark, S. L.: 1974. Epidemiology and community medicine, Appleton-Century-Crofts, New York.

Lucas, A. O.: 1976. Epidemiology and health statistics in the control of communicable diseases, Chapter 14. In White, K. L., and Henderson, M. M., editors: Epidemiology as a fundamental science, Oxford University Press, Inc., New York.

Mack, T. M.: 1974. General epidemiology: a guide to understanding biologic information, Chapter 3. In Kane, R. L., editor: The challenges of community medicine, Springer Publishing Co., Inc., New York.

Winkelstein, W., and French, F. E.: 1972. Basic readings in epidemiology, 3rd ed., MSS Information Corp., New York.

CHAPTER 17

School nursing research: why, how, and what

SUSAN J. WOLD

Like other health sciences, the nursing profession relies on research to justify its practices and to develop new knowledge. Research needs to be done by all nurses in all practice settings; the myth that research belongs in the "ivory tower" must be set aside if nursing is to be a credible profession in its own right. Because the very existence of the school nurse is now threatened by fiscal crises and budgetary cutbacks, research in school nursing is an essential tool for survival.

The purpose of this chapter, then, is to explain *why* research is needed in school nursing, *how* research process is done (in general terms—not as a cookbook approach), and *what* specific research needs have been identified for and by school nurses.

WHY: THE IMPORTANCE OF SCHOOL NURSING RESEARCH
Relevance of research for school nursing practice

Perhaps the biggest problem today's school nurse faces is the lack of research documenting the outcomes of her services. As Chinn (1973) reminds us, there must be *demonstrable benefits* to the learner for *all* services provided in the educational setting if those services are to continue to be funded and maintained. This need to document outcomes is more acute now that budgetary restrictions have forced school districts across the country to reduce or eliminate many services that were once thought to be indispensable. The survival of school nursing services may well depend on the ability of school nurse researchers to document their worth. As Chinn (1973:85) warns:

Unless it can be demonstrated that application of nursing skills in the educational setting enhances or promotes learning in the educational process, justification for retaining the traditional school nurse is certainly questionable.

Hawkins (1971:751) identifies two reasons why school nursing research is of paramount importance. First, school nurses represent "a prominent and consistent public identification of nursing." How they function and how they are perceived by the public *as nurses* can affect the "status, credibility, and public confidence" of the entire nursing profession. Therefore research focused on documenting outcomes, clarifying role expectations, and developing innovative approaches to student health needs can bolster the public image for all nurses as well as improve the quality and cost-effectiveness of services rendered. The second reason for the importance of school nursing research according to Hawkins is related to continuity of care. Hawkins believes that present day school nurses are an important source of information and motivation for the "next generation" of nurses. Thus, through careful research, school nurses can provide important data concerning nursing techniques, approaches, and roles for their successors. The commitment to research as an integral part of their practice can also be a kind of role modeling for future nurses. As nurses (and particularly school nurses) begin to see that research is an important part of ongoing practice in all settings and at all levels of preparation, the credibility and viability of the entire profession, as well as specialties such as school nursing, will be enhanced.

A more specific benefit of research for school nurses identified by Hawkins (1971) is its ability to debunk the all too pervasive limited stereotype of the school nurse. Hawkins believes that research studies which differentiate between preventive, educational, and service activities can help nurses identify appropriate activities for their roles. The obvious benefit of that would be to prevent exploitation of the nurse and underuse of her skills. This should help nullify her image as "temperature taker" and "Band-Aider." Perhaps another facet of this stereotypical view of the school nurse is her willingness to "take orders" and to follow the leadership of others. Like Hawkins, Brand (1972) also believes that research can improve the image of the nurse. However, Brand (1972: 22) also sees the following benefits for the nurse's personal development:

School nurses have carried over the traditional nursing ethic of following directives, but they need to become more emancipated in free thinking, weighing alternatives, and achieving constructive individual decisions for the expansion of their role and providing the best health services to children.

The key to this "emancipation" as she views it is research.

The final justification for expansion of school nursing research efforts is provided by Staton (1963:420), who cautions us to "guard against the easy assumption that because things work, they are best." This is a clear warning against mediocre practice. School nurses cannot afford to complacently sit back grinding out the same old routine programs and services just because "we've always done it this way" and it "makes sense." If school nurses expect to keep pace with the rest of the health sciences and with education, they *must* initiate research studies to test new approaches and concepts.

Definitions of research

Having just established the importance and relevance of research for school nursing practice, it is now prudent to define "research." As Wandelt (1970) somewhat facetiously notes, there are probably as many definitions of research as there are researchers. Webster defines research as "studious inquiry or examination . . . investigation or experimentation aimed at the discovery and interpretation of facts, revision of accepted theories or laws in the light of new facts, or practical application of such new or revised theories or laws." Wandelt (1970: xv) defines it as "a quest for new knowledge pertinent to an identified area of interest (a problem), through application of the scientific process." According to Treece and Treece (1977:3), research "in its broadest sense is an attempt to gain solutions to problems. More precisely, it is the collection of data in a rigorously controlled situation for the purpose of prediction or explanation."

For the purposes of this chapter, a workable composite of these definitions will suffice. Thus *research* may be thought of as a systematic scientific problem-solving process, the purpose of which is to identify new facts and relationships. Research is a systematic process (p. 34) because it consists of a methodical series of actions or operations employed for the achievement of specific results. The "specific results" are the solution of a problem. However, "research" is not just a more sophisticated jargonistic word meaning "problem solving." In fact, some authors (Wandelt, 1970; Notter, 1974) outline specific differences between research and problem solving. As they explain, the fundamental difference between research and problem solving is one of *purpose*. The purpose of research is to produce new knowledge, whereas the purpose of problem solving is to find a solution for a particular immediate problem. Therefore, strictly speaking, the problem-solving process is used to solve a problem related to a particular situation or client, whereas the research process solves problems relating to a broader population so that the results may be generalized to populations beyond the specific group or sample included in the study (Wandelt, 1970; Notter, 1974).

Research can be further classified according to purpose as *basic research* or *applied research*. As Notter (1974) explains, *basic research* focuses on finding new knowledge or facts and developing fundamental theories or "truth," which may or may not have immediate, practical applications. The purpose of *applied research,* on the other hand, is to adapt "truth" derived from basic research to day-to-day situations in clinical practice (Treece and Treece, 1977).

To add to the confusion, research is further classified according to the *method* of investigating the problem (Notter, 1974:19-24):

1. *Descriptive research* describes "what is" and analyzes the findings. It can be a means of "getting the facts" or generating hypotheses for future study. Descriptive studies are important forerunners for experimental research and are the most common type of nursing research.
2. *Historical,* or *documentary, research* provides critical interpretation of known facts. Thus, past events are used to help explain present day problems and their origin and to expand the theoretical base used to solve future problems. This is the least common type of nursing research.
3. *Experimental,* or *explanatory, research* looks for new relationships among facts by hypothesis test-

ing in a controlled situation. This involves manipulation of an independent (experimental) variable and comparison of the results with those in a control group. Experimental studies may be used to explain why something happens, to determine the occurrence of a predicted result following a particular intervention, or as a means of program evaluation.

All three types of research are needed in nursing to enhance the credibility of the profession and to improve the quality of nursing practice.

Deterrents to research

There are undoubtedly many reasons for the failure of nurses generally to be actively involved in research. One reason may be that many nurses feel unprepared academically and experientially to conduct research. This is indeed a problem in a profession like nursing in which practitioners represent a variety of educational backgrounds. Although lack of academic preparation in research methods is a reasonable explanation of the source of the problem, it is not an excuse for continued inaction. Professional nurses have a moral and ethical obligation to seek the knowledge and skills they need to improve their practice and contribute to the growth of the profession. The current national trend toward mandatory continuing education for nursing relicensure may be the incentive needed by nurses to learn research skills and to lobby for development of courses and workshops to achieve that goal.

Another reason for nurses' general inaction in nursing research is their impatience with the research process. Nurses need to realize that planning and executing research is time consuming (Martinson, 1976). For nurses who are accustomed to doing a lot of problem solving about day-to-day patient care problems with immediate results and feedback, research may be frustratingly slow in its production of results. Apparently, some nurses do not believe that the extra time expenditure is worth the wait.

Another deterrent to nursing research, and one that is directly related to nurses' impatience to achieve results, concerns external limitations imposed on the nurse. Specifically, Brand (1972) points out that, especially in school nursing, limitations of time and funding make it difficult for nurses to conduct research, especially studies of a longitudinal or comprehensive nature. This points out the need for nurses, especially those in nonhealth care settings (like schools) to clarify their roles with their administrators so that time and resources for nursing research can be allocated. Ideally, in the not too distant future, the expectation that nurses will do research in their employment setting can be written into their job descriptions. Also, as nurses develop more sophistication in grantsmanship, they will be able to generate additional sources of funding for their research efforts.

Perhaps the single most probable deterrent to nurses' participation in research stems from what Martinson (1976) calls "timidity." Martinson links this to the socialization of nurses into passive, subservient roles and believes this may leave nurses feeling unsure of their abilities, unwilling to take risks, and unable to be assertive in refusing other less important demands on their time, such as committee assignments and other miscellaneous tasks. Because timidity is such an ingrained trait in many nurses, this is probably the most difficult deterrent to counteract. Part of the solution to this problem rests with nursing education; educators need to expand their course offerings to include basic research methods for undergraduate students followed by guided application of research principles in investigating clinical nursing questions. In addition, the socialization of nursing students should emphasize self-actualization, collegial health care team relationships, assertiveness, and risk-taking behaviors. The result should be nurses who are not afraid to initiate research to answer nursing questions and who are willing to work for necessary changes to implement the findings.

Myths about research

In addition to these deterrents to participation in research, there are also some "myths" that interfere with reasonable interpretation and application of research findings. Robinson (1970) exposes several myths that he believes confound researchers in the educational, social, and health sciences. The first myth he discusses concerns the excessive power ascribed to research and researchers in our society. Robinson believes that in our scientifically oriented society, people often regard research as if it were an omnipotent force. This may result in the general belief that research can answer all questions and that its findings are infallible and irrefutable. This kind of public awe for research and researchers can be dangerous; it can tempt researchers to distort their findings, misinterpret their impact, and otherwise abuse this power given them by the public's expectations. Robinson further emphasizes the need for researchers to maintain reasonable expectations for themselves and their work; researchers should not expect to find definitive answers to their research questions and should not regard their findings as "the" ultimate answer. It is vitally important for researchers to remember that the usefulness of their findings depends on the honesty and integrity of the researcher in data gathering, analysis, and reporting of the results. The pressures to "produce" results must not be used as an excuse to falsify data or distort the findings.

Another myth that Robinson (1970) effectively discredits is the belief that some research methods are more "important" and more "honorable" than others. This hierarchical arrangement of research methods inevitably results in placement of experimental research at the "top" in terms of prestige. However, as Robinson points out, many important problems within the educational, social, and health sciences cannot be studied by experimentation! Because these fields concern themselves with humans, it would be unethical to "experiment" in ways that pose risks to the subjects. Therefore descriptive or historical studies may be the most appropriate means for researching many problems involving human subjects.

The last myth about research to be considered here is what Robinson (1970) refers to the "computer mystique." The basic tenet of this myth is that use of a computer for statistical analysis of research data enhances the credibility of the results. It should be obvious that statistical analysis is not improved electronically—unless the human who would otherwise calculate the statistics lacks basic mathematical skills. The computer certainly speeds up the process of data analysis, but the most important part of data analysis is the *interpretation* of the statistical findings, and that interpretation depends on the understanding and skills of the person(s) conducting the study.

HOW: THE RESEARCH PROCESS

Having argued the benefits and importance of research in school nursing, the process of doing research will now be reviewed. Again, the intent in this discussion is to outline the steps in the research process, describing each step in general terms. Individuals with no prior course work and experience in research methods will probably not feel comfortable initiating research studies on completion of this chapter; those per-sons are encouraged to consult the references and to seek expert help through course work and/or consultation with experienced researchers.

The systematic process known as research consists of a series of steps beginning with problem identification and ending with communication of the findings in a research report. Depending on which authority is consulted, the number of steps in the process varies from five (Treece and Treece, 1977) to eight (Notter, 1974) to thirteen (Wandelt, 1970). In this chapter, discussion of the research process will follow the eight-step approach outlined by Notter (1974) (p. 391).

The problem

Simply stated, a research problem is "any question that needs answering" (Treece and Treece, 1977:55). Wandelt (1970) thinks of it initially as an "irritation"—a question or perceived problem that piques one's interest. Researchable problems can be found in many places, including daily encounters with clients and other health care professionals, as well as in the literature.

Identification

Choosing a specific problem to research is an important yet often lengthy process. One of the primary considerations, as Treece and Treece (1977) point out, should be the researcher's interest in the problem. Because of the time, energy, and resources necessary for conducting research, it is essential that the researcher be truly interested in the problem if she is to sustain the commitment needed to complete the project.

Refinement

Once the researcher has selected a problem area of interest for study, the next task is to limit and refine the scope of the problem to a manageable size. Some problems, although they generate a great deal of interest, are simply too large to be researched in one study. An example might be "role effectiveness of school nurses." This is certainly an important and timely topic for study; however, this topic needs to be limited before it can be tackled. In narrowing the scope of that problem, a variety of means could be used; for example, by clarifying "which" and "what kind of" school nurses ("role effectiveness of school nurses in the twenty-four public secondary schools in

---

RESEARCH PROCESS*

The problem
  Identification
  Refinement
  Significance
  Feasibility
  Purpose
Literature review
  Purpose
  Scope
  Method
Hypothesis formulation
Methodology (research design)
  Descriptive study design
  Experimental study design
  Historical study design
Data collection
  Method(s)
  Source (sampling)
Data analysis
  Classification and organization
  Statistical analysis
Findings, conclusions, recommendations,
  and implications
Communicating the findings

*Modified from Notter, L. E.: 1974. Essentials of nursing research, Springer Publishing Company, Inc., New York; Treece, E. W., and Treece, J. W.: 1977. Elements of research in nursing, 2nd ed., The C. V. Mosby Co., St. Louis.

Ramsey County'') the problem becomes more specific. This problem can be further refined by specifying the situation or population that is the object of the nurse's role behaviors; for example, "role effectiveness of secondary school nurses in counseling adolescent diabetics" describes a specific population as the target group for assessing situational role effectiveness. Although further refinement of the sample problem would be needed before a research study could be designed, the point is that the problem area must be reduced in scope to a manageable size. For a problem of the magnitude of school nurses' role effectiveness, planning a series of studies might be the best way to approach the question.

Significance

In addition to looking for a problem that is both interesting and of limited scope, Robinson (1970) emphasizes the need for the problem to be "good" or important. As he points out, if the problem is insignificant, the research will be unimportant as well, regardless of the sophistication of the research design. A search of the literature is one way to establish the importance of a problem. If it has aroused the interest of others, then its importance is enhanced. On the other hand, if a number of studies have already been published that provide the answer to the question or problem, then the importance of studying the problem again merits careful consideration. However, there *is* value in replicating studies already published, unless this has been done many times. Replication can provide additional support for findings from previous studies, enhancing the reliability of the results; if replication fails to confirm the original findings, then that is a significant finding as well and one that should generate further interest in the problem.

Feasibility

In addition to assessing one's interest in the problem and its significance, the feasibility of completing the study must be addressed. The investigator must honestly appraise her qualifications to determine if she has adequate knowledge and skills to complete the study. If the verdict is "no," then the researcher must take whatever corrective action is needed. Another consideration in determining the feasibility of a research project is accessibility of needed resources. If the researcher does not have access to the subject pool and other resources necessary for proper investigation of the problem, then completion of the study by that person at that time is not feasible (Notter, 1974).

Purpose

Once all these hurdles have been overcome and the problem has been selected and refined, the researcher must decide the *purpose* and rationale for completion of the study (Notter, 1974; Treece and Treece, 1977). This helps give the study direction and an identifiable focus (Notter, 1974). The purpose statement explains *why* the research is being done, and the rationale helps justify the usefulness and significance of the study. Hence, there is a close relationship between the "what" (problem) and the "why" (purpose and rationale).

The literature review
Purpose

Review of the literature provides additional background information about the problem and past investigations of it. According to Treece and Treece (1977:72), the following are five practical purposes for reviewing the literature:

1. To determine what, if any, research has already been done on the problem
2. To uncover research methods used by other investigators that may be applicable to this study
3. To locate data and/or other ideas to be used for this study or for another project in the future
4. To identify the specific aspects and variables that must be incorporated into the study's design if previous findings are to be confirmed or refuted
5. To unearth comparative data to facilitate interpretation of the study's findings and conclusions

Treece and Treece (1977) further note that an additional serendipitous outcome of the literature search is the expansion of knowledge, insight, and general scholarship of the researcher; the researcher thus becomes more qualified to investigate and analyze the problem, while simultaneously contributing to his personal growth.

Scope

Treece and Treece (1977) advocate a broad background search of a topic or problem rather than a narrow one so that the investigator develops an overview instead of a specific, limited viewpoint. Thus instead of looking only for studies identical to the one contemplated, all relevant aspects of the problem and methodology should be searched.

Method

Not only should the literature review be broad, but it should also be done *early* in the process of researching the problem, before the study is underway. This eliminates design flaws that are preventable based on the published experiences of others and ensures that the investigator has a full understanding of the problem (within the limits of current knowledge) before the study is launched.

There are many helpful tips for the literature search that describe the actual review process (Wandelt, 1970; Notter, 1974; Treece and Treece, 1977). Among the general suggestions are use of indexes such as *International Nursing Index, Index Medicus,* and *Nursing Research* as sources of studies and abstracts; review of abstracts as a preliminary method of skimming previous relevant studies; consulting the bibliography and reference lists accompanying other articles and studies found in the literature to identify other pertinent sources; and employment of computers (such as MEDLINE or ERIC) to identify and even annotate sources relevant to the topic.

As a final note about the literature search, the researcher is encouraged to allow a fair amount of time for this step in the research process. First of all, locating references may not be easy, and time delays may be encountered while awaiting interlibrary loans for some materials. Also, to cover the problem area adequately, a broad search is needed, as already mentioned; there are no shortcuts for that kind of search—it simply takes time. And last, the literature review should include time to do just that: review the literature sources located. The literature references gathered by the investigator should be read and "digested" before proceeding with the study design.

Hypothesis formulation

A hypothesis may be thought of as a "hunch" or an educated guess about the solution to the problem under consideration. More precisely, a *hypothesis* is a "statement of the predicted relationships between the factors [variables] one wishes to analyze . . . in a study" (Notter, 1974:46). It represents a tentative solution to the problem, derived from such sources as the investigator's own experiences, analysis of the problem, explanations and theories uncovered during the literature review, as well as from the researcher's original "hunch" (Notter, 1974; Treece and Treece, 1977).

Hypotheses flow directly from the problem statement or description and are important because they determine the design of the study and the variables to be included (Notter, 1974). However, Robinson (1970) warns against assigning too much importance to the hypothesis and expecting too much from it. Specifically, he points out that research *never* "proves" a theory or hypothesis; rather, a "successful" theory or hypothesis is one that has survived the testing process without being *dis*proved.

Although hypothesis formulation is an integral step in experimental or explanatory research, an operational hypothesis is not always necessary in other types of studies. In exploratory descriptive studies where the primary purpose may be to generate hypotheses for future study, the emphasis will be on data gathering or fact finding and general exploration of the problem rather than on testing of solutions; hence no hypothesis will be included (Notter, 1974; Treece and Treece, 1977). In addition, Notter (1974) explains that studies whose purpose is to test research instruments to establish their validity and reliability likewise require no hypotheses.

However, for those studies in which hypotheses are to be tested, it is important that they be stated clearly and specifically; this makes them more readily testable and measurable (Treece and Treece, 1977). As a variation, some researchers prefer to state the hypothesis in its null form. Instead of predicting (as in an operational hypothesis) that there *is* a significant difference between the independent variable(s) (manipulated by the researcher) and the dependent variable(s) (observed terminal outcome), the *null hypothesis* predicts that there is *no* statistically significant difference between them.

Statistical significance tests are used to determine the significance of the findings compared with chance occurrence. Thus if the .05 level of significance is selected to test a hypothesis, there are five chances in one hundred that the findings are due to chance; if the .01 level of significance is used, there is one chance in a hundred that the findings happened by chance (Treece and Treece, 1973). Following is an example of an operational hypothesis and its null form:

Operational hypothesis
The student absentee rate (number of students absent per day) at school A will be higher than the student absentee rate at school B.
Null hypothesis
There will be no difference in the student absentee rates of schools A and B.

The researcher arbitrarily preselects the statistical level of significance (such as .05 or .01) to be used in accepting or rejecting the null hypothesis; rejection of the null hypothesis indicates that there *is* a statistically significant difference (Notter, 1974; Treece and Treece, 1973; 1977).

Methodology (research design)

Following problem identification, literature review, and hypothesis formulation, the investigator is ready to determine the research design or methodology (Notter, 1974). As Robinson (1970) reminds us, the research design is only a tool for studying the problem. Therefore the investigator should choose whatever method is most appropriate, efficient, and "respectable" for studying the particular problem.

Based on her experiences, Brand (1972) recommends that the researcher discuss her proposed research design and data-gathering methods with all personnel who may be involved in any part of the study. This enlists their cooperation and helps anticipate any problems or needed revisions in the research design. As noted earlier, three basic designs are used for research in nursing: descriptive, experimental, and historical.

Descriptive study design

The descriptive study, as previously noted, is the most common type of nursing research (Notter, 1974) and has as its purpose the determination of "what is." Among the techniques used in descriptive research is the *pilot study,* which is "a preliminary study designed to help refine the problem, develop or refine hypotheses, or test and refine the data collecting methods" (Notter, 1974:141).

A basic technique for descriptive research is the *survey,* which involves investigation of a particular population or community through such methods as interviewing and questionnaires (Treece and Treece, 1977). Surveys are further classified as follows (Notter, 1974:56):

1. *Correlational,* for which data is collected from the population on more than one variable as a means of estimating the relationship between the variables
2. *Longitudinal,* in which data is collected over a period of time to study the changes over time
3. *Cross-sectional,* for which comparative data is collected simultaneously from two or more population groups at different points in their evolution

Another type of "survey" described by Notter (1974) is the *case study,* in which an in-depth study is made of one subject. Although this method is infrequently used in nursing research, it is a respected and respectable approach.

Experimental study design

Classical experimental design is considered the "strongest" kind of experimental research; this design uses four cells, consisting of a "control" group, an "experimental" group, a "before" test, and an "after" test (Treece and Treece, 1977), and might be used to test new treatments or nursing care approaches. Treece and Treece (1977) describe additional experimental methods that will not be reviewed here.

However, some significant problems do not

lend themselves to experimental study, as Robinson (1970) points out. This is especially true in nursing and other interactional professions where experimentation may be impractical or unethical. In such situations, Robinson (1970) advocates "quasi-experimental," analytical, or descriptive methodologies.

Historical study design

As noted earlier, historical research analyzes past events in its search for truth. According to Notter (1974), the specific design used for a retrospective or historical study will depend on the purposes of the study. The usual approach is documentary, using sources such as manuscripts, correspondence, minutes of meetings, diaries, biographies, or memoirs for data collection (Notter, 1974).

Treece and Treece (1977) discuss the pros and cons of historical research in some detail. Among the advantages they cite are the relative ease and reasonable expense of data collection, the wealth of data usually available, and the insight into problems that such data provides. One of the primary disadvantages they note is that the conditions under which the data was collected are unknown, so that the validity is not certain. Notter (1974) therefore emphasizes the importance of evaluating the authenticity of documents used for historical research and encourages the use of *primary* (providing direct evidence about the event) rather than *secondary* (one or more steps removed from the event) *sources* for data collection. Another complication and disadvantage of this type of research is that testing historical studies is difficult and the ability of the findings to be generalized is less likely (Treece and Treece, 1977). Despite these disadvantages, historical research is important, especially in school nursing where the past (Chapter 1) provides a great deal of insight into the cause and dimensions of current problems in the field.

Data collection
Methods

Obviously, the method of data collection chosen by the investigator depends on the problem studied and the overall research design. Among the data collection methods commonly used in nursing research are observation, interviewing, questionnaires, critical incidents, Q-sorts, diaries, record analysis, and nursing activity analysis (Notter, 1974). These methods may be used singly or in combination within any given study. A brief description of the most commonly used methods follows (Notter, 1974):

observation Data collection via persons (observers) who carefully observe and record an activity or behavior related to the problem being studied; the observers may be disguised or undisguised, and may or may not be participants in the study as well.

interviewing Data collection by means of verbal questioning; interviews may be structured or unstructured and are especially useful in obtaining facts, opinions, impressions, or ideas from respondents (subjects).

questionnaires Data gathering via paper-pencil means; useful for surveying large populations and when interviewing is impossible or impractical; data asked for may include the subject's (respondent's) knowledge, attitudes, observations, experiences, or opinions.

critical incident technique Use of written reports describing the subject's previous experiences or observations; this method relies on the subject's memory or recall of "human activity" incidents.

Q-sort technique Collection of data regarding attitudes via a forced-choice rating by having subjects sort cards with printed statements on them into a specified number of piles; sorting is based on the "importance" rating assigned each printed statement by the subject; this technique is useful in comparing the attitudes and opinions of persons or groups and in detecting changes in their attitudes or opinions over time.

For an in-depth discussion of other aspects of data collection, such as maintaining confidentiality, securing participants' informed consent, and the effects of sponsorship of research on successful data collection, the reader is referred to Notter (1974) and Treece and Treece (1977).

Source(s)

The source for the data will depend on the type and extent of data sought; for example, historical studies require archival, documentary sources, whereas studies of nurse-client interactions could probably use observation and/or interviewing techniques.

Generally, researchers do not include all members of the population (number of units or persons being studied) to be studied in the data collection phase of the research (Treece and Treece, 1977). Including the entire population could be very expensive and time consuming and would not necessarily alter the findings of the study. Most investigators use sampling techniques to simplify their data collection. A *sample* is a representative selected part of the whole (population) (Notter, 1974; Treece and Treece, 1977). Because the data collected for the study will be drawn *only* from the sample(s), the validity of the research findings will depend on how *representative* the sample is of the population from which it was drawn; therefore the investigator must clearly define the population to be studied (Treece and Treece, 1977) and must be sure that all characteristics to be studied are represented in the sample. For example, in a study of the role perceptions of full-time school nurses employed in elementary and secondary schools in the Midwest, the population is defined in terms of employment basis (full- or part-time), employment category (school nurse), type of school (elementary or secondary), and geographic location (Midwest); a sample of this population should thus include nurses from elementary and secondary schools who are employed full time in the Midwest. To further clarify the population before sampling, the investigator would need to define terms such as "school nurse," "full time," "elementary" and "secondary" school, and "Midwest." The specific sampling technique used will depend on the purpose of the study and the nature of the population studied.

Robinson (1970) notes that another prevalent myth about research concerns sampling: many people seem to believe that the bigger the sample, the better the study is. This belief has been vigorously debunked (Robinson, 1970; Treece and Treece, 1977); as stated previously, the important characteristic of a sample is its representativeness, *not* its size. According to Hawkins (1971), sampling has been a particularly thorny problem in school nursing research studies. As he views it, the problem includes inadequate responses and lack of a sampling source representing *all* qualified or employed school nurses.

Data analysis

Throughout this book, the importance of careful planning for programming and other activities has been emphasized. Careful planning is also necessary for research efforts, and particularly with regard to data analysis. Notter (1974) emphasizes the need to decide how the data will be analyzed *before* it is collected; this helps ensure that the researcher will collect all the information needed for the analysis. Treece and Treece (1977) further suggest that the investigator set up the tables to be used in illus-trating the findings before data is collected; this makes it easier to "plug in" the data and may speed the analysis process.

Data classification and organization

Once the data has been collected, the researcher will need to somehow sort and organize it so that she can begin to interpret and understand it. How this is done will depend on the complexity and volume of data collected (Treece and Treece, 1977). Among the means of classifying and organizing data (Notter, 1974; Treece and Treece, 1977) are grouping of data by percentages, mean scores, averages, and rank order, and display of data through graphs and tables.

Statistical analysis

In addition to inspecting, grouping, and tallying data, the researcher may wish to use some form of statistical analysis as well (Notter, 1974). The researcher who is contemplating any statistical analysis but lacks a strong background in statistics should consult with a qualified statistician prior to data collection, at the time of computation, and again when drawing conclusions and deciding how to report the results (Notter, 1974).

Statistical procedures are generally grouped as descriptive or inferential. Descriptive statistics are used to determine characteristics of the data and include frequency distributions, calculation of measures of central tendency (means, medians, and modes), and use of standard deviation and standard scores, as well as rank order correlation (Notter, 1974; Treece and Treece, 1977). Inferential statistics assist the researcher in making inferences or judgments about the data and the level of significance of the findings; inferential statistical methods commonly used include the chi square and the t test (Notter, 1974). Detailed explanations of these methods and how to calculate and use them can be found in basic research texts or statistics books.

Findings, conclusions, recommendations, and implications

The next step in the research process is interpreting the findings, drawing conclusions, making pertinent recommendations regarding implementation of the findings, and identifying implications for further study. The researcher's labors at this step are intended to answer the question "So what?" In other words, the task is to determine what was learned from the study and decide what to do with the newly discovered "truth."

This obviously is a very important undertaking, requiring diligent use of the researcher's gray matter. This process is also a test of the researcher's honesty and integrity. Because of the power and aura that research and science have in our society, researchers must realize that misinterpretation and misapplication of research findings are real hazards that can be best avoided by careful and thoughtful decision making in interpreting research findings. Notter (1974) urges researchers to avoid drawing conclusions that are not based on actual data and to avoid making recommendations that are not justified by the study's results.

Another research myth (Robinson, 1970) that is relevant to this discussion is the too prevalent belief that statistical association implies causation. As Robinson points out, this notion is ridiculous because a statistical association is not necessarily a relevant association! An example he proposes is that even if one could statistically establish a high correlation between drinking milk during childhood and later drug addiction, one would obviously *not* conclude that drinking milk causes drug addiction!

Robinson (1970) suggests that a more reasonable approach to judging causality on the basis of statistical association would be to weigh the consistency, strength, specificity, and logic of that association in reaching any conclusions. In further support of Notter's (1974) pleas for caution at this step in the research process, Robinson (1970) urges researchers not to "overgeneralize" from their data; he recommends that investigators "qualify" their findings when necessary and admit and even point out the flaws in the study, rather than disguising them with elaborate statistical processes.

Communicating the findings
Purpose

For research findings to be incorporated into nursing practice, they need to be disseminated to interested parties. Among those who may be interested in the study's results are other researchers, who may wish to replicate and substantiate the findings or study other aspects of the problem suggested by the findings, and nursing students and practitioners, who may wish to directly implement the study's recommendations.

Method

Sharing or communicating research findings can be done in many ways, formally and informally, including lectures, research conferences and symposia, classroom presentations, formal papers, and published reports. For research findings to reach the largest number of interested persons, publication in a national journal is recommended. This is especially important for nursing in order to facilitate development of a sizable and high-quality professional literature; establishment of an independent, research-based literature is crucial if nursing is to clearly establish itself as a viable health care profession, rather than continuing to be seen as medicine's little sister.

Format

The precise format for a published research report may vary from journal to journal and discipline to discipline, but the general format follows the steps of the research process. Typically, the report begins with an overview of the problem, including the actual problem statement, review of pertinent literature, statement of purpose of the study, and identification of any hypotheses tested. A section on methodology usually follows, and includes details of the study's design, such as method (descriptive, experimental, historical), population studied and sampling procedures, description of data collection procedures (such as questionnaires or interview guides), and description of data analysis methods. This is followed by a section presenting the results or findings, which includes a summary of the data, using tables, graphs, or other illustrations, and any statistical results. Discussion of the results then follows, including interpretation of findings, conclusions drawn, comparison of the results with those of other studies, recommendations for implementation, and implications for further study. The report is followed by a complete list of all references cited in the report plus appendices for samples of forms (Notter, 1974).

Regardless of the method chosen for communication of research findings, whether it be done formally or informally, verbally or in writing, the important thing is that it should be done and should be done as soon as possible. Treece and Treece (1977) point out that there is an inevitable time lag between initiation of a research project and its completion and dissemination of findings; often, this lag can be 1 to 2 years or more. To minimize the delay in communicating results, the researcher could begin writing up portions of the report, such as the problem statement, literature review, hypotheses, and methodology before the study is completed. It might also speed up publication efforts if the researcher contacts journal editorial staffs prior to completion of the study to ascertain their interest in publishing the study and to learn what format they prefer.

To further assist the process of communication of nursing research in general and school nursing research in particular, Brand (1972) encourages the development of a national clearinghouse; she believes this can help reduce needless duplication of research efforts (an obvious exception to "needless" duplication is planned replication, which could be facilitated by this kind of clearinghouse). It is also suggested that nurses who do not feel comfortable with their present skills for verbal presentation or publication of their research findings begin to develop and improve those skills, so that their research findings are available to benefit us all.

WHAT: SCHOOL NURSING RESEARCH NEEDS

Having duly explained the importance of research in school nursing and having described the process for carrying it out, the next question is: What are some of the specific research needs in school nursing today? In the remainder of this discussion, I will identify some of the research needs I have found and some suggested in the literature. This is not intended to be an exhaustive list; rather, its purpose is to stimulate the reader's creative thinking processes, which may lead to development of other innovative and valuable research projects.

The overriding research need in school nursing today is to produce data *documenting* the accountability and "net worth" of school nursing services. Thus any studies that can support the contribution and impact of the school nurse's contributions to the school health program are important. This need is especially acute now, as has been repeatedly noted, because of the budget squeeze affecting virtually all school systems across the country. Again, the facts are unmistakable: those groups within school staffs who can *demonstrate* and *prove* the merits and cost-effectiveness of their services can thereby justify their continued employment within the school; conversely, those groups who cannot or simply do not carefully document the benefits and outcomes of their

services cannot (and should not) be guaranteed unlimited employment.

General research areas suggested in the literature are related to quality of care and overall justification for having school nursing services. Basco (1963) concluded that research to establish the validity of accepted school nursing standards is badly needed. It would also be useful to know how and to what extent those standards are being applied and to study changes in quality of care that may occur when standards are implemented. Believing that all services offered to students should be demonstrably beneficial to the learner, Chinn (1973) advocates development and implementation of studies that explain and justify how school nursing services enhance or promote learning. Indeed, Chinn (1973) also identifies the need for studies clarifying the relationship between health problems and school performance; if there is *no* relationship, then perhaps school health programs are superfluous. Igoe (1977) believes that our increasingly skeptical and taxation-conscious society needs to see evidence demonstrating the importance of health maintenance, preventive care, and health education; she encourages school nurses to provide such data documenting the importance of these preventive strategies. In other words, there is a need to prove (through research) that prevention is better than cure; until that fact is clearly established for taxpayers and school boards, deciding which school health team members should provide those services is a moot point, because budgetary cutbacks may prevent the services from being offered at all.

Research to clarify the role of the school nurse has also been recommended. Staton (1963) suggests completion of studies to identify what exactly the school nurse's role is and to analyze the day-to-day job activities for appropriateness and priority. Another related kind of study would consider the use of nonprofessional assistants to carry out activities currently assigned to the school nurse but which do not require the nurse's skills to complete and are of lesser priority. Staton (1963) also lobbies for cost-effectiveness studies of school nursing activities and procedures. Also, Chinn (1973) supports further research concerning the role of the school nurse, especially as it influences the school's educational goals.

Another research area that is related to the role of the school nurse concerns her relationships with the rest of the school health team.

Following her study of school nurses' perceptions of their school health team relationships, Thomas (1976) concluded that additional research in this area is needed to measure the quality and frequency of school health team interactions and to compare school nurses' perceptions of school health team functioning and communication with those of other team members. Staton (1963) suggests that research to identify the techniques for improving school health team relationships, especially as they affect efforts to follow up student health problems, should be initiated.

In addition, as noted in Chapter 5, there are many research needs related to planning, implementation, and evaluation of school screening programs. Research such as the epidemiological and demographic studies suggested by Ford (1970) can provide useful data about the health needs of the population and changes over time; such data is essential for program planning. Regarding implementation of school screening program planning, data is needed describing the adequacy of screening procedures and other early detection methods. Chinn (1973), for example, questions the advisability of expecting teachers to detect health problems and refer students for follow-up; she suggests that research data concerning the teacher's role in early detection is needed. Finally, as an example of research to evaluate the school screening program, research documenting the long-range effects of the screening program on the prevalence and severity of conditions/diseases for which screening was done is recommended.

Again, these are only some of the research needs in school nursing today; there are undoubtedly many more. In short, the need for research to document the merits of school nursing services is so acute that research is needed in virtually all aspects of school nursing. An imaginative pamphlet entitled *Today's School Nurse Makes A Difference* (School Nurses Organization of Minnesota, n.d.) describes the benefits of school nursing services to students, parents, the school, and community. However, for that byword, ''today's school nurse makes a difference,'' to become a *documented* reality, a large volume of carefully planned and executed school nursing research will need to be done.

REFERENCES

Basco, D.: 1963. Evaluation of school nursing activities, Nursing Res. **12**(4):212-221.

Brand, M. L.: 1972. Action research for problem solving in school health, School Health Rev. **3**(3):21-22.

Chinn, P.: 1973. A relationship between health and school problems: a nursing assessment, J. School Health **43**(2): 85-92.

Ford, L. C.: 1970. The school nurse role—a changing concept in preparation and practice, J. School Health **40**(1): 21-23.

Hawkins, N. G.; 1971. Is there a school nurse role? Am. J. Nurs. **71**(4):744-751.

Igoe, J. B.: 1977. Bridging the communication gap between health professionals and educators, J. School Health **47** (7):405-409.

Martinson, I. M.: 1976. Nursing research: obstacles and challenges, Image **8**(1):3-5.

Notter, L. E.: 1974. Essentials of nursing research, Springer Publishing Co., Inc., New York.

Robinson, G.: 1970. Exploring some myths in research design, J. School Health **40**(7):335-338.

School Nurses Organization of Minnesota (SNOM): n.d. Today's school nurse makes a difference (pamphlet), School Nurses Organization of Minnesota, St. Paul.

Staton, W. M.: 1963. Research needs in school nursing, J. School Health **33**(9):418-421.

Thomas, B.: 1976. The school nurse as a member of the school health team: fact or fiction? J. School Health **46** (8):466-470.

Treece, E. W., and Treece, J. W.: 1973. Elements of research in nursing, The C. V. Mosby Co., St. Louis.

Treece, E. W., and Treece, J. W.: 1977. Elements of research in nursing, 2nd ed., The C. V. Mosby Co., St. Louis.

Wandelt, M. A.: 1970. Guide for the beginning researcher, Appleton-Century-Crofts, New York.

SUGGESTED READINGS

ASHA Research Council's Committee on School Health Research (W. M. Staton, Chairperson): 1974. Evaluative criteria for the critical analysis of school health research and research reports, J. School Health **44**(3):119-121.

Backstrum, C. H., and Hursh, G. D.: 1963. Survey research, Northwestern University Press, Evanston, Ill.

Down, F. S., and Newman, M. A.: 1977. A source book of nursing research, 2nd ed., F. A. Davis Co., Philadelphia.

Lindeman, C. A.: 1975. Priorities in nursing research, Nurs. Outlook **23**(11):693-698.

Parkin, M. L.: 1972. Information resources for nursing research, Can. Nurse **68**(3):40-43.

Pavlovich, N.: 1978. Nursing research: a learning guide, The C. V. Mosby Co., St. Louis.

Wold, S. J.: 1980. School nursing: problems and prospects. In Reinhardt, A. M., and Quinn, M. D., editors: Family-centered community nursing: a sociocultural framework, vol. 2, The C. V. Mosby Co., St. Louis.

CHAPTER 18

Management process: a systematic approach to planning, implementing, and evaluating school health programs

SUSAN J. WOLD

Traditionally, nurses have tended to be "doers" rather than managers. Indeed, as described in Chapter 1, the early physician- and hospital-dominated education and supervision of nurses both encouraged and rewarded such behaviors; nurses were taught specific skills and tasks and were expected to carry them out as ordered. Thus while physicians and hospital administrators retained for themselves the authority and responsibility for major decision making and policy formulation, nurses were expected to conform to those decisions and carry out physicians'/administrators' orders and whatever tasks might be delegated.

Because medicine and hospital and health care administration have been male-dominated fields and because our culture has also been traditionally male dominated, nurses, who are typically female, were slow to challenge the "system" of health care decision making and role definition. However, the revitalization of the women's movement in the late 1960s and early 1970s served partially as a means of raising the consciousness of the women in nursing. No longer were nurses content to "do" and "react": now they wanted increased authority commensurate with the responsibility they had been shouldering for years. In other words, nurses were ready to take charge of their own collective destiny; they realized that numerically they dominated the health care professions and that nursing care was the single most important service provided within hospitals and other acute care settings. The traditionally acknowledged supremacy and leadership of the physician within the health team now was questioned and in some cases directly challenged.

Thus in recent years more and more nurses have been placed in positions of authority and leadership within health care institutions, with the result that nurses have exerted a greater degree of control over health care and nursing care than they originally did. However, nursing education has not been able to fully prepare nurses for these positions and roles of leadership, administration, and management; thus some nurses who are expected to function as managers and leaders within health care organizations lack the requisite skills and theoretical background. The result is that too often these nurses continue to "do" rather than to *manage*.

I believe that *all* nurses in *all* settings and at *all* hierarchical levels need to regard themselves as managers and to behave accordingly. Not only do top-level nursing administrators (such as directors of nursing services in hospitals and school systems) and middle management level nurses (supervisors and head nurses, for example) need to be competent and knowledgeable managers, but staff nurses in all settings also need to be skilled and competent managers as well. Staff nurses who assume responsibility for a group of clients/patients within a hospital or other acute care setting need to be effective managers to efficiently plan and deliver needed nursing care on a day-to-day basis. Likewise, school nurses, who generally serve more than one school, also need to make efficient and effective use of their time; accomplishing that aim depends on careful application of management process and principles. In other words, in addition to having a working knowledge of the nursing process, all nurses need a working knowledge of management theory and process;

399

both of these systematic processes are essential in delivering quality nursing care to clients in all settings.

Because management process provides a rational approach to defining the health needs of a (school) population, developing and implementing plans to meet those needs, and meaningful evaluation of programmatic outcomes, management process is an important systematic process for school nurses to understand and consistently employ within school health programs. Obviously, it is beyond the scope and intent of this book to provide an "instant" crash course in management for school nurses or nursing students; the nursing literature in recent years has practically exploded with books describing and detailing the essentials of management for nurses. In addition, many baccalaureate and graduate nursing programs have begun courses and study programs in management for nurses. Thus, opportunities for students and graduate nurses to increase their knowledge and skills in management and leadership are available elsewhere.

Therefore this chapter will not attempt to provide school nurses with in-depth knowledge and skills for functioning as managers and leaders within the school health program. Rather, the emphasis will be on highlighting the steps of the management process and illustrating their applicability for school nurses. Specifically, in the remainder of this chapter the following will be discussed:

1. Management: what it is and what it is not
2. Management: functions and process
3. Putting management process to work: the school nurse as a manager within the school health program

MANAGEMENT: WHAT IT IS AND WHAT IT IS NOT

As Hersey and Blanchard (1977) are quick to point out, there are probably as many definitions of management as there are management authors and authorities. While these definitions seem generally to differ only semantically, it is important to distinguish between *management* (as it has been variously defined) and other terms, such as *administration* and *leadership*.

Defining management

According to Odiorne (1961:4), management means "making things happen." In other words, management is action oriented. Webster's definition is similar; management is the "judicious use of means to accomplish an end" or "the conducting or supervising of something (as a business)." However, Hersey and Blanchard's (1977:3) definition specifies an additional element that is part of management; as they view it, management is "working with and through individuals and groups to accomplish *organizational goals*." Thus, the end that is sought is an organizational goal, whether that organization is a business, hospital, other health care institution, school, political or community group, family, or other public or private organization.

Stevens (1978:10) agrees with Hersey and Blanchard (1977) that management entails working with and through people to accomplish the organization's goals, but goes a step further in emphasizing the importance of *how* the goals are achieved. Specifically, Stevens endorses a *functional* approach in which the manager performs identified actions or functions that collectively contribute to organizational goal achievement. This functional approach to management is widely discussed and espoused in the literature. However, there is no universal agreement among management authorities concerning the specific number or labeling of management functions (p. 401).

Despite the discrepancies among authorities concerning the precise number and labeling of management functions, the differences among authors are more semantic than substantive. In other words, while authors may use different labels for these functions and may vary as to the number of functions they identify, they are all describing the same behaviors and the same basic process. Thus, as is the case with the nursing process and research process, the literature contains confusing and overlapping terminology in describing management process, although all the authors are discussing and describing basically the same process.

Since the precise choice of terminology seems often to be "arbitrary and capricious," the same prerogative will be exercised in this chapter in selecting a definition of management and listing managerial functions to be discussed. Thus, for the purposes of this chapter, Scanlan's (1974:4)* definition of *management* as "the coordination and integration of all re-

---

*From Scanlan, B. K.: 1974. Management 18: a short course for managers. Copyright © 1974 John Wiley & Sons, Inc. Reprinted by permission of John Wiley & Sons, Inc.

ELEMENTS OF THE MANAGEMENT PROCESS
ACCORDING TO VARIOUS AUTHORS

Newman (1963)
  Planning
  Organizing
  Assembling resources
  Supervising
  Controlling
Scanlan (1974)
  Planning
  Decision making
  Organizing
  Directing
  Controlling
Fulmer (1976)
  Planning
  Organizing
  Leading
  Controlling
Longest (1976)
  Planning
  Organizing
  Directing
  Coordinating
  Controlling

Hersey and Blanchard (1977)
  Planning
  Organizing
  Motivating
  Controlling
Dale (1978)
  Planning
  Organizing
  Staffing
  Direction
  Control
  Innovation
  Representation
Stevens (1978)
  Planning
  Organizing
  Directing
  Control

---

sources (both human and technical) to accomplish specific results" will be used. This definition is functional in that it focuses on the manager's actions needed to "coordinate and integrate" the available resources. For the purposes of this chapter, the managerial functions to be discussed are planning, organizing, directing and heading, and controlling.

Differentiating management from related concepts

In searching through the available literature, it soon becomes apparent that some authors use terms like "management," "administration," and "leadership" interchangeably, whereas others define them as distinct yet related concepts. Because my views agree with the latter position, the remainder of this discussion will focus on distinguishing between these distinct, yet related concepts.

Management versus administration

The distinction between management and administration has been discussed by a number of authors, including Alexander (1978), Odiorne (1961), and Stevens (1975). As Stevens (1975:29) explains, *administration* refers to "a comprehensive executive role including functions of setting divisional goals, policy formulation, and management." Management, on the other hand, is the process of carrying out the organization's work through coordination and integration of human and material resources. In other words, according to Stevens, administration is a more encompassing term than management. Thus all administrators are (theoretically) managers (although not all administrators are *effective* managers), since they must rely on their human and material resources to "get the job done." However, not all managers are administrators; only those managers who have administrative power and authority to participate in organizational goal setting and policy formulation are both administrators and managers. Thus, for example, the school nursing supervisor within a school district is likely to be an administrator as well as a manager, whereas a school (staff) nurse contributing to the goal achievement of one or more individual school health programs will most likely be exclusively a manager.

Another distinction between management

and administration has been made by Odiorne (1961). Odiorne views the key difference between them as being not one of scope but rather one of *method*. Thus in an explanation sure to raise the hackles and blood pressure of administrators everywhere, Odiorne (1961) explains that whereas managers "size up" a situation to determine which actions are appropriate and likely to be most effective, administrators follow "stereotyped patterns" of action, even when they are not effective or appropriate:

In short, management means making things happen; administration means following certain textbook procedures mechanically whether they produce the results desired or not.

While Odiorne's explanation of the differences between the two concepts may outrage some and amuse others, its primary value derives from its ability to illustrate the continuing lack of agreement among authorities concerning the absolute difference (if any) between these two processes. It is therefore important for readers of administration and management literature to determine how each author they encounter distinguishes between these terms. In addition, Odiorne's obvious contempt for administrators should likewise illustrate the point that how one is regarded as an administrator *or* a manager depends greatly on individual behavior and role effectiveness. Therefore administrators who wish to be likewise perceived as effective managers will need to apply management theory and principles in the execution of their role functions.

Management versus leadership

The distinctions between leadership and management have been discussed by many authorities, including Hersey and Blanchard (1977), Stevens (1975), and Stevens (1978). Predictably, these authors do not agree about the differences and relationship between these concepts; thus Hersey and Blanchard view leadership as a broad concept and management as one type of leadership, whereas Stevens (1978) views leadership as one aspect of the larger concept of management. Distinguishing between these terms can thus become a "which comes first—the chicken or the egg?" type of argument, with little likelihood of reaching absolute agreement.

Because one can locate and cite an authority to support either position, it is important to choose a position compatible with one's own

views and make it known. Therefore, for the purposes of this chapter, Stevens' (1978) view of leadership as one of the functions essential for effective management will be adopted. According to this viewpoint, leadership refers to one's ability to influence others to follow or to take direction. For a manager to be successful in carrying out the organization's goals, strong leadership must be exercised. In other words, an effective manager must also be an effective leader, whereas an effective leader may not be and need not be a manager: a leader is a leader as long as there are followers.

Summary

In summary, the concepts of administration, management, and leadership are closely related, yet distinct. Administration is a broader concept than management and refers to an executive role including organizational goal and direction setting and policy formulation. Management entails accomplishing organizational goals through coordination of resources (human and material), and is thus an essential part of administration. Thus, all administrators are managers, although not all managers are administrators. Finally, leadership refers to one's ability to influence others and gain their cooperation and compliance; as such, it is a vital managerial function to be carried out by all administrators and managers.

MANAGEMENT: FUNCTIONS AND PROCESS

As illustrated in Fig. 18-1, there are four basic managerial functions that make up the management process: planning, organizing, directing and heading, and controlling. While each of these functions is discrete and flows logically from the function that precedes it, in actuality there is some overlapping and repetition of these functions during the management process. Thus, while planning is the first step in managing, it may be repeated during the process if the plan needs to be amended or revised. Likewise, organizational elements such as staffing patterns and delegation of responsibilities, and control measures such as reporting mechanisms and budget, may need revision or modification during the management process. In addition, directing and heading are functions that permeate all three of the other functions and hence must be carried out throughout the entire management process. Thus, while the functions are discrete and can be discussed and conceptual-

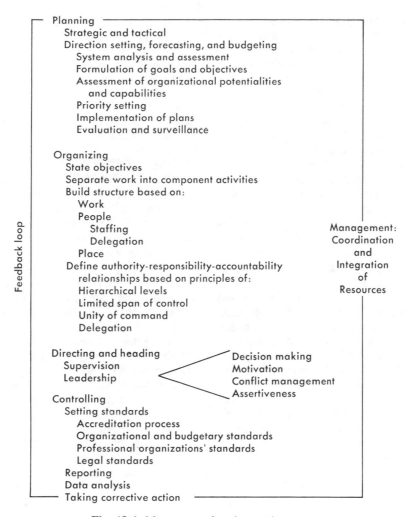

Planning
  Strategic and tactical
  Direction setting, forecasting, and budgeting
  System analysis and assessment
  Formulation of goals and objectives
  Assessment of organizational potentialities
      and capabilities
  Priority setting
  Implementation of plans
  Evaluation and surveillance

Organizing
  State objectives
  Separate work into component activities
  Build structure based on:
    Work
    People
        Staffing
        Delegation
    Place
  Define authority-responsibility-accountability
      relationships based on principles of:
    Hierarchical levels
    Limited span of control
    Unity of command
    Delegation

Directing and heading
  Supervision
  Leadership

  Decision making
  Motivation
  Conflict management
  Assertiveness

Controlling
  Setting standards
    Accreditation process
    Organizational and budgetary standards
    Professional organizations' standards
    Legal standards
  Reporting
  Data analysis
  Taking corrective action

Feedback loop

Management:
Coordination
and
Integration
of
Resources

Fig. 18-1. Management functions and process.

ized in the order presented in Fig. 18-1, there is inescapable overlap and repetition among them. Finally, it should be noted that the outputs of the controlling function are sent back as inputs to the planning function by way of the feedback loop; this allows any needed modifications to be made in the planning, organizing, directing and heading, and/or controlling functions.

Planning

According to Arndt and Huckabay (1980: 66), *planning* is "the act or process of interpreting the facts of a situation, determining a line of action to be taken in light of all the facts and the objective sought, detailing the steps to be taken in keeping with the action determined, making provision to carry through the plan to a successful conclusion, and establishing checks and bal-

ances to see how close performance comes to the plan." Because organizational structure, supervisory and leadership patterns, and control mechanisms all derive from the organization's objectives and plans, planning is necessarily the initial managerial function to be carried out (Scanlan, 1974).

Because careful, thoughtful planning is essential for successful management, the importance of the planning process cannot be overstated. Indeed, many of the problems confronting school health programs and school nurses can probably be traced to inadequate or shortsighted planning. The lack in some school districts of precise *written* school health programming plans with measurable *documented* outcomes has no doubt contributed to an increasing public skepticism concerning tax-supported services, thus resulting in budgetary and personnel cutbacks in school health and school nursing in many communities. Indeed, Jacobsen and Siegel (1971) make an impassioned plea for the importance of comprehensive community health planning, so that the school health program is planned as an integral part of the overall community health plan; they believe that this "partnership" between school and community requires "strong interrelation, involvement, interaction and cooperation" if a viable and comprehensive school health program is to result (1971:157). In sum, planning is a vitally important process, since it is the process by which the organization's purposes and directions are established along with specific means or methods for achieving them; planning is thus the foundation for the remaining managerial functions.

In their discussion of the work of Levey and Loomba, Arndt and Huckabay (1980) describe two basic types of planning: strategic and tactical. *Strategic planning* focuses on determination of the organization's overall goals and basic directions; it is long range in focus and generally depends on allocation of large numbers of resources. In contrast, *tactical planning* results in plans that have a short-range focus, are more detailed, have a narrower scope, require allocation of fewer resources, and therefore are more flexible and more readily modified. An example of a strategic plan might be a decision to gradually expand a district's school health program to provide primary care health services to disadvantaged children; a related tactical plan might be to create a pilot program in one school for 1 academic year to test the feasibility of the strategic plan.

Models for planning abound in management literature and include those proposed by Longest (1976), Stevens (1978), Scanlan (1974), and Arndt and Huckabay (1980). One of the most logical and comprehensive of such models is that described by Arndt and Huckabay (1980). According to their view, planning is a continuous process involving seven interdependent and at times simultaneous stages. Their model is reproduced in Fig. 18-2, and each stage will be briefly highlighted in the remainder of this discussion.

Stage 1: System analysis and assessment

During this initial phase of the planning process, the nurse-manager surveys the existing organization as a whole to determine "where

we are now." This may include a review of current goals and objectives, adequacy and availability of resources to meet the organization's needs, adequacy of the operation of the organization, and evaluation of organizational and subsystem performance outcomes (Arndt and Huckabay, 1980). This kind of overall assessment and analysis is an important first step toward strategic planning.

Stage 2: Formulation of organizational and individual goals (objectives)

During this stage, the question to be answered by the nurse-manager is: "Where do we go from here?" Thus the major task is to determine the desired outcomes or goals/objectives for the organization and a schedule or timetable for their completion. These objectives should include both long-range (strategic) and short-range (tactical) outcomes and most importantly should be stated in behavioral and measurable terms.

Indeed, the paramount importance of behaviorally stated program objectives for school nursing services has been ably described by Dickinson (1971). Dickinson points out that as a result of the current "squeeze" on the educational dollar, support services (pupil personnel services) are being cut back or eliminated. In deciding which of those services to reduce or eliminate *first,* Dickinson believes that those services with what he calls the "haziest relationship" to the school district's educational goals are the most likely choices. As he further points out (1971:533):

It is, therefore, necessary that all services clearly demonstrate their accountability to the educational process, and school nursing services must also join in this accountability process. . . . The writing of behavioral objectives . . . is a necessary first step in showing how the school nurse makes a contribution to educational goals.

Stage 3: Assessment of present organizational potentialities and capabilities

As Arndt and Huckabay (1980) point out, determination of realistic and feasible goals and objectives for an organization depends on careful, thorough assessment of the current capabilities of the organization as a whole. This kind of assessment or inventory requires close scrutiny of the organization's subsystems as well, including departments or other organizational service units. The specific kinds of data to be

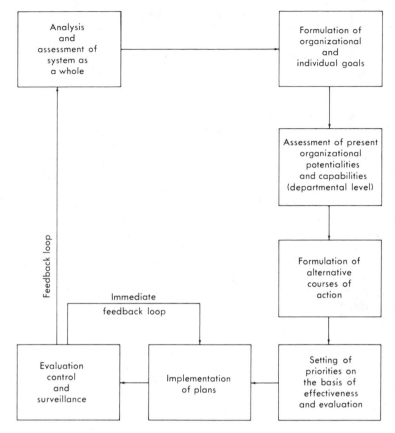

Fig. 18-2. The process of planning. (From Arndt, C., and Huckabay, L. M. D.: 1980. Nursing administration: theory for practice with a systems approach, 2nd ed., The C. V. Mosby Co., St. Louis.)

gathered include (1) available resources (including personnel, equipment, funding, and physical space), (2) strengths and weaknesses (in such areas as communication patterns, staffing, and programming), and (3) environmental (internal and external) constraints and opportunities. The purpose, then, of this step in the planning process is to ensure that the organization's plans are more real than ideal; that is, to ensure that the plans generated are realistic and attainable within the limitations of the organization's resources. Thus if one of the organization's objectives requires more personnel than are presently available, a realistic plan for recruiting additional personnel must be undertaken before that objective can be met; if the prospects for securing the necessary additional personnel seem bleak (for whatever reason), then that objective is not realistic and attainable for that organization at that time. In other words, while such gaps may become the impe-

tus for aggressive organizational resource procurement efforts, they are also a current limitation in terms of organizational capabilities and must be regarded as such.

Stage 4: Formulation of alternative courses of action

During this stage, means or methods for achieving the organizational goals/objectives that were formulated and revised in stages 2 and 3 are identified. It is important to generate *alternative* methods of goal achievement during this stage so that all possible and feasible means for carrying out the plan(s) can be identified and evaluated; this helps ensure that the course of action finally adopted represents the best possible alternative, given the present resources and limitations of the organization. Arndt and Huckabay (1980:70) identify the following specific factors to be considered in evaluating and selecting alternative courses of action.

1. Degree of relevance of the proposed course of action to the organization's purposes and obligations
2. Anticipated cost-effectiveness ratio
3. Acceptability to organizational staff and clientele
4. Time frame needed for completion of the course of action compared with the urgency of solving the problem or meeting the objective
5. The "extra dividend factor," which is the special advantage of one course of action over another; for example, an action for which the necessary groundwork has already been laid previously or by another organization or group would have that advantage over another alternative for which no preparation has been done

This stage also includes formulation of plans detailing the types and amounts of resources needed, how they can be procured, and identification of any additional programs or procedures needed to ensure successful completion of the planned actions.

Stage 5: Priority setting based on effectiveness and evaluation

Because at this stage no action or implementation has actually occurred, the priority setting will have to be done based on the projected consequences of the plans formulated and refined during stage 4. The priorities assigned are thus "educated guesses" based on such factors as the following (Arndt and Huckabay, 1980):

1. Expected impact of the plan on the health status of the organization's clients or consumers
2. The accepted obligations of the health care organization as defined by law and by organizational philosophy
3. Community readiness
4. Public relations impact (acceptability of the plan to the public)
5. Time constraints

While priority setting during this stage is of necessity based on educated guesses or projections, the importance of priority setting cannot be overstated, despite the uncertainty of its accuracy or outcome. The special importance of priority setting by school nurses has been documented and reported by Marriner (1971). The research method used was a descriptive comparative survey, which was administered to the school nurses of one unnamed district (N, or number of respondents, not given) as a pilot study. The respondents were asked which activities were highest priority for them at the time of the study, which activities they believed *should* be highest priority, and which activities were of *lowest* priority but should be *higher* in priority. The detailed outcomes of that survey are reported by Marriner (1971) and will not be repeated here. However, her conclusion is very relevant to this discussion of priority setting as part of the planning process, since she noted that "the higher the priority the school nurse rated on activity, the more likely she was to carry out that function" (1971:420). In other words, then, nurses (and particularly school nurses) need to be conscious of the priorities they set and how those decisions are made, since as Marriner's study implies, assigned priority influences the likelihood that the action will be carried out.

Stage 6: Implementation of plans

During this stage, which Arndt and Huckabay (1980) characterize as the "action and direction" stage, the nurse-manager focuses on the details of implementing the plan(s). Specifically, she must decide *what* resources are needed, *what* actions are to be taken, *who* will be responsible for implementing various aspects of the plan(s), *how* those actions will be carried out, and *when* the actions should begin as well as *when* they should be completed.

Thus at this time it is prudent for the manager to formulate any policies and procedures necessary to facilitate implementation of the plan. As defined by Scanlan (1974:17), a *policy* is a guide for decision making within an organization or a "rule for action"; to be effective, a policy should include a definition of the subject matter covered by the policy, specify lines of authority and approval, be clearly and concisely stated, and, above all, be *communicated* and made known rather than filed neatly away. A *procedure* is a "sequence of steps that should be followed in implementing plans" (Scanlan, 1974:17). While policies are decision-making guides that allow some latitude concerning the precise manner in which the plan will be implemented, procedures, on the other hand, are more specific and detailed and indicate *exactly* what actions (steps) need to be taken and in what order they must be completed. Because policies and procedures are complementary, both are important and useful in organizational planning.

Stage 7: Evaluation and surveillance

Before the planning process can be considered complete, some provision for ongoing surveillance and summative (end) evaluation of outcomes must be planned (Arndt and Huckabay, 1980). In other words, the plan(s) must identify *how* (standards, EOCs), *when* (timing of periodic progress checks plus setting of final completion date), and *by whom* the actual outcomes will be measured and evaluated (compared with objectives or *planned* outcomes). This helps ensure that meaningful and deliberative (as opposed to rote or haphazard) evaluation will actually take place and also helps identify the kinds of data that must be gathered to facilitate meaningful evaluation. Indeed, the importance of planning for the evaluation of outcomes cannot be overstated; if the plan(s) do not specify what data will be needed for the evaluation and who will collect it, it is possible that when the evaluators begin their review of the outcomes they will find crucial kinds and pieces of data irretrievably missing. However, when the plan(s) include thoughtful attention to the prospects and realities of the eventual outcomes and results, the results and recommendations (outputs) of the evaluation process then become inputs for subsequent planning and revision of plans; this "recycling" of evaluation results into planning occurs by way of the feedback loop shown in Fig. 18-2. Thus the feedback process allows the manager to revise plans as needed to ensure that they continue to be appropriate, realistic, and effective.

Characteristics of a "good" plan

To assist managers in assessing the merits of their plans, Arndt and Huckabay (1980) have identified the following list of criteria that they suggest be used to decide if an organization's plans are "good":

1. The plan is based on clearly defined objectives and its intent is clear to all persons responsible for implementing it.
2. The plan is clear and simple, thus avoiding costly errors and delays that could result from ambiguity.
3. The plan should be stable yet flexible; the plan must be adaptable to changing circumstances and needs while avoiding the kind of excessive fluidity that results in chaos, confusion, and distrust.
4. The plan should be realistic and economical regarding the resources necessary for implementing it, and, whenever feasible, it should use *existing* human and material resources.
5. The plan specifies necessary operational details and control (evaluation) measures, including the following:
   a. Realistic and congruent sequencing, scheduling, and coordination of activities and plans.
   b. Appropriate priority setting.
   c. Realistic target dates.
6. The plan realistically anticipates and forecasts the future.
7. The plan is purposeful and rational and can be justified based on organizational and individual objectives.
8. The plan considers and allows for the "unique sociopolitical environment" of the organization.

Assuming, then, that the manager has devised a valid, realistic, and workable plan that can survive the scrutiny of these criteria, the stage is set for focusing on the organizational details and actions necessary for implementing the plans successfully.

Organizing

Once the organization's goals and directions have been set, the next task for the manager is to determine how the plans will be carried out. To accomplish the work of the organization, the manager must employ the process of organizing, which, as shown in Fig. 18-1, is the second managerial function. As defined by Arndt and Huckabay (1980:73), *organizing* is "the process of grouping activities, delineating authority and responsibility, and establishing working relationships that will enable both the institution and the employee to realize their mutual objectives."

Elements of organizing

As Scanlan (1974) further clarifies, the process of organizing is built around three key elements: (1) the *work* to be done, (2) the *people* who will do the work (human resources), and (3) the *place* (including both environmental factors and technical and material resources) in which the work will be done. These three key elements must be considered in the order just presented, and a balance must be achieved among all three.

The work. Because the primary reason for its existence is (or should be) achievement of organizational goals and objectives, the organization should be built around the work to be done, rather than around the people who do the work. This is the *principle of functionalization,* which is vitally important in organizing (Scanlan, 1974). In other words, the work to be done is the most important consideration in organizing. Therefore, instead of building the organization around the talents and skills of particular individuals or groups (workers), the wise manager will develop an organizational structure that is based on a clear definition of the work to be done. In this way, the organization can remain stable and functional despite personnel changes (Scanlan, 1974).

The people. The second element of organizing is the people who will carry out the work of the organization (the workers). While it is not wise to build an organization around specific people or personalities, it is important to achieve a successful match or "fit" between the work or jobs to be done and the individuals or groups who will do the work. Thus the tasks to be done need to be grouped into manageable units or combinations that can be done by one person. The manager must thus consider the educational level, skills, and experience of the workers to realistically estimate what kind of tasks they can perform and how much (quantity or volume) work they can produce. In other words, the abilities, skills, and interests of the people who conduct the work of the organization must be carefully evaluated in delegating work assignments to them, so that maximum effectiveness and efficiency can be achieved (Scanlan, 1974).

The place. In addition to careful attention to the work to be done and the people who will do it, the manager must also consider the place in which the work will be carried out (Scanlan, 1974). That is, the manager must assess and provide for all inanimate or physical elements needed to carry out the work of the organization; such factors include environmental factors (space, heating, lighting, etc.), available technical resources (machinery and equipment), and other material resources (disposable health or first aid supplies, secretarial supplies, etc.). The physical environment must be adequate and suitable for carrying out the specified work of the organization if realistic goal achievement is to occur.

The process of organizing

As previously mentioned, the manager must consider the work, the people, and the place in the order listed and should attempt to achieve a balance among them. Scanlan (1974) suggests that this can be best accomplished by viewing

and conducting organizing as a step-by-step process.*

Step 1: State the objectives. Obviously, before one can organize the resources to accomplish some work, it is necessary to clearly define and state, through outcome-oriented objectives, exactly what the work is expected to accomplish or achieve. Ideally, an outcome of the planning process should be a clear, logical statement of desired organizational outcomes (objectives); however, realistically it may at times be necessary to clarify and further refine the organization's objectives at the beginning of the organizing process.

Step 2: Separate the work into its component activities. During this step, the manager's task is to break down the basic work activities identified in step 1 into "fundamental work activities" (Scanlan, 1974:56). In other words, the work activities should be broken down into their component tasks as a prelude to their subsequent grouping (during step 3) into units or jobs assigned to specific people.

Step 3: Build a structure based on work to be performed, people who must do the work, and the workplace. As explained by Scanlan (1974:56), the manager's task during this step is to build "practical work units" that can be delegated to workers. Thus the work activities defined and broken down during step 2 are now "grouped" into units of activity or *jobs,* which can then be assigned to specific people within the organization. Scanlan suggests (1974) that the manager's primary basis for grouping work activities as a unit or job should be the similarity of the work activities, while her secondary consideration might be the complementarity of the work.

STAFFING. Although Scanlan does not specifically isolate and discuss staffing as a concern of the manager during the process of organizing (presumably because his book is oriented toward private enterprise and not toward health care providers), staffing is an important organizational consideration in health service settings. Careful attention to staffing patterns helps ensure efficient and effective use of the organization's human resources (personnel).

In school nursing, adequate and appropriate staffing has been a consistent and escalating problem. As noted repeatedly in this book, the

---

lack of clear guidelines for assignment of school health and school nursing personnel, differentiating their roles and functions, and establishing meaningful school nurse–student ratios has resulted in wasteful and ineffective use of personnel. School nurses have often felt frustrated and overwhelmed by the nonnursing tasks delegated to them and have been justifiably angered by their resulting inability to devote more time to the provision of high-quality nursing care to their student populations. However, at least part of the responsibility for this inappropriate and ineffective staffing of school health and school nursing services must be accepted by school nurses themselves. Because there is little research data available to support school nurses' (and nursing educators') claims that provision of high-quality school nursing *requires* nurses prepared at particular educational levels or nurse-student ratios of a particular size or the assistance of qualified school health aides, school nurses cannot convincingly argue for larger nurse-student ratios or the addition of clerical and other support personnel to assist them in carrying out their programs. In other words, while school nurses and nursing educators *believe* that school nurses must be prepared at a baccalaureate level or above, and while they *believe* that school health aides can be effective adjuncts for school nurses, more research concerning staffing patterns and outcomes in school nursing needs to be done to confirm and support these beliefs. If school nurses are to retain and possibly expand their funding within the public schools, they will have to *prove* their need for improved staffing ratios and additional support personnel to an increasingly skeptical and fiscally conservative public and to the elected officials who represent them.

Although research to define and evaluate optimal and existing school nursing staffing patterns is unquestionably needed, there are guidelines for nursing staffing patterns that can be used until research data for school nursing staffing patterns is available. As Ramey (1976a) points out, a prerequisite to the development of an appropriate staffing method or formula is the careful articulation of a statement of philosophy regarding the values and beliefs of the organization. This philosophy should identify the role and value of school nursing services within the school, the numbers and desired level of preparation of school nurses and auxiliary personnel

needed to implement the health program, and any additional values or beliefs that influence the manner in which staffing decisions are made within the school district or institution.

Armed with that philosophy, the nurse-manager is ready to assess the needs of the client population as a further input into decision making about staffing. The importance of assessment of the needs of the client population cannot be overstated, since "the success of any staffing pattern rests upon having the correct number of appropriately prepared personnel to meet the needs of patients [clients]" (Ramey, 1976a:211). In the case of school nursing, this assessment will include data from student health records, census data concerning the age distribution, income, and educational level for the community and school population, and data concerning the community's health status, such as vital statistics concerning communicable diseases and other morbidity and mortality. As noted earlier, this kind of client needs assessment followed by appropriate goal and priority setting is part of the planning process for the nurse-manager. The organizational goals and priorities that result are the basis on which staffing decisions can be made. To determine precise staffing needs to meet the goals, the nurse-manager may wish to adapt for her setting and use staffing formulas like those proposed by Ramey (1976a) and Arndt and Huckabay (1980); ideally, however, school nurses need to secure research data specific to their practice setting so that such decisions can be made intelligently and defensibly.

DELEGATION. Another important concern of the nurse-manager during the process of organizing is delegation. Delegation refers to the manager's effective use of personnel to accomplish specific results (work); that is, *delegation is the process of getting things done through other personnel* (Volante, 1976). Following are some of the advantages of delegation:

1. Delegation contributes to the "growth and development" of employees in an organization by allowing them to gain experience and increased confidence through their successful handling of gradually increased responsibility (Scanlan, 1974).
2. Use of the organization's available skills, knowledge, and expertise through appropriate delegation of responsibility is cost-effective. For example, when a school nurse occupies her time with tasks that could be carried out by a nonprofes-

sional assistant (school health aide), the costs of the service rendered are needlessly increased. By delegating responsibility to the appropriate person at the appropriate level of the organization's hierarchy, such "hidden" costs are eliminated and cost-effectiveness is enhanced (Volante, 1976).

3. Delegation frees the nurse-manager to "manage." The manager's primary concern must be to get things done through the efforts of others, rather than "doing" everything herself. The manager who insists on doing everything herself, even when there are others capable of carrying out the task, will not have time to carry out her managerial functions of planning, organizing, directing and heading, and controlling. Thus the irony is that while she is busy with tasks that others could accomplish, she is likewise unable to carry out her own job responsibilities. In short, delegation is essential if the manager is to have the time and energy to "manage" (Scanlan, 1974; Volante, 1976).

However, while there are notable advantages to delegation, it is also important to point out what delegation is *not*. First, delegation is not "dumping" (Scanlan, 1974). To be successful, delegation requires that the employee have a clear understanding of what he is to accomplish (expected results) and that he receive whatever support, assistance, or "coaching" may be needed to carry out the delegated responsibility. In addition, Scanlan (1974) points out that the responsibilities delegated to the employee should be meaningful to the person expected to carry them out; he should know the job is important to the organization and to the manager and should receive positive feedback on its completion.

Delegation must also not be construed as "abdication of authority" (Scanlan, 1974:197). This means that while the subordinate or employee is given some freedom to make decisions and take action, he does so within clearly defined guidelines, such as the policies and procedures that are set forth during stage 6 of the planning process. However, Scanlan points out the hazards of an overabundance of policies and procedures (commonly referred to as "red tape"); if the organization's policies require that the subordinate "clear" every decision with the manager then there is no actual delegation of responsibility taking place, and the structure is self-defeating. Likewise, a plethora of rules and regulations may frustrate employees' efforts and willingness to accept and carry out delegated tasks and functions. Instead, the nurse-manager should create a climate in which

subordinates can function as fully as their skills and experience allow.

Third, delegation does not result in "loss of control" by the manager (Scanlan, 1974). The manager, through periodic review or "progress checks," maintains control and creates the opportunity to provide support and guidance to her subordinates. Finally, contrary to the opinion of managers who are reluctant to delegate, delegation is *not* "avoiding decisions." As Scanlan points out, delegation allows the manager to make the decisions that are most important and require her skill and expertise, whereas many of the detailed day-to-day operational decisions can be made by those who are best informed about situational details.

Having defined what delegation is and what it is not, it is now appropriate to consider *how* delegation can be accomplished. As Scanlan (1974) describes it, delegation is a three-step process. The first step is to *assign responsibility*. This entails both providing an adequate job description listing the tasks or duties for the worker and specifying the expected results or outcomes of the worker's performance. In addition to clarifying the tasks to be performed and the specific results expected, the manager should also clearly identify for the subordinate the areas of his job in which he is accountable or responsible for achieving results and the manner in which performance or accountability will be measured.

The second step in the process of delegating is *granting authority* (Scanlan, 1974), which includes both a "preliminary planning phase" and a "continuing support phase." During the planning phase, the subordinate is asked to share his ideas concerning alternative strategies and plans for accomplishing the desired results and to anticipate and propose solutions for any foreseeable problems; following dialogue with the manager, a mutually determined course of action is adopted. The continuing support phase, as its name implies, is devoted to provision of any needed assistance or counsel by the manager to help ensure the successful accomplishment of the desired results.

The third step in the process of delegating is *creating accountability* (Scanlan, 1974). The "end product" of delegation is the accountability of the subordinate or person to whom a task is delegated, without which true delegation does not exist. Unless the person to whom responsibility and authority have been delegated is held accountable for the results (good or bad) of his actions, then the delegation process is incomplete, ineffective, and will result in the manager having no control over the outcome; in that instance, insubordination and chaos are possible outcomes.

Step 4: Define clearly the authority-responsibility-accountability relationship. It is also important to *clearly* establish and effectively communicate the downward flow of authority and responsibility and the upward flow of accountability within the organization so that each employee is aware of his position within the organizational structure and clearly understands his relationship with other employees in the hierarchy (Scanlan, 1974).

At times, managers who are unclear about the distinctions between the terms authority, responsibility, and accountability may tend to view and use these terms interchangeably, resulting in conflict and confusion for their subordinates. It should be noted that all three concepts are important for managers in effectively and efficiently organizing; however, since the usefulness of these concepts depends on the accuracy of their application, Scanlan's (1974: 53)* definitions of each concept follow:

authority "The right to issue valid instructions which others are expected to follow" (1974:53). Authority is *formal* (granted by the organization) and is attached to a specific position within the organizational hierarchy. Its success depends on the willingness of subordinates to follow instructions (implied consent).

responsibility "The group of activities, tasks, or duties that have been assigned to a person," and "the obligation to secure desired results" (1974:53-54). Therefore responsibility has two aspects: (1) the obligation to carry out assigned duties to the best of one's ability and (2) to *account* to a higher authority for the outcome of those assigned duties.

accountability "The obligation to account to a higher authority for the degree of success achieved in performing assigned tasks" (1974:53).

As these definitions indicate, authority and responsibility flow downward, while accountability flows upward.

To facilitate the nurse-manager's delegation of work to others, the importance of delegating *authority commensurate with the responsibility* needs to be emphasized. If an employee is to be held responsible and accountable for a job, task, or decision, he must be given the neces-

sary *authority* to act or carry out the job. In other words, an employee can only be held accountable within the limits of the authority or decision-making power delegated to him (Scanlan, 1974). This means that managers (including nurse-managers) must be willing to relinquish or share their authority with subordinates if responsibility is to be successfully delegated. A nurse-manager who "delegates" responsibility to a subordinate (such as a school health aide), but attempts to retain the authority to make pertinent decisions, is *not* delegating in the true sense and cannot therefore hold that person (health aide) accountable for completion of the assigned responsibility. Such reluctance to delegate authority commensurate with responsibility is one factor preventing efficient and cost-effective use of nursing personnel in all settings, including schools.

ORGANIZATIONAL STRUCTURE AND LINES OF AUTHORITY. In addition to delineation of clear job descriptions for all persons within the organization, clear definition of the authority-responsibility-accountability relationship can be accomplished by preparation and dissemination of an organizational chart illustrating the structure of the organization and the relationships among individuals and positions.

According to Stevens (1975:36), an *organizational chart* is a "graphic representation of the organizing process." As she points out, organizational charts are usually *positional* in that they are organized by position and rank. Figs. 18-3 and 18-4 are examples of such positional organizational charts.

Within any organizational chart, two basic types of relationships can be identified: *line* and *staff. Line functions* are part of the organization's formal chain of command and include three basic functions that are necessary regardless of the type of organization studied: (1) creation, (2) distribution, and (3) financing of the product or service offered by the organization (Scanlan, 1974). Using Fig. 18-3 as an example, the "health service head nurse" is part of the line structure, most likely based on her involvement with *creation* and *distribution* of health services. In contrast, *staff functions* are those which are auxiliary or supportive to the line or formal structure of the organization; they are generally advisory in nature and often arise as an organization becomes large and complex, thus requiring the assistance of others, including specialists or those with expertise within a particular knowledge area (Scanlan, 1974; Ste-

---

*Copyright © 1974 John Wiley & Sons, Inc. Reprinted by permission of John Wiley & Sons, Inc.

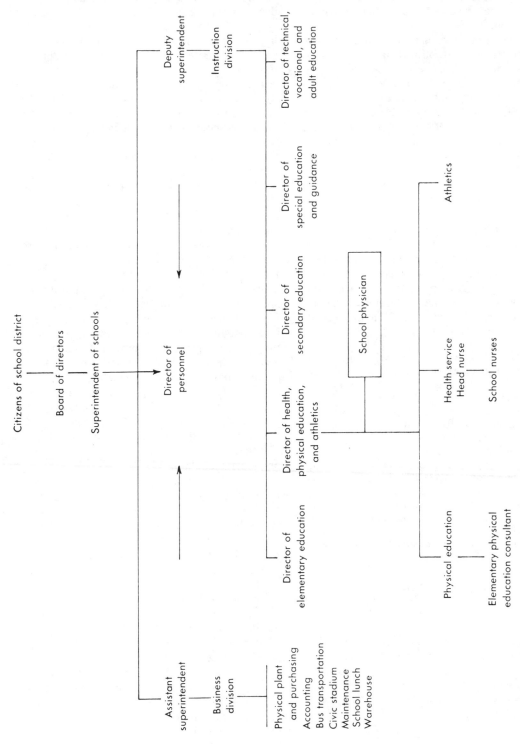

Fig. 18-3. Organizational structure pattern of a school district—variation A. Organization of staff in the line-staff type of administrative control found in many medium-size school districts. (From Mayshark, C., Shaw, D. D., and Best, W. H.: 1977. Administration of school health programs: its theory and practice, 2nd ed., The C. V. Mosby Co., St. Louis.)

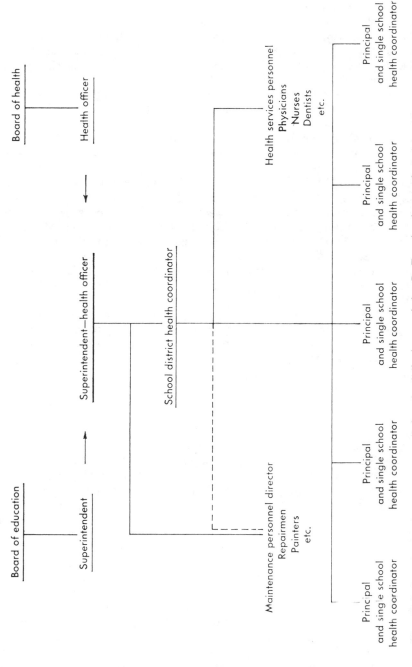

Fig. 18-4. Organizational structure pattern of a school district—variation B. Functional type of administrative control in which the board of education and the board of health share responsibility for the school health program in a school district. With this administrative pattern, the district health coordinator has authority over the single school health coordinator in matters pertaining to school health. (From Mayshark, C., Shaw, D. D., and Best, W. H.: 1977. Administration of school health programs: its theory and practice, 2nd ed., The C. V. Mosby Co., St. Louis.)

vens, 1975). In Fig. 18-3, the "school physician" is a staff or advisory function.

If an organizational chart is properly constructed, all members of the organization should be able to identify the lines of authority or "chain of command" (Stevens, 1975). That is, each employee should know to whom she reports directly and be able to trace the lines of authority from herself all the way to the top of the organization's hierarchy. For the organization to function smoothly, all members should respect those hierarchical lines in the chain of command and should not "go over the head" of their immediate superiors to a higher authority until or unless they have first attempted to resolve their problems or concerns with their superiors; this avoids the additional problem of undermining the authority of the persons who have been passed over (Stevens, 1975). Organizations typically have policies and procedures for handling problems or grievances and moving them "up the line" when necessary for resolution; employees should familiarize themselves with these processes and operate within those guidelines in seeking assistance further up the line to avoid generating further conflict and problems with their immediate superiors.

PRINCIPLES OF ORGANIZATION. Finally, the outcome of defining the authority-responsibility-accountability relationships is affected by the application of certain classic principles of organizing. Nurse-managers should understand and apply these in their efforts to design and sustain a workable organizational structure.

The first of these organizational principles is the *principle of hierarchical levels,* which states that an organization with more than five (or, at the extreme, seven) levels of employees is "top heavy" with administration. According to this principle, an organization should incorporate the fewest possible number of employee levels necessary to carry out the work of the organization as a means of minimizing the "distortion between management goals and the actual work done" (Stevens, 1975:38).

A second important principle of organizing is the *principle of limited span of control* (Longest, 1975; Stevens, 1975). According to Longest, *span of control* is defined as "the number of subordinates reporting directly to a superior" (1976:112).* This principle is based on recognition of the fact that there is a limit to the number of subordinates that a manager can *effectively* supervise; hence, there is a need to limit a manager's span of control. There are no "magic" formulas or ratios for determining the ideal or optimal number of subordinates that a manager can supervise. Rather, the optimal span of control for a manager requires assessment of such factors as the manager's level within the organizational hierarchy, the "abilities and availabilities" of the manager, and the nature of the work to be done (Longest, 1976: 113).

A third important organizational principle is the *principle of unity of command,* which states that each individual in an organization should report to one boss and *only* one boss to avoid presenting conflicting demands or expectations (Stevens, 1975; Longest, 1976). However, as Longest notes, this principle does not always work in health care organizations. Indeed, the school nurse finds herself generally confronted with violations of this principle: she is accountable to the principal in each of her schools and to the person/department within the school district responsible for school health and/or pupil personnel services. Thus, while the district's school nursing supervisor might view the nurse's primary responsibility as being health promotion and primary prevention, the building principal may expect her primary function to be that of "Band-Aider" or "attendance checker."

The fourth and last organizational principle to be mentioned in this discussion is the *principle of delegation* (Stevens, 1975), which is also referred to by Longest (1976) as the *principle of delegation of routine matters.* According to this principle, tasks and decision making should be delegated down to the lowest possible organizational level that is still consistent with valid and reliable or "good" decisions. This prevents the wasteful and costly expenditure of employee time on tasks or decisions that could be handled by someone further down in the organization with less education, skill, or experience, and at the same time frees that higher level employee to make decisions and carry out functions for which he is uniquely qualified (Stevens, 1975; Volante, 1976). Armed with her commitment to its importance, the nurse-manager can practice this principle through application of the three-step process of delegation.

Directing and heading

The third managerial function and, according to Longest (1976), the most complex is direct-

---

*Reprinted with permission of Reston Publishing Company, Inc., A Prentice-Hall Company, 11480 Sunset Hills Road, Reston, Virginia.

ing and heading. As defined by Longest (1976: 149-150), *directing* means "the issuance of orders, assignments, and instructions that permit the subordinate to understand what is expected of him, and the guidance and overseeing of the subordinate so that he can contribute effectively and efficiently to the attainment of organizational objectives."* Thus directing and heading includes both the delegation or assignment of responsibilities to another person (subordinate) and concurrent provision of guidance and support for the subordinate in carrying out those responsibilities.

Although a person often formally becomes a "director and header" by virtue of her position in the organizational hierarchy, such as "Director of School Nursing Services," successful implementation of the directing and heading role requires application of principles of *supervision* and *leadership*. In other words, although a person may be formally regarded as a "director," successful directing and heading requires something more than mere status or position: one must consciously strive to direct and head effectively, drawing on appropriate theory and principles. In the ensuing discussion, principles and theory that I believe are "appropriate" will be highlighted. However, the reader is cautioned that the scope of the discussion is purposely limited; the reader is encouraged to consult the References and Suggested Readings at the end of the chapter for more in-depth discussion.

Supervision

Following minor modifications of Fulmer's (1976) definition of "supervisor," a workable definition of supervision emerges. According to this definition, *supervision* may be thought of as "directing the performance of one or more workers so that organizational goals are accomplished" (Fulmer, 1976:4). Arndt and Huckabay (1980) suggest that the obligation of a supervisor is to obtain "maximum performance" from subordinates.

Elements of supervision. Thus, based on these two viewpoints, supervision can be regarded as a function requiring both *directing and motivating* activities on the part of the manager or supervisor. More specifically, the following three primary elements of effective supervision can be identified:

1. *Motivating subordinates to achieve their*

---

*Reprinted with permission of Reston Publishing Company, Inc., a Prentice-Hall Company, 11480 Sunset Hills Road, Reston Virginia.

fullest potential; although motivational theory will be discussed more fully later in this chapter, it is important to note at this point that a key corollary goal to successful motivation of subordinates is to help them become aware how their *personal* objectives and needs can be satisfied through their work and participation in achieving *organizational* goals (Scanlan, 1974; Arndt and Huckabay, 1980).

2. *"Coaching and counseling"* activities (Scanlan, 1974:6); because the intent of these actions is to stimulate the subordinate to perform at his optimal level, coaching and counseling activities are obviously related to employee motivation; however, if *periodic performance appraisal* (employee evaluation) is included as a basis for realistic and helpful counseling and coaching, then these two elements (motivating and coaching and counseling) can be appropriately regarded as separate but related elements of supervision.

3. *Emphasis on staff development and continuing education,* which Arndt and Huckabay (1980) consider to be vital aspects of supervision, especially when the "supervisees" are professionals, such as school nurses. This element entails the supervisor's emphasis on providing subordinates with "continuing education and experience, rather than expending energy to give orders and keep people 'under control' " (Arndt and Huckabay, 1980: 99).

Supervisory styles. The manner in which a manager carries out these elements of supervision with her subordinates reflects her particular style of managing/supervising. That is, supervisors and managers generally adopt (consciously or unconsciously) a consistent approach or pattern of supervising/managing, which can be thought of as their "style."

Among the more interesting, innovative, and widely respected efforts at identifying managerial or supervisory styles is the work by Blake and Mouton (1978) who developed a tool called the *New Managerial Grid,*® which they view as the key for mobilizing human effort and for getting the maximum performance results of which people are capable (Fig. 18-5).

To preface the following brief descriptions of the five basic managerial styles included in the grid, it should be noted that Blake and Mouton (1978) are committed to the belief that regardless of which grid position or style a manager

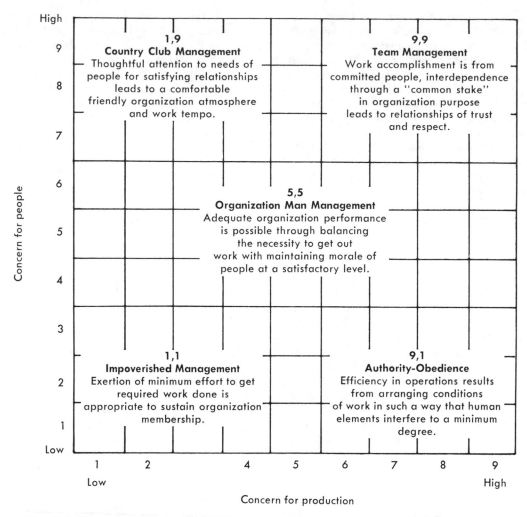

Fig. 18-5. The managerial grid. (From Blake, R. R., and Mouton, J. S.: 1978. The new managerial grid, Gulf Publishing Co., Houston.)

occupies or exhibits according to the self-survey report, that style or position *can be changed*. In other words, a manager is not "stuck" with her initially identified grid position, but can in fact modify that consciously. Indeed, a large portion of their book is devoted to detailed discussion of the intricacies of the grid positions and ways in which managers can begin to move toward a more productive and effective position.

As illustrated in Fig. 18-5, the *Managerial Grid* is constructed with two axes. The horizontal axis represents the manager's *concern for production* or "getting the job done"; it

ranges from a low of 1 to a high of 9, indicating the manager's *degree* of concern for that dimension. The vertical axis represents the manager's *concern for people* or healthy, mature work relationships and also includes a range of degree of concern from a low of 1 to a high of 9 (Blake and Mouton, 1978). Thus, in reporting and describing each of the five basic grid positions or styles, Blake and Mouton (1978) use a two-digit label, reflecting the relative concern for production and people. To avoid confusion (since the numbers 9 and 1 are used in describing four of the five basic styles), in the numerical configuration of each style, the *first* number *always* refers to the concern for production (horizontal axis), while the *second* number *always* refers to the concern for people (vertical axis). Thus, for example, "9,1" describes a style that is high on concern for production and low on concern for people, while "1,9" refers to a style with a high concern for people and a low concern for production.

THE 9,1 "AUTHORITY-OBEDIENCE" MANAGER. The 9,1 position in the lower right corner of the grid represents the *authority-obedience manager,* who is characterized as a "driver" concerned only with high productivity (Blake and Mouton, 1978). The 9,1 manager maintains tight supervision over her subordinates, demanding unquestioning obedience. The 9,1 style is autocratic and emphasizes "getting results"; therefore the 9,1 manager resists decentralization of decision making and delegation of other responsibilities, preferring to make all the decisions herself. This managerial style results in one-way, downward communication and very little upward communication; upward communication is limited to reporting back to the boss about work completed or unexpected results. Because direct communication with the manager or boss is discouraged, the workers are unable to discuss problems with the boss; therefore an active grapevine is likely to develop among the subordinates.

Blake and Mouton (1978) found that the 9,1 manager has two basic assumptions about people: (1) people inherently dislike work and (2) subordinates are not as capable as she is of effectively planning and organizing their work. Thus the 9,1 manager believes she must coerce and punish her workers, much like a parent figure, to keep them producing maximally. This (9,1) pattern yields between average and outstanding productivity; morale is generally low (except for those individuals who *prefer* a controlling boss), as is job satisfaction, and turnover is high. This manager actively *suppresses* conflict; indeed, as Blake and Mouton (1978) note, the motto for the 9,1 manager seems to be "nice guys finish last."

THE 1,9 "COUNTRY CLUB" MANAGER. A great contrast to the 9,1 task manager is the 1,9 *people-oriented,* or *country club, manager,* who assumes that if you keep people happy, they will be productive. Thus she tries to create a "country club" atmosphere, complete with lengthy coffee breaks and long lunches (1978). In short, the atmosphere is like that of "one big happy family," in which conflict is suppressed

to maintain the "family's" harmony. This suppression of conflict hurts the organization, since discordant yet potentially innovative ideas and approaches are forcibly restrained, resulting at times in "bitching" by employees. As a result of the 1,9 manager's lack of emphasis on productivity or getting the job done, decision making often does not occur at all. In addition, because the subordinates sense the manager's lack of organization and control, productivity is low and morale and job satisfaction are only average (Blake and Mouton, 1978).

THE 1,1 "IMPOVERISHED" MANAGER. The third basic grid style is the 1,1 position located in the lower left-hand corner of the grid. This *impoverished manager* is low in her concern for both task and people; thus this style may be thought of as "management by default." The apparent goal of this manager is *survival;* she wants to maintain her position and is willing to do what she is told. Therefore the 1,1 manager wants to know "the rules" of the organization and wants to find out "who *really* has power" so that she knows exactly whom to please.

The 1,1 manager fears conflict and will go to almost any lengths to avoid it, such as avoiding attending meetings where conflict is expected or throwing away memos to which a definite reply is expected. When she is unable to physically avoid conflict, the 1,1 manager will use "double-talk" to avoid committing herself to a position, preferring instead to maintain "overriding neutrality"; indeed, Blake and Mouton describe this person as "slippery" because she is impossible to pin down. The 1,1 manager tends to be aloof and allows her staff to "do their own thing" as long as their performance does not jeopardize *her* security or position within the organization; typically she ignores employees' mistakes, unless she is called on personally to account for them, in which situation she would fix the blame on somebody else. Thus the 1,1 manager can be characterized as a "psychological dropout" or a person who is "present, yet absent" (Blake and Mouton, 1978:105). Predictably, subordinates of the 1,1 manager (with the exception of those who *prefer* to be "left alone" by their supervisor) have low productivity, low morale, and low job satisfaction, and turnover is high.

However, interestingly enough, Blake and Mouton (1978) found that 1,1 managers are *not* necessarily uncommitted and uninvolved individuals in other spheres of their lives. Indeed, many of them are actively involved in civic or political activities, often holding positions of responsibility and leadership within other organizations, and/or are involved in creative endeavors. Blake and Mouton (1978) speculate that perhaps such individuals have gravitated toward the 1,1 position at work for any or all of the following reasons:

1. They previously took risks in the organization and got hurt or perhaps were repeatedly passed over for promotions.
2. They may dislike the job, perhaps seeing it as boring, nonchallenging, or "dead-ended," while at the same time they find the fringe benefits, such as salary, vacation benefits, and prestige, very attractive.
3. Their work may be secondary to their personal interests or hobbies, thus reducing their commitment.
4. For any or all of these reasons they do not feel fulfilled in their work, yet they are too close to retirement and too "trapped" by the system's inducements (such as tenure or pension) to be able to quit or find a new job.

Thus, in a sense, 1,1 managers are the product of personal and organizational failure.

THE 5,5 "ORGANIZATION MAN" MANAGER. The fourth supervisory style included in the *Managerial Grid* is the 5,5 position in the center of the grid—the *organization man,* or *compromise,* manager (Blake and Mouton, 1978). The 5,5 position is based on an assumed conflict between an organization's concern for productivity and its interest in meeting the needs of its people; thus instead of resolving the conflict by swinging the pendulum to either the 9,1 or the 1,9 position, the 5,5 manager "dampens" the pendulum by seeking workable, compromise, middle-ground solutions. In other words, the 5,5 manager tries to "balance" concern for task or production (getting the job done) with concern for people or morale.

The 5,5 manager tends to seek practical versus ideal solutions to problems and relies on "tried and true" traditional approaches or precedents within the organization, which are often regarded as "sacred cows." When conflict arises, the 5,5 manager's approach is to first allow the involved parties to "cool down" and then attempt to resolve the issue by "splitting the difference," an approach that results from her belief that "half a loaf is better than none." The 5,5 manager is not overly aggressive in setting production goals or in prodding people to meet them; as a result, both productivity and morale are merely average. Furthermore, because the 5,5 manager is traditional in her thinking and orientation to problem solving, creativity is effectively stifled. Thus the long-range consequence of the 5,5 managerial style is maintenance of the status quo.

THE 9,9 "TEAM" MANAGER. The fifth managerial/supervisory style depicted on the grid is the 9,9 position, located in the upper right-hand corner. The 9,9 manager is high on concern for *both* productivity and people and is described as a *team manager* or participative manager. The 9,9 manager achieves "effective integration of people with production . . . by involving them and their ideas in determining the conditions and strategies of work" (Blake and Mouton, 1964:142). Thus a primary goal of the 9,9 manager is to "promote the conditions that integrate creativity, high productivity, and high morale through concerted team action" (Blake and Mouton, 1964:142). The 9,9 manager values "sound and creative" solutions to problems; to obtain them, she actively solicits the input and contributions of her human resources (subordinates and peers). Thus the 9,9 manager succeeds in obtaining employees' involvement in the commitment to the organization by encouraging their active participation in setting goals, planning strategies, and evaluating results. She is committed to the "team" approach, in which the whole is viewed as more than the sum of its parts, and the contributions of individuals at all hierarchical levels are valued and sought. Because she recognizes the value of subordinates' contributions and the extent of their abilities, the 9,9 manager believes in delegation and decentralized decision making. When mistakes occur, the 9,9 manager's typical reaction is not to blame or castigate, but rather to ask: "What can we learn from this mistake and how can we avoid this kind of error in the future?" (1964: 148). Open, direct communication among subordinates and between subordinates and the manager is encouraged, and free-flowing, two-way communication throughout the organization or unit therefore occurs as a result of the 9,9 managerial style. Conflict is viewed by the 9,9 manager as inevitable and potentially growth producing. Therefore, unlike the other four managerial styles, the 9,9 manager *manages* conflict through open *confrontation;* that is, conflict is brought out into the open where it is subject to scrutiny and direct resolution so that *optimal* (versus expedient) solutions can be found. Thus, because this style emphasizes maximal concern for both production and people and yields high productivity and morale, Blake and Mouton (1978) view the 9,9 managerial/supervisory style as the preferred or "ideal" style.

As noted earlier, Blake and Mouton emphasize the feasibility of changing one's managerial grid position to a more effective pattern or style, with 9,9 hailed as the ultimate goal. The reader is referred to their book, *The New Managerial Grid* (1978), for discussion of strategies for accomplishing such a change.

Leadership

Another important element in successful directing and managing is leadership, because "excellent planning can often occur with the development of a well-conceived organizing process, but if the appropriate leadership cannot be brought to bear on the operations of the organization and unit, much of the anticipated effectiveness cannot be realized" (Stevens, 1978: 123-124).

Defining leadership. According to Douglass (1977), *leadership* is essentially a *relationship* between an appointed (designated) or emergent leader and the persons or constituencies with whom she collaborates to achieve goals. Leadership is both a science and an art, since it is based on scientifically derived empirical research data and yet also requires the skill (art) to implement those scientific "truths" (Douglass, 1977). A *leader,* then, is "one who influences people through processes and guides others to the realization of a definite goal or goals" (Douglass, 1977:1).

However, perhaps the most specific and useful definition of leadership is that advanced by Hersey and Blanchard (1977:84) following their search of the literature; they conclude that the most nearly universal definition views leadership as "the process of influencing the activities of an individual or a group in efforts toward goal achievement *in a given situation.*" Thus, based on this definition, Hersey and Blanchard (1977) conclude that the leadership process (L) is a function (f) of three groups of variables: those related to (1) the *leader* (l), (2) the *follower* (f), and (3) the *situation* (s) as represented with the equation: $L = (l, f, s)$. Hersey and Blanchard (1977) are quick to point out that while this definition includes situational variables, it does *not* specify particular types of organizations in which the definition would or would not apply; this is because they believe

that in any situation or organization, such as a business, hospital, school, or family, in which someone attempts to influence the behavior of others, leadership is occurring. Likewise, the use of the words "leader" and "follower" does not necessarily indicate a *hierarchical* or boss-subordinate relationship. Instead, the definition implies that any person in any situation who attempts to influence someone else's behavior is a "potential leader," and the person being influenced is the "potential follower," regardless of the situation or setting in which the "leading" occurs or the nature of the relationship between the parties (such as employer-employee, peer-peer, or family member–family member).

Leadership as an element of directing and heading. The skillful application of leadership principles contributes to effective directing and heading in two basic ways. First, leadership is a key element of direct supervision of subordinates in an organization, because while a manager may occupy a position of authority and formal power within the organizational hierarchy, she will be unable to effectively supervise subordinates and encourage them to attain the organization's goals *unless* she can gain their cooperation, commitment, and involvement. That is, to be *maximally* effective as a manager/supervisor with regard to the directing function, a manager must obtain the respect of subordinates so that they will view her as a leader, be receptive to her guidance, and be responsive to her delegation of responsibility to them. In other words, designation of oneself as a *formal* leader with legitimate authority in an organization is not enough to ensure successful directing and heading; to be successful, the formal leader must be regarded as such by her subordinates. Indeed, in organizations in which formally designated leaders do *not* command the respect and cooperation of their followers, the emergence of an *informal* leader from the ranks of those who do *not* have legitimate (granted by the organization) authority is possible and even likely. Thus, it is important to recognize that leadership does *not* reside in a position within an organization, but is an interactional process among people, requiring application of science and art by the would-be leader and a favorable, supportive, accepting response by the supposed followers.

The second basic way in which leadership is a vital contributor to successful directing and heading concerns the overall direction setting and guidance for the department, unit, or organization as a whole. That is, in addition to exercising leadership in direct supervision of employees or subordinates, the manager must likewise be able to "lead" effectively if she expects to direct and "head" the organization in creative, innovative, and growth-producing ways. In other words, on a grander scale than the usual one-to-one boss-subordinate relationships, the directing and heading function requires the manager to focus her attention on the organization as a whole, including planning creatively for the future (strategic planning) and continually (especially in nursing and other health care professions) seeking new and expanded funding sources to support and facilitate the organization's ability to meet its goals.

Leadership styles or patterns. Since the publication of their article "How to Choose a Leadership Pattern," the work of Tannenbaum and Schmidt (1958) has been widely quoted and cited. Among their achievements was the identification of a *continuum of leadership behavior,* ranging from a highly autocratic or "boss-centered" style at the extreme left to a highly democratic or "subordinate-centered" style at the extreme right. Their schema, as modified by Hersey and Blanchard (1977), is illustrated in Fig. 18-6. As Tannenbaum and Schmidt (1958) explain, the continuum represents the range of possible leadership behaviors from which a manager can choose. The actions or styles to the far left indicate a high degree of *managerial control,* whereas the actions toward the right indicate increasing *subordinate freedom.*

Another schema for conceptualizing leadership patterns or styles is the managerial grid, which was discussed previously. Indeed, the grid bears a strong resemblance to the continuum of leader behavior described by Tannenbaum and Schmidt (1958). For example, the leader behavior at the far left of the continuum, "makes decision and announces it," is like the 9,1 task manager described by Blake and Mouton (1978); the leader behavior at the far right of the continuum, "permits subordinates to function within limits defined by superior," closely approximates the 9,9 team manager position on the grid. Therefore either of these conceptual approaches might be used to identify or label one's leadership style or pattern.

However, a key difference between the Blake

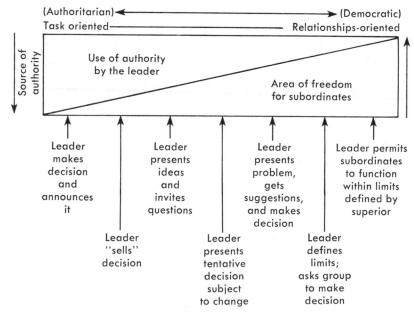

Fig. 18-6. Continuum of leader behavior. (From Hersey, P., and Blanchard, K. H.: 1977. Management of organizational behavior: utilizing human resources, 3rd ed., Prentice-Hall, Inc., Englewood Cliffs, N.J. Reprinted by permission of the Harvard Business Review. Exhibit modified from "How to Choose a Leadership Pattern" by Robert Tannenbaum and Warren H. Schmidt (May-June, 1973). Copyright © 1973 by the President and Fellows of Harvard College; all rights reserved.)

and Mouton (1978) approach and that of Tannenbaum and Schmidt (1958) and Hersey and Blanchard (1977) concerns their philosophical orientation to leadership styles. While Blake and Mouton describe the 9,9 team manager as the "ideal" leadership pattern, Tannenbaum and Schmidt (1958) and Hersey and Blanchard (1977) do not believe that an "ideal" leadership pattern exists which is universally appropriate and effective. Rather, they emphasize the importance of the *interaction* among leader, follower, *and situational* factors, and the need for the leader to be flexible enough to modify her style as the situation requires. Thus, as with other topics addressed in this book, there is no universal agreement in the literature concerning the existence of an "ideal" leadership style.

Additional principles integral to successful directing and heading

At the beginning of the discussion of the directing and heading function, the point was made that successful completion of this function depended on careful and scrupulous application of principles of supervision and leadership. Having discussed both supervision and leadership, the reader might reasonably conclude that coverage of the directing and heading managerial function is now complete. However, some other "hidden" concepts and principles that also contribute to successful directing and heading within the realm of supervision and leadership are (1) decision making, (2) motivation, (3) conflict management, and (4) assertiveness.

Decision making. *Decision making,* which may be defined as "making a choice between two or more alternatives" (Longest, 1976:84),* is almost universally regarded as a key element in management. However, there is some difference of opinion regarding the placement of decision-making process within the management schema; some authors (Scanlan, 1974) view decision making as a free-standing managerial function, while others (Longest, 1976) view it as part of the planning function of the manager. These differences of opinion are largely semantic, in my opinion, because as long as decision making is regarded as an essential aspect of managing, precisely *where* it is

placed within management process is relatively unimportant. Thus, while discussion of decision making in this chapter has been arbitrarily placed within the context of directing and heading, it is important to recognize that the decision-making process permeates *all* aspects and functions of management at all hierarchical levels.

Models and systematic processes for making decisions have been widely proposed in the literature by a variety of authors (Odiorne, 1961; Drucker, 1967; Scanlan, 1974; Bailey and Claus, 1975; Longest, 1976). The decision-making process as conceptualized by these authors and others is basically the same, although the semantics used to describe decision making vary by author and professional orientation; that is, authors who are professional management or business consultants may use different jargon from professional nurse-managers or hospital and health care administrators, and yet all are describing essentially the same process. Likewise, it should be noted that decision making closely parallels other systematic processes discussed in this book, including nursing process, planned change process, and even management process. Thus decision making is not some alien "new" process, but is a logical outgrowth of the systematic problem-solving process applied with a slightly different emphasis.

Drucker (1967) describes decision making as a sequential six-step process* as follows:

1. Classification of the problem
2. Definition of the problem
3. Specifications to be satisfied by the problem's solution
4. Deciding what is "right" versus what is "acceptable" in meeting the "boundary conditions" (specifications)
5. Building into the decision the action to carry it out
6. Feedback to test the decision's validity and effectiveness against the "actual course of events"

His approach is simple, direct, and readily applicable.

During the first step of the decision-making process, *classification of the problem,* the "effective decision maker" needs to ask whether the situation or problem is "a symptom of a fundamental disorder or a stray event" (1967:

---

*Reprinted with permission of Reston Publishing Company, Inc., A Prentice-Hall Company, 11480 Sunset Hills Road, Reston, Virginia.

*Reprinted by permission of the Harvard Business Review. Excerpt from "The Effective Decision" by Peter F. Drucker (January-February, 1967). Copyright © 1967 by the President and Fellows of Harvard College; all rights reserved.

93).* If the conclusion is that the problem is fundamental or *generic,* then a rule or principle will be needed to solve it; if, on the other hand, the problem is believed to be a unique or isolated event, then it must be handled as such.

The second step of the decision-making process, *definition of the problem,* focuses on determining the nature and scope of the problem and its key elements. Drucker (1967) points out, however, that this may seem deceptively easy to do; in fact, the hazard of this step is the possibility that the definition of the problem may be *incomplete,* which is more of a risk than making a wrong definition. To counteract the possibility of incomplete problem definition, Drucker (1967) advises would-be decision makers to check and recheck their problem definition against *all* observable and known facts, summarily reject *any* definition that fails to account for *all* of them, and rediagnose the situation if necessary.

The third step, *identifying the specifications or "boundary conditions" the decision must satisfy,* is also an important part of the decision-making process. Indeed, Drucker (1967:95) believes that a decision which fails to satisfy the boundary conditions (including attainment of the "minimal" goals and satisfaction of certain "conditions") is "worse than one which wrongly defines the problem . . . [because] it is all but impossible to salvage the decision that starts with the right premises but stops short of the right conclusions."* As he further points out (1967:95), "clear thinking about the boundary conditions is needed to know when a decision has to be abandoned."* In other words, for a decision to be effective, it must not only "make sense," but it must also satisfy the boundary conditions.

The fourth step of the process entails *deciding what is "right" versus what is "acceptable" for meeting boundary conditions.* Drucker believes (1967) that the effective decision maker should *start* with what is "right" or ideal, recognizing that she will probably have to compromise in the end. However, being able to make the *right* compromise will depend on the manager's (decision maker's) knowledge of ex-

actly what is needed to satisfy the boundary conditions (specifications). In other words, if the decision maker *begins* by asking what is *acceptable* instead of what is *"right,"* in the process of answering that question she "usually gives away the important things and loses any chance to come up with an effective—let alone the right—answer" (1967:96).*

The fifth step involves *activating the decision.* Drucker (1967) identifies four questions that must be answered to translate the decision into action: "Who has to know of this decision? What action has to be taken? Who is to take it? What does the action have to be so that the people who have to do it *can* do it?"*

The sixth and last step in Drucker's decision-making process is *building in feedback mechanisms to test the validity and effectiveness of the decision.* Without belaboring the importance of feedback in *any* systematic process, suffice it to say that two basic questions need to be answered during this step: "How is the decision being carried out? Are the assumptions on which it is based appropriate or obsolete?" (1967:93).* The answers to these questions can then become inputs back to the beginning of the process.

Motivation. An essential aspect of directing is being attentive to the motivations of one's subordinates or employees. Everyone has personal goals or objectives (whether stated or unstated, conscious or unconscious) that he or she tries to accomplish. The manager's challenge is to be aware of her subordinates' objectives so that she can help find ways of satisfying them within the context of the organization or work setting. This requires effective *communication* between the manager and subordinate and also requires that the manager try to create what Scanlan (1974:7) calls a "motivation-producing climate." In other words, a manager who is truly interested in achieving high productivity or "getting the job done" will be attentive to the needs and motivations of her employees or subordinates and will be interested in assisting employees to meet their needs at work.

Motivation can be defined as "the way in which needs (urges, aspirations, desires) control, direct, or explain the behavior of human

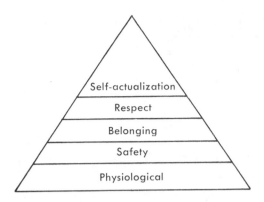

Fig. 18-7. Maslow's hierarchy of needs.

beings'' (Longest, 1976:156).* Psychologists and management theorists have long been interested and involved in exploring human motivation, and many interesting theories have emerged as a result. However, for the purposes of this chapter, only the work of three men will be discussed: Abraham Maslow, Frederick Herzberg, and Douglas McGregor.

MASLOW'S HIERARCHY OF NEEDS. Maslow's theory, as published originally in 1943, is that man's needs can be arranged in a hierarchy based on their order of importance or priority in guiding or motivating behavior and that behavior is goal directed toward satisfaction of these needs. As illustrated in Fig. 18-7, man's basic needs can be arranged in five hierarchical levels, which, beginning from *lowest* or most basic to highest, are as follows (Maslow, 1943):

1. *Physiological needs* for food, water, shelter, sexual gratification, and clothing
2. *Need for safety,* including both physical and economic security
3. *Need for belonging* or membership in groups and the need for friends and social acceptance
4. *Need for respect,* including self-esteem, status, recognition, and prestige
5. *Need for self-actualization,* or self-fulfillment, which results from achievement of one's potential

This hierarchy is viewed as dynamic (nonstatic) and subject to change. Only when the lower four levels of needs are fairly well satisfied will they cease to be motivating for the individual,

*Reprinted with permission of Reston Publishing Company, Inc., a Prentice-Hall Company, 11480 Sunset Hills Road, Reston, Virginia.

and only then will the individual be able and motivated to work toward self-actualization or achievement of his potential.

HERZBERG'S MOTIVATION-HYGIENE CONCEPT. Herzberg is a psychologist who studied motivation of people to work. His original study, carried out in Pittsburgh during the 1950s, involved interviews with more than two hundred engineers and accountants concerning events or incidents at work that had made them feel exceptionally *happy* and exceptionally *unhappy* with their jobs (Herzberg, 1964). This study was later replicated by others, including Myers (1964).

Herzberg's primary finding was that levels of job satisfaction, motivation, and productivity were closely related to the following two groups of factors:

1. *Dissatisfiers,* which are factors that describe a person's relationship ''to the context or environment in which he does his job'' (Herzberg, 1964:4); such factors include salary, company policy, and work conditions. When these factors are adequately satisfied or taken care of, they *prevent dissatisfaction* and are therefore also referred to as preventive or ''hygiene'' factors. However, these factors are not highly motivating when they are improved, although their deterioration does result in *dis*satisfaction (Herzberg, 1964; Myers, 1964).

2. *Motivators,* or *satisfiers,* which are factors that describe a person's relationship to *what* he does and that serve ''man's basic and human need for psychological growth; a need to become more competent'' (Herzberg, 1964:5). These motivators include achievement, responsibility, growth, the work itself, advancement, and ''earned'' recognition (Myers, 1964). When these factors are present, they are generally highly motivating.

The thirteen factors on Herzberg's list of motivators and dissatisfiers (hygiene factors) are illustrated in Fig. 18-8. When the dissatisfiers or hygiene factors are adequately taken care of, the worker is brought to a *neutral* state (represented by the ''0'' at the center of the figure), in which he is neither dissatisfied nor motivated. For true motivation to occur, some of the motivators, or satisfiers, must be present.

Herzberg's suggestion that the factors which contribute to motivation and job satisfaction are

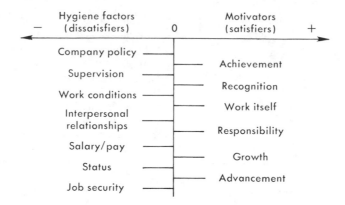

Fig. 18-8. Herzberg's motivation-hygiene concept. (Modified from Herzberg, F.: 1964. Personnel Administration **26**(1):3-7; Myers, M. S.: 1964. Harvard Bus. Rev. **42**(1):73-88.)

separate and distinct from the factors which result in job *dis*satisfaction was both innovative and controversial. Specifically, his suggestion that salary or pay is *not* a motivator has been challenged and disputed in management circles (Myers, 1964), since money has been traditionally used and regarded as an employee motivator. Perhaps the most reasonable conclusion concerning the motivating powers of money is that while *automatic* (such as annual) pay increases or raises are *not* motivating, money that is given in recognition of an individual's achievement (such as incentive pay for salespersons) *can* be motivating. This is an area for continuing research.

Based on Herzberg's (1964) research and replications by others (Myers, 1964, 1966), the following conclusions can be drawn:

1. Factors in the work situation that *motivate* employees are *distinct* from factors that dissatisfy them.
2. Effective job performance requires the satisfaction of *both* motivation and maintenance (hygiene) needs.
3. A job environment with many opportunities for meeting motivation needs encourages and leads to motivation-seeking behaviors, while a job setting in which *few* motivation opportunities exist encourages worker preoccupation with maintenance factors (dissatisfiers).
4. Therefore when motivation needs are *satisfied,* the maintenance factors exert *little* influence as either satisfiers or dissatisfiers; *however,* when the motivators are *not* taken care of, the individual becomes "sensitized" to the environment and may become hypercritical of maintenance fac-

tors, such as low salary or crowded work conditions.

5. *Therefore, motivation is facilitated by management actions that provide conditions of motivation and satisfaction.*

INTERFACE OF HERZBERG AND MASLOW. As shown in Fig. 18-9, the seven dissatisfiers, or hygiene factors, identified by Herzberg correspond with the lower four levels of Maslow's hierarchy; the motivators *all* relate to the "self-actualization" level of Maslow's hierarchy. Therefore these two frameworks are complementary, since Herzberg's motivation-hygiene concept is an expansion and extrapolation of Maslow's work.

MCGREGOR'S THEORY X AND THEORY Y. McGregor (1960) was one of the first authorities to recognize and acknowledge the effect of a *manager's* attitudes about people and their motivations on her style of managing and motivating employees or subordinates. McGregor concluded that there are basically two philosophies or sets of assumptions about human nature that a manager might have: "Theory X" and "Theory Y."

According to McGregor (1960), a Theory X manager believes that the average person inherently dislikes working and would avoid it altogether if he could. For this reason, most workers must be "coerced, controlled, directed, and threatened with punishment" to get them to put forth adequate effort to meet organizational objectives. Furthermore, the Theory X manager believes that most people *want* to be directed and told what to do, would like to *avoid* responsibility, have little ambition, and are primarily interested in security. Therefore a Theory X manager tends to supervise closely, set

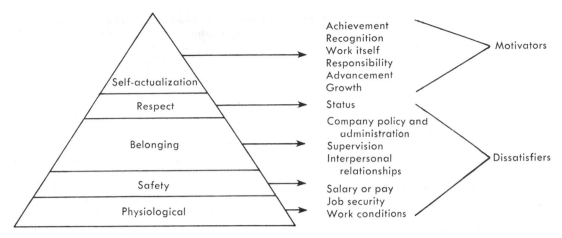

Fig. 18-9. Interface between Maslow's hierarchy of needs and Herzberg's motivation-hygiene concept.

goals and objectives *for* subordinates (rather than allowing them to participate or to set their own goals), and to plan work assignments in detail (Veninga, 1973b).

In contrast, the Theory Y manager believes that the average person does *not* dislike work, but regards work as a natural part of life. The Theory Y manager also believes that when workers are *committed* to carrying out certain objectives, they will work toward them in a self-directed manner without threats of punishment or imposition of other external controls. The Theory Y manager recognizes that workers' commitment to objectives depends on the rewards to be gained from their achievement and realizes that the most significant of such rewards are those related to self-actualization. The Theory Y manager does not believe that people want to avoid responsibility; rather, she realizes that when conditions are right, people will not merely accept responsibility but will actively seek it. Likewise, she believes that avoidance of responsibility, laziness, and concern for security are *learned* characteristics resulting from one's experience. Furthermore, the Theory Y manager believes that creativity, imagination, and ingenuity are prevalent characteristics in the general population, although the intellectual potential of the average person (worker) is only partially used (McGregor, 1960; Veninga, 1973b). Thus a Theory Y manager allows subordinates to have input concerning organizational goals and objectives, allows and encourages subordinates to assume re-

sponsibility, and allows and encourages self-direction (Veninga, 1973b).

When Theory X predominates in an organization, McGregor (1960) believes that not only is employee motivation low or absent, but that this style of directing and heading is actually antagonistic. Therefore a Theory Y orientation is recommended for managers who are concerned about motivating their subordinates to obtain maximum productivity.

ROLE OF THE MANAGER/LEADER IN MOTIVATING SUBORDINATES. It seems appropriate at this point to identify some specific recommendations or suggestions for managers who wish to help motivate their subordinates. These suggestions are based on the work of Maslow (1943), McGregor (1960), Herzberg (1964), Veninga (1973b), and Blake and Mouton, (1978) and are as follows:

1. The manager needs to regard her role as two dimensional; she must attend to satisfaction of maintenance (hygiene) needs, while providing conditions conducive to motivation.
2. The manager who gravitates toward McGregor's Theory Y position is more likely to successfully motivate subordinates than will a Theory X manager.
3. The Theory Y manager will hopefully also operate from the 9,9 managerial grid position (the team or "participative" manager).
4. As a 9,9 team manager, the following day-to-day behaviors should be evident in motivating subordinates:
   a. Provision of necessary job information and descriptions for employees

b. Maintenance of high performance standards

c. Encouragement of goal setting and exercise of employees' independent judgment

d. Maintenance of an atmosphere of approval in which mistakes and failures are regarded as bases for growth and not for recrimination

e. Provision of jobs with a future, that is, jobs that are not seen as "dead-ended"

f. Provision of enough money (through salary and incentives) to eliminate dissatisfaction and meet basic needs

g. Offering of personal support regarding work-related or personal problems (because the boss or manager is regarded as a "significant other" by subordinates)

h. Provision of awards and recognition for work achievements

i. Most of all, providing *challenging work* that allows the individual to grow and achieve his potential

Conflict management. Another area in which the nurse-manager needs to develop both comfort and skill is conflict management. Conflict is virtually inevitable in work and life situations and may result from actual or perceived differences in such variables as values, goals, personality, and status (Litterer, 1965). Conflict may be intrapersonal (within an individual), interpersonal (between two or more individuals), intraorganizational (within an organization), or interorganizational (between two or more organizations). This discussion will be limited to conflicts that are primarily interpersonal and intraorganizational—that is, conflicts occurring between people within an organization.

Conflict can be viewed as both destructive and constructive. Conflict can be *destructive* if it is poorly or inadequately resolved, which may lead to hostility, strained work relationships, and possibly decreased productivity. On the other hand, conflict may be *constructive* if (1) it arises as nonconformity with *traditional* ways of thinking and doing things, (2) it challenges outmoded patterns of action, and (3) it stimulates development of innovative, creative approaches to problem solving.

Referring again to the *Managerial Grid* (Blake and Mouton, 1970, 1978), five basic styles of approaching conflict resolution can be identified, which correspond with the five basic managerial styles identified on the grid. These grid styles and conflict approaches as previously described are summarized in Table 18-1. Obviously, Blake and Mouton (1970) regard the 9,9 "confrontation" approach as "ideal" in resolving conflicts, although confrontation is

Table 18-1. Managerial Grid styles with corresponding conflict resolution approach

Managerial Grid style	Conflict approach
9,1 Authority-obedience manager	Suppression: win or leave
1,9 Country club manager	Smoothing over
1,1 Impoverished manager	Overriding neutrality
5,5 Organization man, or "compromise," manager	Split the difference (compromise)
9,9 Team manager	Confrontation

more easily contemplated than carried out.

However, Veninga (1973a) has the following specific suggestions for direct conflict resolution that would be consistent with a 9,9 approach:

1. Determine the "right" moment to attempt conciliation; timing is critical, so it is important to know what "orientation" the parties bring to the conciliation talks. If both parties are convinced that they are right and are unwilling to consider modifying their point of view (the "win-win" orientation), chances of successful resolution of their conflict are *minimal*. If one party is determined to "win," while the other is willing to discuss and negotiate (the "win-compromise" orientation), chances of resolving the conflict are fair. If both parties are committed to finding the *best* solution to the conflict, (the "compromise-compromise" orientation), chances for resolution are good.

2. Arrange the confrontation meeting in a *neutral setting,* away from distractions and interruptions and allow enough time for the discussion.

3. Open the discussion/interview with statements designed to avoid creating or increasing defensiveness and that help put the person/subordinate at ease; that is, avoid blaming and adopt an attitude of mutual responsibility and a commitment to mutual problem solving.

4. To help strengthen the person's self-esteem, convey your continuing feelings of acceptance and respect early in the discussion, such as by asking for his opinion.

5. Follow through as promised with agreed-on action to resolve the conflict.

In other words, rather than avoiding, suppressing, smoothing over, or splitting the difference (which some might view as a "lose-lose" situation), the nurse-manager should directly *con-*

front conflict, so that it can be *managed* and can become a basis for growth and learning.

Assertiveness. With the resurgence of the women's movement in the early 1970s came an expanded interest in assertiveness training. Women (and men who felt taken advantage of) were encouraged to begin viewing themselves as persons of worth and to stand up for their rights. Thus each female was encouraged to become *The Assertive Woman* (Phelps and Austin, 1975), was assured that this was *Your Perfect Right* (Alberti and Emmons, 1974), and was duly admonished *Don't Say Yes When You Want to Say No* (Fensterheim and Baer, 1975).

For women in general, who have been successfully socialized to *believe* they are less important, less capable, and less deserving of fulfillment than men, this movement toward more assertive behavior was a whole new style of relating to the world and was both scary and exhilarating. For women in the health care professions (especially nurses), who have nonassertively allowed predominantly male groups such as physicians, administrators, and politicians to devise and perpetuate an abominably self-serving health care "system" able to "strip [clients/patients] of everything from their dignity to their life savings" (Chenevert, 1978: vii) while at the same time repeatedly demeaning women as both clients/patients and as colleagues, the need for assertiveness training and resocialization as assertive persons is especially acute. Indeed, as Chenevert (1978:viii) points out:

We have to take the initiative. Women have waited long enough for permission to speak up and to share our experiences, observations, and insights with the men who regulate and control care-giving systems. Whenever a patient receives less than satisfactory care, speak up. Whenever a patient is treated in an unkind manner, speak up. By failing to speak up, we are condoning current practices.

Whether women and nurses elect to become more assertive through formal assertiveness "training" workshops or courses, or whether they choose to adopt a self-help approach, the time to begin is *now,* and the place to begin is by developing an understanding of what assertive behavior *is.*

DEFINING ASSERTIVENESS. According to Alberti and Emmons (1974:2), *assertive behavior* is that which "enables a person to act in his own best interests, to stand up for himself without undue anxiety, to express his honest feelings comfortably, or to exercise his own rights without denying the rights of others." That is, an assertive action is (1) *problem-centered* as opposed to *person*-centered and thus avoids creating defensiveness in the other person, (2) *clear* and *direct* in its communicated message, (3) an *expression of* the person's real and *honest feelings,* and (4) does *not interfere with the rights of others* (Phelps and Austin, 1975).

OTHER COMMUNICATION STYLES. Phelps and Austin describe other typical styles of relating and communicating with others that are too often used in place of assertive behavior. The first is *nonassertion,* or *passivity,* which entails allowing others to disregard one's thoughts and feelings without challenging them or "fighting back"; the nonassertive person thus constantly seeks others' approval at all costs, puts herself last and others first, fears and avoids conflict, views herself as "not OK," and can be represented by "Doris Doormat" in Table 18-2.

According to Alberti and Emmons (1974), nonassertiveness can be either situational or generalized. *Situational* nonassertiveness occurs in persons who are usually able to communicate adequately about their needs and wishes but who, in certain anxiety-producing situations, become nonassertive. *Generalized* nonassertiveness, on the other hand, is the typical style for persons who are often described as shy or reserved and is used by them in almost all circumstances.

In significant contrast with the nonassertive communication style, the *aggressive* person (exemplified by Agatha Aggressive in Table 18-2) stands up for her rights and wishes without regard for the rights and feelings of others (Phelps and Austin, 1975); thus, she tends to "put herself up by putting others down" (Alberti and Emmons, 1974:21). She is generally viewed as obnoxious by others and often alienates herself from other people as a result (Phelps and Austin, 1975). Her apparent outlook on the world is "I'm OK and you're *not* OK." As with the nonassertor, the aggressive person may be either situationally or generally aggressive (Alberti and Emmons, 1974). Aggressive behavior may reflect the person's true outlook on life and other people, or it may be a confused, misguided attempt at becoming assertive—an overreaction of sorts.

While Agatha Aggressive represents a person who is overtly and directly aggressive, Iris Indirect (Table 18-2) is an example of *indirect aggression,* or getting one's way through indirect

Table 18-2. Nonassertive, aggressive, indirect, and assertive communication styles*

Selected typical characteristics	Doris Doormat	Agatha Aggressive	Iris Indirect	April Assertive
Point of view	I'm not OK	You're not OK	You're not OK, but I'll let you think you are	I'm OK and you're OK
Dominant role Sample games	Inhibited underdog "If it weren't for you," "Kick me," and "Why does it always happen to me?"	Underdog in bear suit "Now I've got you!"	Mad dog in lamb's suit "I'm smiling while stabbing you in the back"	Top dog "Let's play tennis"
Self-sufficiency	Low	High or low	Looks high but is usually low	Usually high
Decision making	Others choose for her	Chooses for others and they know it	Chooses for others and they don't know it	Chooses for herself
Significant other	Agatha, Iris, or April	Doris	Agatha, April, and/or Doris	Herself
Feedback she gets from others	Guilt, anger, frustration, disrespect	Hurt, defensive, humiliated	Confusion, frustration, feels manipulated	You respect me and I respect you
Social pattern	Puts herself down	Puts herself up by putting others down	Appears to put others up while putting them down	Puts herself up
Defensive pattern	Flees or gives in	Outright attack	Concealed attack	Evaluates and acts
Action pattern	Underreacts	Overreacts	Acts indirectly	Acts directly
Success pattern	Lucks out	Beats out others	Wins by manipulating others	Wins honestly
Potential for	Suicide, alcoholism, drug abuse, other withdrawals	Committing crimes, homicide	Being murdered, provoking retaliation	Peaceful, active life

*From Phelps, Stanlee, and Austin, Nancy, THE ASSERTIVE WOMAN. Copyright © 1975 Impact Publishers, Inc., San Luis Obispo, Calif. Reprinted by permission of the publisher. The idea for this chart was modified and adapted from the "Characterological Lifechart of Three Fellows We All Know," presented by Gerald Piaget at the Institute on Assertive Communication, American Orthopsychiatric Association Convention, San Francisco, April, 1974.

or "sneaky" means (Phelps and Austin, 1975). Iris' life position is "You're not OK, but I'll let you think you are" (1975:11). She tends to be manipulative and may be thought of as passive-aggressive.

The assertive style, as defined earlier, is represented in Table 18-2 by April Assertive, who believes "I'm OK and You're OK." As a person of high self-esteem, April feels free to *choose* how she will conduct her life and how she will respond in any situation. She does not feel pressured to adopt a particular life-style or career pattern or to make "socially acceptable" choices; rather, she is true to herself.

For the nurse-manager, assertiveness is an important component of successful directing and heading. The manager who is unable to assert herself in documenting the needs of her organization or department or in dealing with internal or external conflicts will find leading and directing very difficult and frustrating. Again, whether she opts for a formal course or workshop or the do-it-yourself approach, the method is immaterial; what matters is that all nurses, but especially those at middle and upper level management positions, begin *now* to become truly assertive and fully functioning persons.

Controlling

The last managerial function to be discussed is *controlling,* which can be defined (Longest, 1976:202) as "the regulation of activities in accordance with the requirements of plans."* Stated more simply, controlling is "ensuring that events conform to plans" (Scanlan, 1974:85). Thus, by definition, controlling is directly related to planning. While exactly "what" is controlled depends on the nature and purpose of the organization and its objectives, most health care organizations are concerned with controlling the quality of care they deliver and the costs incurred in the process (Longest, 1976).

Although controlling is usually the last managerial function included in any list or model of management, it is nonetheless one of the most important managerial responsibilities; indeed, Scanlan (1974:85) refers to controlling as the "essence of management" and describes it as the "function which gives meaning and depth to all other functions." Thus development and

implementation of an effective and appropriate control system are critically important aspects of management and help ensure that the organization's objectives are met. The essential elements of such a control system include (1) setting standards, (2) reporting, (3) interpreting and evaluating information (data analysis), and (4) taking corrective action (Scanlan, 1974).

Setting standards

Simply defined, *standards* are "criteria against which to judge results" (Longest, 1976:203).* In nursing, a standard is defined as "a model or example established by authority, custom, or general consent . . . [specifying] a criterion and a level or degree of quality considered proper and adequate for a specific purpose" (Ramey, 1976b:79). For the nurse-manager, the EOCs specified during the planning process are standards indicating desirable planned outcomes or quality of care. However, other sources of standards also must be considered by the nurse-manager.

One important source of standards for nursing is voluntary accreditation of health care institutions and schools of nursing, such as the accrediting procedures of the Joint Commission on Accreditation of Hospitals (JCAH) and the National League for Nursing (NLN). These organizations develop and communicate standards with which institutions and organizations desiring accreditation must demonstrate compliance. Hospitals that are awarded JCAH accreditation will, it is hoped, be providing safe effective patient care, and schools of nursing accredited by the NLN presumably will graduate competent and safe nursing practitioners. Although such accreditation is voluntary, institutions who do not seek or obtain accreditation often are unable to get funding from governmental and other endowment bodies; hence "voluntary" accreditation is a powerful source of standard setting and enforcement.

Standards may also be imposed on an organization-wide basis, such as through a hospital's nursing services department. The policy and procedure manuals used in hospitals and other nursing settings, including schools and public health nursing agencies, are potential sources of nursing standards. Thus, for example, a school nursing policy manual that describes the ex-

---

*Reprinted with permission of Reston Publishing Company, Inc., a Prentice-Hall Company, 11480 Sunset Hills Road, Reston, Virginia.

*Reprinted with permission of Reston Publishing Company, Inc., a Prentice-Hall Company, 11480 Sunset Hills Road, Reston, Virginia.

pected school nurse actions in carrying out screening procedures and following up defects within a school vision screening program provides some standards concerning acceptable vision screening for that population and institution. Likewise, the procedure for obtaining informed consent from prospective surgery patients in hospitals comprises a standard of sorts for ensuring that patients' rights are safeguarded.

A third potential source of nursing standards is professional organizations, such as the ANA, ASHA, and the National Association of School Nurses (NASN) to name a few. These organizations, among their many other functions, attempt to define and communicate standards for practice that will ensure provision of quality care to the pertinent client populations. Thus the ANA (1973) has written and published standards for nursing care in general (Chapter 14), in addition to developing standards for a number of nursing specialty areas as well. Unfortunately, the major problem with setting standards for nurses and other health care professional groups is that there are so many organizations vying for the right to represent each group of professionals that standard setting becomes lost in a political jungle. This problem is especially knotty for school nurses, who are caught in the crossfire between warring nursing and education organizations.

A fourth potential source of standards for the nurse-manager is the legal arena. Specifically, this refers to laws governing nursing, such as states' nursing practice acts, and the legal granting by states of individual licensure to nurses. Such legal restraints define (more or less clearly) what nursing practice is construed to be, by whom it may be practiced, and what kinds of nurse conduct (including morals and ethics) are acceptable. This is indeed an area about which many nurses are both naive and uninformed, and yet these legal standards are binding on all nurses.

Reporting

The second element of a control system (Scanlan, 1974) is development of a reporting mechanism whereby the manager can be sure that she receives necessary data and feedback at the appropriate intervals. Controlling must be oriented in the *present* so that needed changes can be made before it is too late. Therefore the reporting mechanism must be designed in such a way that the manager receives needed data at the right time—finding out at the end of the fiscal year that the budget has been exceeded is not helpful, since corrective action can no longer be taken. Scanlan (1974) further cautions managers to devise a *practical* reporting system, eliminating unnecessary and complicating detail. The reporting interval will need to be established in accordance with the particular situation.

Interpreting and evaluating information (data analysis)

This third step, data analysis, is critical, because it becomes the basis for taking corrective action during the fourth step of the control process (Scanlan, 1974). Obviously, it is important that the manager have available the data needed to evaluate the success of the plan, since absence of or failure to collect pertinent data will greatly complicate (or even thwart) the manager's decision-making process. The exact nature and quantity of data needed for evaluation of the success of a plan will of course depend on the nature of the plan. Possible sources of data to be used in deciding what, if any, corrective action is needed are (1) client data, such as from health records, survey forms, and clinics; (2) financial data, including itemized expenditures and sources and amounts of income, to be compared against the original budget plan (developed as part of the planning function) as a means of measuring cost-effectiveness; (3) employee appraisal (performance evaluation) data, gathered as part of the directing and heading function (supervision); (4) chart/health record audit data and peer review data; and (5) research data, a source that is increasingly important in nursing in general and school nursing in particular as a means of measuring effectiveness and validity of nurse actions and approaches.

Taking corrective action

Based on the manager's analysis of the data gathered in step 3, some specific decisions have to be made at this point. The manager must decide what, if any, corrective actions are needed, and how to go about implementing them. As Scanlan (1974) points out, this requires excellent decision-making and critical thinking skills on the part of the manager and the exercise of strong leadership in accomplishing the changes. The manager's decisions concerning corrective actions to be taken become, by way of the feedback loop (Fig. 18-1), inputs to the planning process in which the details of the implementation can be worked out. Examples of possible corrective actions that may be taken by the nurse-manager or a higher authority (such as an accrediting body, a state board of nursing, or a court), include (1) counseling or conferring with involved parties to discuss improving performance and outcomes; (2) scaling down or revising planned outcomes or revising the means for achieving them; (3) modifying pertinent policies or procedures; (4) revising the budget to reflect actual costs; (5) disciplining involved individuals or groups by means of fines, suspension, or revocation of accreditation or licensure; or (6) planning continuing education or in-service programs to improve staff's compliance with expected performance norms. These are just a few examples of the many possible courses of corrective action available to the nurse-manager.

Conclusion

Before terminating this overview of management process, it is appropriate to reiterate the importance of management process for nurses at all hierarchical levels in all organizations and settings. All nurses, and especially those who are particularly vulnerable right now (such as school nurses), must become knowledgeable and competent managers within their particular nursing sphere. Nurses must become more actively involved with *planning—including planning the budget*—within their employment settings and must likewise concern themselves with the *directing and heading* function if nursing is to ever take charge of its own destiny and break out of the pattern of being a "silent majority" (Chenevert, 1978) within the health care system.

PUTTING THE MANAGEMENT PROCESS TO WORK: THE SCHOOL NURSE AS A MANAGER WITHIN THE SCHOOL HEALTH PROGRAM

In Chapter 2, one of the basic roles identified for the school nurse was that of *manager of health care;* the corollary goal that was identified for her as manager was: "To participate in planning, implementation, and evaluation of a school health program." At that time, the point was also made that while the school nurse must become a more vocal and active participant in carrying out that goal (especially the planning and evaluation aspects), she should not be expected to *be* the school health program in and of

herself nor be expected to plan, implement, and/or evaluate the health program without benefit of the input and assistance of others. Chapter 2 also included discussion of suggested ways in which the school nurse might participate in planning, implementing, and evaluating the school health program. The remainder of this chapter will consider suggested involvement and actions for the school nurse in more fully operationalizing each of the managerial functions: planning, organizing, directing and heading, and controlling.

Planning

Repeatedly throughout this book the need for conscious and conscientious planning has been emphasized; specifically, the need for planning *programs* instead of merely offering "services" (as in the case of various kinds of screening) has been emphasized. In short, the intended message has been that "If you don't know where you're going, how will you know when you get there?" Perhaps a more important point is that made by Adams (1978:569), who warns that: "If you don't know where you're going . . . you may wind up somewhere else."

For school nurses, there is an acute need to be represented at the school district level in the determination of school health program goals and objectives, which of course should be developed only after careful and thorough assessment of the health status and needs of the school community. Whether this participation by school nursing representatives in district-wide program planning is provided by a school nursing administrator or by a qualified staff nurse is less important than simply ensuring *active and vocal participation by some school nursing representative*. If school nurses wish to have a hand in shaping their own destinies, this is an important place to begin.

Another vitally important area for involvement of school nurses concerns the allocation of resources for the district's school health program. Specifically, this suggests that school nurses need to participate more fully in the budget-setting process, which involves "assigning dollars to goals" (Adams, 1978:569). According to Arndt and Huckabay (1980:228), a *budget* is "a predetermined standard of performance in terms of the controllable costs for any given volume of service covering a specific time period." In other words, a budget is a kind of financial plan for carrying out the organization's goals and objectives and is also a standard used during the control process to measure adequacy of financial resources for meeting those goals (Longest, 1976; Arndt and Huckabay, 1980). While it is beyond the scope and intent of this book to explain the process of developing a budget, a working knowledge of the budgeting process is important for nurses in all settings—and especially in schools, where the budget has become the "ultimate control measure." For discussion of the budgeting process, the reader is encouraged to consult Stevens (1975), Alexander (1978), and Arndt and Huckabay (1980). School nurses, then, need to familiarize themselves with the process of budgeting (including the politics of getting one's "pet" programs funded) and need to *actively* participate in this process to ensure that school health objectives for which they have responsibility are adequately funded. If a school health program includes certain high-priority objectives, then there *must* be adequate funds budgeted to carry out those objectives, or the likelihood of accomplishing them is small. Nurses, particularly school nurses, must stop being so naive about how and by whom important decisions about funding are made; if school nurses are committed to the achievement of particular goals or objectives, they must make their views known and obtain funding for their preferred goals.

Organizing

As indicated during discussion of the organizing function earlier in this chapter, the primary organizing problems for school nurses and school health programs are staffing and delegation. For school nurses themselves, a major problem often is the high student-nurse ratio. That is, one school nurse may be expected to serve three or more schools, with student populations totaling several thousand or more. Under those circumstances, being able to actually function as a school nurse and accomplish *anything* beyond the stereotypical expectations of administering first aid or filling out records is nearly impossible. Research to identify rational methods for staffing schools and for determining workable student-nurse ratios is sorely needed—and it will have to be initiated by nurses themselves, since they are the group needing relief.

In addition, school nurses also need to address the sticky and troublesome area of delegation of responsibility *to them* by others, including administrators (principals), teachers, coun-

selors, and others, including secretarial and clerical personnel. School nurses are too often expected to carry out highly inappropriate functions, such as answering the telephones for the principal while the secretary is on a coffee break or telephoning the homes of all absent students to discover the reasons for their absence. In part, these abuses of her good nature are due to poor understanding of her actual role within the school and its health program. Sometimes, attention to improving her "public relations" with faculty and staff members on an informal basis (such as over coffee in the faculty lounge) will effectively clarify others' perceptions of her role and lead to more appropriate expectations of the school nurse. In situations where these informal "chance" encounters are not enough to improve her image and visibility within the school, the nurse may want to formally clarify her role for faculty, staff, and parents by delivering a presentation describing her role and functions at a faculty or PTA meeting. She may also wish to formally present herself to the students at homerooms, other classes, or during all-school assemblies. But the point is, that if the school nurse wishes to "change her image" from Band-Aider, record keeper, attendance checker, and all around *nice* person (and you know where nice guys usually finish), she will have to actively clarify her role and at the same time begin to assertively refuse to accept delegated tasks that are not within her role or realm. If ever there was a "right" moment to haughtily announce that "I *don't* do windows!" (which I fervently hope has never been expected, although many equally inappropriate tasks *have* been), this is it!

The debate concerning the use, nonuse, and abuse of nonprofessional assistants or school health aides is another aspect of organizing that is presently unresolved and in need of attention from the school nurse in her role as manager. There have been numerous articles in the literature concerning the role of nonprofessional assistants in school health, including those by Tipple (1964), Bryan and Cook (1967), the ASHA Subcommittee on the Role of the Nonprofessional Assistant in School Health Services (1968), Randall et al. (1968), and Lum (1973). These articles point out both the problems and potential benefits of employing nonnurse assistants in the school health program. The problems include the possible confusion of administrative and school personnel about the role and functions of school health aides as compared with the role and functions of the school nurse, which some authors, including Tipple (1964), fear might result in *replacement* of school nurses by school health aides. Unfortunately, this has already happened in many districts.

Another possible problem concerning employment of school health aides (nonprofessional assistants) is the failure of school nurses to use them as fully as possible and to take advantage of the "extra" time nurses recapture when they delegate nonprofessional tasks to their nonprofessional assistants. Indeed, the studies by Bryan and Cook (1967) and Randall et al. (1968) indicate that while school nurses may have more time *available* for public health school nursing when a nonprofessional assistant is available to relieve them of mundane, nonnursing tasks, the nurses may need help (in the form of guidance or in-service education) to use that time wisely. Nurses may also need to work on improving their supervisory and delegation skills if they are to benefit maximally from the presence and availability of their nonnurse assistants. Despite these potential and actual problems, which may result from employment of nonprofessional assistants in the school health program, such auxiliary personnel are a necessary component of school health services, since without them, school nurses will continue to be frustrated and overwhelmed by the nature and volume of the many nonnursing tasks that usurp their time and prevent them from truly practicing as school nurses.

The challenge for the school nurse as manager with regard to nonprofessional assistants is to (1) participate in development of clear and appropriate job descriptions for auxiliary personnel; (2) encourage recruitment of qualified and motivated school health aides or assistants; (3) participate in development of guidelines for delegation of specific responsibilities to the school health aide, (4) by incorporating elements of the directing and heading function, provide appropriate orientation for school health aides and provide adequate supervision and "coaching"; and (5) document through research the efficiency (cost-effectiveness) and impact of employment of school health aides in freeing nurses to practice high-quality school nursing.

Directing and heading

After the lengthy discussion of directing and heading that has already appeared in this chapter, it may seem that the topic has been exhausted. However, because the lack of both leadership and assertiveness on the part of school nurses has been pathetically evident, perhaps a few more words on the subject will not be construed as "overkill."

The absence of leadership in nursing in general, and school nursing in particular, has been widely documented and discussed in the literature for some time now. Most authorities in nursing who have published their views within the forum of professional journals seem to agree with McBride (1972:1445):

Nursing's contribution to the development of a more responsive and competent system of health services is directly related to the quality of leadership the profession can provide through its practitioners, educators, and researchers.

However, despite the recognized importance of leadership by nursing "authorities," McBride (1972) asserts that most nurses (presumably those who are not considered "authorities") *neither want to be* leaders *nor are educated to be* leaders.

McBride (1972:1445) continues the attack by pointing out a major curricular flaw of most nursing education programs:

We devote hours of classroom time to scrutinizing nursing care plans, but scarcely mention how an institution's organizational plan may crush any efforts on the part of nursing to be innovative. Leadership of the nursing team may be discussed, but lobbying for legislation that will improve nursing care, deciding what to say to an angry community member who wants nursing to get involved in improving the local school system, or understanding what it means to take on functions previously only in the doctor's domain—these are issues rarely discussed in any but general terms.

In other words, (school) nurses need to begin to regard themselves as leaders—and they need the educational preparation to back them up.

For school nurses to begin to take charge of their destinies and exert power over the almighty school budget (as it affects school health) will require not only educational preparation in leadership theories and principles and a commitment to apply them, but will also require skill and persistence in assertive communication. School nurses cannot afford to sit idly by, waiting for some (presumably male?) messiah or Prince Charming to come along and rescue them from inertia and the consequent and pervasive threats of extinction. As Chenevert (1978:28) warns:

Instead of pining away, waiting to be rescued, we had better uncover, develop, and mobilize our own resources if we want to save ourselves and our professions. There are no knights in shining armor, and kissing toads will only lead to warts.

Controlling

The managerial function of controlling has been perhaps the weakest link in the management process for school nurses. One of the primary problems has been the lack of accepted, communicated, and enforceable standards of practice for school nursing; without such standards, it is difficult to recognize quality school nursing and practically impossible to measure it. With so many professional organizations in the running to be "the" representative for school nurses, such as the ASHA, ANA, NASN, and APHA, development of standards that are acceptable to each organization and to the school nurses they represent becomes a very difficult, although nonetheless essential, task.

A related area of controlling that merits the efforts and energies of school nurses is development of reasonable and appropriate school nurse certification requirements and procedures. Certification is a way of controlling who is allowed to practice school nursing by limiting the field to nurses who are judged educationally and/or experientially qualified and credible to practice in the school setting. Certification is a means also for ensuring that school nurses are educationally on a par with other school faculty members, which should increase their acceptance and status. States in which no certification requirements have been set need to begin now to rectify that omission; in states where the certification criteria are inappropriate or vague, the time is ripe to revise them. Once the criteria have been developed, approved, and implemented, the next challenge will be to *enforce* them, by whatever means are deemed appropriate, including dismissal of nurses who, after a reasonable time for compliance, are unable or unwilling to meet the criteria and become certified.

In addition to development of practice standards and certification criteria, school nurses individually can begin to emphasize other means for upgrading their practice. One means of so doing would be to either plan and deliver their own continuing education offerings or to petition existing continuing education providers, such as colleges, foundations, or privately-run continuing education firms to offer programs or courses on topics of interest to school nurses in a particular region. Suggested topics for such sessions include health assessment techniques, assertiveness training, or research methods. A second way of upgrading individual practice might be development of some system of peer review among the school nurses within a particular district or those sharing a particular interest and expertise, such as care of adolescents. While peer review is a relatively recent concept in nursing and one with both disadvantages and advantages (Ramphal, 1974), it provides a useful source of performance feedback for school nurses.

Finally, to reiterate a point emphasized throughout this book, school nurses *must* become more vociferous and sophisticated in their quest for funding within the school health program, using *documentation of* their client *outcomes* and *cost-effectiveness of their services,* which requires painstaking *record keeping* and generation of *research* concerning school nursing and its outcomes. However, even the effectiveness of these measures will be diminished unless school nurses have the presence of mind and the savvy to "tell the right people" (Adams, 1978) about their accomplishments.

In sum, the management process is one of the most important keys to the future of school nursing. If we expect to survive the budgetary curtailments and begin reshaping our public image, we had better stop "doing" and start "managing."

REFERENCES

Adams, R. M.: 1978. If you don't know where you're going . . . you may wind up somewhere else, J. School Health **48**(9):569.

Alberti, R. E., and Emmons, M. L.: 1974. Your perfect right, 2nd ed., Impact Publishers, Inc., San Luis Obispo, Calif.

Alexander, E. L.: 1978. Nursing administration in the hospital health care system, 2nd ed., The C. V. Mosby Co., St. Louis.

American Nurses' Association: 1973. Standards: nursing practice, American Nurses' Association, Kansas City, Mo.

American School Health Association Subcommittee on the Role of the Non-Professional Assistant in School Health Services (Helen Brion, Chairman):1968. The non-professional assistant in school health services, J. School Health **38**(5):278-282.

Arndt, C., and Huckabay, L. M. D.: 1980. Nursing administration: theory for practice with a systems approach, 2nd ed., The C. V. Mosby Co., St. Louis.

Bailey, J. T., and Claus, K. E.: 1975. Decision making in

nursing: tools for change, The C. V. Mosby Co., St. Louis.

Blake, R. R., and Mouton, J. S.: 1964. The managerial grid, Gulf Publishing Co.

Blake, R. R., and Mouton, J. S.: 1970. The fifth achievement, J. Appl. Behav. Science 6(4):413-426.

Blake, R. R., and Mouton, J. S.: 1978. The new managerial grid, 2nd ed., Gulf Publishing Co., Houston.

Bryan, D. S., and Cook, T. S.: 1967. Redirection of school nursing services in culturally deprived neighborhoods, Am. J. Public Health 57(7):1164-1176.

Chenevert, M.: 1978. Special techniques in assertiveness training for women in the health professions, The C. V. Mosby Co., St. Louis.

Dale, E.: 1978. Management: theory and practice, 4th ed., McGraw-Hill Book Co., New York.

Dickinson, D. J.: 1971. School nursing becomes accountable in education through behavioral objectives, J. School Health 41(10):533-537.

Douglass, L. M.: 1977. Review of leadership in nursing, 2nd ed., The C. V. Mosby Co., St. Louis.

Drucker, P. F.: 1967. The effective decision, Harvard Bus. Rev. 45(1):92-98.

Fensterheim, H., and Baer, J.: 1975. Don't say yes when you want to say no, Dell Publishing Co., Inc., New York.

Fulmer, R. M.: 1976. Supervision: principles of professional management, Glencoe Press, Beverly Hills, Calif.

Hersey, P., and Blanchard, K. H.: 1977. Management of organizational behavior: utilizing human resources, 3rd ed., Prentice-Hall, Inc., Englewood Cliffs, N.J.

Herzberg, F.: 1964. The motivation-hygiene concept and problems of manpower, Personnel Administration 26(1): 3-7.

Jacobsen, R. F., and Siegel, E.: 1971. Comprehensive health planning in the space age: the role of the school health program, J. School Health 41(3):156-160.

Litterer, J. A.: 1965. Managing conflict in organizations, Proceedings of the Eighth Annual Midwest Management Conference, Business Research Bureau, Southern Illinois University, Carbondale, Ill.

Longest, B. B.: 1976. Management practices for the health professional, Reston Publishing Co., Inc., Reston, Va.

Lum, M. C.: 1973. Current concepts in the use of nonprofessional assistants in school health services—a selected review, J. School Health 43(6):357-361.

Marriner, A.: 1971. Opinions of school nurses about the preparation and practice of school nurses, J. School Health 41(8):417-420.

Maslow, A. H.: 1943. A theory of human motivation, Psychol. Rev. 50(7):370-396.

McBride, A., Diers, D., Slavinsky, A., Schlotfeldt, R., Christman, L., and Kibrick, A.: 1972. Leadership: problems and possibilities in nursing, Am. J. Nurs. 72(8): 1445-1456.

McGregor, D.: 1960. The human side of enterprise, McGraw-Hill Book Co., New York.

Myers, M. S.: 1964. Who are your motivated workers? Harvard Bus. Rev. 42(1):73-88.

Myers, M. S.: 1966. Conditions for manager motivation, Harvard Bus. Rev. 44(1):58-71.

Newman, W. H.: 1963. Administrative action: the techniques of organization and management, 2nd ed., Prentice-Hall, Inc., Englewood Cliffs, N.J.

Odiorne, G. S.: 1961. How managers make things happen, Prentice-Hall, Inc., Englewood Cliffs, N.J.

Phelps, S., and Austin, N.: 1975. The assertive woman, Impact Publishers, Inc., San Luis Obispo, Calif.

Ramey, I. G.: 1976a. Eleven steps to proper staffing. In Stone, S., Berger, M. S., Elhart, D., Firsich, S. C., and Jordan, S. B., editors: Management for nurses: a multidisciplinary approach, The C. V. Mosby Co., St. Louis.

Ramey, I. G.: 1976b. Setting nursing standards and evaluating care. In Stone, S., Berger, M. S., Elhart, D., Firsich, S. C., and Jordan, S. B., editors: Management for nurses: a multidisciplinary approach, The C. V. Mosby Co., St. Louis.

Ramphal, M.: 1974. Peer review, Am. J. Nurs. 74(1):63-67.

Randall, H. B., Cauffman, J. G., and Shultz, C. S.: 1968. Effectiveness of health office clerks in facilitating health care for elementary school children, Am. J. Public Health 58(5):897-906.

Scanlan, B. K.: 1974. Management 18: a short course for managers, John Wiley & Sons, Inc., New York.

Stevens, B. J.: 1975. The nurse as executive, Contemporary Publishing, Inc., Wakefield, Mass.

Stevens, W. F.: 1978. Management and leadership in nursing, McGraw-Hill Book Co., New York.

Tannenbaum, R., and Schmidt, W. H.: 1958. How to choose a leadership pattern, Harvard Bus. Rev. 36(2):95-101.

Tipple, D. C.: 1964. Misuse of assistants in school health, Am. J. Nurs. 64(9):99-101.

Veninga, R.: 1973a. The management of conflict, J. Nurs. Adm. 3(4):13-16.

Veninga, R.: 1973b. Unpublished material (lecture notes and course materials) from Public Health 5-070, University of Minnesota, Minneapolis.

Volante, E. M.: 1976. Mastering the managerial skill of delegation. In Stone, S., Berger, M. S., Elhart, D., Firsich, S. C., and Jordan, S. B., editors: Management for nurses: a multidisciplinary approach, The C. V. Mosby Co., St. Louis.

SUGGESTED READINGS

Anderson, C. L., and Creswell, W. H.: 1980. School health practice, 7th ed., The C. V. Mosby Co., St. Louis.

Beyers, M., and Phillips, C.: 1974. Keys to successful leadership, Nurs. '74 4(7):51-58.

Creighton, H.: 1975. Law every nurse should know, 3rd ed., W. B. Saunders Co., Philadelphia.

Creighton, H., and Squaires, G. M.: 1974. School nurses: legal aspects of their work, Nurs. Clin. North Am. 9(3): 467-474.

Derr, C. B.: 1972. Conflict resolution in organizations: views from the field of educational administration, Public Administration, Sept./Oct., pp. 495-501.

Edwards, L., and Kelly, E.: 1977. A three-level school health program, Nurs. Outlook 25(6):388-391.

Filley, A. C., and House, R. J.: 1969. Managerial process and organizational behavior, Scott, Foresman & Co., Glenview, Ill.

Grissum, M., and Spengler, C.: 1976. Womanpower and health care, Little, Brown & Co., Boston.

Hanlon, J. J., and Pickett, G. E.: 1979. Public health: administration and practice, 7th ed., The C. V. Mosby Co., St. Louis.

Hover, J., and Zimmer, M. J.: 1978. Nursing quality assurance: the Wisconsin system, Nurs. Outlook 26(4):242-248.

Humes, C. W.: 1975. Who should administer school nursing services? Am. J. Public Health 65(4):394-396.

Jenne, F. H., and Greene, W. H.: 1976. Turner's school

health and health education, 7th ed., The C. V. Mosby Co., St. Louis.

Kron, T.: 1976. The management of patient care: putting leadership skills to work, 4th ed., W. B. Saunders Co., Philadelphia.

Kruckel, K.: 1973. The name of the game is accountability, J. N.Y. State School Nurse-Teachers Assoc. **5:**29-31, Fall.

Long, G. V., Whitman, C., Johansson, M. S., Williams, C. A., and Tuthill, R. W.: 1975. Evaluation of a school health program directed to children with history of high absence: a focus for nursing intervention, Am. J. Public Health **65**(4):388-393.

Mayshark, C., Shaw, D. D., and Best, W. H.: 1977. Administration of school health programs: its theory and practice, 2nd ed., The C. V. Mosby Co., St. Louis.

McCool, B., and Brown, M.: 1977. The management response: conceptual, technical and human skills of health administration, W. B. Saunders Co., Philadelphia.

Miller, D. F.: 1970. Recent litigations relating to the school health services, J. School Health **40**(10):526-527.

Morgan, M. K., and Irby, D. M.: 1978. Evaluating clinical competence in the health professions, The C. V. Mosby Co., St. Louis.

Murchison, I., Nichols, T. S., and Hanson, R.: 1978. Legal accountability in the nursing process, The C. V. Mosby Co., St. Louis.

The non-professional assistant in school health services: 1968. J. School Health **38**(5):278-282.

Patterson, J.: 1969. Effectiveness of follow-up of health referrals for school health services under two different administrative patterns, J. School Health **39**(10):687-692.

Peter, L. J., and Hull, R.: 1969. The Peter principle, William Morrow & Co., Inc., New York.

Public Law 93-380, Section 438, amended August 12, 1974 (Buckley Amendment), J. N.Y. State Nurse-Teacher Assoc. **6:**6-7, Spring.

Richards, M. D., and Nielander, W. A.: 1974. Readings in management, 4th ed., South-Western Publishing Co., Cincinnati.

Rubin, I. M., Fry, R. E., and Plovnick, M. S.: 1978. Managing human resources in health care organizations: an applied approach, Reston Publishing Co., Inc., Reston, Va.

Schaefer, J.: 1974. The interrelatedness of decision making and the nursing process, Am. J. Nurs. **74**(10):1852-1855.

Shortell, S. M., and Richardson, W. C.: 1978. Health program evaluation, The C. V. Mosby Co., St. Louis.

Stone, S., Berger, M. S., Elhart, D., Firsich, S. C., and Jordan, S. B.: 1976. Management for nurses: a multidisciplinary approach, The C. V. Mosby Co., St. Louis.

Tuthill, R. W., Williams, C., Long, G., and Whitman, C.: 1972. Evaluating a school health program focused on high absence pupils: a research design, Am. J. Public Health **62**(1):40-42.

White, H. C.: 1971. Perceptions of leadership styles by nurses in supervisory positions, J. Nurs. Adm. **1**(2):44-51.

Wohlking, W.: 1970. Organizational conflict and its resolution: implications for supervising nurses, Superv. Nurse **1**(10):17-30.

Yura, H., Ozimek, D., and Walsh, M. B.: 1976. Nursing leadership: theory and process, Appleton-Century-Crofts, New York.

CHAPTER 19

Planned change: the importance of legislative/political savvy

SUSAN J. WOLD

Although change has been an acknowledged part of life since time began, the rate at which significant changes occur has accelerated. As a result, many people have difficulty adjusting to change and consequently experience what Toffler (1970) calls "future shock." Indeed, the changes resulting from man's ingenuity during the twentieth century alone are incredible. For example, during this century man has created and refined the automobile; learned to fly in increasingly sophisticated aircraft; explored outer space and walked on the moon; and successfully united a human egg and sperm in a test tube, implanted the developing embryo inside the mother's uterus, and delivered an apparently normal, healthy baby as a result. Many of these changes have created new moral and ethical dilemmas that may intensify future shock.

Changes affecting the health care system in general and the nursing profession in particular are likewise occurring at a dizzying pace. For example, in recent years, basic educational preparation for nurses has shifted away from the hospital-based diploma program and toward associate and baccalaureate degree programs in institutions of higher learning; it has been proposed that by 1985 entry level into nursing be a baccalaureate degree, thus eliminating diploma or nondegree programs altogether. Other significant changes in educational preparation for nurses have included the movement away from the early "training" of nurses by physicians toward nursing education provided by qualified nurse faculty members. In addition, some schools have developed baccalaureate nursing curricula that have built-in specialization in contrast with the traditional and customary generalized preparation; in such nursing programs, a student may elect to pursue an emphasis in episodic (acute care) nursing or in distributive (wellness- and prevention-oriented) nursing practice.

Another significant area of change for nursing involves the structure or organizational pattern in which nursing care is delivered to clients. For many years, the team concept was popular; under team nursing organization, the client/patient received nursing care from personnel of different preparation and skill levels, each one contributing according to her abilities. However, the result of this pattern was that the person who often provided most of the direct nursing care to the client was the least-prepared or skilled person on the team—the nurse's aide or nursing assistant. The registered nurse found herself in the role of an administrator or "paper pusher" with little or no direct client contact. The frequent result was frustration for both the nurse and client. The team concept has been modified and even eliminated in some institutions and replaced by primary nursing, in which a client or patient is assigned one nurse who plans and coordinates his care and serves as his personal advocate while he is receiving care. This system helps ensure that nursing care plans are devised and modified by qualified registered nurses who know the client/patient well enough to assess his needs and plan acceptable, effective interventions.

Changes have also occurred in the settings in which nurses are employed and in the roles they carry out. In addition to the more traditional nursing settings such as hospitals, physicians' offices, clinics, public health agencies, and schools, nurses are now located in day care centers and preschools, industrial settings, and hospices. Nurses' roles have changed from the original "physicians' handmaidens" to more active and responsible participation in health care delivery. Nurses now may seek advanced preparation to become nurse practitioners in such specialty areas as adult health and geriatrics, pediatrics, and school nursing (the school nurse practitioner, which is described in Chapter 20). Indeed, some nurses have expanded their horizons beyond even these roles, choosing to establish and maintain an independent nursing practice; such practices have been set up in both rural and urban areas.

While these are by no means an exhaustive list of changes in nursing, they are examples of the many and rapid changes confronting nurses today. In fact, confrontation with change often awaits the new graduate at her first job in nursing. This is because changes in the "real world" of nursing practice often occur at a disparate rate with nursing school curriculum revisions. Thus, for example, students prepared to work within the structure of a nursing "team" may find as new graduates that team nursing is "out" and primary nursing or some alternative structural pattern is "in." Or, students from particularly innovative and progressive nursing schools may graduate with expectations of true collegial relationships with physicians and commitment to provision of truly client-centered nursing care at an unhurried pace. For new graduates who are eager to practice this kind of professional nursing as they learned it in school, the realities of day-to-day practice (as they soon discover) may result in what Kramer (1974) describes as "reality shock."

The obvious conclusion to be drawn from all these examples is that change is inevitable in nursing and is occurring at a frenetic rate. Since change cannot be avoided, nurses must therefore learn to deal with it effectively, including how to initiate or *plan* change so that there is some control over the outcome and some opportunity to adjust and accept it. The purpose of this chapter is to assist nurses to cope more effectively with change by presenting a very basic discussion of the following:

1. The nature of change
2. The process of planned change
3. Strategies and principles for effecting planned change
4. The importance of legislative/political savvy

THE NATURE OF CHANGE

According to Webster, to *change* means to "make different in some particular" or modify.

Beyond this basic definition, there seems to be little agreement in the literature concerning the types or classification of changes. Some authors (Schaller, 1972) classify changes as structural, technological, behavioral, or attitudinal. Others (Hersey and Blanchard, 1977) describe changes of knowledge, behavior, attitudes, and organization performance. Bennis et al. (1961) present a more elaborate typology of change, including coercive change, indoctrination, technocratic change, interactional change, socialization change, emulative change, natural change, and planned change. However, for the purposes of this book, a simpler classification of change, based on the work of Bennis et al. (1961, 1969) and Gerlach and Hine (1973), will be briefly described. Specifically, four types of change will be highlighted: developmental change, revolutionary change, evolutionary change, and planned change.

Developmental change

Developmental change can be thought of as both a personal internal process and a social interactive process. In the former instance, *developmental change* is defined by Webster as a process of "gradually unfolding," such as the expected growth and development of an infant into an adult. Although the process of human growth and development generally follows a predictable series of stages, the development of professional persons such as school nurses may *not* be predictable and will not necessarily occur in an ordered sequence. Thus the historical development of the school nurse role (Chapter 1) has been somewhat haphazard and unguided and has resulted in the current lack of unity among school nurses as well as lack of agreement about future roles and functions appropriate for their practice.

Instead of focusing on the developmental changes that occur within individuals as just described, Gerlach and Hine (1973) direct their attention to developmental change within social systems. According to their point of view, *developmental change* is synonymous with "reform" and refers to change that attempts to reduce the society's internal conflicts by adding to or somehow improving the existing social system. In other words (1973:12), developmental changes ". . . help the society adjust, incrementally, to the changing situations it faces." Thus developmental change is a gradual process by which a society adapts to the stresses or changing situations it faces. And, as Gerlach and Hine (1973) note, developmental change does *not* require a "radical shift" in the society's goals and values; rather, developmental change is often initiated by persons who want those goals and values implemented more effectively. In other words, "developmental social change elaborates on or brings to full realization all the potentials of a basic social pattern" (Gerlach and Hine, 1973:13).

Revolutionary change

A second type of change is *revolutionary change*, which Gerlach and Hine (1973:24) define as "radical alteration of fundamental social structures, a change in the direction of basic social patterns." However, as they caution, the fact that revolutionary change entails a "radical" shift in social structure does *not* necessarily mean that such change is "bad" or based on violence and bloodshed. In addition, although some basic distinctions between developmental change and revolutionary change are immediately apparent, in actuality, distinguishing between the two is not always easy (Gerlach and Hine, 1973).

Table 19-1 summarizes the key differences between developmental and revolutionary change as described by Gerlach and Hine (1973). As depicted in Table 19-1, there are four key differences between those two types of change. The first distinction concerns the social balance, or equilibrium. In developmental change, the society maintains its "dynamic equilibrium" so that societal elements such as social, religious, political, and economic institutions are "more or less complementary and mutually reinforcing" (Gerlach and Hine, 1973:12). In contrast, revolutionary change disrupts the status quo or "workable balance" of the social system, thus hurling the system out of its established equilibrium (Gerlach and Hine, 1973).

The second important distinction between developmental and revolutionary change concerns the effect of each on social goals and values. As noted earlier, developmental change does *not* require a radical shift in the society's goals or guiding and motivating values; instead, the emphasis is on finding more effective ways to implement those goals and values. Revolutionary change, on the other hand, involves "fundamental transformations" in the societal structure and setting *new* social goals and directions (Gerlach and Hine, 1973:13).

The third area of contrast between these two types of change involves the perceptions of those persons affected by and participating in the change effort. In the case of developmental change, the reaction of persons holding positions of social, economic, or political power is, typically, to regard the change as "challenging" and as evidence of "progress" (Gerlach and Hine, 1973). However, those same powerful persons are likely to view revolutionary change as threatening to them and their positions. In addition, revolutionary change can be threatening to other elements of the society as well. For example, using the "trinity of class distinctions" colorfully described by Alinsky in his widely quoted *Rules for Radicals* (1971), which is intended to be a "pragmatic primer for realistic radicals," there are three basic social strata: (1) the "Haves," or upper class, who possess power, money, status, luxury, and security and who therefore wish to maintain the status quo, unchanged; (2) the "Have-Nots," or lower class, who are characteristically impoverished and "politically impotent" (1971: 18) and thus are eager to *get* what the Haves

Table 19-1. Comparison of developmental and revolutionary change

Developmental change	Revolutionary change
System is in "dynamic equilibrium"	Disruption of the system's "workable balance"; *no* equilibrium
No radical shift in social goals or values	"Fundamental transformations" in social structure; *new* societal goals and directions
Reactions of persons holding positions of social, economic, or political power: developmental change viewed as "challenging" and thought of as "progress"	Reactions of persons holding positions of social, economic, or political power: revolutionary change seen as "threatening" by those in power and may also threaten those who propose it
Achieved using existing problem-solving and decision-making procedures and rules	Rejects "conventional" problem-solving strategies; violation of the "rules" and use of unpredictable and unexpected methods

want to keep; and (3) the "Have-a-Little, Want Mores," or middle class, who are torn between hanging on to what they have (and the status quo) and seeking change to get more, an ideological struggle that, according to Alinsky (1971:19), transforms them into "social, economic, and political schizoids." Revolutionary change may be threatening for all three groups: the Haves may fear loss of their material wealth and power; the Have-a-Little, Want Mores, while they may want to "get" more, nonetheless may view revolutionary change as jeopardizing what little they have; and the Have-Nots may prefer the certainty of their present situation to the uncertainty (and potentially *worse* situation) that may result after the change. Thus, while both the Have-Nots and the Have-a-Little, Want Mores may benefit from revolutionary change, they also must consider the possibility that the change would be detrimental to them.

The fourth major distinction between developmental change and revolutionary change, as characterized by Gerlach and Hine (1973), concerns the strategies of achieving each. Thus, while developmental change is achieved by employing *existing* problem-solving and decision-making procedures and rules, such as the judicial system, revolutionary change entails *rejection* of "conventional" problem-solving strategies. Since proponents of revolutionary change obviously do not believe in the existing system with its goals and institutions, they likewise summarily reject its rules. Indeed, changing the rules may become an end in itself, with disruption of the existing decision-making process as an alternative goal (Gerlach and Hine, 1973). Thus, initiators of revolutionary change are likely to violate the rules by substituting unpredictable and unexpected methods, such as "sit-ins" and other kinds of public demonstrations.

In concluding this discussion of the similarities and differences between developmental and revolutionary change, it is important to note that sometimes a change which seems to be developmental ultimately results in fundamental or radical change(s) in the social system and thus is actually a *revolutionary* change (Gerlach and Hine, 1973). In addition, contrary to popular belief, such revolutionary changes are *not* necessarily initiated by "antiestablishment" forces, nor is bloodshed a prerequisite. In fact, many revolutionary changes begin as developmental changes or may at least *appear* initially

to be developmental changes and are often brought about by persons in positions of social, political, or economic power in the society or "establishment" (Gerlach and Hine, 1973). In other words, whether a particular change is viewed as developmental or revolutionary may depend on its long-range outcome and extent of its impact on the existing social order.

Evolutionary change

As defined by Webster, *evolution* is "a process of continuous change from a lower, simpler, or worse to a higher, more complex, or better state" and is synonymous with "growth" and "unfolding." Thus evolutionary change is a gradual process. Although evolutionary change is commonly thought of as the long-term outcome of developmental change, Gerlach and Hine (1973:26) define *evolutionary change* as an "interweaving" of *both* developmental and revolutionary change. As they point out, periods of developmental change are generally followed by what they term a *revolutionary breakthrough* that permanently changes the social structure. The revolutionary breakthrough results in destruction of the old pattern or social structure and is accompanied by construction of the new. When the net effect of the destruction of the old (revolution) and construction of the new (development) is a change to a "higher, more complex, or better" state, then the change is considered to have been evolutionary. In other words, evolutionary change is the outgrowth of both developmental and revolutionary changes.

Planned change

The fourth type of change to be highlighted in this discussion is *planned change,* which has been defined as "a deliberate and collaborative process involving change-agent and client-systems . . . brought together to solve a problem or . . . to plan and attain an improved state of functioning in the client-system by utilizing and applying valid knowledge" (Bennis et al. 1961: 11). Thus planned change entails mutual goal setting and an equal power ratio (between client and change agent) and "deliberativeness" of both parties.

As previously discussed, planned change is a process with which nurses in all settings and at all hierarchical levels must become comfortable and adept. If nursing is to evolve into a respected and freestanding profession, nurses must actively participate in the planning and implementation of appropriate changes affecting nursing practice. This is especially true for school nurses, who are continually faced with the threat of elimination from the school setting. For school nurses to achieve needed changes affecting their practice, such as improved educational preparation, meaningful certification regulations and procedures, and realistic nurse-pupil ratios, will require carefully planned and executed changes. For that reason, careful attention to the process of planned change is encouraged.

THE PROCESS OF PLANNED CHANGE

As with some of the other systematic processes discussed in this book (specifically, the nursing process and research process), there is no absolute agreement in the available literature concerning the precise number and labeling of the steps in the process of planned change. Some authorities (Lewin, 1947) describe a three-step process; others (Longest, 1976) describe planned change as a six-phase process that closely parallels the problem-solving process. Still other researchers and authorities (Lippitt et al., 1958), through research that expanded the three phases ("unfreezing," "moving," and "refreezing") of Lewin (1947), characterize planned change as a seven-step process. In addition, Schaller (1972) briefly highlights several other planned change models located during his review of the literature, each

of which incorporates a different number of steps, the labels for which are unique to the particular philosophy and professional orientation of the author(s).

As a result of his literature search concerning models for planned change, Schaller (1972) came to two conclusions: (1) there is no one "right" model of planned change that will be universally appropriate for all change agents in all situations and (2) each person initiating planned change (also referred to as a *change agent*) will need to select the model she is most comfortable with and modify it as needed for her particular needs, personality, and circumstances.

Schaller's conclusions seem to be both reasonable and pragmatic. For that reason, the model or process of planned change presented in this chapter has been adapted from the models and processes described by three sources: Lewin (1947), Lippitt et al. (1958), and Longest (1976). The process of planned change below includes six distinct steps (eight, if the two subphases of step 3 are included). Although I have arbitrarily determined the precise sequencing and labeling of the steps in the process, I have attempted to illustrate the similarity and congruence between the process of planned change and the nursing process. For further clarity, my view of the congruence of the two systematic processes is depicted in Table 19-2. Ideally, if nurses can accept the notion that these pro-

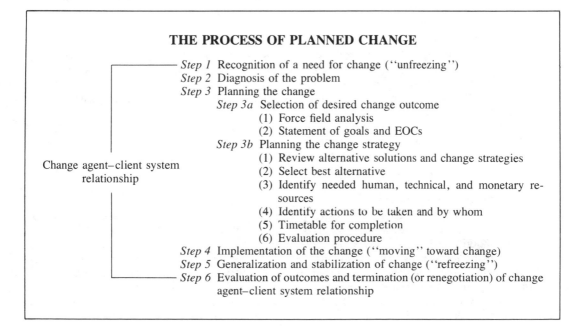

THE PROCESS OF PLANNED CHANGE

Change agent–client system relationship

Step 1 Recognition of a need for change ("unfreezing")
Step 2 Diagnosis of the problem
Step 3 Planning the change
    Step 3a Selection of desired change outcome
        (1) Force field analysis
        (2) Statement of goals and EOCs
    Step 3b Planning the change strategy
        (1) Review alternative solutions and change strategies
        (2) Select best alternative
        (3) Identify needed human, technical, and monetary resources
        (4) Identify actions to be taken and by whom
        (5) Timetable for completion
        (6) Evaluation procedure
Step 4 Implementation of the change ("moving" toward change)
Step 5 Generalization and stabilization of change ("refreezing")
Step 6 Evaluation of outcomes and termination (or renegotiation) of change agent–client system relationship

Table 19-2. Congruence of nursing process and planned change process

Nursing process	Planned change process
Step 1 Assessment Data collection Nursing diagnosis	*Step 1* Recognition of a need for change ("unfreezing") *Step 2* Diagnosis of the problem
Step 2 Planning	*Step 3* Planning the change *Step 3a* Selection of desired change outcome *Step 3b* Planning the change strategy
Step 3 Implementation	*Step 4* Implementation of the change ("moving")
Step 4 Evaluation	*Step 5* Generalization and stabilization of change ("refreezing") *Step 6* Evaluation of outcomes and termination (or renegotiation) of change agent–client system relationship

cesses are both similar and congruent, they may be more inclined toward and less hesitant about participation in planned change efforts to improve the process and outcomes of nursing practice.

Identity of change agent and client system

In addition to the divergent opinions in the literature concerning the number, sequencing, and labeling of the steps in the planned change process, there is likewise no agreement concerning the identity of the change agent or her relationship with the client system. Thus a working definition of change agent must be arbitrarily chosen. Therefore, for the purposes of this chapter, the definition of change agent proposed by Bennis et al. (1976:5) will be used; according to their definition, the term *change agent* refers to "the helper, the person or group who is attempting to effect change." In further discussion of their definition, Bennis et al. (1976) emphasize their belief that the change agent may be *either* a person or group found *within* the organization *or* a person or group brought in from *outside* the client system or society. In contrast, Lippitt et al. (1958) argue that the change agent must be a person or group from *outside* the organization, which is a philosophical position that Bennis et al. and I have rejected as being too narrow. The *client system* is the recipient of the change agent's assistance and may be a person or a group such as a family, organization, or society (Lippitt et al., 1958; Bennis et al., 1976).

Role of the change agent

Using the definition of change agent proposed by Bennis et al. (1976), the role of the change agent is to act as a "helper" to assist the client system (individual or group) to plan, implement, and evaluate the outcomes of a planned, deliberate change effort. Thus the change agent may be any helping person, such as a health care professional, or may be a "professional" change agent—that is, a person or group who specializes in assisting groups and organizations to initiate change. Although to many people the term change agent connotes a person specializing in organizational change, it is important for all helping professionals, especially nurses, to view themselves as change agents. Indeed, until nurses (and school nurses in particular) begin to view themselves as change agents who can improve health care delivery and begin to act on that perception, nursing will continue to be dominated and controlled by other more powerful groups and coalitions within the health care system.

Lippitt et al. (1958) believe that regardless of professional affiliation and background, every change agent operates on the basis of assumptions she has made (consciously or unconsciously) concerning the following:

1. The nature of the client system
2. How the client system got into trouble—that is, how the problem developed
3. The nature of the problem
4. The actions or processes that will solve the problem or relieve the trouble

5. The ways in which the change agent can personally intervene to help bring about the desired change

Because of these individual differences in values, assumptions, and perspective, there can be no one "right" role for a change agent or helper. One must adopt a helping style and approach that is compatible with her values and assumptions. Indeed, such individual differences have resulted in a number of theories and approaches to helping (a few of which are discussed in Chapter 11) from which professional helpers may either select one particular theory/approach or eclectically adopt scientific elements of several theories/approaches.

In addition to individual variations in assumptions and approaches to their roles, change agents likewise may differ in the manner in which their relationship with the client system is initiated. Lippitt et al. (1958) describe three basic ways in which the change agent and client system may be brought together. First, the change agent may observe or hypothesize the existence of a problem within the client system and may either offer to help correct it or may try to stimulate the client system's own awareness of the problem. An example of this might be the school nurse who believes that because teachers in her school have a limited and stereotyped view of her role, they only refer students to her who are sick or in need of first aid. Acting as change agent in this example, the school nurse might plan to discuss her role and her conception of appropriate referrals at an upcoming faculty meeting. The second way in which the change agent-client system relationship may be initiated is through the intercession of a third party, who somehow becomes aware of the problem and brings the two (change agent and client system) together. An example of this might be the teenage girl who, suspecting that her best friend may be pregnant, refers her to the school nurse for counseling and assistance with decision making. The third method of initiating the change agent-client system relationship, and according to Lippitt et al. (1958) the most common, is for the client system to recognize its own problem and seek help directly. Thus, the troubled adolescent who is struggling with peer relationships and the task of identity formation may refer himself to the school nurse for help in sorting out his feelings.

Regardless of the manner in which change agent and client system are brought together, their relationship is critically important in determining the outcome of the change effort. Therefore, as with any helping relationship, it is important for the change agent and client system to establish rapport, build trust, and maintain congruence of purpose if their planned change is to be achieved and ultimately stabilized. Maintenance of an effective working relationship between them may be enhanced by use of the contract-setting process (Chapter 14); through overt contracting, they can thus determine not only what they are trying to accomplish (goal) but also how they are going to work together to achieve it (process). Since their relationship must remain viable until after the stabilization of the change (p. 441), the importance of open and effective communication between them throughout the change process cannot be overstated.

Planned change: a systematic process

Having described the nature and reiterated the importance of the change agent-client system relationship, it is now appropriate to discuss the process of planned change. On p. 441, as well as within the context of this discussion, six distinct steps in the planned change process are represented. These steps will be discussed in the chronological order given on p. 441, although the reader is cautioned that in reality, these steps may overlap to varying degrees and may repeat themselves (Lippitt et al., 1958).

Step 1: Recognition of a need for change ("unfreezing")

Before any change can be planned, a particular need or problem must arise. This need may be a minor "irritation" or a major problem with far-reaching consequences. However, before planned change can be initiated, the "irritation" or need must be translated into what Lippitt et al. (1958:131) call "problem awareness." That is, the client system must be consciously aware of the problem, actively desire to change the status quo to solve or ameliorate the problem, and want the assistance of a change agent.

If the client system is a group or society, the degree of problem awareness will probably not be uniform throughout the system's subparts. In other words, some members of the client system may be acutely aware of the problem and strongly motivated to change, whereas other system members may be unaware of the problem, apathetic about it, or ambivalent. Thus, at least initially, the change agent may find herself working with only a fraction of the total client system (Lippitt et al., 1958).

In addition to being aware of the problem, the client system needs to believe that change is possible and that things can get better. This kind of hope allows the client system to risk the change process and to be optimistic about its outcome. If the client system has repeatedly tried to change without success, it may feel discouraged and defeated and be reluctant to try again (Lippitt et al., 1958).

Assuming, then, that the client system is aware of the problem, desires to change, believes that change is possible and desirable, and is willing to work with a change agent, the next consideration is initiating the change agent–client system relationship. A potentially major problem that may arise is availability of suitable and qualified change agents (Lippitt et al., 1958). Sometimes, especially in isolated or remote communities, qualified change agents may not be available or accessible. Even in well-populated metropolitan areas the number of qualified change agents may be inadequate to meet the demand. In the case of the school nurse as a change agent, the numbers of schools each nurse is expected to serve plus the overwhelmingly large student–school nurse ratios with which she must contend conspire to minimize the nurse's availability and effectiveness. In areas where qualified change agents exist both within and without the client system, locating the change agent may be a problem. Indeed, for the client seeking a physician as change agent for a particular health problem, the complexity and consequent specialization that characterize contemporary medical practice nearly require that the client diagnose his problem as a means of locating the appropriate specialist!

This developing problem awareness and recognition of a need for change constitute what Lewin (1947) calls "unfreezing." Again, as described earlier, this awareness typically occurs in one of three ways: through the observation or hypothesis of a change agent, through the intervention of a third party, or through the client system's recognition of its own problem (Lippitt et al., 1958).

However, regardless of the way in which "unfreezing" occurs, the change agent–client system relationship is critically important in determining the outcome of the change effort. For that reason, the change agent and client system

need to reach early accord concerning the nature of their relationship. During step 1, their helping relationship is established, and the contracting process (Chapter 14) is begun following development of problem awareness and recognition of the need for change. Although the change agent may come from within or without the client system, in either case the client seeks a change agent who identifies with the client system's values and empathizes with its needs and yet at the same time is neutral enough to be objective in assessing and analyzing the client system's problem (Lippitt et al., 1958).

Step 2: Diagnosis of the problem

The task during step 2 is to further clarify and delimit the problem (Longest, 1976). Since it is possible that the "irritation" which precipitated the client system's awareness of the need for change is only a symptom of the real problem, it is essential for the change agent and client system to identify and agree on the nature of the true problem. If this step is not carried out, the change agent and client system may find themselves working at cross purposes, each convinced that he is addressing the real problem.

As shown in Table 19-2, this step is analogous to the assessment phase (step 1) of the nursing process. In both processes, definition or diagnosis of the problem depends on adequate data collection from all sources relevant to the problem. Depending on the type of problem area under investigation, such data may come from health records, other kinds of records including vital statistics and other statistical sources, or from persons knowledgeable about the client system and its needs (including the client system itself). As with the nursing process, it is important that the data collection be thorough and painstaking to ensure that all relevant information is amassed. Following data collection, the change agent and client system collaboratively review the data to determine the precise nature of the problem. Their "output" at the conclusion of this second step, then, is a clear statement of the true nature of the problem.

Step 3: Planning the change

Once the change agent and client system have determined the nature of the problem, they are ready to begin planning the actual change to correct or ameliorate it. This third step (planning the change) includes two subphases: (1)

selection of desired change outcome and (2) planning the change strategy.

Step 3a: Selection of desired change outcome. Following diagnosis of the problem (step 2), the change agent and client system need to consider the realistic potential for change or improvement in the situation. That is, they must decide whether the outcome they desire is realistic and attainable. Failure to select a realistic outcome may doom the change effort to certain failure and may reduce the client system's willingness to again risk changing at a later time. A conceptual tool that is useful in assessing realistic change potential within a client system is Lewin's (1947) "force field analysis."

FORCE FIELD ANALYSIS. According to Lewin (1947), the likelihood of change or no change in any situation or environment depends on the dynamic interaction of two sets of forces: driving forces and restraining forces. These two groups of opposing forces constitute a "force field" in which the length of the arrows indicates the relative strength of the forces; thus, the longer the arrow, the stronger the force (Fig. 19-1). (NOTE: Although the arrows in Fig. 19-1 are equal in length, thus indicating forces of equal strength, in actuality, the forces in the force field may be of varying strengths.) The *driving forces* are those factors within the situation which favor and "drive" the system toward change. In contrast, the *restraining forces* work in opposition to the driving forces and thus "restrain" the system by providing resistance to change (Lewin, 1947; Watson, 1969). When the driving forces and restraining forces are equal in strength, a state of *quasi-stationary equilibrium* exists (Lewin, 1947; Arndt and Huckabay, 1980). As Lewin (1947) further explains, this quasi-stationary equilibrium is a dynamic balance that can be altered at any time by modifying either set of forces.

Force field analysis can be used both to determine realistic planned outcomes for the change effort, based on careful "diagnosis" of the forces in the situation, and as a means of selecting a change strategy. In this latter context, change is facilitated by (1) adding driving forces, (2) removing or reducing restraining forces or resistance factors, and (3) transforming restraining forces into driving forces (Lewin, 1947; Benne and Birnbaum, 1960).

STATEMENT OF GOALS AND EOCs. Following careful analysis of the driving and restraining forces, the change agent and client system can proceed with negotiation of mutually acceptable goals (planned outcomes) for their contract. By this time, if their force field analysis was thorough and unbiased, they should be able to set goals that are realistic and measurable. To be useful, EOCs must be stated in specific, measurable (observable and/or quantifiable) terms (Chapters 13 and 14). EOCs represent the breakdown of individual goals (planned outcomes) into individual component parts or behaviors, which, when collectively achieved, equal attainment of the overall goal. For the change agent and client system, EOCs that are collaboratively determined and agreed to facilitate both the process of change (by specifying *exactly* what the intended outcomes are) and the evaluation of their mutual efforts.

Step 3b: Planning the change strategy. The second subphase of step 3 is planning the strategy to be used in effecting the desired change. As classified by Chin and Benne (1976), change strategies generally fall into one of three groups: (1) power-coercive, (2) empirical-rational, and (3) normative-reeducative. These strategies will be discussed in some detail later in this chapter.

REVIEW ALTERNATIVE SOLUTIONS AND CHANGE STRATEGIES. One of the first tasks during step 3b is to generate as exhaustive a list as possible of the alternative solutions and change strategies that could be used to solve the current

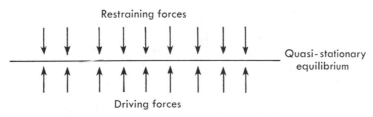

Restraining forces

Quasi-stationary equilibrium

Driving forces

Fig. 19-1. Lewin's force field analysis. (Modified from Lewin, K.: 1947. Human Relations **1**(1):5-41.)

problem facing the client system. Use of techniques such as "brainstorming," in which *all* possible alternatives are listed without prior evaluation of their plausibility or practicality, is suggested. Indeed, if the change agent and client system can break away from the usual logical thought process, which Gerlach and Hine (1973) describe as "vertical thinking," and can instead indulge in the kind of tangential, nonlogical "lateral thinking" proposed by Gerlach and Hine, then perhaps the possible alternatives they identify will be not only exhaustive but also highly creative.

SELECT BEST ALTERNATIVE. Following generation of a list of possible alternative solutions, the change agent and client system are ready to select what they believe is the *best* alternative from their list. To accomplish this, they will need to review each suggested course of action, carefully weighing the "pros" and "cons" of each. This is a point at which their value judgments will be clearly evident, since what may be viewed as a "pro" to one person may be seen as a "con" to another. Lippitt et al. (1958) point out that at this stage in the change process, the client system may get "cold feet." That is, during the process of generating and subsequently choosing solutions for the problem, the client system may begin to realize, perhaps for the first time, that it will have to change its behavior or practices in some way. At this point, the client system may begin to resist and may wish to terminate its relationship with the change agent; to prevent such preliminary termination of their relationship, the change agent will need to employ motivational and human psychology concepts to renew the client system's commitment to the change effort.

IDENTIFY NEEDED HUMAN, TECHNICAL, AND MONETARY RESOURCES. Once a particular strategy has been chosen, the change agent and client system must determine what resources they will need to carry out their plan. As with the contracting process described in Chapter 14, they will need to identify and assess the range of resources each of them (change agent and client system) brings to the relationship. The kinds of resources needed may be human (knowledge, skills, personnel), technical (machinery and equipment), and monetary (including their budget). If resources are needed beyond those which are available from the change agent and client system, some decision must be reached concerning what other resources are needed, where they can be procured, and who will obtain them.

IDENTIFY ACTIONS TO BE TAKEN AND BY WHOM. The next step in the contracting process between the client system and change agent is the division of labor, or deciding who is going to do what. This includes not only decisions concerning who will obtain other needed resources, as discussed in the preceding step, but also decisions concerning exactly what kinds of actions must be carried out to implement the change strategy and who will carry them out. Again, it is important that the division of labor be specific *and* that both parties agree to its terms. Failure to reach agreement and commitment to their plan at this stage could sabotage the entire change effort.

TIMETABLE FOR COMPLETION. Following assembly of needed resources and careful division of labor, the next task is to determine the timetable for completion of the change effort. Depending on the magnitude of the proposed change effort, it may be advisable to set both long-range and short-range time limits or deadlines. If the change is to be carried out in phases or stages, then time limits for each phase could be set. Again, it is important that the timetable, like other aspects of the change effort, be realistic and not overly ambitious. If the time allotted for each phase is too short, the client system may become frustrated and discouraged and be disinclined to complete the change process.

EVALUATION PROCEDURE. The last specific area included in step 3b is determination of the procedure to be used in evaluating the success of the change effort. The outcome of the change effort will of course be measured through use of the EOCs developed during step 3a. At this step, then, the task is to determine *who* will assess the attainment of the EOCs, *how* that assessment will be done, and *when* that evaluation will take place. This, of course, is another area to be considered within the division of labor between the client system and change agent and should be clearly spelled out within their contract.

Step 4: Implementation of the change ("*moving*" toward change)

By the time the change effort is implemented, the change agent and client system should have finalized their helping contract and thus have a clear sense of purpose and process. If their mutual planning has been carefully and completely done, then implementation of the change strategy should proceed smoothly.

This step is obviously crucial to the outcome of the change effort, since it represents the actual movement toward the change. By this time the client system has moved beyond mere planning and into the action phase. For the client system, this step may be seen as the crux of the change process. Because of the importance of this step to the client system, two critical factors must be provided to prevent the client from becoming discouraged and quitting: support and feedback (Lippitt et al., 1958). The client needs support and encouragement to proceed with the change effort at the beginning of the working, or implementation, phase. This support should come from the change agent as a means of reinforcing the client system's desire to change. However, as Lippitt et al. (1958) point out, the client system will be more likely to persevere in its change efforts if it also receives support from other subparts of the client system. Thus, in the case of an organizational change, if the subparts of the organization lend their support, encouragement, and cooperation to those subparts who have been contracting with the change agent, the chances of undermining and sabotage are lessened and the active members of the client system will be more likely to continue their change strategy efforts. However, in addition to the need for support from the change agent and other members of the client system, the client system also depends on feedback from others concerning the impact of its efforts. Indeed, Lippitt et al. (1958) describe situations in which the client system, having received no feedback concerning the effects of its change efforts, became erroneously convinced that the strategy did not work and prematurely abandoned a workable and succeeding plan. Thus, during this critical phase of implementation, the likelihood that the client system will persist in its change efforts and enjoy moderate success will be enhanced if adequate support and feedback are provided.

It would be both naive and misleading to discuss implementation of change strategies without acknowledging the possibility of resistance to change. As implied in the discussion of force field analysis, resistance to change in the form of restraining forces may be present before any change effort is undertaken. However, it is also possible that resistance to a proposed change may not surface until the change strategy is well underway. Although it is not possible to predict

with any certainty the likely sources of resistance within any given client system, Watson (1969) has identified a number of sources of resistance that can be considered if and when resistance is encountered.

One of the first sources of resistance to change cited by Watson (1969) is fear of the unknown. It is this fear or anxiety that causes people to cling to behaviors they know are ineffective in preference to adopting other behaviors, the consequences of which are largely unknown or uncertain. This kind of fear of risk taking could be due to insecurity or could be the result of past risk-taking efforts that failed.

A second possible source of resistance to change might be the pressure to adhere to group norms within an organization. Thus, the usual and customary ways of behaving may be so strongly ingrained and accepted that individuals within the system are unable to change them. In this instance, in order for meaningful and lasting change to occur, the norms will have to be changed throughout the organizational system, rather than through the efforts of one or two persons (Watson, 1969).

A third source of change resistance cited by Watson (1969:494) is what he calls "systemic and cultural coherence." Basically, this means that because the client system *is* a system (a fact which is more readily apparent when the client system is a group or organization), any change in one part will affect other parts of the system as well. Therefore a change that is viewed as positive by some members of the client system may be seen as threatening to others, who will then actively resist its implementation. For this reason, it is important for the change agent and the pro change elements or members of the client system to try to predict the outcome of the proposed change effort on other persons and groups beyond themselves, so that resistance can be anticipated and plans for counteracting it can be formulated.

A fourth possible source of resistance to change rests within the vested interests of various elements of the client system or other groups and organizations who are likely to be affected by the change (Watson, 1969). Thus, for example, school nurses who are graduates of hospital diploma programs cannot realistically be expected to overwhelmingly support a proposal requiring all school nurses to have baccalaureate degrees, since such a stance would likely cost them their jobs. Unless persons or groups believe that their vested interests will be protected (or viable substitutes provided), they are likely to strongly resist the change efforts. Thus the change agent may need to show them how the change will benefit them if their cooperation is to be obtained.

A fifth source of resistance to change efforts described by Watson (1969) concerns those elements of a culture, society, or organization which are considered "sacrosanct," or untouchable. Thus practices and rituals that have been traditionally carried out may persist. Perhaps this is nowhere more evident than in the nursing profession, where many archaic patterns have been rigidly perpetuated "because we've always done it this way."

Finally, another important source of resistance to change described by Watson (1969) concerns rejection of "outsiders." Often, individuals and groups are suspicious of persons and ideas imported from outside their society, culture, or organization and may be outright hostile. As Watson notes, research findings have documented the nearly universal occurrence of this phenomenon among primates as well as humans. The apparent antidote to this reaction, according to Watson (1969), is to obtain the support and participation of "local" persons or insiders so that the change effort cannot be dismissed as a "foreign" affair.

Probably the best defense against resistance to change is careful planning, including anticipation of likely sources of resistance and development of contingency or backup plans to counteract any resistance that may occur. Again, because the implementation step is crucial in determining the outcome of the change effort, it is important to minimize and overcome any serious resistance that may develop during the change process, so that movement toward change can be unobstructed.

Step 5: Generalization and stabilization of change ("refreezing")

After the change has been implemented during step 4, the next step in the process is to ensure the stability or permanence of the change (Lewin, 1947; Lippitt et al., 1958). Lewin (1947) was the first to emphasize the importance of this step, describing the need to "freeze" (or "refreeze") the changed behavior or pattern at the new level. As Lippitt et al. (1958) point out, stabilization of the change is essential to prevent backsliding into the previous behaviors or patterns; without conscious efforts to reinforce the change, they say, the cli-

ent system will likely slide back into its former ineffective ways, and the change effort will have failed.

An important factor in ensuring the stabilization and permanence of the change is the degree of generalization (Lippitt et al., 1958). That is, the greater the degree or extent of spread of the change to other subparts of the client system or to neighboring systems, the more likely it is that the change will endure. Thus if a school nurse who has implemented a problem-oriented recording format for her pupils' health records can succeed in getting other school nurses within her district to adopt the same format, then the likelihood that this change in procedure will persist is enhanced.

Stabilization of the change or "freezing" can also be facilitated through provision of positive feedback concerning the effects of the change (Lippitt et al., 1958). If those persons or system subparts affected by the change can identify benefits from the change, they are more likely to follow through with it and support it. However, in addition to expressions of the value of the change, it is also essential that "hard" objective data be available to *measure* the impact of the change on the client system. Therefore it is important to devise (during step 3a) EOCs which are meaningful, relevant, and measurable so that the impact of the change can be objectively determined.

The change agent will need to be especially vigilant during this step of the process, since the client system may become prematurely complacent about the outcome of the change effort, not realizing the importance of and need for stabilization efforts. The change agent as the "expert" will need to assist the client system in efforts to generalize the change (facilitating its spread to other subparts or systems) and stabilize it through collection and evaluation of positive feedback (both subjective and objective data). The change agent may wish to schedule periodic follow-up sessions with the client system over an extended period of time to monitor the stabilization process and to provide support for the client system as it adapts to the change.

Step 6: Evaluation of outcomes and termination (or renegotiation) of change agent–client system relationship

The last step in the change process includes two primary elements: evaluation of the outcomes of the change effort and termination or renegotiation of the helping relationship between the change agent and client system.

Although evaluation is an ongoing process that is appropriate throughout the change effort, a summative or terminal evaluation at the conclusion of the change process is especially important in determining the relative success of the change strategy and any need for further change (Longest, 1976). The procedure to be used for this final evaluation is the one planned during step 3b and should be based on the EOCs developed during step 3a. Both the change agent and client system should participate in this evaluation process, with other persons or groups included as appropriate.

Depending on the outcome of the evaluation process, the relationship between the change agent and client system may be terminated (Lippitt et al., 1958) or renegotiated. As with other kinds of helping relationships, it is important for the change agent and client system to begin planning for the termination of their relationship almost as soon as it is initiated. Their mutual contract should therefore identify *when* the relationship will terminate or be evaluated. In addition, it may be prudent for the change agent to periodically remind the client system of their upcoming termination as the relationship progresses; otherwise, the client system may "forget" that the relationship will end and may become overly dependent on the change agent (Lippitt et al., 1958). If the termination of the change agent–client system relationship is not handled effectively, the permanence of the change may be jeopardized and both parties may be left feeling dissatisfied. If the client system is left with unresolved or negative feelings about the relationship, then it may be less willing to risk changing in the future. In contrast, if the client system has learned problem-solving techniques or developed other mechanisms to bolster its confidence and independence, then it may adapt quite readily to termination of the change agent–client system relationship. If for some reason the objectives of their contract have not yet been achieved, the change agent and client system may decide to renegotiate their contract for a specified period of time to finish their task. However, whether their decision is to terminate or renegotiate their contract, because of the critical importance of their relationship in determining the outcome of the change effort, their decision-making process should be both conscious and collaborative.

As described in this discussion, planned change is a systematic process involving explicit collaboration and cooperation between a change agent and client system to plan, implement, and evaluate a specific desired outcome. Having described the process of planned change, it is now appropriate to move on to discussion of strategies and principles for effecting change.

STRATEGIES AND PRINCIPLES FOR EFFECTING PLANNED CHANGE
Strategies for changing

According to Chin and Benne (1976), planned change strategies can be grouped into three major categories: empirical-rational, normative-reeducative, and power-coercive strategies. Depending on the nature of the planned change, any one of these strategies may be appropriate, or a combination of two or more strategies might be used. However, for the purposes of this discussion, each of the three categories will be considered separately.

Empirical-rational strategies

As characterized by Chin and Benne (1976), the underlying premise of empirical-rational strategies is that man is a rational being and will act in his rational self-interest once it has been revealed to him. Thus these kinds of strategies focus on demonstrating to the persons whom the proposed change will affect, how they can expect to benefit from the change—that is, how (rationally) the change will serve their self-interest. Empirical-rational strategies thus assume that once the potential benefits are rationally documented, the change will be adopted (Chin and Benne, 1976).

Among the examples of empirical-rational strategies they cite, Chin and Benne (1976) point out that basic research and the application of its findings depend on rational thought processes and empirical methods. Thus to the extent that research studies are carefully designed, rigorously controlled, and truthfully reported, the application of their findings to actual planned change efforts represents an empirical-rational strategy. Another example of an empirical-rational strategy cited by Chin and Benne (1976) is education, particularly educational efforts in which facts and data are disseminated and their applicability is discussed. In this sense, then, educational efforts in which new information is presented or new relationships among known facts are clarified can become the rational basis for a change in behavior.

Normative-reeducative strategies

As described by Chin and Benne (1976), the underlying premise of normative-reeducative strategies is that man is motivated not only by rationality and intelligence but also by sociocultural norms and his commitment to them. These norms are supported by man's value system and attitudes; therefore change in one's pattern of behavior depends on changing the "normative orientations" to previous patterns and developing commitment to new patterns. Thus change in normative orientations involves changes in the client system's attitudes, values, skills, and/or significant relationships (both internal and external).

To further clarify the nature of normative-reeducative strategies, Chin and Benne (1976: 32-33) identify the following five elements that are common to all strategies of this type:

1. An emphasis on *involvement of the client system* in articulating its problem and developing programs for change and improvement
2. Recognition of the *importance of alteration or reeducation* concerning the client system's values, norms, attitudes, and relationships
3. *Mutual and collaborative intervention* by the change agent and client system in defining and solving the problem
4. An emphasis on *bringing into conscious awareness the "nonconscious elements"* which may be hampering the change effort, so that they may be examined and "reconstructed"
5. *Reliance* by the change agent and client system *on behavioral science concepts and methods* in solving the problem

In other words, normative-reeducative strategies are predicated on the belief that "clarification and reconstruction of values is of pivotal importance in changing" (Chin and Benne, 1976:33).

In their discussion of specific applications of normative-reeducative strategies, Chin and Benne (1976) identify two basic approaches that are typically used. The first focuses on improving the client system's problem-solving processes, which might be accomplished through organizational development programs. The second normative-reeducative approach they describe focuses on fostering growth and self-actualization among the individuals who make up an organizational, group, or community client system; methods used include psychotherapy, laboratory training sessions, and group training experiences described as "therapy for normals" (Chin and Benne, 1976:36). Although there are some differences between these two approaches, there are two important similarities: both often use "temporary systems" such as a residential laboratory experience or a workshop to produce growth in client system participants, and both emphasize the importance of "experience-based learning" in producing lasting change within human systems (1976:37).

As a final comment concerning normative-reeducative strategies, it should be noted that normative-reeducative strategies are similar to empirical-rational strategies (discussed previously) to the extent that both use knowledge to help effect change. However, there is a key difference between these two groups of strategies as well: whereas empirical-rational strategies attempt to effect change through presentation of "knowledge, information, or intellectual rationales for action and practice" (Chin and Benne, 1976:23), normative-reeducative strategies are based on the belief that improvement in knowledge is not enough to effect change; rather, meaningful and lasting change is presupposed to depend on normative reorientations or values' clarification. Because these two groups of strategies are complementary, change agents may at times wish to employ a combination of both strategies; this might entail an initial workshop to present some new information, followed by an experiential session or training laboratory to apply that new knowledge and to clarify and reconstruct attitudes and values.

Power-coercive strategies

The third major category of planned change strategies described by Chin and Benne (1976) is power-coercive. Power, which is the ability to influence others, is an ingredient of all change efforts and strategies to some extent (Chin and Benne, 1976). However, in this group of strategies, wielding power is vital to the success of the change effort. The power may be political, such as use of the legislative process to pass important laws to correct problems within a society, or the power may be economic, as exemplified by federal programs in which distribution of monies to groups or communities may be restricted or withheld pending compliance with federal regulations regarding its use or regulations requiring that specific conditions be satisfied. Economic power is therefore coercive, in that it forces individuals or groups to comply under threat of economic losses. Another kind of power that may be used for change is moral power (Chin and Benne, 1976), in which the change agent(s) may try to play on feelings of shame and guilt; this is often the basis for some forms of child punishment and discipline and was part of the power used by Viet Nam War protesters, who were convinced that the war was immoral.

In addition to classifying power-coercive strategies on the basis of their power source (political, economic, or moral), these strategies can also be grouped according to whether their use of power is legitimate, based on legal or administrative authority, or simply coercive and/or antiestablishment in nature (Chin and Benne, 1976). Thus if the federal government issues a grant to a university for nursing education while at the same time placing some external controls over the curriculum in which the money is to be used, that action represents both use of legitimate (legally sanctioned) and coercive (controlled compliance) power. If, on the other hand, students registered in a nursing program that is federally funded (as in the preceding example) initiate a boycott of classes and sit-in demonstrations to convince university administrators to improve or modify that curriculum, then their tactic is clearly coercive and not legitimate (administratively sanctioned). Thus, in some instances the goal may be for those who have the power and control to maintain it, while other persons or groups (such as the Have-Nots or Have-a-Little, Want Mores) seek to gain power and control.

Power-coercive strategies as used in real life situations may be either violent or nonviolent. Violent coercive strategies rely on use of physical force to achieve the change goal and thus use physical power as well as the other power sources already discussed. Perhaps one of the most shocking and dramatic examples of the use of violent power-coercive strategies in this country was the kidnapping of newspaper heiress Patty Hearst by the avowed radical group the Symbionese Liberation Army (SLA) during the early 1970s. Although other kidnappings of famous persons had also attracted national attention and provoked outrage among many Americans (such as the kidnapping of the Lindbergh baby in 1932), the Hearst kidnapping was particularly shocking because the SLA was an unknown group and seemed to lack organization and a clear sense of purpose, despite their

demand that as one condition for Miss Hearst's release her family must donate money and supplies to groups designated as poor and disadvantaged by the SLA.

Tactics like those of the Symbionese Liberation Army have generally been associated with other countries and continents and not with the United States or other stable democracies. Thus, because of the perpetual strife in such areas of the world as the Middle East, the overthrow of the Shah of Iran in 1979 was not a complete surprise. However, the deposition of the Shah by the forces of the Ayatollah Khomeini illustrated a surprising combination of power sources. Khomeini invoked economic power by seeking and, to the amazement of many, getting compliance with his request for a general strike or shutdown of the country's stores, factories, and businesses for an indefinite period. Khomeini also was able to successfully combine religious, or moral, power (his Islamic faith) with political power and the use of physical armed force in working toward his goal of forming an Islamic republic.

There are likewise many examples of use of nonviolent power-coercive tactics for achieving planned change. One of the most obvious and prominent examples in recent history was civil rights leader Martin Luther King, Jr., who led hundreds and at times thousands of blacks (and sympathetic whites) on peace marches throughout the South during the blacks' 1960s struggle for racial equality. Although these marches and the other tactics employed by King and his followers were intended to be nonviolent displays, they were often turned into violent and bloody confrontations by angry and fearful whites.

Because of the economic fluctuations and uncertainty in contemporary America, many groups seeking nonviolent power-coercive changes have found economic sanctions to be very effective. For example, during the early 1970s the American housewife openly rebelled at soaring meat prices in supermarkets; organized and encouraged by a vocal group of housewives, American families across the country successfully forced down meat prices by boycotting meats and substituting cheese, poultry, fish, and other sources of protein into family meals.

Another kind of nonviolent power-coercive strategy that relies on economic power to some extent is work stoppage or striking by workers or employees to gain greater salaries, better working conditions, and additional employee benefits. Although such tactics have tradition-ly been associated with blue collar workers and labor unions, in recent years these tactics have been successfully used by groups that have generally been esteemed as "above" such tactics and too "professional" to strike. Thus, amid the howling protests of the public and some governmental bodies, physicians, nurses, teachers, and other "indispensable" services workers such as police and firemen, have gone on strike to achieve their change goals. Indeed, groups that have never before considered unionism appropriate or desirable, such as college professors and nurses, are, in many institutions and settings, organizing themselves as unions to improve their power base and bargaining position.

As a final example of effective use of economic sanctions, in this case based on a political and moral ideology, the policy of some women's groups, including professional nursing organizations, to avoid scheduling major meetings and conventions in states that have not ratified the Equal Rights Amendment (ERA) illustrates employment of economic sanctions in a manner which repeatedly has sparked intended controversy. Although women have traditionally been viewed (both by men and by themselves) as politically weak and ineffective, their use of methods which directly affect the economy of individual states and communities has proved that women can indeed effectively use economics to increase their political clout.

The final group of power-coercive tactics to be discussed is political activism. An example of the use of legitimate political power to effect change in government is voters' rights, or the capability of the electorate to maintain some control over their government by "controlling" who gets elected to public office. Although voters at times seem to be apathetic about exercising their voting privileges, apparently believing that their votes "don't really make a difference," in actuality voters have made some very powerful decisions. For example, under the sponsorship and leadership of a previously unknown citizen named Howard Jarvis, California voters overwhelmingly approved a controversial bill referred to as Proposition 13, which reformed the entire budgeting process for the state government. This voters' victory became known as the "taxpayers' revolt" and has spread to other states as well.

Another example of the power of voters' rights occurred in the state of Minnesota during the 1978 general elections. Dissatisfied with a lengthening tradition of high taxes, excessive governmental spending and waste, and lack of responsiveness of elected officials to their constituency, the voters surprised the then controlling Democratic-Farmer-Labor (DFL) party by resoundingly defeating many of their candidates, thus disrupting their control of both legislative houses and sending two Republicans to the United States Senate. Although no cries of "power to the people" were heard, no doubt that was the message that DFL party officials received.

In addition to the exercise of one's prerogative to vote, political activism also includes influencing the legislative or law-making process, which will be discussed later in this chapter. As Chin and Benne (1976) point out, both laws and judicial decisions to interpret them are means of effecting change. However, according to Chin and Benne, a frequent mistake of change agents who use legislative process to achieve their goal is their apparent assumption that once the law has been passed, the change has been made. Chin and Benne (1976) suggest that a more effective strategy would be to apply normative-reeducative strategies to encourage acceptance and assimilation into actual practice of the changed law; this would be an example, then, of use of multiple strategies for effecting planned change.

Principles of changing

To help ensure the success of whatever planned change strategies the change agent selects, application of change principles may be useful. From their experiences and observations within educational institutions, Benne and Birnbaum (1960:287-292)* have derived seven such principles for use in effecting and stabilizing planned change in institutions and organizations. Each of these principles will be briefly discussed.

The first principle of changing discussed by Benne and Birnbaum (1960) follows:

To change a subsystem or any part of a subsystem, relevant aspects of the environment must also be changed.

This implies, as they note, that during step 2 of the planned change process (diagnosis of the

---

*Reprinted from "Change Does Not Have To Be Haphazard" by K. D. Benne and M. Birnbaum, in The School Review. Copyright 1960 by The University of Chicago.

problem) the likely impact of the change on other elements or subsystems of the organization should be diagnosed. If the diagnostic process reveals that success of the proposed change depends on changes in other aspects or subsystems of the organization or institution, then those additional changes must be addressed as part of the primary change effort. Interpreting this principle literally, an example of its application might be a school district's efforts to mainstream handicapped children into regular classrooms. Since many handicapped children require extra assistance with personal care as well as with classroom activities and assignments, pupil-teacher ratios would become an important consideration in planning such a change; unless teachers were given reduced class sizes and additional supportive services from the school nurse and other school personnel, the mainstreaming effort might not succeed. In addition, in that example, if the handicapped students being mainstreamed are placed in schools that are not environmentally conducive (that is, having ramps, elevators, and barrier-free bathroom facilities), then their integration into the school will be jeopardized.

The second principle of changing described by Benne and Birnbaum (1960) follows:

To change behavior on any one level of a hierarchical organization, it is necessary to achieve complementary and reinforcing changes in organization levels above and below that level.

An example of the use of this principle might be a decision to increase the efficiency and role effectiveness of school nurses in a particular school district by providing the assistance of school health aides. Probably one of the first tasks to be completed to ensure success of this plan would be to educate the nurses regarding the capabilities and limitations of school health aides and to encourage delegation of appropriate tasks to aides. To further reinforce and complement the change, some change in attitude and behavior on the part of the building principals might be indicated. Thus, perhaps through use of normative-reeducative strategies, the principals can be assisted to better understand the scope of the nurses' role and encouraged to allow nurses the necessary freedom (such as the freedom to leave the building at their own discretion for meetings, conferences, and home visits) to carry it out. At the same time, the aides themselves may need some initial and periodic normative-reeducation regarding their role, to be sure that they are functioning within their capabilities and limitations (legal and individual). Finally, if the job description for the school health aides includes taking over some of the typing and filing that had previously been done by other clerical and secretarial personnel in the school, then the job descriptions and roles for those personnel may also need to be changed as a result of the reduction in their workload.

The third principle of changing proposed by Benne and Birnbaum (1960) is as follows:

The place to begin change is at those points in the system where some stress and strain exist. Stress may give rise to dissatisfaction with the status quo and thus become a motivating factor for change in the system.

In other words, the change agent should identify the leverage point and initiate the change there. Again citing the example used to illustrate the second principle of changing, the movement toward employment of school health aides illustrates this third principle as well. Although many nurses may feel uneasy and threatened by the trend toward incorporation of health aides into the school setting, fearing that the aides may be viewed by administrators as a low-cost substitute for the nurse in the school, the increased workload and demands on nurses' time due to the ever-increasing pupil-nurse ratios may conspire to increase nurses' dissatisfaction with the present situation and thus increase their receptivity to the notion of employment of school health aides.

The fourth principle of changing according to Benne and Birnbaum (1960) is related to the third:

In diagnosing the possibility of change in a given institution, it is always necessary to assess the degree of stress and strain at points where change is sought. One should ordinarily avoid beginning change at the point of greatest stress.

In other words, one should begin at a point where *some* stress and strain exist, but *not* at the point of *greatest* stress. A likely reason for this principle is the fact that at points of maximum stress and strain in an organization there are likely to be persons with vested interests and a great deal "at stake." Thus, the outcome of the situation may be seen as crucial, and the pressure and stress may become more intense. If the change effort does not succeed, the participants may be worse off than they were before the change effort was initiated and may be less willing to risk changing again in the future. Thus, if the point of greatest stress and friction among school nurses in a particular district in carrying out their role effectively is their perceived conflict with school social workers regarding the prerogative and responsibility for making home visits to follow up student health problems, then that conflict should *not* be the first target for the change agent's efforts at improving the nurses' role effectiveness and job satisfaction, since the result could be increased stress and friction between the nurses and social workers.

The fifth principle of changing offered by Benne and Birnbaum (1960) is as follows:

If thoroughgoing changes in a hierarchical structure are desirable or necessary, change should ordinarily start with the policy-making body.

As Benne and Birnbaum point out (1960), the approval of the policy-making or governing body helps legitimize the change, which tends to strengthen support for the change effort. Thus if school nurses in a particular district plan to expand or redefine their role, they would be well advised to begin by presenting their changes to the district's policy-making body, which is probably the school board. This would be especially important if their proposed changes entail modifications in the structure of the school health program and the lines of authority to be used in carrying out the program's objectives.

Following is the sixth principle for effecting planned change as described by Benne and Birnbaum (1960):

Both the formal and the informal organization of an institution must be considered in planning any process of change.

Benne and Birnbaum refer to the well-documented fact that all organizations have both a formal and an informal power structure. The formal power structure includes persons in authority, such as supervisory and administrative personnel, whereas the informal power structure often includes small cliques or social networks formed by the rank and file. Change agents who fail to realize or to heed this fact and who focus their efforts only on the formal power structure of the organization will probably not achieve lasting change. If, for example, a school nurse is concerned about what she perceives to be inappropriate referrals she receives from teachers, such as referral of children for minor first aid that teachers are equipped to handle within their classrooms, she might approach the building principal and ask

him to remind teachers of existing first aid policies. This would illustrate use of the formal authority or power within the school. However, it is possible that this approach alone would not solve the problem; to increase the likelihood that change in the teachers' behavior would occur and be stabilized, the nurse could meet informally with those teachers known to be influential or informal leaders among their peers and try to "sell" them on the importance and necessity of the change.

The seventh principle of changing identified by Benne and Birnbaum (1960) follows:

The effectiveness of a planned change is often directly related to the degree to which members at all levels of an institutional hierarchy take part in the fact-finding and the diagnosing of needed changes and in the formulating and reality-testing of goals and programs of change.

As Benne and Birnbaum explain (1960), participation in the planning of change by those who are to be affected by it increases the chances that new insights will be discovered and that the goals of the change effort will be accepted. For example, if school administrators believe that the student population served by their schools is undergoing demographic changes as indicated by available data, they may decide that some basic revisions in the district's school health program are warranted. To successfully implement this change, the administrators would probably need to solicit participation and input from all personnel and concerned persons affected by the health program, including nurses, pupil personnel services workers, teachers, administrators (including principals), parents, students, and any other groups or individuals who will be affected by the change.

These seven principles, then, when used in conjunction with one or more of the planned change strategies discussed earlier in this chapter and within the context of the planned change process, help ensure the success of any planned change effort.

THE IMPORTANCE OF LEGISLATIVE/POLITICAL SAVVY

As noted in the introduction to this chapter, nursing, like many other professions and disciplines, is undergoing rapid and continuous change. To assist nurses (particularly school nurses) to understand and more effectively cope with change, this chapter has described the general process of planned change efforts. From the numerous examples cited throughout the discussion, it should be obvious that there are settings and situations in which those ideas and processes can be readily applied to improve nursing practice. However, there is one setting or arena for planned change in which nursing has not as yet fully and thoughtfully participated—the legislative/political sphere. Because the importance of legislative/political involvement for nursing cannot be overstated, the remainder of this chapter will attempt to describe political savvy, including how to get it and how to use it.

Nurse power: why it is needed

Despite recent estimates that nearly one million registered nurses are employed in this country (ANA, 1977) and that nurses constitute the largest group of health care professionals in the United States (Bowman and Culpepper, 1974), nurses have exerted relatively little influence on major decision making and policy formulation within our so-called health care delivery "system." Indeed, as Bowman and Culpepper (1974:1056) note:

For too long nurses have underestimated the power they have in being the largest group of health professionals in the nation. If nurses as a group mobilized for patient advocacy, they could radically change the picture of health care delivery in the United States.

The fact that many nurses view themselves (individually and collectively) as powerless is not surprising to Ashley (1973:638), who describes nursing's entire history as

. . . A power struggle: the struggle to obtain a proper education though opposed by more powerful groups, the struggle to throw off the burden of oppression imposed by those groups, the struggle for the freedom to practice without numerous and professionally extraneous restraints and restrictions. Finally, all of us, at one time or another, have struggled with the need to convince others of the value of nursing and its place in the health care scheme.

The problem seems to be that nurses have been their own worst enemy. Despite our potential impact on the health care delivery system based on sheer numbers of nurses, the nursing profession has been hampered by our political naivete and inexperience. Thus, while we too frequently succumbed to the temptation to blame medicine for "taking over" nursing's power and rights of self-determination, in actuality, nursing has allowed its unequal and subservient status to continue by cooperatively functioning

as a "silent majority" that threatens and challenges no one (Ashley, 1973).

The precise roots of powerlessness in nursing are inextricably tied to the historical development and socialization of women in general and particularly women in health care (Ehrenreich and English, 1973; Lieb, 1978). Traditionally, women, including nurses, have been effectively socialized to be passive, dependent, and compliant individuals. Indeed, this "gender-role socialization" has been so successful that even well-educated women have been found to lack "achievement motivation" and to therefore underperform and underachieve within the work world (Lieb, 1978).

Powerlessness has been an especially prevalent and crippling problem for school nurses in recent years. One problem has been their relatively limited and unimaginative job descriptions, which have often included expectations that the nurses considered inappropriate, unrewarding, and at times menial; such expectations have included first aid, record keeping, and attendance monitoring. These limited job descriptions have encouraged school nurses to be doers and not managers, with the result that many nurses have had little direct input into overall planning for the school health program; consequently, school nurses have been primarily involved with implementing programs and services largely designed and planned by others with little or no nursing input. It is thus no wonder that school nurses have felt underused, unimportant, and powerless to effect changes in the system.

The solution to the problem of powerlessness in nursing seems fairly obvious: nurses must learn to recognize and harness the latent power they already possess by virtue of their sheer numbers within the health care delivery system and must actively seek ways to increase their power base and to use their power and influence to advance the status and credibility of the profession as a whole. In other words, as Novello (1976:1) advises, if nurses "are dedicated to improving health care in this country, it is important that we understand the reality and legitimacy of power and politics if we are to make any meaningful contributions."

Nurse power: acquisition and uses
Definitions of power

Power has been defined by many authorities (Ashley, 1973; Bowman and Culpepper, 1974; Archer, 1975; Deloughery and Gebbie, 1975; Novello, 1976; Claus and Bailey, 1977). With the exception of Claus and Bailey (1977), most authorities apparently equate power with influence. In contrast, Claus and Bailey (1977) make an important and useful distinction between the two concepts; in their view, power is the *source* of influence, whereas influence is the result of the proper use of power.

Having made that distinction, Claus and Bailey define *power* as "the ability and willingness to affect the behavior of others" (1977: 17). In their view, power is comprised of three critical elements: (1) *strength,* or ability; (2) *energy,* or willingness to use one's strength (ability); and (3) *action,* the observable performance-based results or outcomes of using strength and energy to achieve goals. These three elements work together, and, if successfully combined, the result is power, which when appropriately wielded influences others.

Bases of power

For nurses to begin efforts to acquire and use power, they must understand not only the definition of power but also the sources or bases from which it is derived. Although the literature includes a variety of classification systems for power sources and bases, in my opinion none of them is entirely satisfactory for this chapter's discussion of power. Therefore I have summarized the important bases, or sources, of power that may be applicable for nurses (below).

Power bases, or sources, can be divided into two basic groups: formal and informal power. *Formal,* or *authorized,* *power* usually accompanies specific *positions* within an organization or society (Claus and Bailey, 1977); formal power or authority is thus organizationally determined (Arndt and Huckabay, 1980). One type of formal power is *coercive power,* which encourages compliance based on fear of punishment or retribution (French and Raven, 1959). An example of coercive power is government's enforcement of existing federal and local laws; police enforcement of laws is an authorized formal power. Another example of use of coercive power is the Theory X manager described in Chapter 18; as noted in that discussion, Theory X managers believe that employees or subordinates *must* be punished and coerced to make them work, since they allegedly are not self-directed or motivated. The opposite of coercive power is *reward power;* by possessing the ability to positively reward others' behavior, the person using reward power obtains compliance with his wishes (French and Raven, 1959; Arndt and Huckabay, 1980). Thus if a subordinate in an organization sees that compliance with his boss's wishes is rewarded through praise, salary increase, promotion, or other *means which are valued by that worker,* he will comply in order to get those rewards. To some extent, coercive and reward powers are also used by many parents as a means of shaping their children's behavior into parentally and socially acceptable patterns.

The third type of formal power base illustrated below is *legitimate,* or *position,* *power.* Legitimate power is generally associated with management positions within organizations (Arndt and Huckabay, 1980) and may include coercive and reward powers as well. It is important to realize that legitimate power is tied to a position or a job title within an organization and is independent of the personal characteristics of the manager. In other words, the power is vested in that *position,* such as principal of a school or school nursing coordinator for a district, and does *not* depend on personal traits or characteristics of the principal or school nursing coordinator; whoever occupies that particular position within the organization, then, possesses the legitimate power granted by the organization to that position.

In contrast with the organizational derivation of formal power, *informal power* is based on personal traits, characteristics, or skills possessed by an individual (Claus and Bailey, 1977; Arndt and Huckabay, 1980). One type of informal power is *expert power,* which is one's ability to affect the behavior of others based on credibility derived from expertise or special knowledge and skills in a particular field or area (French and Raven, 1959; Arndt and Huckabay, 1980). Thus a teacher or researcher who

---

Bases of Power

Coercive power
Reward power
Legitimate, or
   position, power
} **Formal**

Expert power
Referent power
Charismatic power
Traditional power
} **Informal**

is viewed as especially knowledgeable or skilled in some field or specialty (such as school nursing) can influence others to comply with his wishes because his ideas are viewed as credible and worthy of others' respect.

Another base of informal power is *referent power,* which is derived from the admiration of an individual by others (French and Raven, 1959; Arndt and Huckabay, 1980). The individual who possesses referent power is admired for one or more of his personal characteristics and may be looked to as a role model for others. Thus nursing students or graduate nurses who are inexperienced or otherwise in need of guidance in carrying out their roles and responsibilities may identify with one or more nurses (including both practitioners and educators) whom they admire and respect and may consciously or unconsciously emulate the behavior of these role models. Because students and others who have not yet fully developed their own philosophy and "style" for nursing practice may be very impressionable and may be likewise unable to fully discriminate between highly competent and less effective role models, nursing educators and others responsible for orientation and staff development of nursing personnel in all settings need to be aware of the impact of referent power and take actions that ensure provision of role models who *are* competent and who will exert a positive influence on students and staff.

Closely related to referent power is *charismatic power.* According to Webster, *charisma* is "a personal magic of leadership arousing special popular loyalty or enthusiasm for a public figure" or a "special magnetic charm or appeal." Thus, in a sense, charismatic power is a type of referent power in which the leader's "charm" and personality alone may influence the behavior of others. Political and religious leaders often derive much of their power from charisma; examples include Jesus Christ, John F. Kennedy, Billy Graham, Franklin Delano Roosevelt, and Iran's Ayatollah Khomeini. Of course, if a charismatic leader also possesses other attributes that are generally admired and respected, such as skill and expertise in some area, then he may thus combine expert power, referent power, and charismatic power and may therefore increase his sphere of influence.

The last type of informal power to be mentioned in this chapter is *traditional power,* which is based on time-honored and accepted practice and behaviors. This is the basis for the argument "But we've always done it this way." Traditions and other social norms are more influential and tenacious than we sometimes realize, especially in nursing, which is why research data to support or refute these practices and traditions is needed. While traditional power within an organization can be a stabilizing influence, it can also be counterproductive if it results in a tendency to cling to past "tried and true" behaviors despite the existence of data documenting the ineffectiveness or hazards of such behaviors and policies. Therefore all nurses need to be especially vigilant about the traditional power that may be in operation in their work settings, whether it be evidenced by the school nurse who refuses to try "new" methods or by organizational policies and procedures which are clearly outdated, and should initiate whatever planned change may be indicated.

As a final comment in this discussion of power bases, it should be noted that contrary to popular and uninformed opinion, formal power is not necessarily "better" than informal power. Indeed, a common yet sometimes fatal mistake made by persons occupying positions of formal power in an organization is to assume that their formal authorized power will exert a stronger influence over the behavior of their subordinates or employees than will the informal power of subordinate individuals or groups. Informal power networks within an organization can either support or undermine the formal power in an organization. A leader or manager who wishes to be successful needs to at least avoid alienating individuals who have informal power and ideally should try to enlist their support.

Acquiring and using power through legislative/political action
Is politics a dirty word?

Although *politics* is often defined as the "art or science of government," Mullane (1976:45) believes that definition is too narrow and suggests that politics be defined instead as "the art of using influence to bring about change." Probably as a result of some of the highly publicized and shocking revelations of corruption and dishonesty in government in recent years (such as the Watergate and Abscam bribery scandals), "politics" often connotes images of scheming politicians, "shady" deals, ruthless ambition, corruption, and fiscal irresponsibility. This negative image of politics and politicians is unfortunate because it provides a further rationalization for many persons and groups (including some nurses) to remain uninvolved. This attitude is not only irresponsible, but it is also self-defeating, especially for groups like nurses. Nurses need to accept the reality that political decisions affect (both directly and indirectly) health care and nursing (N-CAP, nd). We cannot afford to persistently bury our heads in the sand—we cannot continue our blithe and unrealistic assumption that "someone else" will look out for our professional interests. Thus, even though there *are* corrupt politicians and flagrant abuses of power within our political system, that is not sufficient justification for branding *all* politicians and *all* political action as "bad" or "dirty." However imperfect the system may be, it is nonetheless a powerful system. The question we in nursing should be asking ourselves now is not *"Should we become politically involved?"* but rather, *"How* can we become politically involved and active?"

Readiness for political action

As Claus and Bailey's definition of power (1977) indicates, power includes not merely a capability to influence others but the willingness and actions to follow through and obtain results. Thus, to effectively wield political power, these three elements (ability, willingness, and action) are essential. However, Novello (1976) believes that effective use of political power depends on one's readiness or preparedness to become politically powerful, and she identifies five actions that are prerequisites for political action readiness.

The first prerequisite for political action readiness according to Novello (1976) is *establishment of goals*. In other words, the individual or group must decide *why* political power is to be sought and *how* it will be used; that is, *specific goals* and motivations for obtaining and wielding political power must be clearly identified. This is important in giving direction to the political efforts of the group (or individual) and will also affect the specific strategies and tactics chosen to accomplish the goals. This identification of goals for action has been a problem in nursing according to Novello (1976). At times, as she notes, we have failed to be completely honest with ourselves concerning our true motivations and purposes for political action; thus we may have insisted that our purpose was "better health care and nursing care for

clients," while our "hidden agenda" was actually the "enhancement and advancement" of the nursing profession.

Once specific and clear goals for action have been set, the next step toward political action readiness according to Novello (1976) is *analysis of the situation*. This analysis of the present situation may be accomplished through use of the force field analysis concept described earlier in this chapter. At this point, it is advisable to weigh "what is" against "what should be," determine the feasibility of the goals, and assess the availability of suitable resources to accomplish them.

The third prerequisite for becoming politically powerful is *establishment of a willingness to use power* (Novello, 1976). In other words, there must be a *conscious decision* to use power, which in turn is based on a strong conviction that "power is an essential component of today's politics" (Novello, 1976:5). For women, and especially nurses, willful exercise of power has traditionally been regarded as "unfeminine" and even "unprofessional." However, as noted earlier, it is time for women and nurses particularly to accept the inevitability of political power and to resolve that we will actively acquire and responsibly use it, rather than merely react to its use by others.

The fourth prerequisite action for becoming politically powerful is *developing faith in one's ability to effect change* (Novello, 1976). This, too, is a problem for women and nurses, who have traditionally been socialized to believe that they are powerless and have no control over their destiny. However, *believing* in one's ability to effect change sparks the confidence needed to carry through and achieve the political action goals of the individual or group.

The final prerequisite action for political involvement readiness according to Novello (1976) is *setting aside large blocks of time for political involvement*. Novello reminds us that political activity is, like other worthwhile activities, time-consuming. The problem for many nurses has been that political involvement has been a low priority activity, probably because nurses have been politically naive and have viewed themselves as powerless pawns in the system. However, as Novello (1976:5) points out, this political inaction is both shortsighted and fiscally foolish, because while "nurses on the average spend approximately one-quarter of their time on the job earning money to pay their taxes . . . [they] spend virtually no time over-seeing the spenders of those taxes."

Guidelines for political behavior

Taking some liberties with the original adage, it should be noted that in politics it isn't only whether you win or lose that is important (and winning is clearly preferred!), but how you play the game. Indeed, in politics how you play the game may well determine whether you win or lose. Therefore, in this discussion suggested guidelines or ground rules for political action will be proposed.

Novello (1976:6-7)* proposes seven guidelines for political behavior:

1. *Identify and cultivate the players*. Again, remembering the earlier discussion of formal and informal power, it should be obvious that the important "players" in the political arena are *not* necessarily the elected officials.
2. *Do your homework*. It is important to be fully knowledgeable about whatever issue you are addressing and to take a position or stand for which you are aware of all the possible ramifications and outcomes.
3. *Learn the art of timing:* there is both a right and wrong time to act.
4. *Learn to compromise*. Since, as Novello points out, "half a loaf is better than none," decide what you absolutely have to achieve and what you can live without and be prepared to relinquish the nonessentials.
5. *Deal from strength*. Cultivate your strength and use it (e.g., votes) to enlist the cooperation of others (candidates).
6. *Resist the temptation to openly humiliate or take unfair advantage of others*. Humiliation and unfair manipulation of others are the kinds of actions that have given politics its negative image. Also, these behaviors are not likely to achieve positive or lasting results and may instead backfire; consequently, legitimate causes and issues that you support may be defeated simply because your tactics were offensive and ineffective.
7. *Learn how to win and, more importantly, how to lose*. The realities of life are such that it is not reasonable to expect to always win. Therefore one must behave in socially accepted ways following both victories and losses.

As an alternative (or perhaps adjunct) to Novello's guidelines, Mullane (1976:51) has identified qualities that she believes nurses need to be politically successful; she describes these qualities as the "four Cs":

1. *Consistency*, which refers to the importance of nurses' consistent support of *all* issues relevant to nursing as a whole and not just those of a special interest group.
2. *Credibility*, which is based on nurses' demonstration to the public and to legislators that they can identify political goals and follow them through to completion; this credibility thus inspires public and legislative confidence in the nursing profession and its purposes.
3. *Constituency*, or a "critical mass in membership and support" without which success is impossible.
4. *Courage*, which depends on having the strength to follow through with a political action despite all obstacles until the goal is achieved.

These four qualities, coupled with Novello's seven guidelines for behavior, should provide the basis for effective political involvement and action. The next issue is, what activities are appropriate for nurses and how and where do we start?

Legislative/political action: getting started

As Novello (1976) points out, an important first step toward becoming politically powerful is to get involved with the political process at the local or community level. One obvious and prominent way to become involved in local politics is to participate in political campaigns. The Nurses Coalition for Action in Politics (N-CAP, nd) suggests five specific ways for nurses to participate in political campaigns:

1. *Endorse candidates;* endorsement not only assists the candidate to get votes from other nurses and their relatives, friends, and other colleagues, but it also often results in good press coverage for the endorser (in this case, nurses). In other words, endorsements of candidates by nurses benefit both the candidates and nurses.
2. *Donate money;* even small contributions for a candidate can be helpful, since financial contributions can be used to buy media time and coverage, thus increasing the candidate's visibility.
3. *Volunteer time;* most campaigns need more volunteers than they actually get, and usually have enough variety of jobs and tasks that there should be something of interest for nearly anyone who can donate time.
4. *Educate other nurses about candidates and health issues;* by informing other nurses about candidates' voting records, their position on various health issues, and their qualifications to represent nursing's concerns and viewpoints within the legislative arena, nurses can help ensure that their fellow nurses vote intelligently based on adequate information.
5. *Get involved;* this includes attending precinct

---

*Copyright © 1976 National League for Nursing.

caucuses, serving as convention delegates, planning and participating in events at which nurses (and other voters) can meet the candidates, encouraging other nurses to register and vote, and encouraging qualified nurses to run for office themselves.

Following the election of the candidate(s) supported by nurses, the job is not finished. Nurses must maintain contact with their legislators throughout their respective terms in office and keep them informed about nurses' viewpoints on health-related issues. Nurses are the most qualified experts to speak for the nursing profession and must accept and act on their responsibility to do so. While personal face-to-face contacts with legislators are probably more effective than other less direct means, such encounters are not always possible. Other effective methods of communicating with legislators include telephone calls, telegrams, and letters. To make personal visits with legislators or letters sent to them most productive, compliance with Fleischhacker's (1977:153-154) list of basic "dos and don'ts" is advisable. Among her specific suggestions are the following:

1. Discuss only one concern or bill per visit or per correspondence.
2. Obtain basic background information about the issue and/or bill before contacting your legislator so that your opinion sounds informed; when discussing or referring to a specific bill, identify it by its correct number.
3. Indicate concretely how you want your legislator to vote on the bill or issue and cite specific reasons and data for your stance.
4. Time your visit or letter carefully and be sure your contact occurs at least several days ahead of any scheduled vote on the bill or issue.
5. When writing to legislators, express your thoughts and concerns using your own words rather than a form letter; letters that are thoughtfully written and that clearly articulate and explain your position have greater impact than standardized form letters.
6. During face-to-face or telephone contacts do not try to impress the legislator with your credentials.
7. Observe basic social amenities, including thanking the legislator for his time (following personal meetings or telephone calls), writing thank you letters if he votes as you requested, sending written letters to follow up or reinforce personal visits or telephone contacts as needed, and writing to let him know when you think he is doing a good job. It is important to be courteous and thoughtful because legislators are also human and are motivated by positive feedback and "stroking" like other people. Also, because legislators serve for a

period of years (usually) you may need to deal with them repeatedly; it therefore is not wise to alienate them.

Finally, an important way in which nurses can become politically powerful is through active participation in professional organizations concerned with health and nursing (Novello, 1976).

Acquiring and using power through membership in professional organizations

Probably one of nursing's biggest political faux pas has been our failure to get organized and to amass a sizable base of support. While individual political involvement and commitment are also needed to help nurses to achieve their political goals, there can be no doubt that lawmakers and other powerful persons and groups are impressed by the strength of numbers. For special interest groups like nursing who can enlist the support and involvement of large numbers of persons, political clout or power will be more tangible.

Unfortunately, while nurses are arguing and debating the question of which organization "really" represents nursing, nurses suffer from a lack of unity and a corresponding lack of collective political clout. Consequently, nurses' concerns and viewpoints may not be heard by the appropriate politicians or officials, and even if they are heard, the messages from various groups of nurses may conflict, thus increasing the confusion and diluting nurses' power and influence.

Recognizing the political importance of strength in numbers, it is likewise unfortunate that many nurses do not belong to professional organizations. Indeed, as Miller and Flynn (1977) report, only approximately 20% of all employed registered nurses are members of the ANA. Although nurses do not yet have one professional organization that is accepted by all nurses as representing them and their concerns, the importance of political involvement and representation for nurses has not gone unnoticed. In fact, in 1974 the ANA provided seed money to launch the Nurses Coalition for Action in Politics (N-CAP). N-CAP is considered to be the "political action arm" of the ANA, and has as its primary functions the political education of nurses and support for candidates who are dedicated to improving health care (Schorr, 1974).

In addition to N-CAP, there are other or-

Table 19-3. Professional organizations that may benefit school nurses

Organization	Address
American Nurses' Association (ANA)	2420 Pershing Road Kansas City, Missouri 64108
American Public Health Association (APHA)	1015 Fifteenth Street N.W. Washington, D.C. 20005
American School Health Association (ASHA)	1521 South Water Street P.O. Box 708 Kent, Ohio 44240
National Association of School Nurses, Inc., (NASN), an affiliate of the National Education Association (NEA)	1201 Sixteenth Street N.W. Washington, D.C. 20036
Nurses Coalition for Action in Politics (N-CAP)	Suite 408 1030 Fifteenth Street N.W. Washington, D.C. 20005
National League for Nursing (NLN)	10 Columbus Circle New York, New York 10019

ganizations that can advance the cause of nursing and school nursing in particular. To expedite school nurses' efforts to become involved with these organizations, their names and addresses are supplied in Table 19-3.

Although school nurses have suffered to some degree from their unclear professional affiliation, which in turn has resulted in competition for school nurses' allegiance by organizations representing nursing, education, public health, pediatrics, and school health in general, this confusion concerning the "true" professional affiliation among all these groups may have been a blessing in disguise; with so many varied groups vying for the affection and loyalty of school nurses, it should be possible for school nurses to obtain political support and assistance from those organizations, thus increasing their political power and influence. Therefore it seems logical that if school nurses would join and actively participate in one or more of these organizations, their ability to get their views and concerns translated into political action would be enhanced.

Even nurses who have managed to become involved in professional organizations, however, have not necessarily been able to translate their unity into actual planned political change outcomes. According to Bowman and Culpepper (1974:1055), this is due to the fact that "as an organized group, nurses have been *re*active rather than active. Positions are taken, but action does not follow." As they point out, nursing groups too often wait until they perceive an external threat to their domain, such as the evolution of new health care personnel (physicians' assistants, for example), before taking action and asserting themselves. The problem is compounded by the additional fact that there are competitive cliques among nurses and nursing leaders that dissipate the potential power of nurses as a group (Bowman and Culpepper, 1974).

In her discussion of nursing organizations as political pressure groups, Bowman (1973) identifies some group characteristics that affect the relative success of such groups in influencing political decision making. The first factor that affects the relative political strength of organizations is *wealth;* a wealthy organization can convert its financial strength into other resources in the form of paid lobbyists and public relations personnel. A second important factor is the *size of the membership;* membership size reflects voting power, so the larger the membership, the greater the respect the organization may command from legislators and other elected officials. A third factor that affects the relative political strength of an organization is the *degree of organizational cohesiveness;* a highly cohesive group can increase its lobbying strength by presenting a "united front." The last factor affecting an organization's relative strength as a political pressure group according to Bowman (1973) is the *importance of the organization to the social system;* an organization or group that has high social status and whose positions are popular and congruent with the society's needs has political strength because of that popularity. Because access to high-quality, low-cost health care plus other health care issues are important to most members of society today, nursing and other health care professionals can expect broad consumer support for many of their professional organizations' positions regarding health issues.

Bowman (1973:76) believes that these factors all contribute to some extent to an organization's "degree of access to public decision-makers." And, she believes, access to key points in the political decision-making process is critically important and is therefore the "primary goal" of all political pressure groups. According to Bowman (1973:76-80), then, the following three basic techniques are used by organizations to develop and improve their access to the decision makers:

1. *Use of propaganda to shape public opinion;* this usually takes one of two forms: a defensive effort to counteract a perceived immediate threat or a long-range effort to improve the organization's public image and public relations; specific methods used include television and radio broadcasts, press releases, pamphlets and brochures, commercials and advertisements, speeches, and bumper stickers.
2. *Electioneering,* or working for the election of a candidate or political party; methods may include attempts to influence party platform committees and powerful party members, threats of voter retaliation against nonresponsive incumbents, financial contributions, "voter mobilization" drives, and informing others regarding candidates' records.
3. *Lobbying,* or attempting to influence public officials (especially legislators) to pass legislation and/or take other actions that advance the organization's purposes and goals; the most important function of lobbyists is to provide both technical and political information to legislators; methods of lobbying include direct contact with legislators and their aides, testifying at public or legislative committee hearings, preparation of legislation proposals and seeking a legislator to introduce and/or sponsor the bill, mobilizing support for the bill within the legislature, and consulting with members of the executive branch (including agency administrators responsible for implementing legislation and policies) to provide information and advice.

While nursing organizations have increased their use of these techniques in recent years, there is still room for improvement and expansion of their efforts to gain political recognition and power.

CONCLUSION

Within the past decade, competition for health care dollars has become very keen. Throughout our nation's economy—especially within our health care system—money has become scarce, and budgets have tightened. This problem has become especially acute within our schools and has resulted in reduction or elimination of school nursing positions. If school nurses are to retain their place within the school, they will need to begin to view themselves as change agents and increase their knowledge and skills in planning and implementing planned change. School nurses will also need to regard themselves as politically powerful and will need to develop enough political/legislative savvy to be able to work within the political arena as a means of implementing planned change. As Ashley (1973:641) warns:

Nurses, individually and collectively, need to recognize and cultivate the power they do have and exercise that power in an intelligent and organized fashion. The conditions in which we practice our profession in the future depend on it.

REFERENCES

Alinsky, S.D.: 1971. Rules for radicals, Vintage Books, New York.
American Nurses' Association: 1977. Facts about nursing 76-77, American Nurses' Association, Kansas City, Mo.
Archer, S. E.: 1975. Politics and economics: how things really work, Chapter 7. In Archer, S. E., and Fleshman, R.: Community health nursing: patterns and practice, Duxbury Press, North Scituate, Mass.
Arndt, C., and Huckabay, L. M.: 1980. Nursing administration: theory for practice with a systems approach, 2nd ed., The C. V. Mosby Co., St. Louis.
Ashley, J. A.: 1973. This I believe about power in nursing, Nurs. Outlook **21**(10):637-641.
Benne, K. D., and Birnbaum, M.: 1960. Change does not have to be haphazard, School Rev. **68**(3):283-293.
Bennis, W. G., Benne, K. D., and Chin, R.: 1961. The planning of change, Holt, Rinehart & Winston, New York.
Bennis, W. G., Benne, K. D., and Chin, R.: 1969. The planning of change, 2nd ed., Holt, Rinehart & Winston, New York.
Bennis, W. G., Benne, K. D., Chin, R., and Corey, K. E.: 1976. The planning of change, 3rd ed., Holt, Rinehart & Winston, New York.
Bowman, R. A.: 1973. The nursing organization as a political pressure group, Nurs. Forum **12**(1):73-81.
Bowman, R. A., and Culpepper, R. C.: 1974. Power: Rx for change, Am. J. Nurs. **74**(6):1053-1056.
Chin, R., and Benne, K. D.: 1976. General strategies for effecting changes in human systems. In Bennis, W. G., Benne, K. D., Chin, R., and Corey, K. E.: The planning of change, 3rd ed., Holt, Rinehart & Winston, New York.
Claus, K. E., and Bailey, J. T.: 1977. Power and influence in health care: a new approach to leadership, The C. V. Mosby Co., St. Louis.
Deloughery, G. L., and Gebbie, K. M.: 1975. Political dynamics: impact on nurses and nursing, The C. V. Mosby Co., St. Louis,
Ehrenreich, B., and English, D.: 1973. Witches, midwives and nurses: a history of women healers, 2nd. ed., The Feminist Press, Old Westbury, New York.
Fleischhacker, V.: 1977. Writing your legislator: some dos and don'ts, MCN **2**(3):153-154.
French, J. P. R., and Raven, B.: 1959. The bases of social power. In Cartwright, D., editor: Studies in social power,

University of Michigan Press, Ann Arbor, Mich.

Gerlach, L. P., and Hine, V. H.: 1973. Lifeway leap: the dynamics of change in America, University of Minnesota Press, Minneapolis.

Haley, J.: 1969. The power tactics of Jesus Christ and other essays, Avon Books, New York.

Hersey, P., and Blanchard, K. H.: 1977. Planning and implementing change, Chapter 10. In Management of organizational behavior: utilizing human resources, 3rd ed., Prentice-Hall, Inc., Englewood Cliffs, N.J.

Kramer, M.: 1974. Reality shock: why nurses leave nursing, The C. V. Mosby Co., St. Louis.

Lewin, K.: 1947. Frontiers in group dynamics: concept, method, and reality in social science; social equilibria and social change, Human Relations **1**(1):5-41.

Lieb, R.: 1978. Power, powerlessness and potential—nurse's role within the health care delivery system, Image **10**(3):75-83.

Lippitt, R., Watson, J., and Westley, B.: 1958. The dynamics of planned change, Harcourt, Brace & World, Inc., New York.

Longest, B. B.: 1976. Managing change: the management imperative, Chapter 10. In Management practices for the health professional, Reston Publishing Co., Inc., Reston, Va.

Miller, M. H., and Flynn, B.C.: 1977. Current perspectives in nursing: social issues, and trends, vol. 1, The C. V. Mosby Co., St. Louis.

Mullane, M. K.: 1976. Politics begins at work, RN **39** (7):45-51.

N-CAP: nd. We can make a difference . . . and we must (pamphlet), National Coalition for Action in Politics, Washington, D.C.

Novello, D.J.: 1976. People, power and politics for health care. In People, power, politics for health care, NLN Publication Number 52-1647, National League for Nursing, New York.

Schaller, L. E.: 1972. The change agent, Abingdon Press, Nashville, Tenn.

Schorr, T. M.: 1974. Nurse power (editorial), Am. J. Nurs. **74**(6):1047.

Toffler, A,: 1970 Future shock, Random House, Inc., New York.

Watson, G.: 1969. Resistance to change. In Bennis, W. G., Benne, K. D., and Chin, R.: The planning of change, 2nd ed., Holt, Rinehart & Winston, New York.

SUGGESTED READINGS

American Nurses' Association Government Relations Division: 1977. Communicating with Congress, ANA Publication Code: GR-3 2M 5/77, American Nurses' Association, Kansas City, Mo.

Grissum, M., and Spengler, C.: 1976. Womanpower and health care, Little, Brown & Co., Boston.

Huxley, A. L.: 1946. Brave new world, Harper & Row, Publishers, Inc., New York.

Lysaught, J. P.: 1974. Action in nursing: progress in professional purpose, McGraw-Hill Book Co., New York.

Nathanson, I.: 1975. Getting a bill through congress, Am. J. Nurs. **75**(7):1179-1181.

National League for Nursing: 1976. Coping with change through assessment and evaluation, Publication Number 23-1618, National League for Nursing, New York.

National League for Nursing: 1976. People, power, politics for health care, Publication Number 52-1647, National League for Nursing, New York.

N-CAP: 1977. A how-to-do-it fundraising book, Nurses Coalition for Action in Politics, Washington, D.C.

N-CAP: 1977. Know your congresspeople: a how-to-do-it book on researching their public record, National Coalition for Action in Politics, Washington, D.C.

Rodgers, J. A.: 1976. Theoretical considerations involved in the process of change. In Stone, S., Berger, M. S., Elhart, D., Firsich, S. C., and Jordan, S. B., editors: Management for nurses: a multidisciplinary approach, The C. V. Mosby Co., St. Louis.

VerSteeg, D. F.: 1975. The political process, or, the power and the glory, Chapter 13. In Bullough, B.: The law and the expanding nurse role, Appleton-Century-Crofts, New York.

PART VII

Future perspectives on school nursing

CHAPTER 20

Expanding the role of the school nurse: the school nurse practitioner

SUSAN J. WOLD

The fact that the American health care "system" is cumbersome, costly, inaccessible to many, often ineffective in solving health problems and meeting the needs of consumers, and above all, grossly inefficient, is no secret. Probably one of the most damning criticisms of our health care system is that by concentrating decision making and prestige in one health care provider group (physicians), the education, talents, and skills of other health team members have been underused; the net effect has been to fragment health care, while at the same time increasing its costs and increasing the level of dissatisfaction among nonphysician health team members.

THE SCHOOL NURSE
PRACTITIONER ROLE

Among the consequently underused and clearly dissatisfied groups of health care providers are nurses. Based in part on the recognition that nurses can contribute more fully and cost-effectively to health care delivery than custom and policy had thus far dictated, during the 1960s the University of Colorado developed the first expanded role for nurses: the nurse practitioner (Silver, 1971b). The original focus in role development was on the pediatric nurse practitioner, whose envisioned role included provision of "augmented and improved direct health care for our child population" in two basic settings: public health facilities and private physicians' offices (Silver, 1971b:62).

Evolution of the school nurse
practitioner role

The school nurse practitioner role, then, evolved from the original pediatric nurse practitioner role, representing a kind of specializa-

tion. As described by Dr. Henry Silver (1971b:64), one of the founders of the first school nurse practitioner (SNP) program at the University of Colorado (established in 1970), the SNP program was an attempt "to rectify a major loss in the present health-care system: the failure to utilize fully the skills and services of the 16,000 school nurses in the United States." Thus the focus of SNP programs has been to adapt the successful role expansion of the pediatric nurse practitioner (PNP) to meeting the needs of school-age children and youth; the result is the emergence of the school nurse practitioner, who is a kind of PNP "headquartered" in the school setting.

Defining the school nurse
practitioner role

The working definition of a *school nurse practitioner,* as suggested by Silver et al. (1977:598), is that she is a registered nurse who has "acquired advanced knowledge and clinical skill in providing health care and services through successful completion of a four-month (or longer) organized course of study that, ideally, has been developed jointly through the collaborative efforts of nursing, medicine, and a school system." Because the SNP role is a clear departure from the "traditional" school nurse role of Band-Aider and record keeper, its successful implementation in any school or school district *requires* not only a highly motivated and well-educated SNP, but also the support and confidence of school administrators and faculty (Barbour et al., 1970). For that reason, it is not uncommon for SNP programs to require prospective students to furnish proof (by means of a letter of support and endorsement from pertinent school officials) of their school administration's support for their proposed role expansion as a means of ensuring that those students accepted into the program have a reasonable chance of being able to actually implement their newly expanded role in their particular schools.

The intent of the SNP role, then, is to increase the availability and accessibility of health care for children and youth (ANA, ASHA, DSN/NEA, 1978) by expanding the traditional school nurse role and by using the school setting to provide a "significant portion" of their health care (Silver, 1971a). More specifically, school nurse practitioners are expected to be able to identify and assess the factors that may operate to produce learning disorders, psycho-socio-educational problems, perceptive cognitive difficulties and behavior problems as well as those causing physical disease" (ANA, ASHA, DSN/NEA, 1978:265). SNPs are expected to establish collaborative relationships with physicians, other health care professionals, educators, and parents to provide "comprehensive assessment and remedial action" (ANA, ASHA, DSN/NEA, 1978:265) and are accountable for their actions to the extent of their educational preparation.

THE SNP ROLE: THE COLORADO EXPERIENCE

With the preceding overview as a common frame of reference, the major portion of this chapter will be devoted to more detailed discussion of the SNP's educational preparation and role. Although the discussion is based on the "Colorado experience," which seems fitting, since that is where the concept and role originated, the educational preparation and role described herein are broadly applicable. Indeed, as a means of ensuring that SNPs across the country will, despite regional or individual philosophical differences, deliver quality nursing care, standards of practice for SNPs are now being developed (ANA, ASHA, DSN/NEA, 1978). Recognizing, then, the University of Colorado's School Nurse Practitioner Program as an acclaimed and fully accredited prototype of such programs, in the remainder of this discussion Judith B. Igoe will describe the educational preparation and role of the SNP based on the Colorado experience.

The educational preparation and role of the school nurse practitioner

JUDITH B. IGOE

Although regular official visits for comprehensive health care occur frequently in most families throughout infancy and preschool years, this custom often disintegrates once the child reaches school age. Specifically, a significant deceleration in the child's use of such traditional health facilities as physicians' offices and community health centers takes place at this time. It is estimated, for example, that 13 million children and adolescents between the ages of 5 to 18 (or 30% of this segment of the population) rarely come to the attention of a health care professional (National Academy of Sciences, 1976; Igoe and Silver, 1977). Generally, the limited health care that is provided to this group is more often than not fragmented and usually associated with serious complaints of illness or injury. Under these circumstances, preventive health services, including immunizations, early disease detection efforts, nutritional surveillance, repetitive developmental evaluations, and health maintenance counseling, are neglected or of secondary importance. Obviously, this is because treatment of the immediate health problem takes precedence. Furthermore, for too many of these boys and girls, emotional disturbances and learning disabilities originating from unsuspected health conditions will go unattended until the symptoms reach crisis proportions, even though good professional care is available.

Despite the urging of health care professionals that all children and adolescents should receive ongoing comprehensive health care (preventive, curative, and restorative services), one third of the families with school-age youth disregard this advice. Why? Often the physician's office or clinic is not readily accessible. Frequently, the high cost of health services discourages parents from seeking health care once the basic immunizations are provided and their child appears to be developing normally, or it may be that the family is generally dissatisfied with the quality of health care available and therefore confines their use of health services to dire emergencies. Just as important a factor contributing to the lack of health services requested by parents for their school-age children and adolescents is the American society's tendency to discredit and slight health maintenance activities in favor of more commonplace treatment of illness practices.

In all likelihood, all of these factors contribute to the failure of children and adolescents to receive the full complement of recommended health services during school years. Regardless of the cause, however, the outcomes are for the most part the same. Opportunities to experience the benefits of preventive health care services never materialize; underlying quiescent health problems persist; and another generation of illness-oriented health consumers come into being who have neither the knowledge nor the interest needed to engage in meaningful health maintenance practices.

A practical and effective method for expanding and improving health care to school-age children is through the use of the school as a legitimate site for the delivery of health care services. Schools are where the children and adolescents are, and here exists the opportunity to detect and modify the course of important health problems, especially for those children who have inadequate access to health care elsewhere. For this reason many school health programs are in the process of significant change (Cronin and Young, 1977). What this change reflects is a transition from the longstanding "hands off" policy adopted by most school districts concerning actual delivery of any health care services, except general screenings for vision and hearing and minor first aid measures. Replacing this antiquated model of school health is a more clinically oriented program that provides on site a variety of health care services, including counseling and education to children and adolescents in need. Of particular importance is the fact that the newer school health model has the potential to capture health dollars for financial support from a variety of sources, whereas the traditional nondelivery-oriented school health program continues to depend on the shrinking education dollar for subsistence.

Many school officials, health care professionals, private foundations, and the federal government have expressed interest in and support for the concept of the school as a site for the delivery of meaningful health care services. The Robert Wood Johnson Foundation, for example, has currently funded experimental school health projects in Colorado, New York, Utah, and North Dakota to determine the extent to which use of the school setting enhances the health care available to boys and girls of school age (Chestnutt, 1978). The Division of Nursing of the Department of Health, Education, and Welfare has financed training programs so that health care professionals within schools could be adequately prepared to function. Various professional organizations, including the ANA and ASHA, have also endorsed this concept of school health (ANA, ASHA, and DSN/NEA, 1978). In the minds of many, therefore, it seems important to establish the school health office as a setting where the health care given will go far toward meeting the health care needs of the school-age child.

Over the past 10 years, the University of Colorado (as well as other educational institutions) has been able to demonstrate that much of the health care and services required by children and adolescents in schools can be given by school nurses who have been specially educated as school nurse practitioners (Igoe, 1975; Silver et al., 1976).

EDUCATION OF SCHOOL NURSE PRACTITIONERS IN COLORADO
Overview

The School Nurse Practitioner Program at the University of Colorado began in 1970 under the joint sponsorship of the University of Colorado Schools of Medicine and Nursing and the Denver Public Schools. Graduates of this continuing education program are prepared to deliver primary health care services to children in schools and other health facilities. Ninety-four percent of these nurses are now employed by schools in thirty states. Fifty percent of the participants in the School Nurse Practitioner Program have had their master's degree prior to enrollment to the program. Nine and four tenths percent of the graduates come from minority groups. In 1978, seventy additional nurses enrolled in the program from throughout the United States and Europe, thirty-five of whom completed their training in the summer of 1979, with the remainder graduating in 1980.

The school nurses enrolled in the Colorado program participate in a 16-month course that is evenly divided between classroom instruction and closely supervised clinical practice. The overall educational goals for the program are threefold (Igoe, 1978):

1. To increase the nurse's skill in the evaluation and enrichment of the physical, cognitive, and psychosocial health status of

school-age children/adolescents for the purpose of providing comprehensive primary health care services and health education to children who fail to use traditional health facilities
2. To improve the screening and referral procedures for any child/adolescent in school with complaints of illness and injury
3. To increase the nurse's skill in the evaluation and management of the health status of children/adolescents experiencing developmental disabilities

Building on previous nursing experience and education, the curriculum for this program is intended to increase the participant's pediatric knowledge as well as clinical skills to improve judgment abilities and develop the capability for greater health care responsibilities. Specifically, the nurses learn improved interviewing techniques and become expert in performing the essentials of a physical examination, including the basic skills of inspection, palpation, and auscultation as well as the use of such tools as the stethoscope and otoscope. They learn about (1) physical, psychosocial, and personality processes and development; (2) variations of growth patterns; (3) various aspects of parent-child relationships; (4) perceptual, physical, and cognitive assessment using various screening procedures; (5) the essentials of nutritional needs for the older child; (6) cultural, economic, and ethnic factors affecting health; and (7) the appropriate management of a number of common acute and chronic problems in childhood, including those in neurology, dermatology, allergy, otorhinolaryngology, gynecology, ophthalmology, orthopedics, and dentistry. Proficiency is developed in counseling parents in childrearing practices and various physical, emotional, and personal problems. Special techniques for direct health counseling with students are also significant aspects of the nurses' learning.

On completion of the program, the nurse is ready to perform competent health evaluations, identify and manage various health problems in consultation with a physician, develop and implement directly health maintenance plans, and appropriately refer children requiring the services of other health and educational specialists.

Curriculum

Approximately 3 months prior to the onset of classes in Denver, all program participants receive a packet of review materials. The packet includes information relative to anatomy and physiology, general principles of growth and development, the philosophy of adult education, common problems of school-age children and adolescents, and the constituent activities that are incorporated in a standard history and physical examination.

The learning derived from the review materials and activities constitutes the first step toward role development in the School Nurse Practitioner Program. Because these review materials are largely self-instructional, the responsibility for learning is placed directly on the learner from the start. Experience over the past 10 years has shown that this approach not only stimulates the nurses' confidence in their own abilities, but it also introduces the concept of continued self-directed learning as a necessary aspect of their new role (Hall and Weaver, 1977).

Denver-based study is 16 weeks long and is completed over the course of two summers. In addition to the 3-month review period and 4 months of study in Denver, there is a 9-month period of home-based instruction involving full-time clinical practice, a preceptorship with a physician, and self-instructional materials for continued learning. The following sequence is typical for most nurses who are chosen to participate in this program: review → summer session I (Denver, 2 months) → home-based instruction (September-June) → summer session II (Denver, 2 months).

The following general areas are included in the curriculum of the Colorado School Nurse Practitioner Program:

1. *History taking and counseling* (150 hours). Theory and practical experience in systematic collection of physical, developmental, social, nutritional, dental, and general health information. The basic approaches to counseling pupils and their parents, including use of psychotherapeutic behavior modification, anticipatory guidance, play therapy, and crisis intervention techniques are taught.
2. *Physical diagnosis* (36 hours of didactic and 50 hours of clinical sessions conducted concurrently with history taking session). Systematic assessment of physical status and the recognition of the range of normal for school-age children.
3. *Neurological status* (24 hours). Theory and practical experience with the neurological evaluation of children.
4. *Common childhood problems* (32 hours). Theory and practical experience in the assessment of physical, perceptual, cognitive, mental,

and psychosocial growth and development of school-age children.

5. *Health education* (26 hours). Preparation of nurses to instruct children to become more knowledgeable and responsible health consumers. Includes preventive health maintenance services and disease and accident prevention.

6. *Developmental disabilities* (240 hours). Seminars focusing on the physical, emotional and environmental factors that influence a child's ability to learn. Particular attention is given to the prevention, early identification, and remediation of perceptual handicaps, psychoeducational difficulties, and physical handicaps of school-age children, including mental retardation. Nurses in clinical settings assess academically impaired children and participate in developing a mental health maintenance program for the child.

7. *Creative nurse management.* Techniques designed to assist nurses with the development and implementation of health care plans to alleviate health problems and promote well-being.

8. *Role development* (32 hours). Examination, clarification, and strengthening of the role of the nurse in the school setting. Training in assertiveness skills, stress management, and team development are emphasized. The staff for this seminar includes nursing and medical faculty from the School Nurse Practitioner Program, representatives from the school system, a special education teacher, and a child psychiatrist.

9. *Family dynamics.* The attitudes that affect member interactions and the critical periods in family life and the effect of family dynamics and sociocultural patterns on health are stressed. This study is integrated throughout the program.

10. *Community resources and delivery of child health care services.* Recognition of community resources, health delivery systems, and the referral process. This study is designed to increase the collaboration between school and community in the delivery of health services.

11. *Clinical application and experience in the school.* Planned field experiences and practice in schools and other settings under the direction of competent nursing and medical instruction and practitioners to allow an orderly transition from theory to clinical application.

12. *Cultural concepts.* Integrated throughout all aspects of the curriculum.

The multidisciplinary faculty who participate in the School Nurse Practitioner Program are current practitioners in nursing, pediatrics, other medical specialties, psychology, special education, nutrition, health education, dentistry, physical therapy, occupational therapy, audiology, and speech pathology. Several faculty members have joint appointments in two disciplines such as nursing and medicine.

In addition to didactic classroom presentation, a variety of community facilities are available for clinical practice. The University of Colorado, in collaboration with a nearby school district and health department, operates a children's clinic in which health services and education are provided to more than 500 pupils. This clinic provides ample opportunity for supervised practice of the School Nurse Practitioner Program participants. Furthermore, a unique health education center is part of this clinic and offers the nurses a special experience in health education designed to increase the children's participation in and responsibility for their own health care. This health education is under the general direction of a group of specially trained adolescents who are responsible for orienting the clinic patients to the concept of participation.

Other available clinical practice sites include the University of Colorado Medical Center pediatric outpatient clinics, Department of Child Psychiatry's Center for Children with Psycho-Educational Problems, John F. Kennedy Developmental Center, the Denver Public Schools, private physician's offices, mental health centers, and public health clinics.

To optimally use the time during which participants are in Denver, various activities that have been hypothesized to be suitable to the school nurse practitioner role have been field tested by the nurse practitioner faculty prior to the actual incorporation of these experiences into the curriculum. Field testing helps to preserve the relevance of the didactic and clinical material provided to program participants.

Nurse participants who successfully complete the program may earn up to thirty-four hours of undergraduate and Bureau of Classroom Instruction credit and a total of sixty-four Continuing Education Units for the semester. The University of Colorado School Nurse Practitioner Program received full accreditation in 1977 from the ANA.

SNP PRACTICE

The SNP functions may be categorized into group and individual health services and education. For those SNPs who function in schools where they are responsible for the entire school health program, the number of health services and education to classrooms or groups of students is much greater than for SNPs whose model of practice is different. Generally the SNP who manages the overall school health program does not have a caseload in excess of

1400 students or more than two school buildings to attend. In addition to his/her appointments with individual students for health care and counseling, this SNP must coordinate health care plans, provide consultation (and some teaching) in the area of health education, supervise mass health screenings as well as conduct other functions customary to the school nurse role. Contrary to the understanding of some school officials, school nurse practitioners continue to perform many of the functions that they had previously handled, especially those activities directly related to the evaluation and management of a student's health status. However, clerical administrative functions (e.g., basic record keeping, relieving secretaries, routine truancy follow-up, playground duty, etc.) have been delegated to a clerical assistant. This health clerk also makes appointments and triages simple conditions following the nurse's instruction.

The types of individual health services provided by school nurse practitioners include the following: (1) annual checkups for the well child/adolescent, (2) the illness/injury visit, and (3) the developmental disabilities workup. Components of each of these areas are included in the following lists:

Annual checkup—
well child/adolescent

1. Vision, hearing, dental screening.
2. Urinalysis and hematocrit values (depends on sex, age, and other indicators).
3. Health history (includes gathering data pertinent to developing health maintenance plans jointly with the child and family).
4. Physical examination, including neurological evaluation.
5. Formulated nursing diagnosis.
6. Collaborative health maintenance plan developed, and workup recorded on health record.
   a. Health counseling using special programs such as behavior management techniques, structured doll play, Dusco, etc.
   b. Use of health maintenance materials, such as SNP stress management programs.
   c. Referral for special anticipatory guidance programs, such as bike safety course.
   d. Immunizations.

   e. Dietary surveillance and/or growth monitoring.
7. Evaluation of the health maintenance plan; ANA Standards of Nursing practice are the basic criteria used.

Illness/injury visit

1. Present illness history, SNP's knowledge of growth and development enables them to appropriately question and involve child as well as teacher and parent.
2. Regional examination as indicated by the history.
3. Laboratory tests as indicated. Many health offices at school are equipped to handle urine and throat cultures, stool specimen analysis, pregnancy tests, etc.
4. Formulate nursing diagnosis.
5. If required, prepared a detailed written referral for further evaluation.
6. If not done sooner, contact the teacher and parent if indicated.
7. Treatment at school. The following measures exemplify the curative health services presently available in some schools employing SNPs:
   a. First aid measures.
   b. Management of iron deficiency anemia with dietary instruction and therapeutic doses of ferrous sulfate.
   c. Antibiotic treatment for bacterial infections.
   d. Use of over-the-counter medicines to alleviate upper respiratory tract infections and allergic conditions.
8. Evaluation of the treatment plan (ANA Standards).

Developmental disabilities workup

1. Review previous health records.
2. Obtain health history with particular attention to the developmental section. SNPs have their own developmental history that assists the nurse in determining the child's strengths as well as weaknesses.
3. Perform a health evaluation physical examination and, if indicated, neurological assessment (including the Boston neurological developmental tool) and additional developmental screenings (Slosson, Peabody, Beery, Riley, and Buttons). These screenings enable the nurse to clarify which other professionals should see the child and when.

4. Formulate a nursing diagnosis.
5. Collaborative health maintenance plan developed; workup recorded; referrals and reports prepared. This plan includes development of a mental health maintenance plan. After identification of a child's abilities, the SNP prepares a behavior management program designed to reinforce the positive aspects of a child's functioning in an effort to prevent the development of a poor self-concept, which is a common occurrence among children with academic difficulties.
6. Participation as a member of the school's resource team for evaluation of the child with learning problems. In this capacity, the school nurse practitioner not only provides information about the child's physical health status but also serves as the child's advocate by reminding other team members of the child's capabilities.
7. Evaluation (ANA Standards of Practice).

For the school nurse practitioner who is responsible for the entire school health program, all of these functions would be performed. In light of the additional activities and responsibilities, this SNP's schedule is normally more structured than previously. Furthermore, many nurses who are responsible for the entire school health program have instituted designated sick-call periods in their schools (except for emergencies) as another method for improving the organization of the school health office.

There are two other patterns of SNP practice in schools. One is for the nurse to float from school to school to evaluate students in need of health appraisals. Follow-up and management services become the responsibility of the regular school nurse or ancillary personnel who attend that school on a regular basis. The last pattern is the least common type of practice for SNPs in schools. This involves stationing the SNP in the school district's diagnostic and treatment clinic where the nurse will work primarily with children/adolescents experiencing academic difficulties, many of which are health related.

Not all SNPs work in schools. Some are employed in correctional institutions, physicians' offices, health department clinics, and college health services. In all of the facilities, SNPs have a significant contribution to make because of their in-depth knowledge of the health and learning needs of school-age youth.

Representative sites in which SNPs function

SNPs are functioning in fifty states. Several school sites are described to further illustrate the role of the SNP (Silver, 1978)*:

Since 1972, the school system in Gary, Indiana, has utilized school nurse practitioners to increase and improve the health care available to school-age children in that city. Faced with the problem of a projected primary care physician-to-population ratio of 1:20,000, school nurse practitioners have been utilized as a vital resource for the health care delivery system. Under physician supervision, school nurse practitioners are responsible for much of the health assessment and primary health care needed by a significant proportion of the child population of Gary. As part of their expanded role, school nurse practitioners assess and manage a wide variety of acute and chronic health problems, and give preventive care. They do a variety of screening tests including those for sickle cell disease and hypertension, serve as members of the diagnostic team for children with learning disabilities on whom they perform physical and neurological evaluations and administer learning disability screening tests, monitor schools for health hazards, prescribe medications, care for various types of traumatic wounds, evaluate and treat athletic injuries, and provide prenatal service and education to pregnant students who continue to go to school.

Another type of exciting new health care program has been initiated by the communities of Posen and Robbins, suburbs of Chicago. Both Posen and Robbins are economically deprived (ranking 197th and 201st out of 203 suburban communities in the Chicago area). Recently they have begun using school nurse practitioners in a clinic arrangement in remodeled classroom space in one of the schools in Robbins. In this clinic school nurse practitioners offer primary (including diagnostic, preventive, and ongoing) health care and provide treatment in cases which previously might have been limited to visits to an emergency clinic in hospitals outside these communities (or received no care at all). Among other functions and activities, the school nurse practitioners identify problems and arrange for follow-up on those problems previously identified but for which nothing had been done.

In a third setting, the Commonwealth of Pennsylvania, through the effective utilization of school nurse practitioners, has changed school health from a health care system of limited value to a dynamic one capable of providing extensive health care to children. Thus far, more than 100 of the 505 school districts in Pennsylvania are involved in the change. These districts are concentrated around Pittsburgh, Philadelphia, and Harrisburg with planning to in-

---

*From Silver, H. K.: 1978. Testimony prepared for Senator Edward M. Kennedy's Child Health Hearings, Denver, Colorado, November, 29.

volve rural school districts now underway. It has been found that an expansion of the role of the school nurse to that of a school nurse practitioner provides the key by which a school district (or any other unit providing school health) can develop a purposeful system of health care for school-age children. Under the new system, the nonprofessional activities of the traditional school nurse, which may consume up to 75% of her time, are provided by a trained nonprofessional health worker under the supervision of the school nurse practitioner who is then able to take over a large part of the role of the school physician and, in addition, add a number of new services including improved history taking, assessment and management of problems, provision of anticipatory guidance, diagnosis and treatment of acute health care problems, and the coordination of community and educational resources. School physicians, no longer needed for screening physical examinations which formerly took up much of their time, are employed more effectively and for fewer hours in the professionally demanding role of consultant in medical-pediatric matters to the school nurse practitioner.

The unique role of the SNP as a health educator

The University of Colorado course for SNPs involves an unusual approach to health education. As a result of their special preparation, SNPs are training children in classrooms as well as during visits to the health office to assume new assertive roles as health consumers (Igoe, 1977). Through the use of specially designed comic books, age-appropriate health history records, child-oriented appointment sheets, and games with an emphasis on decision making, SNPs are helping children/adolescents learn how to implement the behaviors known as the Participatory Health Consumer Role; these behaviors are as follows:

1. Asking questions for the purpose of clarification and improved understanding
2. Personally communicating information about one's own health
3. Acquiring pertinent health information simultaneously with the delivery of service
4. Participating in the decision-making activity with regard to one's own health at the time health services are rendered
5. Assuming responsibility for certain tasks related to the maintenance of one's own health

During their own course of instruction, SNPs also learn new ways to equip and organize their health offices so that the participatory health consumer role is positively reinforced at every opportunity.

EFFECTIVENESS OF THE SNP

Although studies of the functions and effectiveness of the SNP have been limited up to this time, it is anticipated that within 5 years, the results of a number of studies will provide a fairly definitive answer to the following questions: Should schools serve as health care delivery sites? How well do SNPs serve as primary health care providers in school settings?

In the meantime, the following findings constitute what is already known about SNPs (Hilmar and McAtee, 1973; McAtee, 1974). Between 1970 and 1974, the University of Colorado School Nurse Practitioner Program functioned as a research demonstration project. Evaluation studies to compare the performance of the program graduates with "regular" school nurses indicate the following:

1. SNPs devote a much larger proportion of their time with patients and do thorough extensive assessments and in-depth appraisals of health problems, whereas "regular" school nurses are occupied primarily with brief and essentially superficial patient encounters.
2. SNPs manage a significantly greater proportion of health problems of schoolchildren and are less likely to refer pupils inappropriately to physicians or others for consultation or care.
3. SNPs exclude (dismiss from school) half as many pupils as do "regular" school nurses because nurse practitioners can recognize and manage health problems in the school setting.
4. SNPs counsel parents with more sharply focused and specific recommendations about their children's health problems. These more sharply focused recommendations are better understood by parents so that children sent home from school are more likely to receive needed medical attention.
5. SNPs spend twice as much time as "regular" school nurses providing direct patient care.
6. SNPs have tripled the number of daily contacts with parents of students to discuss emotional, physical, learning, or other student problems.
7. School health aides, teacher's aides, and parent volunteers are an important asset in

permitting SNPs to practice in their expanded role.

8. Use of SNPs has significant financial benefits for medical care, school systems, and for parents.

SUMMARY

SNPs are school nurses who have received additional training to provide improved health care to the 30% of school-age youth whose health needs are generally neglected (Silver et al., 1977). The school is the site from which the SNP provides much of this health care. The following activities constitute the meaningful role played by the SNP:

1. Assumes basic responsibility for identifying and managing many of the health problems of children.
2. Delivers well child care to school-age children who fail to use other community health facilities.
3. Performs necessary evaluative procedures such as a complete health history, basic physical examination, and variety of special procedures.
4. Assesses the overall condition of an ill child as to the acuteness and severity of disease and decides what problems she can handle herself and which ones will need referral to other resources.
5. Provides skillful management of childhood emergencies until additional assistance is available.
6. Determines the presence of significant emotional disturbance in childhood and adolescents and assists in management or arranges for adequate referral.
7. Participates and assists in assessing and managing specific problems relating to perceptually handicapped children of school age.
8. Contributes significantly to the health education of pupils by applying methods designed to increase the pupil's responsibility for his own health care.
9. Collaborates with teachers and other school personnel to interpret pupil health status and suggest appropriate management techniques.
10. Counsels parents regarding parent-child relationships and various emotional and health problems.
11. Coordinates health care plans between family, school, and community settings

to enhance the quality of child health care and to diminish both fragmentation and duplication of services.

THE SNP AND THE FUTURE OF SCHOOL NURSING

From the foregoing discussion it is apparent that the SNP can contribute a great deal to the success and effectiveness of the school health program. Indeed, some proponents of the SNP role envision, as a result of more effective use of school nurses' skills through this expanded role, "a major modification" of the present health care system in this country, since as a consequence of school nurses' role expansion, the school could become "the setting where a significant proportion of total health care of children would be provided" (Silver, 1971a: 1333). In fact, The Robert Wood Johnson Foundation awarded grants totaling $4.8 million to four states (selected from 30 that applied) for the purpose of "broadening and strengthening" the clinical skills of school nurses by preparing them as SNPs, placing them in schools serving children with limited access to health care, and evaluating the impact of the services provided by these SNPs (Four grants announced to expand school nurses' roles, 1978). The planned, independent evaluation of the outcome of this project (to be carried out by the University of California, Los Angeles) is expected to document the following:

1. The extent to which children's health care accessibility is enhanced
2. The SNP's productivity and her ability to follow up children referred to other resources for care
3. The nature of the health problems identified and followed up within the participating communities in the four selected states
4. The cost (actual and comparative) of providing these more complete school-based health services

Although it is still far too early to expect results from these grants, which were awarded during 1978, the idea of using schools as a site for provision of primary health care has been and continues to be controversial. Among the arguments *against* such use of schools for health care delivery is the fear that this practice may encourage parents to abdicate their responsibility for the maintenance of their children's health and may precipitate a return to the practice of the 1930s and 1940s of having the school provide "routine" periodic inspections (cursory examinations) of children. Such practices are believed by many to be both costly and ineffective in improving children's health and health-related behaviors. It should be noted, however, that while these are valid concerns, the intent of the SNP role is to encourage families *and* children to become more involved and responsible in health maintenance and disease prevention. Furthermore, the SNP role is intended to improve the accessibility of health care for children and to decrease the number of inappropriate referrals of children to community health care resources through improved assessment of their health needs. In other words, the SNP is viewed as a supplemental health care resource for children, not as a substitute for the existing health resources in the community.

However, despite the many positive outcomes predicted for the SNP role, unless school nurses can be relieved of duties not requiring their professional knowledge and skill (such as administration of first aid), they will be unable to expand their roles. For that reason, it is critically important that nurses have qualified school health aides or other nonprofessional assistants, including secretaries/clerks and volunteers, to free them to carry out their expanded roles (Silver, 1971a). And, obviously, school nurses, especially those functioning in the expanded SNP role, must be willing to delegate all tasks that do not require their education and skill and must provide appropriate supervision for the aide. It is one thing to receive assistance; it is another to know how to use it.

In looking to the future of school nursing, then, the school nurse practitioner may be expected to remain viable. It seems likely that, based on differences in local needs and available resources, the precise role of the SNP may vary. In communities where there are no physicians or other health care resources, she may indeed continue to be a primary health care provider. On the other hand, in locales where there are many primary health care providers readily accessible, the SNP's role may emphasize continuity of care through appropriate referral and follow-up. Whatever her particular role may become, the school nurse practitioner will be able to contribute competently and confidently to the success of the school health program.

REFERENCES

ANA, ASHA, and DSN/NEA: 1978. Guidelines on educational preparation and competencies of the school nurse practitioner, J. School Health 48(5):265-268.

Barbour, A., Ager, C., and Sundell, W.: 1970. A survey of Denver public school nurses to explore their concepts related to expanded role functioning, J. School Health 40(10):546-548.

Chestnutt, J.: 1978. Judy Igoe talks about school nurse practitioners, Am. J. Nurs. 78(9):1418-1446.

Cronin, G., and Young, W. M.: 1977. Posen/Robbins: a model school health care project, Nurse Pract. 2:22-24, Sept./Oct.

Four grants announced to expand school nurses' roles: 1978. J. School Health 48(7):416.

Hall, J. E., and Weaver, B. R.: 1977. A systems approach to community health, J. B. Lippincott Co., Philadelphia.

Hilmar, N. A., and McAtee, P. A.: 1973. The school nurse practitioner and her practice: a study of traditional and expanded health care responsibilities for nurses in elementary schools, J. School Health 43(7):431-441.

Igoe, J. B.: 1975. The school nurse practitioner, Nurs. Outlook 23(6):381-384.

Igoe, J.: 1977. A program to expand the role of the adolescent health consumer, narrative of grant proposal submitted to the Office of Consumer Education, Department of Health, Education, and Welfare, Washington, D.C. Funding awarded June, 1978.

Igoe, J. B.: 1978. Educational preparation for SNPs offered by the University of Colorado Medical Center, Schools of Nursing and Medicine, Curriculum Handbook, Nov.

Igoe, J. B., and Silver, H. K.: 1977. Improving health care in the school setting, Nurse Pract. 2:7-9, Sept./Oct.

McAtee, P. A.: 1974. Nurse practitioners in our public schools: an assessment of their expanded role as compared with school nurses. Clin. Pediatr. 13:360.

National Academy of Sciences: 1976. Toward a national policy for children and families, National Academy of Sciences Printing and Publishing Office, Washington, D.C.

Silver, H. K.: 1971a. The school nurse practitioner program: a new and expanded role for the school nurse, J.A.M.A. 216(8):1332-1334.

Silver, H. K.: 1971b. The utilization of allied health professionals, Superv. Nurse 2(8):62-70.

Silver, H. K.: 1978. Testimony prepared for Senator Edward M. Kennedy's Child Health Hearings, Denver, Colorado, Nov. 29.

Silver, H., Igoe, J., and McAtee, P.: 1976. The school nurse practitioner: providing improved health care to children, Pediatrics 58(4):580-584.

Silver, H. K., Igoe, J. B., and McAtee, P. R.: 1977. School nurse practitioners: a concise descriptive definition of their functions and activities, J. School Health 47(10):598-599.

SUGGESTED READINGS

Blust, L. C.: 1978. School nurse practitioner in a high school, Am. J. Nurs. 78(9):1532-1533.

DeAngelis, C.: 1978. Robert Wood Johnson Foundation School Health Project, J. School Health 48(10):619.

Lampe, J. M.: 1972. A new approach to delivery of health care to school children as instituted by Denver, Colorado Public Schools, J. School Health 42(5):272-274.

Lewis, C. E., Lorimer, A., Lindeman, C., Palmer, B. B., and Lewis, M. A.: 1974. An evaluation of the impact of school nurse practitioners, J. School Health **44**(6):331-335.

Nader, P. R., Conrad, J., Williamson, M. C., McKevitt, R., and Berrey, R.: 1978. The high school nurse practitioner, J. School health **48**(1):649-654.

Silver, H. K., and Nelson, N.: 1971. The school nurse practitioner program: a new concept in providing health care, J. Nurs. Adm. **1**(3):4-6.

Williamson, M. C.: 1978. Staff development for the school nurse practitioner, J. School Health **48**(8):471-473.

CHAPTER 21

School nursing: surviving and thriving

SUSAN J. WOLD

The first twenty chapters of this book have traced the historical role development of the school nurse and identified and discussed problems that have plagued school nurses, frustrating their role development and threatening their very existence. In addition, a conceptual framework, believed to provide a sound basis for school nursing practice, has been identified and proposed.

Because these discussions have centered on topics that are broad, far reaching in their consequences, and often very complex, readers may by now be left with feelings of confusion and powerlessness concerning the future of school nursing. Therefore, at this point it is appropriate to summarize the major problems confronting today's school nurse, identify goals for them, and propose strategies for achieving those goals.

CONTEMPORARY SCHOOL NURSING: PROBLEMS/NEEDS, GOALS, AND STRATEGIES

In attempting to identify problems or needs confronting as large and diverse a group as today's school nurses, one risks overgeneralizing. Inevitably, there will be those school nurses who insist that some or all of these alleged "problems" and "needs" do not apply to them—and they may be right. However, in assessing the problems and needs confronting school nurses and school nursing *in general,* the list presented and discussed in this chapter is applicable and may even be seen by some as too narrow or limited in scope. Readers are encouraged to critically appraise this list, deciding which problems affect and impede their own practice and which, if any, of the suggested strategies they can employ.

I have summarized the problems/needs confronting contemporary school nursing and

nurses in Table 21-1. They are arranged in what seems to me to be a logical order for discussion; this sequencing does *not* necessarily indicate priority of the problem or need. Indeed, all the problems included in this discussion are important and in need of immediate and continuing efforts to solve them.

Role confusion and ineffectiveness

Throughout this book, evidence has been presented to document school nurses' persistent problems with role confusion and consequent ineffectiveness. As previously discussed, these problems have resulted from confusion on the part of the nurses themselves, as well as from the misperceptions and conflicting expectations of others in the school and community. However, school nurses' persistent role confusion and ineffectiveness seem to be attributable to four specific, basic problems: (1) school nurses' limited role perceptions, (2) school nurses' failure to regard and conduct themselves as managers and leaders within the school health program, (3) ineffective school health team relationships and communication patterns, and (4) infrequent and inappropriate use of nonprofessional assistants. In the remainder of this discussion, each of these problems will be briefly addressed.

School nurses' limited role perceptions

As previously noted, while many problems confronting school nurses are in part due to others' misperceptions of their skills, preparation, and role within the school's health and educational programs, restrictive perceptions of their roles held by many school nurses have contributed to their role confusion and ineffectiveness. As described in Chapter 1, to some extent nurses' restrictive perceptions of their roles and functions may be due to the influence of the

Table 21-1. Problems/needs confronting school nursing/nurses with suggested goals and strategies

Problem/need	Goal	Strategy
Role confusion and ineffectiveness due to the following:		
School nurses' limited role perceptions	School nurses will adopt distributive (health promotion and disease prevention) rather than episodic (disease- and crisis-oriented) focus	Revise and expand school nurses' own role perceptions and expectations through the following: Values' clarification and support group services for school nurses Continuing education, including SNP preparation, for qualified and receptive nurses to upgrade their school nursing skills Improved baccalaureate education for *all* nurses, with emphasis on managerial, leadership, and research skills.
	School nurses will carry out five roles discussed in Chapter 2: Manager of health care Deliverer of health services Advocate for children's health rights Counselor for health concerns of children, families, and school staff Educator for school/community health concerns	Improve and expand school nurses' public relations skills and efforts through one-to-one conferences with students, parents, and school personnel, and speaking before groups such as classes, faculty meetings, school boards, and parent-teacher association (PTA)
School nurses' failure to function as managers and leaders within school health program	School nurses will, in their role as manager of health care, participate fully and appropriately in planning, implementation, and evaluation of school health program	Apply management process and principles, and planned change theory and process
Ineffective school health team relationships and communication patterns	Establish and maintain effective school health team relationships and communication patterns	School nurses must clarify and interpret their roles to other health team members, both formally and informally Take advantage of opportunities for team and interdisciplinary participation Develop broad base of school and community involvement
Infrequent and inappropriate use of nonprofessional assistants	Delegate to nonprofessional assistants all tasks not requiring school nurses' professional skill and judgment	Critically review and evaluate school nurses' job descriptions and current range and frequency of activities to assess time use Recruit appropriately qualified nonprofessional assistants Educate school nurses to improve their willingness and ability to delegate and to supervise their nonprofessional assistants
Duplication of and/or gaps in children's health services	Integrate school health program into overall community health program	Develop and maintain relationships with community health care professionals and organizations Establish school health program planning committee that includes not only school health care professionals (including nurses) and administrators, but also includes representatives from community

Continued.

Table 21-1. Problems/needs confronting school nursing/nurses with suggested goals and strategies—cont'd

Problem/need	Goal	Strategy
Varied and often inadequate educational preparation of school nurses	School nurses will improve their academic preparation to levels comparable to teachers and other school health team members	Convince school nurses of importance of advanced and continuing education through values' clarification sessions If relevant continuing education courses (including SNP programs) are not available, petition area schools of nursing to offer them School nurses must be professional and self-directed enough to continually seek available and appropriate means, including workshops and courses, to maintain and enhance their clinical skills
Need for increased documentation of practice outcomes	School nurses will become accountable for their practice through the following:	
	Consistent planning and evaluation of school health programming outcomes	Use management process, especially planning and control, to guide program efforts and evaluate results Use behavioral objectives and EOCs Improve *documentation* of those objectives and outcomes in student health records
	Conduction of ongoing research to validate practice interventions and outcomes	Improve education for (school) nurses regarding research methods Formation of research support and self-help groups Improve nurses' priority-setting skills and their assertiveness in communicating their priorities to others Initiate and maintain ongoing research, which is needed in virtually all areas of school nursing
	Effective communication of outcomes	School nurses should document everything they do, keeping detailed records of numbers of individuals served by program category plus outcomes of those services; daily activity logs and program data sheets are possible means Increase visibility of school nurses through attendance at and participation in PTA, faculty, school board, and other meetings School nurses need to consistently, conscientiously *publish* their research findings and other practice outcomes in professional journals *and* need to seek local media coverage of their activities
Inadequate quality assurance Lack of mandated standards for school nursing practice	School nursing standards will be developed and adopted	Form national task force to review current school nursing practices, philosophies, national, state, and local standards, guidelines, and policies, and research data and to then develop acceptable, meaningful, and appropriate school nursing standards

Table 21-1. Problems/needs confronting school nursing/nurses with suggested goals and strategies—cont'd

Problem/need	Goal	Strategy
Inadequate quality assurance—cont'd		Publish and disseminate standards
		Hold workshops and values' clarification sessions to assist school nurses in applying standards and evaluating their success
		Involve school administrators and other relevant persons in planning for implementation of standards and to encourage their use for annual performance review of nurses
		Secure endorsement of proposed school nursing standards by professional organizations, especially ANA, ASHA, and NASN
Disparity among states regarding school nurse certification	All states will *require* school nurses to be certified and will adopt meaningful, appropriate, and comparable certification criteria and procedures	Each state should begin by developing school nurse certification requirements with input from all groups affected by their implementation
		Establish national task force to review states' certification requirements and procedures and to recommend nationwide certification standards

traditional hospital-based education received by many nurses and the male-dominated health care system in this country, within which nurses have traditionally occupied a subservient, powerless position, subject to the scrutiny and control of others—usually, males. As a consequence of this hospital-based education and experience, many nurses have learned to focus on pathology and episodic nursing care, rather than on health promotion and disease prevention. Nurses with this kind of orientation, when employed in a school setting, may experience understandable difficulty in redirecting their focus and nursing actions toward health promotion and disease prevention. Even for those nurses who may value and understand the importance of health promotion and disease prevention, the rigid role expectations of the administrators and other school personnel with whom they must work may effectively limit the scope of their practice. Too often, the result is an overemphasis on *visible* functions such as first aid and emergency care, transportation of sick children, and record keeping, at the expense of less tangible health promotion and disease prevention activities.

Obviously, the goal for the problem of restrictive role perceptions should be to expand those perceptions. Specifically, there is a need for the focus of school nurses to become less episodic (disease and crisis oriented) and more distributive (health promotion and disease prevention oriented). In addition to adopting a distributive focus, another worthwhile goal for school nurses is to carry out the following five roles discussed in Chapter 2:

1. Manager of health care
2. Deliverer of health services
3. Advocate for children's health rights
4. Counselor for health concerns of children, families, and school staff
5. Educator for school/community concerns

Because these goals represent such a great shift in focus and action for school nurses individually and as a nursing specialty group, they will not be quickly achieved. However, it is suggested that school nurses, individually and collectively, begin by identifying both strategic (long range) and tactical (short range) plans for meeting these goals.

While problems of restricted perceptions of school nurses' roles are partly due to the misperceptions and misconceptions of others, the lion's share of the responsibility for this problem rests with school nurses themselves. For that reason, the primary corrective actions must likewise begin with school nurses. Revising and expanding school nurses' own role perceptions thus become a primary strategy, which can be accomplished through several means. One important method of helping school nurses modify their own role perceptions is to organize and provide support group services for nurses as they begin the process of redirecting the focus of their practice toward health promotion activities such as health education and health counseling and away from others' expectations that nurses emphasize first aid and record keeping. Such support groups allow nurses to share their ideas as well as to actively support each other's efforts, thus increasing their motivation to persist in their role change. Within these support groups or as an adjunct to them, values' clarification workshops could be held; such workshops would help individual nurses identify their own values and role expectations, perhaps reaffirming their commitment to the change process as well.

Another important means for helping school nurses revise and expand their role perceptions and expectations involves continuing education for currently employed school nurses. As discussed in Chapter 2 all school nurses are encouraged to complete course work in public health and public health nursing, child growth and development, educational theories and methods, school health administration, psychology, sociology, and health assessment. For those school nurses whose basic nursing education did not include any or all of those courses, continuing education is an important and viable means of correcting those deficiencies. In addition, school nurses need to develop knowledge and skills in the areas of management theory and practice, leadership, assertiveness, change theory and process, political dynamics, and research methods and process. These topics, too, can be studied through continuing education courses. Finally, another viable and important means for school nurses to upgrade their educational preparation and to expand their role is to seek preparation and certification as SNPs. As discussed in Chapter 20, for receptive, qualified nurses who have administrative support, preparation to become SNPs is an important and highly recommended option. School nurses residing in areas where no relevant or useful continuing education programs are offered and/or who do not have ready access to accredited SNP programs will need to petition collegiate schools of nursing to address these needs.

In addition to focusing on currently practicing school nurses, it is essential to begin reshaping the expectations and perceptions of *future* school nurses; in other words, the role perceptions of nursing students must also be addressed. Students should be provided opportunities to visit with and observe the interactions of school nurses who are positive role models. In addition, students who are interested in becoming school nurses should be advised to obtain appropriate academic preparation and should be urged to complete a carefully supervised school nursing practicum. Furthermore, recognizing that baccalaureate education does not usually produce a practitioner who has adequate preparation in such areas as research and management, students who are seriously contemplating a career in school nursing should be encouraged to seek graduate courses and/or an advanced degree.

Although school nurses' restrictive role expectations are largely a problem of their own creation, the influence of others' opinions—especially administrators'—cannot be overlooked or readily dismissed. It seems likely that others' opinions concerning appropriate and expected roles for nurses in general and school nurses in particular depend, at least partially, on their impressions and observations of nurses they may have previously encountered. Thus, principals and teachers who may have previously encountered nurses who prefer limiting their activities to first aid, record keeping, and attendance monitoring may be expected to doubt the worth and cost-effectiveness of school nursing services.

Therefore, in addition to revising and redirecting their own perceptions and role expectations, school nurses must help redirect and expand the perceptions of "significant others" such as parents, students, teachers, administrators, other school personnel, and professional and lay community members. While there are undoubtedly many ways of accomplishing this, including strategies such as one-to-one conferences with students, parents, and school personnel and speaking before groups such as classes, faculty meetings, school boards, and the parent-teacher association (PTA), one thing is clear: nurses—particularly school nurses—must improve and expand their public relations skills and efforts. Only when school nurses and their significant others achieve congruent role perceptions and expectations will school nurses be able to function fully and effectively within the school setting.

School nurses' failure to function as managers and leaders within the school health program

A second problem contributing to school nurses' role confusion and ineffectiveness is their failure to regard themselves as managers and leaders and to conduct themselves accordingly. Too often, nurses, especially school nurses, have tended to react rather than act and follow passively rather than lead assertively. As a result, school nurses have too often been expected to *implement* the school health program, following minimal (if any) input into program *planning*.

As shown in Table 21-1, the goal for amelioration of this problem is that school nurses will, in their role as manager of health care, participate fully and appropriately in planning, implementation, and evaluation of the school health program. To achieve this goal, nurses must apply management process, including the managerial functions of planning, organizing (including staffing and delegation), directing and heading (including principles of supervision and leadership), and controlling (including standard setting, budgeting, and corrective action). (See Chapter 18.)

In addition to consistent application of management process and principles, school nurses must begin applying planned change theory and process if they are to succeed as leaders within the school health program. As discussed in Chapter 19, this means that nurses must eliminate their political naivete, actively pursuing changes in legislation and budgeting that they believe are vital to the well-being of schoolchildren and school nurses. As discussed in Chapter 19, school nurses must become actively involved in the political process at all levels if their goals are to be realized; nurses must commit their funds and their time to lobbying, testifying, and otherwise supporting legislation they favor. Ultimately, this approach should result in development of the kind of school nurse leaders described by Ford (1970: 23) as *statesmen* "whose stature and skill in public policy arenas guide and influence the direction of the field and who speak eloquently for the nursing of children in school settings."

Ineffective school health team relationships and communication patterns

A third problem, which, along with school nurses' limited role perceptions and failure to think and act as managers and leaders, contributes to their role confusion and ineffectiveness, is the ineffective interpersonal relationships and communication patterns that too often characterize the school health team. While this problem may be partially a consequence of nurses' limited self-perceptions and expectations and others' (principals, teachers, students) misconceptions and misinformation about school nurses and school nursing, miscommunication is undoubtedly involved as well.

Igoe (1977) suggests that misperceptions of the school nurse's role may be at least partly attributable to differences in communication styles of health care professionals (including school nurses) compared with those of educators. Thus, while educators generally learn to communicate in a style that allows them to maintain classroom control and order, nurses generally learn communication skills designed to elicit the client's perceptions, which requires more "give and take." These differences in style may result in teachers labeling school nurses as "too easy" on students, while nurses may regard teachers as authoritarian or "too strict." Once this type of "labeling" begins, the communication style differences escalate into relationship problems within the school health team, often manifesting themselves as territoriality battles between and among school nurses and teachers, administrators, social workers and psychologists, and other professionals. Obviously, when school health professionals and educators expend their energies and time waging territorial battles and building their respective empires, the health and well-being of the students whom they serve receives less attention and effort.

Therefore, to meet the needs of students, it is critically important for school health team members to "bury their hatchets" and adopt the goal of establishing and maintaining effective school health team relationships and communication patterns. An important first step toward achieving that goal is for school nurses to clarify and interpret their roles to other health team members, both formally (such as at faculty and PTA meetings) and informally (through one-to-one conferences or during coffee and lunch breaks).

Another means for helping achieve improved

team relationships and communication patterns is for school nurses to become more vocal and assertive (*not* aggressive!). As noted in Chapter 1, school nurses have traditionally had difficulty with teamwork (Thomas, 1976), often finding themselves at the bottom of the decision-making pyramid. Reiterating the importance of interdisciplinary teamwork in providing comprehensive care to school-age children, Hill (1971) supports movement away from a pyramidal team relationship structure, in which power and decision making are concentrated within a few individuals or positions, and toward the "pie" concept, which emphasizes shared decision making. By participating fully and assertively in all "team" meetings, school nurses can help eliminate counterproductive casteism and elitism among school health team members, thus facilitating the shift toward the "pie" division of labor.

Finally, in addition to clarifying and interpreting their roles and adopting a direct, assertive communication style, Fricke (1972) urges school nurses to improve their school health team relationships and communication patterns by taking advantage of *all* opportunities for interdisciplinary team participation. Fricke believes that nurses should be free to align themselves not only with pupil personnel services team members, but also with other "teams" in the school and community, because this broad base of involvement provides "a larger range of opportunity for meeting the child health needs and promoting positive mental health" (1972: 205).

Infrequent and inappropriate use of nonprofessional assistants

The fourth specific problem contributing to school nurses' role confusion and ineffectiveness is their infrequent and often inappropriate use of nonprofessional assistants within the school health program. This problem is obviously inextricably tied to the previous three problems: (1) because many school nurses have limited perceptions and expectations for their own roles, they become caught up in activities, such as first aid, that do not require their professional expertise; (2) since many school nurses are operating within restricted roles, they do not apply management concepts and process, including principles of staffing and delegation, thus perpetuating those limited roles; and (3) due to ineffective communication patterns and relationships with health team members, school

nurses may fail to understand or appreciate the potential benefits of collaboration with other health team members and school personnel (including clerical and secretarial staff). The result is that many school nurses spend much of their time carrying out tasks (such as first aid and some record keeping) which could be more cost-effectively completed by nonprofessional assistants, thus freeing school nurses for activities requiring their professional skill and judgment.

An appropriate goal for resolving this problem, then, is for school nurses to delegate to nonprofessional assistants all tasks not requiring nurses' professional skill and judgment. No doubt, this proposed goal will be acutely threatening to those school nurses whose hours are typically spent carrying out tasks that do not actually require their skills and judgment; such nurses may rightly perceive that this kind of delegation would force them to either expand their focus or look for alternative employment. However threatening it may be, incorporation of nonprofessional assistants into the school health program seems like an effective means for extending and redirecting school nursing services and is especially fiscally attractive given the current financial crises facing many school districts and the resultant increase in the pupil-nurse ratio.

Thus, despite debate concerning their impact and fears that they may "take over" the school nurse's position within the school, nonprofessional assistants are a necessary and important means for improving the efficiency and effectiveness of the school nurse. As previously suggested, to use such assistants effectively, school nurses must be willing to delegate all tasks not requiring their knowledge, skill, and judgment (Fricke, 1972) and must be willing and able to provide direct and continuing supervision for the assistant or aide (American School Health Association, 1974). For that reason, delegation and supervision are critically important managerial skills to be developed and *used* if school nurses are to use their increasingly limited time more productively and for more potentially satisfying and rewarding activities (Chapter 18).

To begin incorporating nonprofessional assistants into the school health program, school nurses will need to first critically review and evaluate their own job descriptions and present range and frequency of activities to determine exactly where and how they are spending their time; a time study, accounting for all the hours worked by nurses over a period of time such as 2 weeks or 1 month, might be one means of collecting pertinent data. Next, the data should be analyzed to compare *actual* percentages of school nurses' time spent on particular program objectives and activities (such as vision screening) with projected and *desired* time percentages. Thus, if vision screening and follow-up are found to occupy 30% of a nurse's time, while the school health program's objectives and budget only estimated a 10% time commitment, that nurse is spending 20% more time on one program activity or objective than planned and is therefore probably failing to devote adequate time to some other valued activity, such as health education or teacher consultation. Data from this kind of time and activity study can also be analyzed to determine which activities do not require the direct and continuing skills, attention, and judgment of school nurses. In other words, which activities, however "familiar" and "comfortable" they may be for the nurse to complete, are actually "nonessential" and hence able to be delegated to a qualified nonprofessional assistant?

Determining which activities can be safely and legally delegated to nonprofessional assistants requires familiarity with the nurse practice act and other relevant laws in the particular state in question, plus knowledge of school district and building policies, as well as plain common sense. Because nurse practice acts and other legal and administrative standards and policies vary widely throughout the country, the question concerning which tasks can be delegated must be answered by individual states and/or school districts. Once those decisions have been reached, recruitment of appropriately qualified nonprofessional assistants can begin. Depending on the nature of the tasks to be delegated, and the availability of funding, nonprofessional assistants for the school health program may be drawn from older students, salaried school clerical or secretarial personnel, salaried school health aides (who are specially trained in such areas as first aid and clerical skills), or even unpaid adult volunteers from the community.

However, a third vital component of this strategy to incorporate nonprofessional assistants into the school health program is educating school nurses to be able and willing to delegate to and supervise these aides. In their study of the effect of employment of health office clerks on the amount of time spend by school nurses in following up children with health defects, Randall et al. (1968) found that use of clerical nonnurse personnel did *not* seem to make a significant difference in the numbers of children receiving follow-up care. In other words, more helpers do not necessarily accomplish more work. Randall et al. (1968) speculated that school nurses may not know how to use clerical and other nonprofessional help effectively and may also need to develop their supervisory skills.

In contrast, Bryan and Cook (1967) found that, when relieved by nonnurse assistants of tasks not requiring their skills, school nurses *will* use that released time for activities requiring their expertise—although the *extent* to which they will use released time varies from nurse to nurse and depends in part on nurses' willingness to give up "familiar," although nonessential, activities. To avoid such pitfalls, in school districts planning to incorporate nonprofessional assistants, it may be prudent to plan in-service education meetings concerning (1) the role of nonprofessional assistants, (2) the art of delegation, and (3) principles of supervision.

One thing seems clear, however: nonprofessional assistants are here to stay in the school health program; the only negotiable point is whether they will supplement or supplant school nurses—and that is a decision which school nurses themselves will make, either through action or inaction.

Duplication of and/or gaps in children's health services

As illustrated in Table 21-1, a second major problem confronting school nurses and school nursing involves duplication of community health services for children and/or the creation of gaps in services. An example repeatedly cited throughout this book (Chapters 5 and 13) is screening. School-age children are, unfortunately, too often screened needlessly, inconveniently, and certainly expensively for conditions that are not readily detectable by screening, do not generally require or respond to treatment, or may not even apply to their community population. This screening may take place at the urging of well-intentioned, although underinformed or misinformed, adults and may be included in the school health program at their urging. Worst of all, if the community's medical and other health care professionals are not aware and supportive of the program, they may consciously or unconsciously sabotage screening and follow-up efforts, resulting in fragmented, expensive, and largely ineffective health "care" for the children.

While screening is only one example of overlapping, uncoordinated health services, it does point out the hazards of such services. As suggested by such authorities as Jacobsen and Siegel (1971) and Newman and Mayshark (1973), the goal for resolving this problem should be integration of the school health program into the overall community health program. This requires coordination and joint planning efforts and open communication between school health care professionals and community health care professionals. If joint planning is not already part of the process of setting up the school health program, school nurses can and should help initiate this kind of coordinated planning.

Selection of strategies for dealing with duplication of services and/or gaps in health services depends on assessment of the nature and extent of the problem(s) within a particular community or school district and on adequacy and availability of material, monetary, and human resources for resolving the problem(s). Within those limitations, however, two basic strategies may be useful. The first is that school nurses and other school health care professionals and administrators need to develop and maintain relationships with community health care professionals and organizations, such as health departments, health boards, and nursing and social service agencies. These kinds of relationships promote understanding among and between health care professionals, agencies, and school health personnel, thus reducing the likelihood and severity of conflicts among them regarding health programming for children. In addition, such relationships are a source of community support for school health programming efforts, since health care professionals and agencies are more likely to support and willingly participate in school health services and programs (such as vision and hearing screening) if they understand and accept the need for the program or service, and if their input and cooperation have been actively sought. In other words, effective public relations are important to the success of the school health program as an arm of the overall community health plan.

A second strategy for resolving these kinds of problems is to establish a school health program planning committee that includes not only school nurses and other school health care professionals and administrators, but which also includes representatives from the community (parents, physicians, and other health care professionals), representatives from selected community agencies (social services and welfare), and specialized organizations (such as the local hearing society, pediatric specialists, ophthalmologic or optometric societies), based on local needs. The precise role of such a committee or planning group will of course be determined according to local school district policies and customs; thus in some communities this kind of group might be given line authority (Chapter 18), while in other locales, this group might be given a staff or advisory role. Regardless which option is selected, solicitation of community input for school health program planning is strongly recommended as a means of more fully integrating the school's health program into the overall community health program, thus minimizing threats of costly duplication, gaps, or sabotage of programming efforts.

Varied and often inadequate educational preparation of school nurses

A third major problem confronting school nursing and school nurses is the great variation among nurses in educational preparation for their jobs. School nurses, as is the case with most nursing specialty groups, possess a variety of academic credentials, ranging from hospital school diplomas, with an education focused on episodic, acute care, to associate degrees in nursing, to baccalaureate, master's, or doctoral degrees in nursing or related fields (Marriner, 1971; Fricke, 1972). Obviously, these wide variations in academic preparation and focus create problems in setting and enforcing standards of care. However, in addition to that problem, these educational disparities create credibility problems for school nurses—especially for those possessing less than a baccalaureate degree—because their credentials are often below those of the teachers and other school staff members with whom they must develop collegial, working relationships. The result often is that school nurses with a diploma or associate degree have less status (and salary) than teachers in their schools and therefore may experience difficulty securing support and cooperation for their programming ideas and innovations within the school.

In addition, for those nurses whose educational preparation is hospital based and focused on acute, episodic illness, developing and implementing health promotion and disease prevention programs may be a low priority; even those diploma and associate degree nurses who value disease prevention and health promotion strategies may be handicapped, however, since their educational programs may not have prepared them for devising and implementing such programs. Thus those nurses may understandably focus on first aid and care of the sick, which would effectively limit the scope of the school health program.

Clearly, then, there is a need to standardize educational preparation for school nurses. An appropriate goal would be for school nurses to improve their academic preparation to levels comparable with those of the teachers and other school faculty and personnel with whom they must work. As discussed in Chapter 2, minimal academic credentials for school nurses should include a bachelor's degree in nursing plus eligibility to become certified as a public health nurse and as a school nurse. More specifically, school nurses should have had courses in public health nursing, school nursing, plus a supervised clinical experience in both areas; in addition, school nurses need academic background in child growth and development, educational theories and methods, school health administration, leadership and management, psychology, sociology, health assessment, and research methods.

Ideally, the kind of academic preparation just described should serve as a minimal standard. Because baccalaureate nursing programs prepare their graduates to be nursing generalists, and because those programs offer students only limited opportunities for clinical practice, it is highly unrealistic to expect a baccalaureate graduate to function fully and effectively as a school nurse without additional preparation. For that reason, it is strongly recommended that school nurses obtain graduate credits beyond their basic baccalaureate degrees, with an emphasis on related fields such as public health, pediatrics, management, health assessment, and developmental psychology. Indeed, school nurses would be well advised to seek graduate degrees in school nursing or public health nursing, and/or to seek education and certification as SNPs.

An important initial strategy for accomplishing the goal of educational parity is to convince school nurses themselves that such preparation and credentials are needed. This might be accomplished through small group meetings or values' clarification sessions. Unfortunately, even when nurses are convinced that advanced and continuing education is important, they may experience difficulty upgrading their knowledge and skills, simply because the kinds of courses needed are not readily available. If courses or programs of study (such as SNP programs) are *not* available, then school nurses will need to petition area schools of nursing to offer such courses. Like many teachers, school nurses may need to get in the habit of spending part or all of their summers taking necessary courses to upgrade their practice and may need to dissipate whatever resentment they may feel at having to spend "vacation" time going to school themselves—after all, being professional includes the expectation of maintaining and enhancing one's clinical skills, through whatever means are available and appropriate. While nursing registration standards and procedures used in many states currently mandate completion of a specified number of hours of continuing education, nurses should be professional and self-directed enough to seek needed courses without coercion from their employers or state boards of nursing.

Need for increased documentation of practice outcomes

Another recurrent theme throughout this book has been to deplore school nurses' failure to *demonstrate* their worth (Ford, 1970), which has contributed to the escalating cutbacks in school nursing positions around the country. Apparently believing that their contributions to successful school health programs are obvious, school nurses have not taken the initiative to "sell" the merits of their services to school boards, administrators, or even to their consumers: students and their families. By thus failing to demonstrate to the public that school nursing services are worth the cost, school nurses must accept partial culpability for their current status as an "endangered species" within the school.

No doubt, school nurses' failure to sell themselves and their services is related to traditional socialization of women to be passive, reticent, unworldly, and politically naive. While that helps *explain* school nurses' present predicament, it does not *excuse* present or future inaction. Indeed, continued inaction will certainly eradicate school nursing and may jeopardize the future of all school health services as well. Clearly, school nurses must act *now* to meet the need for increased documentation of their practice outcomes and to thereby *demonstrate* their worth and their cost-effectiveness.

In meeting this need for increased documentation of school nursing practice outcomes, a three-pronged goal is suggested:

1. Constant planning and evaluation of school health programming outcomes
2. Conduction of ongoing research to validate practice interventions and outcomes
3. Effective communication of outcomes

The first prong of the goal, that school nurses will become accountable for their practice through consistent planning and evaluation of school health programming outcomes, means that school nurses must use management process, especially planning and control, to guide their program efforts and to evaluate results. This will require that school nurses write behavioral objectives for both total program efforts (such as screening programs) as well as for individual nursing care plans used in working with students and families. In addition, EOCs for measuring the outcomes of total programs and individual care plans need to be developed to *measure* results of nursing interventions. While many nurses have not yet learned how to write specific and measurable behavioral objectives and EOCs, their continued survival in the school setting depends on their willingness and ability to correct that deficit.

A second strategy for achieving the goal of consistent planning and evaluation of school health programming outcomes concerns documentation of client (student) outcomes on an individual basis. In addition to writing behavioral objectives and EOCs for each care plan, school nurses need to improve their documentation of those objectives and outcomes in student health records. Too often students move through their 12 years of public education, accompanied by a health record that is, for all practical purposes, blank. It seems unlikely that all those children have *never* had a health problem for which the school nurse and other school health team members intervened. A more likely explanation for those blank health records is that school nurses did not have the time for completely recording their interventions and outcomes concerning students' health, or that they did not fully comprehend the importance of doing so. In addition, due to fear of the consequences of the open record law, nurses may

hesitate to write down their judgments and actions, lest they be verbally and/or legally challenged.

Such hesitation characterizes too many nurses today; often insecurity and fear of taking and defending a position or stance causes nurses to couch their judgments and assessments in cautious disclaimers like "seems" and "appears." Despite their hesitations or insecurities, nurses—especially school nurses—need to actively assert their judgments and accept ownership of their actions if they are to establish and maintain a credible position in health care; nurses can and should begin by carefully documenting their interventions with individual students.

The second prong of the goal for meeting this need for increased documentation of school nursing outcomes is that school nurses will become accountable for their practice through conduction of ongoing research to validate practice interventions and outcomes. The dearth of meaningful, relevant, and well-designed research in school nursing has been acknowledged and discussed repeatedly. As previously noted, possible reasons for this lack of research include nurses' failure to fully appreciate the importance of such studies, their seeming inability to place research high enough on their list of priorities—especially when other school personnel drain school nurses of time and energy by placing inappropriate demands on them—and school nurses' feelings of inadequacy and insecurity about conducting research, perhaps due to inadequate educational preparation in the area of research methodologies and issues.

Whatever the reasons behind the appalling lack of research to support school nursing interventions and to document their outcomes, there is an acute need for *immediate* action to correct the problem. It is no longer adequate or prudent for school nurses to aver that school nursing services "obviously" make a difference in children's abilities to learn effectively; if the school nurse is to remain a viable part of the school program, she must present *data* documenting her effectiveness (Chinn, 1973). For many school nurses, additional academic preparation in research methods, coupled with supervised application of research methods, may be necessary. A second action would be for school nurses within a school district or geographic area to form their own research support and self-help groups. Such groups would encourage members in their research efforts, provide a resource for problems with research design or implementation, and also provide a forum for sharing research findings (although optimal dissemination of research findings requires that they be *published*).

Another strategy necessary for improving the volume and adequacy of school nursing research is for school nurses to improve their skills of priority setting. Nurses must regard research as a priority that will benefit themselves, through economic survival in the school setting, and that will also benefit schoolchildren, through improved school nursing practice. In addition, once nurses begin to highly value school nursing research, they will need to be assertive in communicating their priorities to others, such as administrators and other school personnel, so that pressures for school nurses to spend their time on first aid and other activities that can be delegated, will lessen. School nurses need to resist others' attempts to structure their practice; rather, they must actively define their roles, using research data to explain and justify their actions and judgments.

Following review of available school health and school nursing literature, one is forced to conclude that research is needed in virtually all aspects of school nursing. Ford (1970) emphasizes the need for epidemiological and demographic studies to identify and prioritize the health needs of target populations within the school and community, from which strengths can be identified and delivery of health services can be planned. Basco (1963) concludes that research establishing the validity of accepted school nursing standards is badly needed as well. Furthermore, it would be useful to know how and to what extent those standards are being applied and to study changes in quality of care that may occur when standards are implemented.

Chinn (1973) advocates development and implementation of studies that explain and justify how school nursing services enhance students' learning and otherwise contribute to the school's achievement of its educational goals. Chinn also notes that studies to clarify the relationship between health problems and school performance are needed; if there is *no* relationship (an improbable conclusion), then perhaps school health programs and school nursing services are superfluous. The point is that data to support and document these relationships must be gathered and communicated if school health programs are to maintain their funding and support.

Igoe (1977) further points out that today's increasingly skeptical and taxation-weary society also needs to be convinced that preventive strategies, such as health maintenance and health education, are important, more effective, and cost-effective as compared with curative, episodic services. In other words, the burden of proving that prevention is indeed better than cure lies squarely with the providers of those services.

As discussed in Chapter 17, research clarifying the role of the school nurse is also needed. Staton (1963) recommends completion of studies to identify precisely the role of the school nurse and to analyze her day-to-day activities for appropriateness and relative priority. For those activities found to be inappropriate for the school nurse and/or which do not require her skills and knowledge, studies exploring their delegation to nonprofessional assistants could be undertaken.

In addition to studying the role of the school nurse, Thomas (1976) recommends research studies to analyze school health team relationships. Specifically, she concludes that studies measuring the quality and frequency of school health team interactions and comparing school nurses' and other school health team members' perceptions of team functioning and communication are needed. The results of such studies could be applied in efforts to improve school health team communication and relationships—areas that have already been identified as problematic.

As discussed at length in this book, the entire area of school-based screening programs needs to be studied; research exploring planning, implementation, and evaluation of screening programs is desperately needed. The epidemiological and demographic studies suggested by Ford (1970) would be helpful in identifying populations to screen and health conditions or problems for which screening would be done. With regard to implementation of screening programs, research testing the adequacy, appropriateness, and cost-effectiveness of screening tools and procedures is also needed. Likewise, studies of the efficacy and efficiency of follow-up methods are needed. Finally, with regard to evaluation of screening programs, research is needed not only to assess the efficiency and effectiveness of the evaluation methods themselves, but is also needed to document long-range effects of the screening program on the prevalence and severity of the conditions for which screening is done.

Again, some of the more pressing areas needing to be researched by and for school nurses have merely been highlighted; undoubtedly, there are many, many other areas of school health and school nursing to be carefully researched. School nurses are encouraged to begin their research efforts now, starting with areas and methodologies with which they are familiar and comfortable and proceeding to larger, more difficult studies as their skills and confidence increase.

The third prong of the goal for meeting the need for increased documentation of practice outcomes is that school nurses will become accountable through effective communication of their outcomes. Because of the ever-tightening squeeze on the educational dollar, it is no longer adequate for school nurses merely to improve their programming, document changed client/student behaviors, and to research and validate their practice interventions and outcomes. Unless those outcomes and research findings are *communicated* to the appropriate persons and groups—that is, to those who control the purse strings—erosion of financial and other support for school health and school nursing services will continue and may result in the eventual elimination of school-based health programs. In other words, if school nurses expect to survive efforts to trim educational budgets, they must not only do a terrific job of program planning, implementation, and evaluation, but they must also be sure that everyone knows it. To ensure that they have adequate information and data to communicate to others, school nurses would be well advised to begin by documenting everything they do. This means that nurses should keep detailed records for themselves of the numbers of individuals served by program area and the achieved outcomes of their services. A daily activity log is one way of accomplishing this. In addition, data sheets or record forms for each school health program objective could be developed, which would simplify summative program evaluation at the end of the school year. Coding systems that would minimize the need for lengthy, handwritten entries could also be developed. Such records could also be used by individual nurses to evaluate their priority setting and the effectiveness of their time use. For those nurses who may view such record keeping as one more useless and time-consuming bit of paperwork, it may be helpful to point out that keeping records to account for one's time and to document one's accomplishments is actually *less* time consuming and frustrating than job hunting.

Effective communication of practice outcomes also requires that school nurses increase their visibility through such methods as attending and participating in PTA, faculty, school board, and other meetings. While such meetings provide a forum for school nurses to clarify their roles and build relationships with influential members of the school community, including parents, teachers, administrators, and board members, they also provide opportunities for school nurses to share and discuss their health programs and statistical outcomes. When nurses take advantage of these opportunities to share and discuss their activities and suggestions for future programming, they may be not only documenting their accountability, but they may also be unconsciously laying the groundwork for continuing or increasing financial and administrative support for their services.

As intimated in the preceding discussion, however, effective communication of research findings is critically important for the continued survival and growth of school nursing. Therefore, in addition to carefully documenting their outcomes and becoming more visible and active within the school community, school nurses must consistently, conscientiously *publish* their research findings and other practice outcomes in professional journals. All outcomes, both successes and failures, are important and should be published. At the same time, school nurses must attend to their public image. For that reason, it also recommended that school nurses seek local coverage of their activities on television, radio, and in newspapers and other tabloids. This may entail writing their own press releases and telephoning local reporters with features and "stories" illustrating that today's school nurse indeed makes a difference in the lives and education of children. While some nurses may pale at the very thought of actively seeking publicity, it is naive to believe that nursing can grow and thrive without public support—which depends, of course, on public awareness. Physicians, lawyers, and other professionals have long recognized the importance of "good press" and have actively courted it; it is past time for nurses to stop being demure and start being self-assured and in control of their public image. If nurses want public recognition for their contributions and achievements, they will have to actively seek it. If, instead, they sit back and wait for someone to take notice, they may be sitting and waiting for a long, long time.

Inadequate quality assurance

The final school nursing problem to be discussed in this chapter is the inadequacy of school nursing's quality assurance measures. This problem has its roots in many of the problems already discussed, including (1) inadequate research documenting appropriate school nursing practices, educational preparation, and standards for care; (2) role confusion; and (3) administrative or managerial problems such as misuse (or disuse) of nonprofessional assistants and inadequate program planning and evaluation. This overall problem of inadequate quality assurance in school nursing can be separated into two specific problems: (1) lack of mandated standards for school nursing practice and (2) disparity among states regarding school nurse certification.

Lack of mandated standards for school nursing practice

The lack of mandated, accepted standards of practice is a problem throughout nursing. Even in those areas or specialties within nursing for which the ANA has developed and published standards, such as psychiatric/mental health nursing and community health nursing, those standards may not be widely known, accepted, or applied by nursing practitioners. For school nursing, the problem is more acute; with the variety of nursing and other professional organizations that have vested interests in children, public health, school health, education, and nursing, merely deciding who has the authority to set and enforce standards is a sticky problem. Probably the closest existing approximation to school nursing practice standards are the ASHA *Guidelines for the School Nurse in the School Health Program* (1974). However, it is unlikely that these guidelines are widely known or applied; hence the problem persists.

The goal for correcting this problem of lack of school nursing practice standards is, obviously, that school nursing practice standards will be developed and adopted. One strategy for accomplishing this is for a group of school nurses, ideally including representatives from pertinent professional organizations such as the ANA, ASHA, and NASN to form a national task force to review (1) current school nursing practices; (2) school nursing philosophies; (3) national, state, and local school nursing standards, guidelines, and policies; and (4) research data as a prelude to development of acceptable, meaningful, and appropriate school nursing standards.

A second strategy for accomplishing this goal is to *publish* and *disseminate* the outcomes of the task force's work: the standards themselves, an explanation of the relevance and importance of each standard, and discussion of suggested methods of implementing the standards and evaluating this achievement. Following efforts to ensure that all school nurses have access to a copy of the standards, workshops and values clarification sessions may be held to assist nurses in applying the standards and evaluating their success. It will also be important to involve school administrators and other relevant persons in planning for implementation of these standards and in encouraging use of these standards as part of the annual performance and salary review process for individual school nurses. Indeed, if school districts begin to use these standards for performance review of their nurses, instead of the too frequently used forms assessing behaviors such as "punctuality" and "neatness," that in itself will be an improvement. Finally, if school nursing practice standards are to be widely applied, the unanimous endorsement of school nurses' professional organizations—particularly ANA, ASHA, and NASN—will be needed; if, instead, these organizations battle among themselves, the wide variation in accepted quality of school nursing practice across the country will continue.

Disparity among states regarding school nurse certification

The second specific problem contributing to the overall inadequacy of school nursing quality assurance is the disparity among states regarding school nurse certification requirements and procedures. According to the study by Castile and Jerrick (1976), twenty-three of the fifty states have mandatory school nursing certification requirements, ten states have permissive requirements, and four states are in the planning process for certifying school nurses. While those precise statistics may already have changed, they do point out the differences among states. In addition, after scrutinizing the Castile and Jerrick (1976) data concerning the criteria and procedures for school nurse certification across the country, the disparities loom even larger: criteria used for certifying school nurses range from those which are relevant and exhaustive to those which are inappropriate and meaningless (Chapter 1).

In states where school nurse certification is either permissive or nonexistent and/or is based on inappropriate, meaningless criteria, attaining and maintaining high-quality school nursing practice is difficult and may result in recruitment of nurses who are not truly motivated or prepared to function as assertive, health-oriented, energetic, and involved professionals within the school community. As a result, school nursing positions may be filled with persons seeking an "easy" job with "good" hours and summers off and who may unconsciously perpetuate the negative, stereotyped image of the school nurse as a person who sits in her office, hands out aspirins, sends home sick (and sometimes clever "unsick") children, and transcribes health records.

An appropriate goal for resolving this problem is that all states will *require* school nurses to be certified and will adopt meaningful, appropriate, and comparable certification criteria and procedures. Only when *all* school nurses are required to meet certain standards regarding their academic and prior employment experiences will school nursing become a credible, viable professional specialty in nursing and in the school setting. While achievement of such standards and prerequisites obviously will not *guarantee* that school nurses will function competently and appropriately, it will certainly be a step in the right direction. If renewal of school nursing certificates can be tied to completion of certain continuing education and/or other experiential requirements, continual ungrading of school nurses' credentials and capabilities should occur, resulting in delivery of higher quality nursing services to school community populations.

A strategy suggested by the ASHA (1974) is for each state to develop school nurse certification requirements with input from all groups affected by their implementation, such as nurses, educators, community health personnel, and consumers of school health services. To avoid development of very different sets of criteria across the country, it may also be helpful to establish a national task force, perhaps including representatives from the major professional organizations in which school nurses are active, to review the various states' certification requirements and procedures, and to recommend some certification standards that can be adopted nationwide. A side benefit of this strategy is that it may foster a sense of national unity among school nurses, diminishing their feelings of powerlessness while enhancing their collective political clout and credibility.

CONCLUSION

In this chapter, five basic, overriding problems confronting school nurses and school nursing have been identified. Goals and strategies for achieving those goals have also been pro-

Table 21-2. The relationship between school nurses' problems/needs and their failure to function as managers within the school health program

Problem/need	Failed managerial function(s)
Role confusion and ineffectiveness due to:	
Limited role perception	Planning, directing and heading
Failure to regard self as manager/leader within school health program	Planning, directing and heading
Ineffective school health team relationships and communication patterns	Planning, organizing, directing and heading
Infrequent and inappropriate use of nonprofessional assistants	Planning, organizing, directing and heading, control
Duplication of and/or gaps in children's health services	Planning, organizing, directing and heading
Varied and often inadequate educational preparation of school nurses	Directing and heading, control
Need for increased documentation of practice outcomes	Planning, organizing, directing and heading, control
Inadequate quality assurance due to:	
Lack of mandated standards for school nursing practice	Planning, organizing, control
Disparity between states regarding school nurse certification	Planning, organizing, control

posed. As noted near the beginning of this chapter, this list of school nursing problems represents my viewpoint, although others' ideas and writings have influenced its development. Also as noted earlier, these problems will not affect all school nurses, nor will they affect school nurses equally. Furthermore, it is possible that there are other problems confronting school nurses (individuals or groups) that have not been included in this list.

The intent of this chapter has been to identify problems that affect *most* school nurses and are therefore of general interest. As a final note, and as illustrated in Table 21-2, the problems discussed in this chapter can *all* be viewed as "failures" of the school nurse in carrying out a primary role: manager of health care. Each of the problems discussed in this chapter is directly related to one or more of the managerial functions discussed at length in Chapter 18. Therefore one may reasonably conclude that the most important strategy for school nurses in solving the problems which thwart their practice, stifle their professional growth, and jeopardize their very survival is to concentrate their energy and efforts on truly becoming *managers* within the school health program. Once school nurses begin to manage their practice and programs, they can not only *survive* budgetary cutbacks, but can also thrive and grow as accepted, valued members of the school health team.

REFERENCES

American School Health Association: 1974. Guidelines for the school nurse in the school health program, American School Health Association, Kent, Ohio.

Basco, D.: 1963. Evaluation of school nursing activities, Nurs. Res. 12(4):212-221.

Bryan, D. S., and Cook, T. S.: 1967. Redirection of school nursing services in culturally deprived neighborhoods, Am. J. Public Health 57(7):1164-1176.

Castile, A. S., and Jerrick, S. J.: 1976. School health in America, American School Health Association, Kent, Ohio.

Chinn, P.: 1973. A relationship between health and school problems: a nursing assessment, J. School Health 43(2):85-92.

Ford, L. C.: 1970. The school nurse role—a changing concept in preparation and practice, J. School Health 40(1):21-23.

Fricke, I. B.: 1972. School nursing for the '70s, J. School Health 42(4):203-206.

Hill, A. E.: 1971. Educational preparation for school health nursing, J. School Health 41(7):354-360.

Igoe, J. B.: 1977. Bridging the communication gap between health professionals and educators, J. School Health 47(7):405-409.

Jacobsen, R. F., and Siegel, E.: 1971. Comprehensive health planning in the space age: the role of the school health program, J. School Health 41(3):156-160.

Marriner, A.: 1971. Opinions of school nurses about the preparation and practice of school nurses, J. School Health 41(8):417-420.

Newman, I. M., and Mayshark, C.: 1973. Community health problems and the school's unrecognized mandate, J. School Health 43(9):562-565.

Randall, H. B., Cauffman, J. G., and Shultz, C. S.: 1968. Effectiveness of health office clerks in facilitating health care for elementary school children, Am. J. Public Health 58(5):897-906.

Staton, W. M.: 1963. Research needs in school nursing, J. School Health 33(9):418-421.

Thomas, B.: 1976. The school nurse as a member of the school health team: fact or fiction? J. School Health 46(8):466-470.

SUGGESTED READINGS

American Academy of Pediatrics: 1977. School health: a guide for health professionals, 2nd ed., American Academy of Pediatrics, Evanston, Ill.

Brand, M. L.: 1972. The potential of school nursing in the '70s, ANA Clin. Sess. American Nurses' Association, Detroit.

Coakley, J. M., and Parker, J. M.: 1965. Education of nurses for school nursing, Am. J. Nurs. 65(11):84-87.

Coleman, J., and Hawkins, W.: 1970. The changing role of the nurse: an alternative to elimination, J. School Health 40(3):121-122.

Cromwell, G. E.: 1952. Teammates—teachers and school nurses, J. School Health 22(6):165-171.

Cromwell, G. E.: 1964. The future of school nursing, J. School Health 34(1):43-46.

Crosby, M. H., and Connolly, M. G.: 1970. The study of mental health and the school nurse, J. School Health 40(7):373-377.

Dickinson, D. J.: 1971. School nursing becomes accountable in education through behavioral objectives, J. School Health 41(10):533-537.

Eddy, R. M.: 1973. Changing trends in school health services, Thrust for Education Leadership 2(4):17-22.

Forban, O.: 1967. The role and functions of the school nurse as perceived by 115 public school teachers from three selected counties, J. School Health 37(2):101-106.

Fredlund, D. J.: 1967. The route to effective school nursing, Nurs. Outlook 15(8):24-28.

Fricke, I. B.: 1967. The Illinois study of school nursing practice, J. School Health 37:24-28.

Hawkins, N. G.: 1971. Is there a school nurse role? Am. J. Nurs. 71(4):744-751.

Igoe, J. B.: 1975. The school nurse practitioner, Nurs. Outlook 23(6):381-384.

Jerrick, S. J.: 1978. The facts of life in school health, J. School Health 48(5):312-313.

Joint Statement of the ANA, DSN/NEA, and ASHA: 1978. Guidelines on educational preparation and competencies of the school nurse practitioner, J. School Health 48(5):265-268.

Lum, M. C.: 1973. Current concepts in the use of nonprofessional assistants in school health services—a selected review, J. School Health 43(6):357-361.

McAleer, H. S.: 1965. What's new in school nursing, J. School Health 35(2):49-52.

McKevitt, R. K., Nader, P. R., Williamson, M. C., and Berrey, R.: 1977. Reasons for health office visits in an urban school district, J. School Health 47(5):275-279.

Nader, P. R., Emmel, A., and Charney, E.: 1972. The

school health service: a new model, Pediatrics **49**(6):805-813.

Oda, D. S.: 1974. Increasing role effectiveness of school nurses, Am. J. Public Health **64**(6):591-595.

Oda, D. S.: 1979. School nursing: current observations and future projections, J. School Health **49**(8):437-439.

Regan, P. A.: 1976. A historical study of the school nurse role, J. School Health **46**(9):518-521.

Schell, N. B.: 1973. School physicians: a weakening breed, J. School Health **43**(1):45-48.

Stobo, E. C.: 1969. Trends in the preparation and qualifications of the school nurse, Am. J. Public Health **59**(4): 669-672.

Subcommittee on Educational Preparation for School Nurses of the Committee on School Nursing, American School Health Association: 1975. Position paper: philosophy and goals for school nurse educational preparation, J. School Health **45**(7):409.

Tipple, D. C.: 1962. Academic preparation of school nurses: implications for the school nurse practitioner, J. School Health **32**(8):311-315.

Tipple, D. C.: 1964. Misuse of assistants in school health, Am. J. Nurs. **64**(9):99-101.

Troop, E. H.: 1963. Sixty years of school nurse preparation, Nurs. Outlook **11**(5):364-366.

Children with special needs

Chronic illness in the school-aged child: effects on the total family*

BEVERLY A. LAWSON

Chronic illness poses difficulties far beyond the physical symptoms and problems of the specific disease. The affected child, his family, and his nurses must deal with the daily consequences of his illness while he is home as well as in the hospital.

No parents are ever prepared to cope with the myriad problems that confront them with the presence of a chronically ill child in the home. Likewise, few nurses are prepared to deal effectively with the challenge of the chronically ill child and his family in the hospital.

Being chronically ill is vastly different from being acutely ill. It stresses and drains the child and every family member over an infinite period of time. The wonderful resiliency of the human being is stretched almost beyond endurance, especially if there is no prospect of improvement, and even more, if the child deteriorates with the passage of time.(1)

A child with a long-term or chronic illness, also described as being handicapped or disabled, is one who has any disorder "with a protracted course which can be progressive and fatal, or associated with a relatively normal life span despite impaired physical or mental functioning. Such a disease frequently shows periods of acute exacerbation requiring intensive medical care"(2). Although the child is the one

who is physically affected by the disorder, his parents and siblings also require care. Indeed, it has been said that "when one member of a family has a chronic illness, the entire family to some degree becomes ill and requires additional succorance and comfort from one or many sources"(3). Much of the current literature attests to this premise.

Parental reactions to birth

During pregnancy the mother, and I believe the father, prepares for the new baby by fantasizing a perfect "dream" child. When the baby is born manifesting disease or defect, the mother must go through grieving for the loss of the anticipated child and at the same time adjust to an imperfect child before she can begin developing a relationship with the baby(4,5).

Some experts believe that parents with a defective child suffer sorrow throughout their lifetimes as a natural response to a tragic fact. The intensity of the sorrow varies over time but it can be dissolved only with the death of the child. This chronic sorrow is probably more frequently seen in parents whose child has little chance of surviving into adulthood, of getting an education, of marrying, or of raising a family. In such cases the parents are reminded daily of all the dreams never to be fulfilled(6).

A crucial factor in determining parents' acceptance of the situation is their ability to master resentful and self-accusatory feelings over having transmitted or in some way caused their child's disorder. Mattsson cites three main patterns which occur as a result of the way in which parents cope with these feelings:

1. The child is fearful; inactive; markedly dependent on his family, especially his mother; and lacks outside activities. The

*Copyright © 1977, The American Journal of Nursing Company. Reproduced, with permission, from MCN, The American Journal of Maternal Child Nursing, January/February, vol. 2, no. 1.

□Ms. Lawson, R.N., M.S., has developed in her thirteen years' clinical experience in pediatrics a concern for the lack of involvement of the whole family in the child's health care. Having been accepted for full-time doctoral study in counselor education at the State University of New York at Buffalo, she intends to combine the expertise she will gain with her nursing knowledge to treat the total family.

497

SCALE FOR DETECTING FAMILIES AT RISK FOR ADAPTING POORLY TO CHRONIC ILLNESS

Factors	Rating	4	3	2	1	0	Stacy (X)	Lori (+)
1	Age	<20	20-25 X	26-30	31-35 +	>35	3	1
2	Income	<5000	5000-7500 X	7501-10,000 +	10,001-15,000	>15,000	3	2
3	Race	Black		Other		White X, +	0	0
4	Years married	<2 X	2-4	5-7	8-10	>10 +	4	0
5	Strength of marriage	Weak		Average X		Strong +	2	0
6	Number of children	1 X	2	3	4 +	>4	4	1
7	Education level	<High school	High school	1-2 years college X, +	3-4 years college	>4 years college	2	2
8	Religious conviction	None	X	Average		Strong +	3	0
9	Community involvement	None X	One group	Two groups +	Three groups	>Three groups	4	2
10	Support from maternal grandmother	None X		Average +		Strong	4	2
11	Husband/wife experiences with and feelings about chronic illness	Negative X		Neutral		Positive +	4	0
						TOTAL SCORE	33	10

Key: <, Less than; >, greater than

child is passive, dependent; the mother overprotective.

2. The child is overly independent, often daring; engages in prohibited and risk-taking activities. The child uses strong denial of realistic dangers; the mother is oversolicitous and guilt-ridden.
3. Less commonly the child is shy, lonely, and resentful, directing hostility toward normal people. His family usually emphasizes his defect and tends to hide and isolate him. The child develops a self-image of the defective outsider(7).

Yancy describes the most frequently seen response as that of the vicious cycle of the overprotective, overpermissive maternal attitude leading to a dependent, demanding child. The child then elicits maternal resentment, which is usually repressed but leads to periodic outbursts of disproportionate anger. These outbursts, in turn, lead to greater maternal guilt(8).

Parents who successfully adjust to a chronically ill child in the home enforce necessary and realistic restrictions on him and encourage self-care, school attendance, and association with his peers. Such an adjustment seems to be influenced less by the nature of the specific illness than by the developmental level of the family, its coping techniques, the quality of the parent-child relationship, and the family's acceptance of the handicapped member. Also significant is the impact on the family of stimuli from doctors, nurses, neighborhood, and school(9).

While as nurses we must be cautious of generalizations and assess each family individually for strengths and weaknesses, current literature has identified some specific characteristics that seem to indicate families at risk of adapting poorly(1,9-11). Based on these data, I have developed a scale for initially assessing each family. (See Scale for Detecting Families at Risk of Adapting Poorly to Chronic Illness.) By applying it to families for whom I have cared in the past, I have found that indeed it seems possible to predict which families are in greater jeopardy.

Stacy and Lori and their families

Stacy K, 2 months old, was brought to the hospital with bulging fontanels and widening suture lines. Just prior to noticing these symptoms, Stacy's father had been tossing her in play and had accidently bumped her head lightly against a low ceiling. A diagnosis of hydrocephalus was made, and shunting pro-

cedures were undertaken. Stacy was readmitted nearly monthly to the pediatric unit with fevers, seizures, increased intracranial pressure, and other problems. She survived for 2 years. As she disintegrated both physically and mentally, her family crumbled under the burden.

The Ks were an idealistic couple when we first met. Both were 22. He was a part-time student, but they could manage financially if no emergencies occurred. Before she was married, however, Ms. K had worked at a rehabilitation center with children with hydrocephalus and meningomyelocele. She pitied these children and knew that she could never deal with a child of her own with such a defect. When Stacy died, Mr. and Mrs. K divorced.

Lori L came to the pediatric unit frequently between age 6 weeks and 6 years for a multistep repair of a severe cleft lip and palate and dental surgery. The only appealing feature of her face was her deep-set, big blue eyes. She was the fourth child of Mr. and Ms. L, a couple in their early 30s with a strong and healthy marriage, a deeply religious background, and the attitude of "Thank God that Lori's defect is on the outside where it can be fixed, not on the inside." Through the years I knew Lori, she blossomed into an outgoing, loving child nurtured by loving, realistic parents who saw Lori as first of all a child who secondarily had a defect.

Even with the limited information in these two case descriptions, scores on the scale can be obtained for both families. The difference between the scores—Stacy K, 33; Lori L, 10—indicates a difference in the families' abilities to adjust successfully.* I have not actually used the scale in hospital practice but have applied it retrospectively. I would encourage other nurses to try it, modify it, and attempt to determine at what score a family is in jeopardy and at what score they become truly a high-risk family.

Problems for parents

Whether a family is at risk or not, they must face the same difficulties. Among these are *marital stresses*. Sultz et al. reported 9% of the mothers in their study group felt that the ill child was a disruptive factor to their marriages. A total of 26% reported it as a strengthening factor. Problems contributing to weakening of the marriage included avoidance of sex for fear of having another sick child or of being unable

---

*The higher the score, the greater the family's risk for poor adaptation.

to cope with another child along with the ill one; too little time left for each other after caring for the ill child and other children; and anxiety over finances. Disagreement between parents over what to expect from the sick child can also pose a problem(11).

Indications are that suicide and divorce rates are higher in families with chronically ill children than in the general population(9). A divorce rate of nearly 50% was seen in one group of parents with children with meningomylocele(10).

Finances are a major area of concern in many families as well. Additional employment was necessary in 20% of the families in one study after chronic illness was diagnosed in a child(11). In many instances funding or financial assistance is available, but it appears to be white, upper-class families who know of its availability or how to seek it.

Lastly, *social activities* are substantially curtailed in many families with a chronically ill child. Citing difficulty in finding someone competent and willing to accept the responsibility of caring for the chronically ill child and exhaustion of funds after meeting medical expenses, 25% of the mothers in one study reported this to be true(11).

Sibling difficulties

Jealousy, insecurity, and resentment may be problems for the siblings of a chronically ill child. Since most children equate love with attention, it is perfectly normal for them to resent the child who receives more attention from his parents because of treatments, special diets, and hospitalization(3). Furthermore, many parents feel their chronically ill child cannot be held to usual standards of behavior(11).

Again, if healthy siblings see differential treatment given to their ill sibling, they often interpret it as preferential. During angry outbursts at the ill child, siblings often wish the other child dead. If the child is then hospitalized or dies, they experience guilt.

Lastly, chronic illness can cause significant and permanent interference with the physical and emotional growth and development of the ill child himself and with the development of healthy family functioning. A large number of chronically ill children have psychological and social handicaps secondary to their conditions. They exhibit more behavioral deviation, have significantly more problems with eating, bedtime activities, speech, temper, nervous tics, and body management than healthy children.

Basic needs of all children

To grow into responsible human beings and develop normal personalities, children need love, discipline, and opportunities for independence. Chronically ill children are no exception. They are children first and ill second. Love, discipline, and independence operate, according to Homan:

In the three geographical divisions of the child's environment: (1) the home and family, (2) the school, and (3) the neighborhood and social contacts. Thus personality development depends upon love [discipline, and independence] in family, in school, and in neighborhood contacts. . . .(12)

For the child who is repeatedly hospitalized, these needs must be fulfilled in the hospital as well. The fact that the chronically ill child may be more prone to personality disorders because of the increased stresses on him and his family should be considered. He may have an increased level of need in all three areas as a result of such stresses.

Love

Of the three elements, undoubtedly the most important is love. The type of love most important for normal personality development is accepting, uncritical love. "This is the kind of love that builds self-confidence, creates a good self-image, and leads to a willingness to try without fear of the consequences of failure."(13)

Parents of the chronically ill child occasionally react with rejection, ambivalence, or a host of other inconsistent reactions as a result of the child's disease or defect. "These possible unpredictable swings from affection to rejection or to ambivalent behavior do not provide consistent reinforcement patterns for the infant"(14). As a result, scores of children feel unloved, unassured, and unaccepted. And, feeling unloved, they are in return unable to give love. They may also misbehave to get attention from their parents.

Discipline

Teaching a child to follow rules and regulations helps him adjust to the world and behave in a socially acceptable manner(15). "Many children reared in an atmosphere of 'permissiveness' become terribly inhibited. They are simply terrified by their own destructive impulses. They lack adequate internal controls and destroy things right and left''(16).

Independence

When a child is sufficiently content and satisfied at home and feels he can always retreat back to its protection, he becomes willing to venture out into the world. "The only thing that will then prevent the normal development of his independence is to have the opportunity to do things for himself denied by those about him''(17). On the other hand, independence should not develop at the expense of the child's safety or of the property or feelings of others. Like overpermissiveness, overprotection can lead quickly to problem behavior and inhibit normal personality development.

When personality development goes awry

If for any reason the school-aged child has not already developed the firm foundation of a healthy personality, the unique challenges and developmental hurdles he faces between the ages of 6 and 12 become difficult, sometimes impossible. The major task for the school-aged child is that of developing a sense of industry and a strong drive toward accomplishment. If he fails at this, he develops feelings of inferiority and inadequacy.

The child must also grow in independence at this time, moving away from familiar family ties to build new relationships with peers. Furthermore, he should develop a healthy attitude toward himself as a person, learn appropriate social roles, and achieve independence in caring for himself. Finally, the child should learn the fundamental skills of reading, writing, and calculating and develop the coordination necessary for games and activities(18).

For the chronically ill child the foundations for these tasks may be weak or flawed. Moreover, he may be sent off to a special school, removed from the familiarity of his neighborhood and friends. Upon contacting children his own age in school, he may for the first time realize that he is different from others. He eats special foods; he can't run; he takes pills; he can't play contact sports. In addition schoolmates who have overheard their parents discussing the child may announce, "You have a disease and you are going to die."

As the hub of existence for the young child, school, occupying 5 days a week, often brings conflict to the chronically ill child. The demands of learning and those of a chronic illness sometimes collide. Studies indicate that chronically ill children miss at least 6 weeks of school per year. In one study 26% of chronically ill children were below expected grade level, with lag increasing with the number of years in school(11).

Such children also exhibit increased truancy and trouble in school and become increasingly more socially isolated. Often they develop changed perceptions of themselves; their illness leads to feelings of decreased self-worth, and, in turn, to lower self-respect and self-confidence(19). In a recent study chronically ill children showed different responses from well children when tested for achievement behavior, defined as taking pride in successful endeavors.

Children diagnosed as chronically ill from birth attributed both success and failure to external rather than internal variables. They did not see their effort as having much effect on success or failure. Perhaps this is an ego-defensive response—they don't experience the most pride, but perhaps more importantly they avoid experiencing the most shame.(20)

The child in the hospital

When the chronically ill child enters the hospital, like any other child he brings with him his struggle with growth and development tasks (which do not stop just because he's sick); his fears about hospitalization; the coping mechanisms, whether good or bad, that he has learned; his family; and his pain. He also brings some or all of the problems that go with chronic illness—physical, psychological, social, financial, or educational. As a result he and/or his family occasionally create chaos or smoldering resentment on the pediatric unit.

I have observed all of the following reactions to the "problem" chronically ill child and his parents at one time or another:

1. Nurses tolerate any and all behavior as long as possible; then ignore, deprecate, or punish the child inconsistently at their own whim.
2. Parents and child are ignored. The mother is left to care for the child as far as possible.
3. Child is isolated and his parents made to feel unwanted or unneeded on the unit.
4. Perhaps worst of all, if the child is acutely ill, all his demands—reasonable or not— are given in to and no expectations or restrictions are placed on him. The prevailing attitudes seem to be that there will be

time to worry about discipline later or that the parents should handle that situation.

It is imperative that nurses begin to look realistically at what is happening in these families and begin using their nursing intervention skills. Perhaps the major question that comes to mind is: Why intervene? If this is the way the family chooses to live and they are satisfied, why should the nurse attempt to change their behavior?

From the preceding discussion it is clear that many families do not choose to live this way; their life-style has evolved from the various pressures with which they were unprepared to deal. They simply have not the strength, support, or knowledge to lead a better life. If we overlook these facts and fail to intervene, we are remiss. To do nothing is to abdicate our role as responsible nurses.

Goals in treating the chronically ill child

Every child needs to live every day of his life to the fullest to achieve his potential. Even sickness and hospitalization can be learning and growing experiences. As a general rule, however, they are not. Too many children emerge from hospital experiences even short ones, psychologically scarred and/or regressed. The usually healthy child may be able to work through this trauma, relearn, and rebuild. But what of children who are hospitalized more frequently or for longer periods of time? What should the goals be in caring for these children?

I have borrowed from Yancy, whose goals for treatment seem clear, concise, and *essential:*

- Treat the handicap/disease itself through correction of defect, control of symptoms, or arrest of progress.
- Prevent the disease process, treatment regime, and various people involved in the program from interfering with the child's development.
- Prevent the illness, treatment regime, and people involved from disrupting the family(8).

The nurse's role

Nurses have unique opportunities daily to be of help in many areas to the chronically ill child and his family. They can foster family involvement in the child's care which, begun in the hospital, must continue at home. They can evaluate family dynamics and provide guidance, encourage healthy parent-child interactions, and suggest appropriate interventions or referrals if needed. Although medical care is not the only intervention needed by these families, it is essential, and a nurse's efforts to help families realize the benefits of continuous care are important.

Over 45% of families with chronically ill children are not receiving active medical care, visiting doctors only during acute episodes(11). Few families receive continuous, ongoing medical care. Only through continuous care can preventive medicine be practiced, families receive support and guidance, misconceptions and fears be dealt with, and parents and child come to truly comprehend and accept the illness and its ramifications.

The parents are an essential part of the team in caring for the chronically ill child and need to be included in all planning and treatments for the child, which is something which the nurse can ensure. What better way is there for parents to gain confidence in caring for their child at home than through education, demonstration, and supervised practice in the hospital? This certainly points up the advantages of extended visiting hours and rooming-in for parents as well.

Parental counseling should also be made available in the hospital. Parents need an opportunity to express their feelings while they are helped to accept and live with the burden of their child's chronic illness and to approach the situation realistically. They need to know there are no perfect parents; that everyone makes mistakes. They must accept that they may upon occasion forget a treatment, get angry, or feel resentful. Above all, they need help to realize that their own lives must continue, that they must allow time for both parents—individually and together—to get away and have fun.

Parents also benefit from sharing with other parents in similar situations. Thus, a nurse might introduce them to other such parents in the hospital and help them locate lay organizations in the community.

Finally, it is imperative to help parents and children (if they are able) to get their feelings, fears, and concerns out in the open. Accordingly, the nurse must make herself available, must allow questions, must be honest and, above all, supportive and accepting of whatever is expressed. To show shock or dismay is to turn off communication.

Children up to 8 or 10 may attribute illness and injury to their own disobedience or their parents' failure to protect them. They might then blame themselves or other family members for causing their disease. Because of these distorted interpretations, they may be reluctant to ask questions or may vent irrational fears. The nurse can help the child to understand the true nature of the sickness and explain to parents the child's reaction(2).

Throughout the literature parents have said that their major problem is lack of assistance in guiding the development of their chronically ill children. If the child's diagnosis has just been made, the nurse should begin immediately to describe growth and developmental patterns and encourage healthy parent-child interactions. Preventing faulty relationships is easier than correcting them. On the other hand, if faulty dynamics are already present, understanding and support is as essential as teaching better ways of interacting. Otherwise parents may feel guilty or inadequate when the nurse intervenes to help them recognize faulty dynamics and change their behavior.

By setting and reinforcing realistic limits for the child in the hospital nurses can also assist parents in rearing their children. If nurses and family members let up on discipline and rules for their chronically ill child, it is easy to see how the sick role is reinforced and how normally unacceptable behavior becomes routine.

If the child is unused to restrictions and rules, the nurse might start by trying to change only one or two areas of behavior, preferably those most irritating to the staff or those interfering most with the child's care. Parents and the entire staff should be included in the plan to provide consistency. If the child is discharged while behavior modification is ongoing, the family should be referred to a counseling service in the community, which can continue the treatment while offering support to the parents.

In dealing with the child who is mentally capable, the nurse can tell him clearly what his restrictions or expectations are to try to get his cooperation. Meanwhile acceptable behavior can be reinforced with rewards; and undesired behavior discouraged through lack of reward— that is, by ignoring it. Such a program was used with Earl.

Earl, 5, had an inoperable brain tumor in remission. His major problem was his refusal to eat except for sweets. He had learned that if he whined or complained of headache, the nurses would take his tray away, take him to the playroom, and rock him. Then, after he calmed down and the food tray had gone back to the kitchen, he was given soda, ice cream, or candy. Many nurses admitted they had difficulty making Earl do anything he didn't want to do because he would shortly die.

Earl grew weaker from poor nutrition, increasingly whiney, and more demanding in other areas. The nurses held a conference and agreed that they would all follow one plan: after 20 minutes Earl's tray would be removed whether or not he had eaten. Except for nutritious snacks there would be no food between meals. In addition each time Earl ate, he was taken immediately to the playroom. If he didn't eat, the tray was removed, nothing was said, and no special consolations of rocking and treats were given. Very shortly Earl's appetite began to increase and he spent many happy hours in the playroom.

Personality clashes

While it is not realistic to expect every nurse to love every child or every child to love every nurse, nurses can show vitally important acceptance and approval of the chronically ill child while he is in the hospital. Ways of doing this include praising the child more for being than for doing and communicating positive feelings. Simple words such as "It's really fun helping you with your bath," make a child feel good and usually gain his help and cooperation. And when the child misbehaves, the nurse should express disapproval of what he has done rather than of the child himself: "I like you, but your splashing all that water on the floor really makes me angry."

Occasionally the nurse will encounter a child she truly has difficulty accepting and caring for. In such a case it is better for both parties if the nurse accepts the fact and asks for a change in assignment.

Even when nurse and child have a good relationship, treatments and medications often result in scenes. Since frequently treatments will have to be continued at home, often for life, much planning and consideration is warranted. If parents provide or witness treatments in the hospital, they will have a more realistic concept of the time and physical energy that will be required for the job at home. Perhaps then the nurse can help them plan how to incorporate needed treatments into the daily home routine with a minimum of disruption(21).

A matter-of-fact manner is the best approach to treatments; an apologetic approach is a mistake. Treatments and medications should never be used as a bargaining point or threat with a child. Rather, since the school-aged child is seeking increased independence, part of the responsibility for care and treatment can be gradually shifted to him. Many children with diabetes give their own insulin by age 10, and children with meningomyelocele can help apply their braces.

Furthermore, in the hospital and at home the child must constantly be challenged by attainable goals. As nurses we must help parents set realistic goals and thus foster the child's continued education and growth.

All families with a chronically ill child should be referred to a community-based nursing service upon the child's discharge from the hospital. If the family is coping well, they can always use the support and guidance of the professional nurse. If they appear to have multiple problems or to be at risk, such a referral can offer them closer assessment and more effective, ongoing planning and intervention.

It is unfair to release these families unprepared and unsupported into a society that is so often unable to understand or accept them. When this occurs, they simply flounder, seeking only emergency care and often the child is soon readmitted to the hospital. Indeed, in one hospital 50% of the readmissions were for chronic illness(22).

I'm not suggesting that we can prevent readmissions. I am suggesting that we can—through identification of problems, early intervention, and preventive counseling and care—decrease their frequency and tremendous cost in time, dollars, and human suffering for the chronically ill child and his family.

But all the good parents and caring nurses in the world cannot produce a well-adjusted chronically ill child if society pities or rejects him, teachers fail to understand or challenge him, and he must live under the cloud of myths and old wives' tales that still surround many chronic illnesses. Consequently, nurses need to take a more active role in educating the public about chronic illness.

There is no quick or easy solution to the dilemma of the chronically ill child and his family. I am convinced, however, that early counseling and appropriate intervention for problems in growth and development and family dynamics are imperative. Through such efforts the door to a fuller life for the family with a chronically ill child can be opened.

REFERENCES

1. Battle, C. U. Symposium on behavioral pediatrics: chronic physical disease: behavioral aspects. *Pediatr. Clin. North Am.* 22:525-531, Aug. 1975, p. 525.
2. Mattsson, Ake. Long-term physical illness in childhood: a challenge to psychosocial adaptation. *Pediatrics* 50:801-811, Nov. 1972, p. 801.
3. Patterson, Paul. *Psychological Aspects of Cystic Fibrosis.* Albany, N.Y., Albany Medical College, p. 3. (Unpublished Manuscript.)
4. Miller, L. G. Toward a greater understanding of the parents of the mentally retarded child. *J. Pediatr.* 73: 699-705, Nov. 1968.
5. Solnit, Albert, and Stark, Mary. Mourning and the birth of a defective chid. *Psychoanal. Study Child* 16: 523-536, June 1962.
6. Olshansky, Simon. Chronic sorrow: a response to having a mentally defective child. *Soc. Casework* 43:191-192, Mar. 1962.
7. Mattsson, *op. cit.,* p. 806-807.
8. Yancy, W. S. Approaches to emotional management of the child with a chronic illness. *Clin. Pediatr.* 11:64-67, Feb. 1972.
9. Debuskey, Matthew, Ed. *The Chronically Ill Child and His Family.* Springfield, Ill., Charles C Thomas, Publisher, 1970.
10. Kolin, I. S., and others. Studies of the school-age child with meningomyelocele: social and emotional adaptation. *J. Pediatr.* 78:1013, June 1971.
11. Sultz, H. A., and others. *Long-Term Childhood Illness.* (Contemporary Community Health Series) Pittsburgh. University of Pittsburgh Press, 1972.
12. Homan, W. E. *Child Sense: A Pediatrician's Guide for Today's Families.* New York, Basic Books, 1969, pp. 8-9.
13. *Ibid.* p. 13.
14. Holaday, B. J. Achievement behavior in chronically ill children. *Nurs. Res.* 23:25, Jan.-Feb. 1974.
15. Salk, Lee. *What Every Child Would Like His Parents to Know.* New York, Warner Books, 1973, pp. 63-64.
16. *Ibid.* p. 71.
17. Homan, *op.cit.,* pp. 25-28.
18. Scipien, G. M., and others. *Comprehensive Pediatric Nursing.* New York, McGraw-Hill Book Co., 1975, pp. 156-166.
19. Pless, I. B., and Roghmann, K. J. Chronic illness and its consequences: observations based on three epidemiologic surveys. *J. Pediatr.* 79:351-359, Sept. 1971.
20. Holaday, *op.cit.,* p. 29.
21. Reif, Laura. Managing a life with chronic illness, *Am. J. Nurs.* 73:262, Feb. 1973.
22. Steen, Joyce. Liaison nurse: ombudsman for the chronically ill. *Am. J. Nurs.* 73:2101, Dec. 1973.

Chronic respiratory diseases of
school-age children*

JOHN P. McGOVERN, M.D.

Chronic respiratory diseases represent a major health problem within the school-age population and to the school health personnel who must deal with these problems (Fig. 1). The purpose of this paper is to conceptualize for the school health team an understanding of these chronic upper and lower respiratory tract diseases and to point out the steps they can take to help cope with these problems.

Among chronic respiratory diseases afflicting the school-age population, allergic conditions represent, by far, both qualitatively and quantitatively, the greatest problem, as schematically shown in Fig. 2 (National Health Survey, 1970). Various studies have shown that from 10% to 28% of the population suffers from major allergic problems. An additional 40% to 50% has experienced (or will experience) some relatively less severe, frequently evanescent, allergic manifestations, often insufficiently pronounced to require medical attention.[1] Specifically, hay fever, perennial allergic rhinitis, asthma, and other allergies account for one third of all chronic conditions reported for children under 17 years of age (Fig. 2).[2]

Because manifestations of the allergic diathesis represent perhaps the most significant chronic school health problem, the major thrust of this paper will deal with these diseases of allergic origin.

In one national survey,[3,4] the total time lost from school because of chronic affections amounted to approximately 33 million days. Asthma accounted for more than 7.5 million days, and hay fever (usually with perennial allergic rhinitis) and other allergies for another 1.5 million days. Also, an allergic component probably exists in most cases of chronic sinusitis[5] and "chronic bronchitis" with cough,[6,7] along with a significant incidence in hearing impairment,[8] recurrent headache,[9-11] urinary tract problems[12] and tension-fatigue syndrome.[13] By comparison, in the same survey, school days lost each year because of heart disease and diseases of the genitourinary tract were 859,000 and 885,000, respectively.

In the United States an estimated 1,600,000 children through 16 years of age have asthma. In a 1961 survey, asthma accounted for 11.4% of all chronic conditions in children under the age of 17 and for 22.9% of all days lost from school by children from age 6 through 16 because of chronic conditions.[14]

However, incidence of an illness, days lost from school, and the high cause for army rejection do not accurately reflect the total deleterious impact on the individuals involved or the cumulative loss to the nation in terms of aberrations of physical, mental and emotional growth and development of our youth. This is a problem of compelling magnitude, one in which all primary physicians and other members of the health team caring for children can and must play an increasingly more effective role.

It is not my intention, nor would it be appropriate or even possible in this paper, to examine, however so lightly, all aspects of allergy in childhood. Rather, I shall identify and comment upon those salient features which relate directly to the school situation and the school health team.

In dealing with specifics of school health and

*From McGovern, J. P.: 1976. J. School Health **46**(6):344-353, June. Copyright 1978 American School Health Association, Kent, Ohio 44240.
□**John P. McGovern, M.D., F.A.S.H.A.,** Director, McGovern Allergy Clinic; Clinical Professor of Pediatrics (Allergy) and Microbiology, Baylor College of Medicine; Clinical Professor of Medicine (Allergy), University of Texas Medical School at Houston.

505

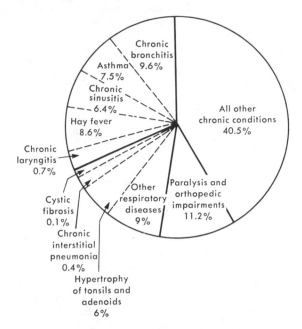

Fig. 1. Distribution of chronic diseases in children 17 years and under.

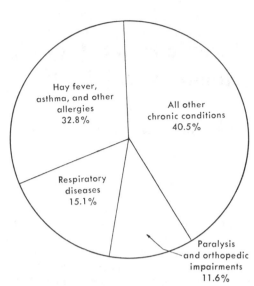

Fig. 2. Hay fever, asthma, and other allergies account for one third of all chronic conditions reported for children under 17 years old.

the allergic child, it is imperative that each involved person be imbued with the concept that every action and the overall goal is to aid in the development of a physically and emotionally mature adult who is capable of functioning as a stable and productive citizen. It is obvious, of course, that with allergy one cannot adequately treat the part without a good knowledge of the whole. Therefore, it is essential for the responsible individuals, not only for direct diagnosis and treatment of allergic children, but also for effective interaction with each member of the health team, to have a clear understanding of the mechanisms, diagnostic approach, and treatment of the allergic diatheses. Early allergy identification should be emphasized; what to look for, how to handle it, when a child should be seen by the primary physician, and when referral to a qualified allergist is indicated.

Also, in recent years there has been continuing abandonment of routine periodic health examinations as a primary school responsibility.[15] This is being replaced by office examinations and follow-up by the child's private physician, or, in some instances, community clinics. Consequently, the bulk of responsibility for school health problems rests with private physicians. Health evaluation by school personnel increasingly has become a responsibility of the teacher who in turn notifies the parents or refers the child to a school nurse and, occasionally, even directly to a private physician. In some instances, a school nurse or physician may refer the child to a health counselor, where one exists. Evaluation of children's health by the school has been relegated to loose screening procedures which, in most cases, are related directly to superficial audiovisual observations or cursory evaluations of athletic capabilities.

HOLISTIC APPROACH AND THE HEALTH TEAM

To insure that health problems of the *whole child* are properly interpreted and effectively managed within the school setting, open lines of communication must exist between his private physician, parents, and the school health team, for asthma and other allergic diseases are classical examples of the need for a multifaceted regimen. In the allergic child's school setting, one must pay particular attention to early symptom recognition and appropriate diagnostic channeling, specific environmental factors, the effects of physical exertion on the disease process, emotional *quanta* involved, problems with medications, and the need for

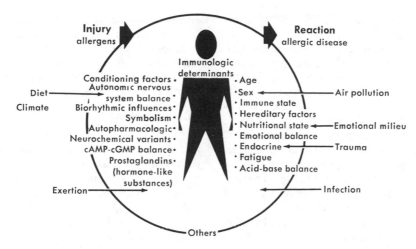

Fig. 3. Allergic disease: reaction to injury. •, Internal factors; ←, external factors.

swift execution of effective emergency care. It is essential, therefore, for each member of the health team to have some direct knowledge of allergies[16] and, within the limits of individual training, some comprehension of the basic concept of a holistic approach[17] to allergic disease (and all diseases, for that matter). This concept, delineated schematically in Fig. 3, shows allergic disease as being a process of "reaction to injury," with many factors both within the body and in the external milieu modifying its expression.[18-20]

Thus, by "holistic approach" we stress the doctrine that the determining factors in nature are wholes, such as organisms, not their constituent parts, and that many changing factors both from within and outside of the body are constantly modifying the disease process. The holistic approach, in diagnosis and treatment, for example, is strongly against fragmenting man into *psyche* and *soma*. Experience repeatedly has shown that the holistic approach to diagnosis and management of allergic patients offers the most effective method of care. Asthma, for example, as might be visualized in Fig. 3, is a much more complicated semichronic disease of a recurring allergic phenomenon than can be understood solely as a manifestation of an antigen-antibody reaction. An allergic child, and thus the allergic reaction, may be conditioned[21,22] by many factors in both the internal and external milieu so that the asthmatic may react with bronchospasm to such diverse stimuli as those from infections, climatic changes, physical exertion, and endocrine and emotional factors, which during early stages of sensitiza-

tion may or may not have had specific meaning.

At this juncture, it might be judicious to define what we mean by the "health team." We regard it as composed of each of the interacting individuals, i.e., teachers, school nurses, health counselors, physicians, parents, and patients, with overall guidance in each case by the child's primary physician.

The chief function of primary physicians, with respect to allergies as they relate to school health problems, is to communicate basic general knowledge and specific medical information when indicated in individual cases to members of the school health team; emphasize early allergy identification—what to look for, how to treat it, and when to refer to the physician; and counsel concerning referral of selected cases to an allergist for specific testing and more comprehensive therapy.

Each member of the school team should be instructed specifically in symptom recognition and diagnostic channeling, environmental control, physical exertion factors, emotional influences, medications, emergency care, and time of referral to a specialist.

SYMPTOM RECOGNITION AND DIAGNOSTIC CHANNELS

Those common symptoms of allergy in the school-age child for which the school health team should be alert are "persistent colds"; stuffy, runny, or itching nose; allergic facial signs[23] (see "Allergic Rhinitis"); sniffing, sneezing, snorting,[24] hacking, or persistent cough[25] which may disturb the class; wheezing, with or without coughing; diminished hearing ability;[26] recurrent headaches;[27-29] itching, watering, and burning of the eyes;[30] itching rash;[31,32] vomiting, diarrhea, and recurrent gastrointestinal cramps.[33] The child may appear pale, have circles under the eyes, breathe through his mouth, seem tired and listless with lack of energy, yet be tense (allergic tension-fatigue syndrome). He may be thought to be anemic because of paleness. For evaluation and therapy for one or more of these symptoms, he may be brought to his primary physician by the mother on her own initiative or upon recommendation by the teacher, school nurse, or health counselor. Detailed history and examination of the child will usually suffice for physician diagnosis and outlining of an appropriate therapeutic regimen. When allergy is suspected, specific allergens with which the child comes in contact at home and in the school environment should be identified. In addition to specific allergens, certain nonspecific factors, such as weather changes, infections, physical exertion, emotional, and endocrine changes, may influence the course of the natural history of this disease.

Once allergy is suspected, it is helpful for the school nurse and the health officer to have at their disposal a history form which can be completed by the parents either at home or at the school office. This is necessary because the child, generally due to age or lack of knowledge, may be unable to competently complete such a form. Most school health forms ask questions related to general symptom categories but request little information about environmental conditions or specific health problems. Once a school nurse or physician is aware that a child is affected by allergy, further specific information should be obtained on a history form.

Once a symptom complex has been evaluated, it is often noted that there may be extreme variations in symptomatology related to the time of day,[34] time of the month,[35] or time of the year (seasonal changes). Correlation of the child's presence in school and marked variations in academic achievement or school athletic performance may be related to allergy exacerbations which can be elicited from a complete history evaluation.

RESPIRATORY ALLERGIC CONDITIONS ENCOUNTERED BY SCHOOL PERSONNEL

Following are some common allergic diseases often seen at school, not only in pupils but also in school personnel, and a brief description and discussion of each. Often overlapping symptom complexes may be seen in the same individual. This is not intended as a comprehensive classification but rather as a handy and practical reference list.

Allergic asthma

Allergic asthma is characterized by wheezing, shortness of breath, and cough occurring in paroxysmal attacks, with symptoms occurring in periods of varying length. Attacks are rarely of such severity as to constitute a real emergency, although, if prolonged, they *can* be (e.g., status asthmaticus). Lower airway obstruction with resultant wheezing can also be almost constant. When considering frequency as well as severity, asthma is the most important of allergic diseases seen in schools, accounting for approximately 23% of all days lost from school by children between ages 6 and 16.[36]

Asthma attacks are often triggered by school activities and environment (see "Exertion"). A teacher or school nurse may be the first person to recognize a child with asthma and should alert the parents or physician.

School personnel should be aware of medications used by pupils and of their possible side effects. Among drugs most frequently used for asthma, alone or in combination, are epinephrine (Adrenalin), ephedrine, and other sympathomimetics. These drugs, used as bronchodilators to relieve obstruction and wheezing, may overstimulate and cause nervousness, talkativeness, or generally hyperactive behavior. Theophylline, another medication used to dilate bronchial airways, may cause nausea or "upset stomach." Barbiturates and other sedatives are often used in combination with the bronchial dilators and may produce excessive sedation, but occasionally, and paradoxically, these medications may have a stimulatory effect.

Corticosteroids and their synthetic analogs act as potent hormones. They should never be used carelessly but, when really indicated, can be valuable in the control of refractory allergic diseases, particularly asthma. Side effects are many but may be minimized by use of the alternate-day therapy technique. Cushing syndrome, "moon" facies, excessive weight, "buffalo hump" fat distribution, abnormal-excessive hair growth and erythematous stress, striae or stretch lines, easy bruising, excessive appetite, collection of edema fluid, slowed growth curve,

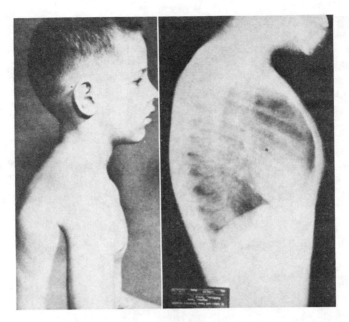

Fig. 4. Increased anterior-posterior dimension of the chest wall ("barrel chest") in asthmatic child. X-ray on right shows hyperventilation with possible early developing emphysema.

altered susceptibility to infection, more labile homeostatic mechanism in the face of extreme stress, susceptibility to peptic gastrointestinal ulceration, and psychological alterations, sometimes with severe psychosis, are some of the possible side effects and complications of prolonged, usually high-dose treatment with corticosteroids. Even with the possible consequences, however, a small percentage of patients may need such treatment for prolonged periods for adequate or life-saving control of the disease process. These children have been labeled "steroid dependent," but newer methods of timing of steroid therapy, along with the holistic approach to overall management, often result in being able to stop the steroids.

One of the complications of persistent and frequent recurrent asthma is evidence of hyperventilation and emphysema with the "barrel chest" contour, as depicted in Fig. 4. Children with severe asthma may evidence growth retardation, be more susceptible to infections, and perform less well in school.

Allergic rhinitis

Whether seasonal ("hay fever") or nonseasonal (perennial allergic rhinitis), allergic rhinitis is the most common of allergic diseases seen in the school. Symptoms vary from primary nasal blocking to include bouts of sneezing with nasal congestion, often associated with itching and nasal mucus discharge. Allergic conjunctivitis with itching, red, and tearing eyes often accompanies allergic rhinitis. If severe, there may be blockage of the ostia of the paranasal sinuses and/or eustachian tubes. These blocked passageways often lead to complications such as "sinus headache," sinus infections, decreased hearing, ear pain, and ear infection. Anosmia and loss of taste acuity also may result from severe nasal congestion. Excessive postnasal drainage may produce a "tickle" in the throat, throat clearing, and intermittent cough. Allergic laryngitis with hoarseness and, rarely, loss of voice may accompany allergic rhinitis. Physical features found in nasal allergy are the "allergic salute" and facial grimacing (Fig. 5), so-called "dark circles under the eyes," or "allergic shiners," horizontal nasal creases (Fig. 6), puffy eyelids, exaggerated and multiple creases of lower eyelids, and adenoid facies (chronic mouth breathing and gaping) (Fig. 7).

Conditions often confused with allergic rhinitis are the common viral cold, bacterial and other viral upper respiratory infections, and vasomotor rhinitis. So-called "common colds" are not chronic, but allergic rhinitis which may appear as "a cold" is frequently of long duration. Usually there is no fever associated with uncomplicated nasal allergy, "hay fever" be-

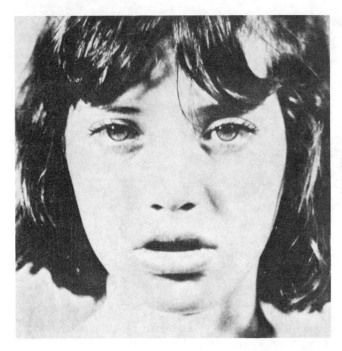

Fig. 5. Typical facial grimacing and "allergic salute" in young child with allergic rhinitis.

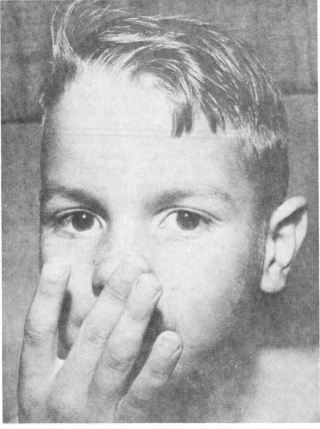

Fig. 6. Permanent transverse nasal crease (McGovern's sign) induced by "allergic salute."

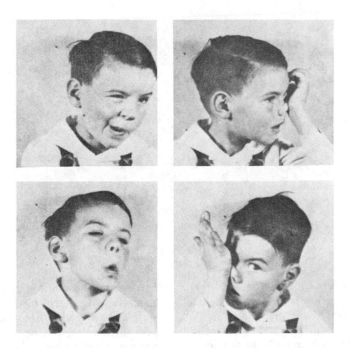

Fig. 7. Typical "adenoid facies" and gaping habitus in child, age 10 years, with perennial allergic rhinitis since infancy. (Courtesy Meyer B. Marks, M.D.)

ing a misnomer, and marked soreness of the throat is almost never found in uncomplicated allergic rhinitis.

Medications often used to treat allergic rhinitis are antihistamines and certain sympathomimetic drugs (e.g., ephedrine), used alone or in combination, either short-acting or long acting. Frequently these drugs cause side effects such as sedation with antihistaminics or central nervous system stimulation with sympathomimetics.

Allergic conjunctivitis[37]

This condition often occurs along with allergic rhinitis but may also occur independently of it. Symptoms are itching, redness, and tearing of the eyes, often associated with puffy and swollen eyelids (Fig. 8). Many times photophobia (sensitivity to light) occurs. These symptoms may often be confused with eye infection and other inflammatory conditions, such as chemical irritations. The presence of itching is often of great help in determining an allergic etiology. Symptoms usually are moderate but may be of such severity as to constitute an almost emergency situation, primarily because of marked discomfort rather than pathology lead-

ing to a permanent damage. Careful conjunctival scrapings by an allergist or ophthalmologist may reveal marked accumulation of eosinophiles.

Medications, and thus side effects, are similar to those mentioned for allergic rhinitis. Some physicians may also prescribe eyedrops, and often a simple cold water compress is helpful in relieving severe symptoms.

Allergic tension-fatigue syndrome

This syndrome may be noted with any chronic respiratory allergic condition and is much more common than formerly realized. Fatigue, lassitude, or being described as "run down" is often the first complaint. In spite of apparent adequate rest, the fatigue may be so severe that the child has difficulty in arising each morning and in performing his usual school and play functions. In addition, irritability, nervousness, and personality upsets may interfere with reasonably expected adjustment to other family members, classmates, and teachers.

The eight most common signs and symptoms of this disorder are (1) accompanying respiratory tract allergy (allergic rhinitis or asthma); (2) abdominal discomfort, frequently with nausea;

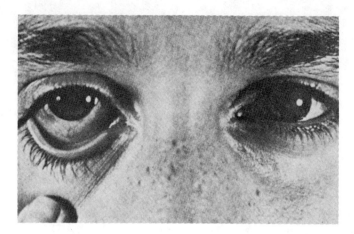

Fig. 8. Allergic conjunctivitis.

(3) recurrent headaches; (4) tenseness and irritability; (5) facial pallor; (6) dark circles under the eyes (so-called "allergic shiners"); (7) tiredness and easy fatigability; and (8) musculoskeletal pains, most frequently in the legs.[38] This condition can usually be alleviated by control of the underlying allergic state, such as avoidance of allergens (often certain foods), hyposensitization to the offending airborne allergens, and appropriate medications.

Allergic cough syndrome

This symptom-complex[39] is characterized by a chronic, dry, hacking cough, as opposed to the congested and productive cough of the posterior nasal drainage in allergic rhinitis, but without associated wheezing. The cough is typically nocturnal and is often accompanied by vomiting and sometimes with weight loss. During the day the cough may often be precipitated by exertion and exposure to inhalant allergens. A combination of various modes of treatment (avoidance, hyposensitization, and appropriate medication) generally is necessary to control the allergic cough syndrome.

Allergic headaches

Headaches of allergic origin[40,41] have many and varied causes, and much concerning the mechanisms involved is still under intense investigation. Various types of recurring headaches may have an allergic basis, and so-called "sinus headaches," particularly when frequent, usually are a secondary complication of perennial allergic rhinitis. This type of headache is more common in later childhood and adolescence and is due primarily to blockage of sinus ostia by the swollen allergic membranes which

line them. Tension headaches and psychogenic headaches also seem to increase in frequency with age. Migraine headaches are one-sided, generally severe, and the typical form is usually not noted until after puberty. Other so-called "vascular headaches," including migraine variants or equivalents, as well as Horton's cluster, or histamine headaches,[42] may be on an allergic basis.

Exertion

It is the responsibility of private physicians to give guidance in structuring exercise programs for asthmatic children. As much as possible, allergic children should be allowed to participate in regular physical fitness programs at school; this gives them added confidence and promotes normal physical as well as emotional growth and development.

Although most asthmatics can tolerate a graded, vigorous exercise program and will benefit from it physiologically and psychologically, the immediate effect of exercise may be temporarily detrimental, with the precipitation of acute bouts of coughing or wheezing.[43] Since exercise may cause initial bronchodilatation with subsequent bronchospasm after moderately vigorous exercise for 5 to 10 minutes, a simple office test of exercise and follow-up observation is often helpful. In the event the child has considerable difficulty with prolonged strenuous exertion, other types of exercise should be suggested that involve shorter periods (3 to 5 minutes) with intermittent spurts of exertion (e.g., shooting baskets with basketball). Swimming is an excellent exercise for allergic children, but diving and underwater swimming should be discouraged for the child who has persistent nasal allergy or recurrent ear infections. In our experience, tennis provides the best of all forms of competitive exercise for the respiratory allergic child; it is generally played outside, not on grass, has built-in intermittent rest periods during retrieval of balls, before serve, at change of courts, and, other than in tournament matches, can be stopped for a rest period whenever desired by one partner without seriously interrupting practice or match play.

Physicians are often asked whether a child with asthma can play in the school band, or, if he is not already proficient with an instrument, which one should be taken up. Of course each case must be evaluated individually, but, for the most part, when moderate to severe respiratory allergy preexists, we tend to discourage the learning of wind instruments or participation in a marching band. The latter frequently exposes the child for long periods to the most inclement of weather and often precipitates attacks.

It should be reemphasized that every child should be allowed to participate in some athletic program, not only for the aforementioned benefits but also so he will not feel too different or set apart from his playmates (see next section).

Emotions

Emotional factors play an important role in allergic disease but the precise mechanistic nature of these influences is still widely debated.[44,45] What *is* definite is the existence of emotional components in many allergic disease reaction patterns. The need exists for a many-sided approach to the problem, one which takes into account not only the environmental milieu of the patient and his primary interpersonal relationships but also the generic imprint of his own unique autonomic nervous system.

If allergic patients are to be managed successfully, it is necessary to give more than lip service to the ancient principle that the mind (psyche) and the body (soma) are one, that they function *interactively* and *interdependently*—a principle which has always guided the wise physician. Plato's words, spoken to the physicians of his day, echo across the centuries and speak to us: ". . . so neither ought you to attempt to cure the body without the mind; and this is the reason why the cure of many diseases is unknown to the physicians of Hellas, because they are ignorant of the whole, which ought to be studied also; for the part can never be well unless the whole is well . . . For this is the great error of our day in the treatment of the human body, that physicians separate the mind from the body.'' We believe these thoughts expressed by that great Greek still have much meaning for us in our so-called ''enlightened age.''

Thus, while helping to control or rid a child of his allergic symptoms, it is most important to understand, allow for, and encourage normal emotional growth and development. Perhaps the key consideration for classroom teachers is: Do not handicap asthmatic children further by excessively protective efforts to be helpful![46] The more normally such children are treated, the better their chances to develop healthy living patterns. Most youngsters with asthma can and should participate in all acceptable activities of childhood.

It is most important to prevent the child from using his allergies for primary or secondary gain. Teachers as well as parents will frequently ask physicians to recommend that an asthmatic child be excused from participating in physical education or other school activities, usually because of an unwarranted degree of anxiety. Often one finds a rather continuously projected apprehension: ''Should we let him participate in such-and-such an activity *because this might precipitate an attack?*'' Needless to say, much of this anxiety spills over to the child.

Actually none of us has a magical crystal ball and, until a child actually tries an activity, we cannot realistically predict the outcome. Thus, we recommend that the allergic child be allowed to participate in any activity acceptable for a ''normal'' child, but we teach what we term the ''baseball theory,'' namely, three strikes and you're out. He should be allowed to participate in the activity in question; if it causes a flare-up, wait a week or 10 days and then try again. Should a pattern of difficulty recur on three consecutive occasions, then that activity should be discontinued for a significant period of time (generally 3 months to a year, depending on the situation) and then tried once again. Much parent and teacher anticipatory worry and anxiety will thus be minimized or ameliorated.

Physicians who treat children with asthma in effect treat the entire family. Hereditary factors in allergic disease may increase parents' feelings of guilt and, subsequently, in many cases add to family conflict, anxiety, and overprotection. These tensions are easily transmitted along with the child to the classroom, where the teacher becomes the mother substitute. Treating the asthmatic child as an acceptable, normal human being makes him less likely to develop secondary emotional problems, most often from loss of feelings of self-worth and self-esteem, that arise when a youngster thinks of himself as different.

Teachers should be instructed to avoid discussing a child's illness or symptoms in the open classroom, to avoid overprotection, and to discourage the child from using his illness for immediate or secondary gain. To do this, they must understand some of the basic psychophysiologic concepts of the child's problem. Effects of conditioning in a school setting as well as concepts of biorhythmic variations[47] should also be considered in the evaluation of a child. Group discussions involving physician, teacher, and parents are often helpful.

Medication

Simple, safe, symptomatic medications, such as antihistamines or sympathomimetic compounds, help most children.[48-50] School personnel should be advised of medications which need to be given during school hours and their possible side effects. The parents or child may be given properly labeled drugs and additional prescriptions, with instructions to leave separate bottles with the school nurse or teacher. Possible side effects should be put on labels when appropriate (e.g., sedation or nervousness). An older child may be allowed to take the prescribed dose to school each day. Many allergic children can be given long-acting antihistamines or sympathomimetic medications in the morning at home, so as to eliminate the burden of taking medicines while at school.

Sometimes a bronchodilator or injectable adrenaline is needed in school for relief of acute coughing and wheezing. If injectable adrenalin is to be administered by a school nurse, the physician should give detailed, printed instructions with the amount of medication and child's name printed thereon.

We do not recommend that an asthmatic child have in his possession for ready use the handy sympathomimetic inhalation sprays. Asthmatic children frequently tend to overuse these gadgets, often develop psychological dependence upon them, and are exposed to the danger of beta-adrenergic blockade when these are used too frequently. This latter event could lead to the life-threatening "locked lung syndrome."

We recommend that allergic children be permitted to attend school when their symptoms are mild to moderate and their oral temperature does not exceed 100° F. Many parents are prone to keep their child home with evidence of only mild symptoms, but in general it is preferable to err slightly on the side of permissive regular school attendance insofar as possible, especially when there is no evidence of infection.

Children who have had generalized or severe local reactions to hymenopteran stings should receive hyposensitization injection therapy, and adrenaline should be immediately available at the school health station in the event of emergency (see "Emergency Care").

Complete immunization (including rubeola, rubella, and mumps) should be given to all allergic children except those who have specific allergies which prevent selected inoculations (e.g., marked egg sensitivity or vaccination in the presence of eczema).

No medication (e.g., aspirin) should be given in school unless ordered by a physician or responsible medical personnel who can refer to the child's health record.

Complications and side effects of medications

Osler has said, "The desire to take medicine is perhaps the greatest feature that distinguishes man from animals." The fact that we are now confronted with a significant problem of drug abuse among our youth attests not only to the truth of this quotation but also to the fact that man, and especially youth, will take drugs for their side effects as well as their primary actions.

It is not unusual for school personnel to notice side effects of medication based on drug intolerance, allergic reactions, or intentional overdosage. The child who is responsible for his own medication at school may sometimes feel that additional dosage may improve symptoms causing him discomfort during school hours. An example is the overuse of inhaler type medication which has created considerable comment in the allergy literature in the past few years.[51] It is suspected, but still unsettled, that misuse of this type of medication leads to increased numbers of deaths among school-age children.

Self-medication is a common occurrence in the school-age child,[52] and all drugs have the potential for side effects. Charney et al.[53] reported that noncompliance also varies with the mother's conception of the seriousness of the illness and that not taking the drug prescribed by the physician is a common occurrence. This would then lead to several possibilities for the ill child in this situation. One is that the child could have a reaction due to medications given by the physician, or to an over-the-counter (nonprescription) medicine, or that the child could have an increase in symptoms due to the fact that the medication was not given. Since the teacher during the school year often sees the child for more hours than the parents, it is necessary for her to recognize symptom-complexes or drug reaction as they arise. These may often vary according to the stress or emotion at the moment. Many allergic children, especially those with asthma, often require two or three times the amount of fluids that normal children do in order to keep their mucous membranes moist and prevent inspissation of mucus. Due to long hours in the schoolroom and the inconvenience of visits to the bathroom, many older allergic children will elect to stay somewhat dry rather than to properly hydrate themselves.

As previously briefly mentioned individually with the various allergic diseases, there are several categories of drugs commonly used by physicians who manage allergic children. These include the antihistamines, sympathomimetics (i.e., adrenaline, isoproterenol, ephedrine, xanthines), sedatives, tranquilizers, and occasionally ACTH, or corticosteroids.

Antihistamines may cause drowsiness, dryness of the mouth, and, occasionally, some difficulty in vision (blurring).

The xanthines (e.g., theophylline preparations) often cause gastric irritation, nausea, refusal of food, and may also produce anxiety or flushing of the skin.

Adrenaline, ephedrine, and isoproterenol may bring about an increase of heart rate, hyperactivity, nervousness, trembling, or agitation.

Barbiturates and other sedatives will generally cause sedation or drowsiness, and, in large doses, can cause an individual to react more slowly. In a few cases, they paradoxically may produce hyperactivity.

Tranquilizers can cause the patient to appear sluggish, mentally dull, or sleepy. Occasionally, depth perception or balance will be impaired.

When children are receiving one or a combination of any of these drugs, they should be closely observed for any sudden change in their academic capabilities or athletic abilities. It is at times necessary to limit participation in contact sports until the child's medication can be regulated. As a general rule, the physician will advise the parents of common side effects; however, it is virtually impossible to predict the effect of any drug on a specific patient. In the event of overdosage, there are almost always side effects. If a teacher is in doubt about the status of a pupil's medication, information regarding the drug should be available. This should be kept on file in the school nurse's office, through a coordinated program between the physician, school nurse, and classroom teacher.

Emergency care

Asthmatic children and Hymenoptera- and penicillin-sensitive children[54] may occasionally present emergency problems[55] that need to be cared for promptly and expeditiously within the school setting. Each school should have at least one person present at all times who knows how to give adrenaline by injection, mouth-to-mouth resuscitation and closed heart massage. Should anaphylactic shock occur or seem imminent, then, because of possible circulatory collapse, adrenaline may be injected directly into the rich venous plexus under the tongue.[56,57]

A communication system should be set up and tested at periodic intervals to insure rapid transportation and physician coverage when needed. For this, cooperation among the school, nearest medical facility, and the physician is most important.

Early comprehensive study of a child with allergy can be a prophylactic measure. Children should never be expected to "outgrow" their allergic symptoms. Some children appear to "outgrow" them but chronic sinusitis or bronchitis may develop later. Buffum urged, "When asthma begins, get it under control quickly. Patients treated early do better."[58] And, to this succinct statement, we could justifiably inject "any severe allergy."

REFERENCES

1. G. D. Barkin and J. P. McGovern, "Allergy Statistics," *Ann Allergy,* 24:602 (1966).
2. C. G. Schiffer and E. P. Hunt, *Illness Among Children,* Children's Bur Publ 405, (Washington, D.C., U.S. Government Printing Office, 1963).
3. Barkin and McGovern, *op. cit.*
4. Schiffer and Hunt, *op. cit.*
5. J. P. McGovern, O. C. Thomas, T. J. Haywood, C. D. Haunschild and H. Gregory, "Respiratory Allergy in Infants and Children: Data from 5,000 Consecutive Cases," *Med Rec & Ann,* 60:444 (1967).
6. *Ibid.*
7. J. A. Murray, S. R. Alexander, B. T. Travis and J. P. McGovern, "Allergic Cough Syndrome," *Sou Med J,* 63:1159 (1970).

8. J. P. McGovern, T. J. Haywood and A. A. Fernandez, "Allergy and Secretory Otitis Media, An Analysis of 512 Cases," *JAMA,* 200:124 (1967).

9. J. P. McGovern and T. J. Haywood, "Headache of Multiple Etiologies and its Holistic Management," *Headache,* 3:78 (1963).

10. J. P. McGovern, "On Etiologic Mechanisms and a New Classification of Allergic Headache," *Headache,* 4:205 (1964).

11. J. P. McGovern and T. J. Haywood, "Allergic Headache." In Frederic Speer, *Allergy of the Nervous System* (Springfield, Thomas, 1970), pp. 47-58.

12. N. B. Powell, P. B. Boggs and J. P. McGovern, "Allergy of the Lower Urinary Tract," *Ann Allergy,* 28: 252 (1970).

13. J. P. McGovern and T. J. Haywood, "Allergic Tension-Fatigue Syndrome with Headache," *Headache,* 2:230 (1963).

14. G. D. Barkin and J. P. McGovern, "What the Classroom Teacher Can Do for the Asthmatic Child." *NEAJ* (November, 1967).

15. K. D. Rogers, "Health Appraisal of School Age Children," *Pediat Clin N Am,* 12:865 (1965).

16. H. G. Rapaport and S. M. Linde, *The Complete Allergy Guide* (New York, Simon & Schuster, 1970).

17. J. P. McGovern and T. J. Haywood, "Holistic Approach to Management of Bronchial Asthma," *Pediat Clin N Am,* 10:109 (1963).

18. H. G. Rapaport and J. P. McGovern, "Factors Involved in the Allergic Diathesis," *Ann Allergy,* 23:447 (1965).

19. J. P. McGovern and T. J. Haywood, "Constitutional and Nonspecific Factors in the Etiology of Atopic Diseases." In *Brennemann's Practice of Pediatrics,* Vol. 2 (Hagerstown, Harper & Row, 1968).

20. J. P. McGovern, "Newer Perspectives in Allergic Disease," *J Nat Med Assn* 61:144 (1969).

21. J. P. McGovern, "On Conditioning Factors of Age in Allergic Disease—Or Why a Special Pediatric Issue," *Ann Allergy,* 23:577 (1965).

22. T. J. Haywood and J. P. McGovern, "Conditioning Factors in Allergic Disease," *Sou Med J* 60:301 (1967).

23. M. B. Marks, "Recognition of the Allergic Child at School: Visual and Auditory Signs," *Journal of School Health* (May, 1974)

24. McGovern, Thomas, Haywood, Haunschild and Gregory, *op. cit.*

25. Murray, Alexander, Travis and McGovern, *op. cit.*

26. McGovern, Haywood and Fernandez, *op. cit.*

27. J. P. McGovern and T. J. Haywood, "Headache of Multiple Etiologies and Its Holistic Management," *Headache,* 3:78 (1963).

28. J. P. McGovern, "On Etiologic Mechanisms and a New Classification of Allergic Headache," *Headache,* 4:205 (1964).

29. J. P. McGovern and T. J. Haywood, "Allergic Headache." In Frederic Speer, *Allergy of the Nervous System* (Springfield, Thomas, 1970), pp. 47-58.

30. Marks, *op. cit.*

31. J. P. McGovern and T. J. Haywood, "Allergic Eczema." In F. Speer, ed., *The Allergic Child* (New York, Harper & Row, 1963), pp. 200-215.

32. T. J. Haywood and J. P. McGovern, "Atopic Dermatitis in Adolescence," *Cutis,* 4:865 (1968).

33. J. P. McGovern and J. I. Zuckerman, "Nutrition in Pediatric Allergy," *Borden's Review of Nutrition Research,* 17:27-46 (1956).

34. R. E. Lee, M. H. Smolensky, C. S. Leach and J. P. McGovern, "Allergy Evaluation: Circadian Rhythm in the Cutaneous Reactions to Antigens," in press.

35. M. H. Smolensky, R. E. Lee, A. Reinberg, and J. P. McGovern, "Circatrigentan Rhythm Secondary to Hormonal Changes During the Menstrual Cycle: Special Reference to Allergology" (Tuxedo, Proc Int Institute for Study of Human Reproduction, in press).

36. Barkin and McGovern, *op. cit.*

37. K. E. Peirce, O. C. Thomas and J. P. McGovern, "Allergy and the Eye." In F. Speer and R. J. Dockhorn, *Allergy and Immunology in Childhood* (Springfield, Thomas, 1973), pp. 673-678.

38. E. G. Weinberg and M. Tuchinda, "Allergic Tension-Fatigue Syndrome," *Ann Allergy* (April, 1973).

39. Schiffer and Hunt, *op. cit.*

40. J. P. McGovern, T. J. Haywood, D. H. Chao and J. A. Knight, "Headaches in Children: Part I, *Headache* (October, 1961); "Part II," *Headache* (January, 1962); "Part III," *Headache* (April, 1962); "Part IV," *Headache* (April, 1963).

41. J. D. Holloman, "Relation of Headaches to Allergy." In R. Patterson, ed., *Allergic Diseases* (Philadelphia, Lippincott, 1972), pp. 509-524.

42. B. T. Horton, "Medicine Symposium: Head and Face Pain," *Trans Am Acad Ophth Otolaryng* (September-October, 1944).

43. L. Stirck, "Breathing and Physical Fitness Exercises for Asthmatic Children," *Pediat Clin N Am,* 16:31 (1969).

44. J. P. McGovern and A. A. Fernandez, "On the Role of Emotional Factors in Allergy, *J Asthma Res,* 1:213 (1964).

45. J. P. McGovern and J. A. Knight, *Allergy and Human Emotions* (Springfield, Thomas, 1967).

46. Barkin and McGovern, *op. cit.*

47. J. P. McGovern, "On the Circadian Cycle in Medicine," *Headache,* 3:127 (1964)

48. Whigham, *op. cit.*

49. J. P. McGovern, "Therapy of Acute Attacks of Asthma in Infants and Children," *JAMA,* 169:20 (1959).

50. J. P. McGovern, T. J. Haywood, and J. T. Queng, "Long-Term Management of the Allergic Child." In F. Speer, R. J. Dockhorn and J. E. Shira, eds., *Allergy and Immunology in Children* (Springfield, Thomas, in press).

51. H. A. Lyons, S. M. Ayres, M. Dworetzky, C. J. Falliers, C. Harris, C. T. Dollery and B. Gandevia, "Symposium on Isoproterenol Therapy in Asthma," *Ann Allergy,* 31:1 (January, 1973).

52. R. J. Haggerty and L. J. Roughmann, "Noncompliance and Self-Medication," *Pediat Clin N Am,* 19: 104 (February, 1972).

53. E. Charney, R. Bynum, D. Edlredge, D. Frank, J. B. MacWhinney, M. McNab, A. Scheiner, E. Sumpter and H. Iker, "How Well Do Patients Take Oral Penicillin? A Collaborative Study in Private Practice," *Pediatrics,* 40:188 (1967).

54. G. T. Stewart and J. P. McGovern, *Penicillin Allergy: Clinical and Immunological Aspects* Springfield, Thomas, 1970).

55. J. P. McGovern and J. A. Knight, *Allergy and Human Emotions* (Springfield, Thomas, 1967).

56. *Ibid.*

57. Queng, Gregory and McGovern, *op. cit.*

58. W. P. Buffum, The Bret Ratner Award Acceptance Speech, unpublished manuscript (1969).

The school-age child with diabetes and the role of the school nurse

JEAN O'LEARY

A school nurse can expect to have at least one and often several diabetic students under her care. The need to provide competent and supportive health care to these juvenile diabetics during the many hours they spend in school is of concern to current health educators (O'Leary and Edwards, 1978).

Diabetes mellitus affects one in 1000 children under the age of 15 and has been said to be the most common chronic endocrine disease (Sussman, 1971). Of the 42 million persons in the United States between the ages of 10 and 19 years, as many as 200,000 have diabetes (Bennett and Ward, 1977).

The Report of the National Commission on Diabetes (1975) to the Congress of the United States indicates a diabetic prevalence rate of 1.3 per 1000 or one diabetic per 768 persons under 17 years of age. Gorwitz et al. (1976) reported an average rate of one per 600 students in their study in two Western counties in Michigan in 1972 to 1973. A later study, conducted in 1975 in Minnesota by Kyllo and Nuttall (1978), reported a prevalence rate of one diabetic per 529 students in the 1771 elementary and secondary schools they surveyed.

PROBLEMS FACING THE SCHOOL-AGE DIABETIC

Entmacher and Marks (1971) have emphasized that a diabetic has a special problem when entering school because "he has to function normally and effectively in a group of healthy children not subject to restrictions imposed by diabetes." A single diabetic in a school of 600 students has a feeling of being different from the other 599. Nondiabetic students do not have to adhere to a specific meal plan by eating at regular intervals. They do not have to do extra planning when participating in sports. They do not have to pack insulin supplies for an overnight outing. The student with diabetes becomes very aware that his day is different from his friends.

Often diabetic students experience a lack of understanding from peers. This may be due to the peers' inadequate knowledge or from their fear of diabetes. Isolation or rejection from classmates can result. Ack (1974) reminds us that our society places great emphasis on physical prowess and beauty. Therefore to be ill is to be different and to be different most often means being inferior. Young people gain perspective about themselves through interactions with others. If these interactions magnify the feelings of being different, their anxiety is increased. Rather than explain why they must order diet soft drinks or why they cannot stay out past dinner time, students with diabetes may simply withdraw from the group.

SCHOOL STAFF RESPONSE TO THE DIABETIC STUDENT

Teachers and counselors are frequently uninformed regarding the symptoms, treatment, and psychological implications of juvenile diabetes. A study by Alvisa et al. (1974), showed that only 36% of teachers had correct knowledge of the nature of diabetes and that only 16% would have been able to offer adequate care in an emergency. These uncertainties cause teachers to fear diabetic reactions in the classroom or on the playground. The apprehension of teachers, especially those teaching in elementary schools, can increase the anxiety of the child with diabetes and alarm nondiabetic classmates. Collier (1969a), in his study of fifty-eight junior and senior high schools in the Minneapolis area, found that even though 156 teachers and 127 counselors appeared to understand what diabetes is, their level of understanding was inadequate regarding physical side effects associated with the control of diabetes. In addition, Collier (1969a) pointed out that teachers and counselors were often unaware of vocational and educational opportunities available to diabetic adolescents, even though good career counseling was available to nondiabetics.

PSYCHOLOGICAL ADJUSTMENT OF THE SCHOOL-AGE DIABETIC

A diabetic student experiences many normal psychological and physiological changes throughout his years in school. Ack (1974:141) emphasizes that the "psychological meaning of an illness (and its psychological management) depends on the age of the child and will change with each developmental stage." The school nurse therefore needs a thorough understanding of emotional adjustment as it parallels physical adjustment.

During infancy and up to about age 5, a mother's reactions and attitudes toward her child's needs will greatly influence the child's later adjustment to this chronic condition (Vandenbergh, 1971). By elementary school age (6 to 10 years), the young diabetic begins to take pride in competence and learns to win recognition by performing a task well. This corresponds with Erikson's (1968) "industry versus inferiority" stage of development. If the home environment favors acceptance of the disease, the young school-age diabetic will follow a diabetic regimen of measuring diet, testing urine, and following schedules with reasonable interest and cooperation. During this developmental stage, praise is a great reinforcer.

During ages 11 to 13 years, a child often questions: "Do I really have diabetes?" "Will I get over it?" Good explanations that are realistic, but not frightening, should be offered to support the student. This is also a time of rapid growth and hormonal changes, and the child's primary concerns are about body image. "How tall will I be?" "How muscular?" "Will I be fat?" There is a great need to feel normal and the student seeks reassurance from same-sex peers (Daniel, 1975). Dietary and medicinal needs, however, can result in feelings of body damage and inadequacy. Because special diets are not required for school friends, the student with diabetes can feel rejected and cheated by life, and the necessity of regular insulin injections, not always understood by others, places undue stress on the young person who needs to be accepted as an equal by peers.

Midadolescents (ages 14 to 16) are concentrating on a struggle for autonomy. Adolescents want to make their own decisions and resent parental authority or concern. They are mortally afraid of being forced by their parents into doing something that would expose them to ridicule from their peers (Erikson, 1968). They are now more aware of the opposite sex and have concerns about dating, popularity, and appearance. A major developmental task at this age is developing one's identity (Erikson, 1968). Rebellion against parents is part of the normal growth pattern. The usual parental misunderstandings and peer group disappointments of this age group simply increase the difficulties of good management (Collier, 1969b). Vandenbergh (1971) states that group psychotherapy is particularly effective because adolescents are more willing to accept criticism and insights into themselves from colleagues than from any adult.

Older adolescents have generally developed independence and appropriate maleness and femaleness. They have learned to relate well to the opposite sex and have an acceptance of themselves. Their concerns now are more future oriented: career, marriage, pregnancy, health, and longevity (Bennett and Ward, 1977). Diabetes may threaten their relationships with dating partners. They wonder if they should tell their dates about their limitations and how their friends' parents will react to their driving a car. They are concerned about what careers or scholarships are open to them and what adjustments may be necessary for college life, employment, or living away from home.

The loss of a boyfriend or girlfriend, a poor self-image, difficulties in school, or misunderstandings with parents, along with the burden of the diabetic regimen, may discourage adolescents from attempting to maintain good diabetic control (Guthrie and Guthrie, 1975). It is the school nurse's responsibility to recognize students' feelings at different stages of development and to assist them toward a healthy adaptation (Crate, 1965).

PSYCHOSOCIAL ADAPTATION OF THE STUDENT

An early defense mechanism following diagnosis of any chronic disease is shock and disbelief, creating panic, anxiety, and helplessness. By the time the student has left the hospital and returned to school, he has probably moved to the stage of denial. He may refuse to accept the diagnosis and so may fail to follow the necessary treatment. This defensive retreat is needed to allow the individual time to return to a state of equilibrium. The school nurse must be understanding and accepting and encourage the student to verbalize his feelings, but being aware of the facts, she must provide the reality that he is not yet able to accept (Crate, 1965).

Anger is another normal stage of adaptation to the illness. Being sick means acceptance of care and dependence on others. Just when a teenager is learning independence, he finds he must turn to others. Bennett and Ward (1977) discuss the anger that can result, which is frequently projected onto others. At this time they say it is best to empathize, because self-anger is only a mask for anxiety, and the person needs reassurance that he is still accepted.

Gradually the denial and anger lessen. The student becomes more aware of what will be expected of him to control the diabetes. The nurse should be gently supportive as the student moves toward acceptance of his newly diagnosed condition.

Maladaptation often occurs when the family does not accept the disease and its implications. Apprehension is noted in both student and parents. When this occurs, the diabetes becomes the center of existing conflict within the family and poor control results (Koski, 1969). Seidman et al. (1980) report a correlation between the child's acceptance and the parents' acceptance. "When the parents cope, the child copes." Parental acceptance allows the child to accept himself and to develop a normal dependence-independence balance; the result is good diabetes control.

PARENTS' ADAPTATION TO THE DIAGNOSIS OF THEIR CHILD'S DIABETES

As parents learn to accept their child's diabetes, they also experience stages of adaptation. Their initial shock and fear can lead to denial. This period of denial, however, can provide parents with some time to accept the reality of the situation. But along with this awareness, anger expressed as "Why" and guilt feelings of "What did I do wrong" often develop. Schiff (1964) states that parental attitudes almost always reflect guilt. These guilt feelings must surface so parents can rid themselves of self-blame.

Parents' reactions can directly affect the child's response. According to Tomm et al. (1977), parents who are fearful convey fear to their child. Likewise, parents who are perfectionistic create a child who, unable to consis-

tently meet such high expectations, becomes rebellious and deceptive, and parents who are overly sympathetic or guilty tend to overindulge the child. Finally, parents who alienate their child cause him to feel lonely and depressed.

Schiff (1964) recommends a tolerant, relaxed approach. In my experience, when a student said, "No big deal, I don't let it (diabetes) run my life," I found a mother who was also relaxed and comfortable. But the young man who said he "didn't want anyone to know" had an apprehensive, overprotective mother with many fears and concerns.

A child who is not giving his own insulin by age 13 is probably still too dependent on the parents, a fact which the Koski study (1969) found correlated with poor diabetic control. This can indicate to the school nurse that family intervention or referral may be necessary.

ROLE OF THE SCHOOL NURSE WORKING WITH DIABETIC STUDENTS

The nurse is the key person in a school setting to promote safe management of students with diabetes and to provide psychological support necessary to facilitate the adjustment of students and their families. Meetings scheduled early in the school year with students and with parents can open lines of communication between home and school, alleviate apprehension, and allow a verbal exchange of concerns. The younger student is usually willing to have his parents meet with the nurse. In addition, the teacher should participate in this conference.

Older adolescent students often resent parental authority or special attention from school staff, and the nurse may have to find subtle ways to reach these older students. One suggestion is to have a confidential session between the adolescent diabetic and the nurse. In a project conducted in a Minneapolis suburban school district, I received good cooperation from the twenty-three junior and senior high students whom I asked to meet individually with me. During those conferences, I gained their commitment to attend a 1-hour group meeting for sharing feelings with other diabetic students in their school.

In addition, I obtained permission to telephone their parents to explain the purpose of the meetings and also to evaluate the family climate and acceptance of their child's diabetes. This provided an opportunity for parents to express some attitudes and concerns and allowed me the chance to provide additional counseling.

The eight junior high students who attended the group meeting with me responded enthusiastically. When asked if they would like to continue meeting at regular intervals, one eighth-grade boy responded, "I sure would—it's good to be able to tell someone else how you feel sometimes." A senior high student with diabetes co-led each of the junior high groups with me; this seemed to add credibility to the meeting and provided the opportunity for junior high students to discuss situations that might occur in senior high.

A 21-year-old nurse, who has had diabetes since age 4, joined us in our senior high meetings. She shared many of the feelings she experienced in high school and answered questions regarding ways one could handle sensitive situations in high school. Students seemed most interested in suggestions of how or if they should discuss their diabetes with a dating partner. They also shared ideas about how to renew a driver's license, how to handle diet and insulin requirements at social events, how to participate in sports or trips, as well as ideas about available careers and scholarships.

Three of the junior high students refused to be identified with the groups. It may be that diabetes was still too threatening to them. Six senior high students had a variety of reasons for not attending, such as not feeling a need for this type of support or having other commitments during the chosen meeting hour. All but three, however, kept their initial individual conference appointments with me.

Yearly conferences and group meetings in every school are suggested so that students with diabetes can develop a level of comfort in discussing their disease as they progress from elementary to junior and senior high school. In sharing feelings with other students who have diabetes, they can improve their own feelings of self-worth and decrease some of the anxiety of differentness through gradual acceptance of themselves.

In addition, when a diabetic student completes the grade level of one school and is ready to progress to a new school, a combined conference involving nurses from each school and the student is recommended. Sharing knowledge helps the student know that others in the school setting are interested and willing to answer questions and provide advice whenever it is needed.

Bennett and Ward (1977) say that the greatest challenge for the diabetic, especially during the teen years, is to accept being different. The Koski (1969) study suggests a confrontation with the student, which allows for the honest admission that he has a chronic disease which makes him different from his peers. It is then vitally important that the nurse extend support to these students and understand what they are experiencing in adjusting to restrictions. A comfortable school climate can help minimize their feelings of "differentness."

All my students agreed that "kids at school," and the public in general, should be educated about diabetes. An understanding of what diabetes is and how one can be a better friend to a classmate with diabetes would greatly increase the chances of a student adjusting to a diabetic regimen. Presently, most school-age diabetics are embarrassed to have attention given to their special needs. But if all classmates shared a common knowledge, much of the stigma could be eliminated, and the condition might be regarded in the same way as students view athletes' special requirements for food, rest, and exercise to maintain physical fitness.

Summer camps for diabetics are also useful. The child improves in self-confidence and self-reliance by being more independent in self-care. It is an opportunity to learn more about diabetes and to see others coping with the exact same needs. The older child with diabetes often resents the label "diabetic camp" and prefers to remain more independent by attending a regular camp elsewhere. This should be encouraged, as long as the physician and family are comfortably certain that the child is mature enough to assume the responsibility. Many young people can also be encouraged to act as student counselors at camps for diabetics, thus increasing their own self-confidence by instructing and encouraging younger children with diabetes.

ROLE OF THE SCHOOL NURSE WITH SCHOOL PERSONNEL

The school nurse is in the best position to organize the support systems within a school setting. She should engage the school social worker, psychologist, and nutritionist (if one is present in the school) to participate in a team approach to assist students with chronic conditions. Parents, teachers, and counselors should also be part of this management team. Whenever a situation requires additional intervention, someone on the team should be qualified to assist. In the absence of school services, the nurse must be alert to all other community resources available for referrals.

An education program for all teachers, food service personnel, custodians, bus drivers, secretaries, and playground supervisors is essential to assist the school staff to better understand diabetes and to recognize the symptoms and treatment of insulin shock. A 20- to 30-minute in-service presentation by the nurse can provide facts and dispel myths about diabetes. This presentation should be inclusive and provide the following information:

1. Common symptoms of insulin shock
2. Treatment of insulin shock
3. Effects of emotional stress and exercise on diabetes

A child who suddenly shows signs of nervousness and weakness, is pale and perspiring, and complains of hunger may be exhibiting the first signs of an insulin reaction. Often the child is irritable, and a personality change is noted. If these first symptoms are untreated, they can progress to a headache, blurred vision, slurred speech, and confusion. Treatment should be administered immediately by giving the child some candy (preferably *not* chocolate, because it absorbs too slowly), some sugar cubes, fruit juice, or regular pop (not diet pop). The child should always carry some form of sugar, but the teacher should also be provided with a simple sugar in the classroom. If the symptoms do not improve within 10 or 15 minutes, the treatment should be repeated and parents notified. Reactose or glucagon can be kept in the nurse's office and given if the student becomes unconscious, and the student should be transferred to a hospital.

The teacher will feel more at ease if he or she has received adequate knowledge about recognizing and treating an insulin reaction. Parents should always be notified, but the student does not always have to leave school if the response to treatment is adequate. Too much attention and apprehension from the teacher or classmates in the event of a mild insulin reaction only cause anxiety for the diabetic student.

It is also important for school personnel to be alerted to the causes of insulin shock. Diet or insulin dosage may need adjusting, but often there are daily stresses that lower the content of the sugar in the blood. These can include an increased amount of physical activity, anxiety before a test or some competition, or any emotional upset that the student might experience. Symptoms may develop, and the student may need to eat or drink some form of sugar to maintain the normal blood sugar level. Scheduling a physical education class after lunch rather than just before is also important for the diabetic student so that adequate food is in the body to balance the insulin taken that morning. Teacher cards available from the American Diabetes Association can be a quick resource for the classroom teacher regarding signs, symptoms, and treatment of insulin shock.

Food service personnel also need to know what substitutes are allowable in providing the proper school lunch for the diabetic student. If the student wishes to supplement from home or bring a bag lunch on certain days, school menus can usually be provided in advance. School treats and parties can be a problem for the elementary student, but if the teacher is familiar with the wishes of the parents, proper snacks can be arranged that will not embarrass the child.

Parents often express concern regarding the safety of their diabetic child (especially the elementary student) during school hours. If the school staff are adequately instructed in supportive procedures for diabetic students, much fear, anxiety, and psychological stress can be eliminated.

For students with diabetes, exercise can be beneficial. Increased exercise decreases extra sugar in the blood, thus proper regulation of diet and exercise is good for the diabetic (Engerbretson, 1977). In the past, some students have been denied athletic endeavors, cheerleading, school trips, or social involvements such as school dances because others feared the possible occurrence of insulin reactions. The diabetic student who is well controlled and has a thorough understanding of diabetes, including the interactions of diet, insulin, and exercise, is able to modify his regimen to compensate for these activities. Engerbretson (1977) stresses the importance of the diabetic student assuming responsibility for his own care, but also notes that the teacher or coach must be aware of the special needs of the diabetic and allow these needs to be met without embarrassment. If the diabetic student feels the need to stop an activity to eat some candy or drink pop, this should be permitted without making the student feel self-conscious. It is equally important that the diabetic athlete not try to stay in the game for the sake of the team; informing teammates of his diabetes and its possible complications and treatment will help them to be more understanding instead of feeling that the diabetic student is letting them down or getting special treatment. However, Engerbretson (1977) points out it is not the coach's duty to inform the team members of the student's diabetes, but that the decision to do so belongs to the individual diabetic. He should be encouraged to explain, but if the student is reluctant, his wishes should be respected.

Likewise, teachers who take diabetic students on a school trip will need to understand the importance of eating meals on time and not taking an extra mile hike just before lunch. But if the students are knowledgeable, psychologically well adjusted, and follow sensible precautions, teachers and parents can comfortably assist these students in planning a normal athletic or social life.

Many studies have been conducted to determine whether diabetes affects students' intellectual abilities. Sterky (1963) found that school achievements were equal in the diabetic and nondiabetic groups of children. In his survey of public school adolescents with diabetes, Collier (1969a:755) reports that "the adolescent with diabetes possesses capabilities for academic achievement which are well within the range of expected normality." Often teachers are unsure of diabetic students' capabilities and may demand too little of them. At the same time it is important for teachers to be alert to possible events that may interfere with students' intellectual functioning. According to Alvisa et al. (1974), in previous studies such causes as frequent absences from school due to hospitalizations, poor metabolic control and inability to concentrate (a symptom of hypoglycemia), or family attitudes that interfere with normal school life have all been noted as reasons for lower academic achievement rather than lack of intellectual ability.

Although researchers are making progress toward better means of controlling diabetes (Feste, 1974), presently there are no known cures. The American Diabetes Association (1978) reports that diabetics are twenty-five times more prone to blindness than nondiabetics, seventeen times more prone to kidney disease, and twice as prone to heart disease. Researchers have concluded that high sugar content in the blood hastens the advent of diabetic complications (Krall and Joslin, 1971). Cahill et al. (1976) report that "the weight of evidence, particularly that accumulated in the past 5 years, strongly supports the concept that the

microvascular complications of diabetes are decreased by reduction of blood glucose concentrations." Therefore school health teams should encourage students to maintain good diabetic management to delay the onset of these complications.

It is vitally important that physicians, families, and school personnel work together to create attitudes that facilitate good management of the school-age diabetic. Tomm (1964:1154) stresses the necessity of continued support as he states that "cognitive development in children includes a very limited capacity to anticipate long-term consequences of present behavior." In addition, a study by Etzwiler and Robb (1972) found that increased knowledge alone did not result in improved control of the disease; rather, the patient must be motivated and supported to carry out proper medical management.

The school nurse provides the link between the home, physician, and school. She must be available in the school to provide this motivation and encourage diabetic students to maintain good management as prescribed by their physician. She maintains open lines of communication between the home and school so that parents' and teachers' concerns can be exchanged. She strengthens the support systems within the school and promotes understanding and acceptance of the student with diabetes and of the limitations imposed by chronic disease. Crate (1965) points out that adaptation is not static but is a generally lengthy and ongoing process. Hearnshaw's (1975) theory is that diabetes is not an illness but instead, a way of life; perhaps with early interventions this theory can be confirmed.

REFERENCES

Ack, M.: 1974. Psychological problems in long-standing insulin-dependent diabetic patients, Kidney Int. (Suppl.) **1**:141-143.

Alvisa, R., Barroso, C., Marquez, A., Guell, R., and Mateo-de-Acosta, O.: 1974. Scholastic situation of the juvenile diabetic, Acta Diabetol. Lat. **11**(3):250-257.

American Diabetes Association: 1978. Fact sheet on diabetes, American Diabetes Association, New York.

Bennett, D. L., and Ward, M. S.: 1977. Diabetes mellitus in adolescents: a comprehensive approach to outpatient care, South Med. J. **70**(6):705-708.

Cahill, G. F., Jr., Etzwiler, D., and Freinkel, N.: 1976. "Control" and diabetes, N. Engl. J. Med. **294**(18):1004-1005.

Collier, B. N., Jr.: 1969a. The adolescent with diabetes and the public schools—a misunderstanding, Personnel Guidance J. **47**(8):753-757.

Collier, B. N., Jr.: 1969b. Comparisons between adolescents with and without diabetes, Personnel Guidance J. **47**(7):679-684.

Crate, M. A.: 1965. Nursing functions in adaptation to chronic illness, Am. J. Nurs. **65**:72-76.

Daniel, W. A.: 1975. Impact of diabetes on adolescents, Tex. Med. **71**:56-60, Nov.

Engerbretson, D.: 1977. The diabetic in physical education, recreation, and athletics, J. Phys. Ed. Rec. **D8**(3):18-21.

Entmacher, P. S., and Marks, H. H.: 1971. Socioeconomic considerations in the life of the diabetic. In Marble, A., White, P., Bradley, R., and Krall, L., editors: Joslin's diabetes mellitus, Lea & Febiger, Philadelphia.

Erikson, E.: 1968. Identity: youth and crisis, W. W. Norton & Co., Inc., New York.

Etzwiler, D., and Robb, J.: 1972. Evaluation of programmed education among juvenile diabetics and their families, Diabetes **21**(9):967-971.

Feste, C.: 1974. Diabetes—a disease requiring self-management, Bond **51**:6. Published monthly by Lutheran Brotherhood, Minneapolis, Minnesota, October, 1974, D. Brostrom, (editor).

Gorwitz, K., Howen, G., Thompson, T.: 1976. Prevalence of diabetes in Michigan school-age children, Diabetes **25**(2):122-127.

Guthrie, D. W., and Guthrie, R. A.: 1975. Diabetes in adolescence, Am. J. Nurs. **75**(10):1740-1744.

Hearnshaw, F. R.: 1975. Learning to live, Queen's Nurs. J. **18**(4):102-103.

Koski, M.: 1969. The coping processes in childhood diabetes, Acta Paediatr. Scand. (Suppl.) **198**:1-56.

Krall, L. P., and Joslin, A. P.: 1971. General plan of treatment and diet regulation. In Marble, A., White, P., Bradley, R., and Krall, L. editors: Joslin's diabetes mellitus, Lea & Febiger, Philadephia.

Kyllo, C. J., and Nuttall, F.: 1978. Prevalence of diabetes mellitus in school-age children in Minnesota, Diabetes **27**(1):57-60.

O'Leary, J. A., and Edwards, R. K.: 1978. A health care model designed to support the school-age diabetic. (Unpublished manuscript.)

Report of the National Commission on Diabetes to the Congress of the United States, vol. III, part I, DHEW Publication (NIH) 76-1021. Bethesda, Md.

Schiff, L. J.: 1964. Emotional problems of diabetic children and their parents, Psychosomat. **5**:362-364.

Seidman, F., Swift, C., and Tarnow, J. D.: 1980. Psychological aspects of juvenile diabetes mellitus. In Traisman, H. editor: Management of juvenile diabetes mellitus, 3rd ed., The C. V. Mosby Co., St. Louis.

Sterky, G.: 1963. Diabetic schoolchildren, Acta Paediatr. Scand. (Suppl.) **144**. In Koski, M.: 1969. The coping processes in childhood diabetes, Acta Paediatr. Scand. (Suppl.) **198**:16.

Sussman, K. E.: 1971. Juvenile type diabetes and its complications, Charles C Thomas, Publisher, Springfield, Ill.

Tomm, K. M., McArthur, R. G., and Leahey, M. D.: 1977. Psychologic management of children with diabetes mellitus, Clin. Pediatr. **16**(12):1151-1155.

Vandenbergh, R.: 1971. Emotional aspects. In Sussman, K., editor: Juvenile type diabetes and its complications, Charles C Thomas, Publisher, Springfield, Ill.

The child with cancer: impact on the family*

MARTHA PEARSE, B.S.

In working with the school-age child with a malignancy, it is important to have an understanding of the changes in family functioning that normally accompany the stresses of progressive disease. The family functions as a unit, no matter who the identified patient is. Family members will each be affected by the disease and in turn have an effect on the adjustment of the other individuals.

The role of teachers and school health personnel is inevitably intertwined in the lives of these young patients and their families, by virtue of the importance of the school in the normal maturation process.

In exploring some of the stresses and joys that affect the family of the child with cancer, it is important to note several underlying considerations that affect the psychological integrity of both the family and school personnel.

First, the school setting is the natural extension of the family in the child's development, both academically and socially. Disruptions in education due to disease or disability have major effects not only on the child and the family, but also on teachers and health personnel.

Second, cancer treatment and its response pose a constantly changing medical and psychological situation. Unlike static disabilities, cancer and its treatment may impose sudden and unexpected turns, remissions and relapses, bodily changes, and psychological, as well as medical, effects of drugs. Even positive changes or sudden improvements require as much if not more adjustment than a decline.[1]

Third, it is unfortunately true that there is still a strong death taboo in our society. Although the treatment of cancer holds increasing promise of long-term control and possible cure, there is a threat of death which must be considered to understand some of the emotional effects of cancer.[2]

Fourth, the family of the child with cancer is an entity representing a spectrum of emotional involvement and reaction.[3-9] There is no effective psychological treatment of the child without consideration of the effects on the family as a whole. The system has an ebb and flow that will revolve around and affect the well-being of the child.

Fifth, the role of school personnel in promoting the growth and maturation of the child is extended.[4] They are involved in the personal lives of their students in a more intense manner than usual. It is important that school personnel resist the notion that school life and home life are separate systems, because in this situation they may overlap more than usual. Although school personnel are not responsible for the primary medical treatment of the child, they are responsible for seeing that the child receives an education and all the normal activities accompanying it. This may require extra effort in maintaining necessary communication with the family.

Sixth, the role of grief will underlie many of the family's adjustments.[2,5,10] Few of us think of grief as an everyday experience, yet it is. We are loathe to call it by name, but we grieve over little things constantly. We may be angered over losing lesson plans or ruining a piece of clothing, and that is grief. Grief is intensified if we lose a leg, or hair, or, ultimately, our hopes and expectations that a child will live a long and normal life. Grief, then, is a normal process, pathological only in rare extremes. Grief and mourning are constant and intensified processes in the family of a child with cancer.[5] It should

*From Pearse, M.: 1977. The child with cancer: impact on the family, J. School Health 47(3):174-179.
□Martha Pearse, B.S., M.A., is a Graduate Student in the Doctoral Program in Somatopsychology and Rehabilitation, Department of Psychology, University of Kansas, Lawrence, Kansas 66044.

be recognized as such, even encouraged, and not dismissed or avoided as a psychological problem requiring the attention of a psychiatrist.

There has been an increasing number of publications in the past few years on children and cancer, children and death, etc. Space limitations prevent reviewing it all, but a selected reference list will be provided for those who wish further reading. It is particularly interesting that more and more attention is directed toward the positive aspects of the psychological management of the disease, such as family involvement and healthy coping mechanisms.[5-7,11] Much of the early literature focused on children's fears, mother's anxieties (fathers only recently have come into recognition), and the psychopathology of grief.

Families, just like individuals, vary in the ways in which they perceive and react to threat. Although the elements of the stress of cancer may be similar, the coping and adjusting mechanisms of one family may be quite different from that of another. It is sometimes helpful to think of the family as a dynamic system in which a change in one individual will necessitate a change in the adjustment of one or more others. The family of a child with cancer is thus in more of a fluid state than is a family of healthy children.

The type of family under our consideration here is one which may appear to an outsider as having a number of unusual living patterns. These patterns of adjustment are not necessarily abnormal; they may be quite facilitative. Their peculiarities are peculiar only because of the threat of relinquishing a child to illness, disability, or death, and with it the family's hopes for continued generations of existence—these are challenges most families do not have to face.

STAGES OF ADJUSTMENT

The family may go through a number of overlapping stages during the course of the child's illness.[12] Kubler-Ross[2] has characterized the stages of death and dying as shock-denial-isolation, anger-rage, bargaining, depression, and acceptance. These stages are experienced by each member of the family, as well as the child. It is important to remember that these stages rarely are sharply defined, nor are they experienced separately, inclusively, or in any particular order.

There are peak times when the emotional concomitants of the disease are intensified.[5,11]

The diagnosis is always extremely difficult. Again, at relapse, especially the first relapse, there is a heightened grief reaction, which perhaps is the most difficult time of all for the child and the family. These are common examples of crisis. Each family will have its own crisis points revolving around its hopes for the future, such as failure to graduate, the surgical removal of reproductive organs, or an amputation that precludes sports activity. Families lose many of their hopes for the future at these times, even though medical control of the disease is hopeful.[3]

The role of denial can be a healthy coping mechanism when it is used to maintain normalcy and hope.[2,3,13] Although occasionally there are families and patients who use denial in the extreme when the threat is too painful to be allowed into awareness, most families will use denial advantageously and in realistic moderation.[12] Few are the families who consistently maintain that the diagnosis is a mistake, or that medication schedules and normal precautions against infection are unnecessary and to be ignored. Few also are the families who succumb to despair, assuming the outcome is too dismally fatal to bother with treatment at all. Denial in moderation allows the family to maintain as full as existence as possible by permitting the hope that, at least for the moment, control of the disease is promising and may be promising again tomorrow.[5,13]

The role of hope in maintaining this and other coping mechanisms is paramount.[2] Initially, there may be hope that the diagnosis was wrong, but, in the face of irrefutable evidence, hope may change to hope for a cure. Later, it may become hope for a long remission, or just one more remission.[5] If the disease progresses toward a fatal outcome, there is hope that the time left will be happy and meaningful, and, at the end, that death will come peacefully. Finally, there is hope that somehow life can go on and there will be peace and joy in the house again.[2,14,15]

The family will be involved in grief processes from the first day, however, and although there will be a heightened stress reaction to each major crisis, a family may well have its grief work finished if the child dies.[3,14-16] Death will bring its own new grief reaction, but it is often faster and less intense than the anticipatory mourning.[2,17] Those on the periphery—friends, teachers, medical staff—may lag far behind.[2]

GUILT

Care of the child with cancer imposes a number of stresses on the family system. Guilt is one of the most pervasive.[2,3,7,8,12-15] There may be guilt that the parents did not seek medical care soon enough, guilt over suspected genetic defects, guilt that financial and emotional resources are diverted from the rest of the family, guilt about the anger the family may feel toward the child for being sick, and guilt that the family is tired of making constant adjustments.[3,6,18]

There are many other kinds of guilt, some rational and some irrational.[2] It is apparent, though, to anyone who works with these families, that guilt is always present whether it is deserved or not. Even in the most devoted, resourceful and stable families, the members, including the sick child, will find something to feel guilty about. Guilt is sly and often out of awareness. It may manifest itself in discipline problems, acting-out behaviors, self-defeating or injurious acts, prolonged mourning, or any number of ways the human mind can find to punish itself.[9,10,19] It is helpful to these families to have an outside perspective, first to allow these feelings to be expressed, then to add the rational perspective that, short of violence, no one person has the power to wreak such havoc on a loved one.

ANGER

Anger is another obvious component in the process. It may be directed toward the disease, doctors, God, or each other. In one of its most destructive forms, anger is directed toward the child for being sick or different, or for dying.[3,12,13,15,20] This type of anger is common, and only malevolent in the extreme. Most family members are relieved if given the opportunity to express their anger and acknowledge it in a nondestructive verbal or physical way. Anger also can be constructive or facilitative if viewed as a source of creative energy. It can be released in outlets such as sports, school activities, gardening, or play. It can be channeled into more direct and intellectual pursuits, such as the local cancer drive, a community project, academic achievement, or hospital work.[20]

Anger that has no outlet is often turned inward, manifesting itself as deep depression or physical illness.[9,12] Whatever its expression or lack thereof, anger is particularly a problem for adolescents. No longer a child and not quite an adult, the adolescent faces what seems like insurmountable barriers to achieving independence and identity.[3,6,20,21] The need for normalcy and the freedom to acquire the skills of adulthood are thwarted at every turn by the demands of treatment or protective families. Normal concerns about sexuality and social skills are compounded by dependency and a different life style.[22]

SENSE OF NORMALCY

An overriding concern of the family is the maintenance of a sense of normalcy and control in everyday life.[3,11,12,14,23-25] This is no small task if the care of the child requires a great deal of attention, which is often the case. In a normal family in which a child has the flu, there will be a disruption in family routine. In the family of a child with cancer, there are constant disruptions due to frequent lab work, trips to the clinic, drug effects, and hospitalizations. If the family is burdened financially or lives some distance from the treatment facility, it only adds to the disruption.[5,7,11,15]

The logistics of cancer care require drastic role shifts within the family.[2,3,11,26,27] Even in the most liberated families in which there is a comfortable sharing and shifting of household responsibilities there is a difficult strain. In traditional families in which the child-caring responsibilities are basically the mother's, there comes a time when mother cannot attend to all the sick child's needs and do all the other things to which her family has become accustomed. In addition, the father may remove himself from the family's activities and direct his energies into his work.[7,12,27-29] Fathers bear a great deal of criticism for this type of behavior, which often occurs at the suggestion of well-meaning professionals. He is directed to go back to work and leave the worry to the doctors and the mother. This is a divisive maneuver, no matter how good the intentions, and is an almost certain way to get families off to a bad start. Most of us, given a chance to escape from a threatening situation, will try to escape. The result is that one parent may be overwhelmed by the needs of the child and family, yet be ahead of the game in grief work. The other parent may avoid this painful daily process, but may be much less able to cope with the child and the disease. This common process increases emotional distance from involved family members and can result in almost total exclusion.

One of the basic indexes of a family's coping mechanism is its pattern of communication, both internally and externally. Parents often respond to the diagnosis as something to be kept from the child.[3] This usually reflects the parent's, not the child's, inability to face the child's disability and possible death.[5,14,15] Moreover, it is not simply a matter of telling or not telling, but of how and when.[2,6,11,20,23,28-33] It is virtually impossible for a child not to realize the seriousness of his or her disease. Even infants respond to the change in a parent's mood, voice, or touch.

Adults and children alike, given partial information, will fill in the rest with fantasy, which may be more frightening than reality. Silence also creates distance and distrust, while honest answers to questions, given with support and realistic hope, dispel unnecessary fears and promote closeness. Few people are comfortable with deceit, and it is rarely in anyone's best interest to conceal such a serious matter. Share's excellent review of the literature and her studies on open family communication are recommended for a more in-depth perspective on this salient topic.[3,5,11,24,26,34]

Communication outside the family also has an important impact on family adjustment. Relatives, friends, and school and business contacts often react with deep fear. The closer the outsiders, the more threatened they become.[10,14,16,35] Friends are suddenly aware of their own and their children's vulnerability to cancer. Medical and school authorities may feel the child's changed status reflects a personal or professional failure, as well as a personal loss. Grandparents may become distant, the car pool may be changed, social contacts may be dropped, playmates no longer want or are allowed to play. At school, children may be excluded from normal activities without adequate reason, ignored in class, asked to use a separate water fountain, teased about their physical appearance, or subjected to other indignities associated with the fear of contagion—emotional or physical.

As a result, families are quickly isolated and stripped of their customary support systems.* It is not just a cliche that in times like this one finds out who one's friends are. Perhaps it is better to be isolated early than to be rejected when the going gets rougher, but that is little solace to lonely families.

In our society, we often equate the unburdening of our souls with a plea to do something. In fact, the plea may be just to stand there. Fami-

*References 3, 11, 13, 14, 20, 26, 29, 36

lies rarely expect miracles from physicians or anyone else, but they do need to know who will listen, and who will stand by them in their hours of need.[11]

It is no wonder in the absence of outside support and effective internal communication that family stresses can be overwhelming. A minor expression of anger can cause major dissension and mutual withdrawal. If parents begin living in their separately invested worlds, the rift widens.[3,5] Father may turn his attention to work; mother may turn hers to the sick child, forming a bond that is impenetrable to the rest of the family. The sick child may become so dependent that he or she cannot bear to be out of the mother's presence, much less go to school.[16,22,29,37] The other children may withdraw into depression or act out to receive needed attention or to express hostility toward other family members.[33] Discipline fails. Sexual problems often abound, as both parents feel impotent and frustratingly unable to exercise normal control in the destiny of their family.[3,13]

The grieving process present from the beginning can grow to difficult extremes if this expression is forbidden or not acknowledged. It is natural to feel sad, angry, and depressed over a real or threatened loss. Grievers can be expected to have bouts of insomnia, inability to concentrate, anorexia, sighing, weeping, vivid dreams, and fantasies of present pain and future hopes that may never be realized. Yet, it is only protracted or unexpressed grief that causes seriou emotional disturbances, physical illness, or long-term problems such as the fear to establish lasting relationships later in life.[3,9,10,17,18,31,37]

When there are lengthy hospitalizations, especially when one parent accompanies the child, the family may finish much of its grieving and learn to live happily without the two of them. A remission or a return to the home may cause major adjustments as the win-lose cycle begins anew.[1,14] Yet, with open support and acceptance of these family dynamics, from within and without, the experience of having a child with cancer can be one of intensified, bittersweet closeness. Long-stifled family interaction can be opened up as the family actively deals with its problems. Mere survival can be difficult, but the threat of a shortened or altered life can sometimes spur a family to spend time, effort, and money on meaningful diversions it previously could "not afford." Life and living take precedence over death and dying. Families with good coping mechanisms use healthy denial at appropriate times to focus on the quality of life so essential to both living and dying. A life fully lived and shared by family and friends is one to be celebrated. A life that is lost will be deeply mourned but still will be celebrated.[2,11]

Families are more resilient than they have been given credit for. In the psychological literature, it is often noted that these stresses result in more than ordinary mental and physical illness, divorce, and separation.[14,18,29,34] In far too many cases it is true, yet statistical evidence is too poorly kept and contradictory to justify labeling these families at any higher risk than any other. The more recent studies, perhaps in response to the grim prognosis of the past, are emphasizing that the family as a whole may have considerable resources to strengthen their bonds, despite tragedy.*

The key, as Kaplan notes in his excellent family-oriented studies, is early intervention. Disruptive patterns can be formed within the first few days or weeks after diagnosis.[5,11] Many of them are not apparent to the family members, except in retrospect when it is too late to change. All professionals who have contact with the family—medical personnel, teachers, ministers, psychologists, social workers—must be willing to accept responsibility for some support and involvement with the family.[5,12,20,39] Compassion is more important than professional training in providing an atmosphere in which the family can do its own work. For those with the courage to take the first step, it can be an immensely rewarding situation.[2,10,28,31]

THE FAMILY AND SCHOOL

School activities for the child with cancer are often the child's most important contact outside the family. It is imperative that the school have good communication with the family about the medical and emotional status of the child, so he or she can have the most meaningful school experience possible.[4,27]

Parents who participate in the care of their child are well informed and usually can be trusted to tell school officials of any special needs or concerns. Likewise, teachers and school health personnel should be trusted to provide the child with as normal a school experience as possible, without fear of parental retribution.

School personnel at times will be expected to

answer questions[4] or respond to demands of anxious parents of the child's friends, including the removal of the sick child from the school situation. Such segregation only reinforces fears of disease and of death for all concerned. If given a chance, children often are more accepting of death and disability than are their parents, although they may understand it at a different level.

In the event of a child's death, classmates may express an interest in attending the funeral or discussing their understanding of death in the classroom. Too often, both these healthy concerns are stifled by adults who feel these are inappropriate activities for younger children. Death has replaced sex as the number one taboo. Yet, children have the need to ask questions and express their grief just as adults do, and perhaps more honestly. By allowing such expression, even if there are no satisfactory answers, teachers can provide an invaluable learning experience and provide good preventive mental health for a child's later and inevitable experience with loss.[10,31,39-42]

REFERENCES

1. Easson WM: The Lazarus syndrome in childhood. *Med Insight* November, 1972, pp. 44-51.
*2. Kubler-Ross E: *On Death and Dying.* New York, MacMillan Co., 1969.
*3. Burton L (ed): *Care of the Child Facing Death.* London, Routledge & Kegan Paul, 1974.
*4. Kaplan DM, Smith A, Grobstein R: School management of the seriously ill child. *J Sch Health* 44:250-254, 1974.
5. Kaplan DM, Smith A, Grobstein R, et al: Family mediation of stress. *Soc Work* 18:61-69, 1973.
6. Taylor G, Sullivan MP, Sutow WW: *Leukemia: A Guide to the Management of the Disease.* Leukemia Society of America, 1971.
7. Debuskey M, (ed): *The Chronically Ill Child and His Family.* Springfield, Ill., Charles C Thomas, 1970.
8. Siegler M, Osmond H: Models of madness: Mental illness is not romantic. *Psychol Today* 8:71-78, 1974.
9. Willis DJ: The families of terminally ill children: Symptomatology and management. *J. Clin. Child Psychol.* 3:32-33, 1974.
10. Krupp G: Maladaptive reactions to the death of a family member. *Soc Casework* 53:425-434, 1972.
11. Schoenberg B, Carr AC, Peretz D, et al: *Psychosocial Aspects of Terminal Care.* New York, Columbia University Press, 1972.
12. Vore DA: The family and loss: Coping with the death of a child. Presented at the American Psychological Association Annual Meeting, Chicago, Ill., 1975.
13. Easson WM: Care of the young patient who is dying. *JAMA* 205:203-207, 1968.
14. Friedman SB, Chodoff P, Mason JW, et al: Behavioral observations on parents anticipating the death of a child. *Pediatrics* 32:610-625, 1963.

---

*References 3, 5-7, 11, 14, 22, 35, 37, 38.

*For further reading.

15. McCollum AT, Schwartz AH: Social work and the mourning parent. *Soc. Work* January, 1972, pp. 25-30.
16. Bozeman MF, Orback CE, Sutherland AM: Psychological impact of cancer and its treatment III: The adaptation of mothers to the threatened loss of their children through leukemia, part I. *Cancer* 8:1-19, 1955.
17. Hodge JR: They that mourn. *J. Religion Health* 11: 229-240, 1972.
18. Moriarity DM: *The Loss of Loved Ones: The Effects of a Death in the Family on Personality Development.* Springfield, Ill., Charles C Thomas, 1967.
19. Cain AC, Fast I, Erickson M: Children's disturbed reactions to the death of a sibling. *Am J Orthopsychiatry* 34:741-752, 1964.
20. Easson WM: Management of the dying child. *J. Clin Child Psychol* 3:25-27, 1974.
21. Moore DC, Holten CP, Marten GW: Psychological problems in the management of adolescents with malignancy. *Clin. Pediatr.* 8:464-473, 1960.
22. Lansky SB, Lowman JT, Vats T, et al: School phobia in children with malignant neoplasms. *Am. J. Dis Child* 129:42-46, 1975.
23. Green M: Care of the child with a long-term life-threatening illness: Some principles of management. *Pediatrics* 39:441-445, 1967.
24. Vernon DTA, Foley JM, Sipowicz RR, et al: *The Psychological Responses of Children to Hospitalization and Illness.* Springfield, Ill., Charles C Thomas, 1965.
25. *The Question of Coping: No. 11: Coping With Chronic and Catastrophic Illness.* Nutley, N.J., Hoffman-La Roche Inc., 1975.
*26. Share L: Family communication in the crisis of a child's fatal illness: A literature review and analysis. *Omega* 3:187-201, 1972.
27. Hamovitch MB: *The Parent and the Fatally Ill Child: A Demonstration of Parent Participation in a Hospital Pediatrics Department.* Los Angeles, Delmar Publishing Co Inc, 1964.
*28. Kaplan DM: The impact of childhood leukemia on patients and families. Presented at the American Cancer Society Science Writers Seminar, March, 1974.
29. Lansky SB: Childhood leukemia: The child psychiatrist as a member of the oncology team. *J Am Acad Child Psych* 13:499-508, 1974.
30. Issner N: Can the child be distracted from his disease? *J Sch Health* 43:468-471, 1973.
*31. Kavanaugh RE: *Facing Death.* Los Angeles, Nash Publishing Co, 1972.
32. Vernick J, Karon M: Who's afraid of death on a leukemia ward? *Am. J. Dis. Child* 109:393-397, 1965.
33. Wright L: An emotional support program for parents of dying children. *J. Clin Child Psychol.* 3:37-38, 1974.
34. Albin AR, Binger CM, Stein RC, et al: A conference with the family of a leukemic child. *Am J Dis Child* 122:362-364, 1971.
35. Cobb B: Psychological impact of long illness and death of a child on the family circle. *J Pediatr* 49:746-751, 1956.
36. Anthony EJ, Koupernik C: *The Child in His Family: The Impact of Disease and Death.* New York, John Wiley & Sons, 1973, vol. 2.
37. Futterman EH, Hoffman I: Transient school phobia in a leukemia child. *J Am Acad Child Psych* 9:477-494, 1970.
38. Lansky SB: Update on psychosocial problems in childhood cancer, in *Cancer Control for the Professional.* Newsletter, American Cancer Society, 3:1-8, 1976.
39. Solnit AJ, Green M: Psychological considerations in the management of deaths on pediatric hospital services. *Pediatrics* 24:106-112, 1959.
*40. Grollman EA: *Talking About Death: A Dialogue Between Parent and Child.* Boston, Beacon Press, 1970.
41. Grollman EA: The way of dialogue on death between parents and children. *Religious Educ* 69:198-206, 1974.
42. Jackson EN: *Telling a Child About Death.* New York, Channel Press, 1965.

Nutritional needs of adolescents*

CAROLYN T. TORRE

Adolescence is a time of rapid physical change. This change and the life situations in which young people become involved as they approach adulthood are reflected in the nutritional needs of this age group.

Adolescence is a period characterized by rapid, recognizable change in the individual's physical makeup. Ironically, the accelerated growth of puberty creates increased nutritional needs at a time when meeting these needs is most difficult because of internal and external factors. Among these factors are a desire to express a developing sense of self and independence through adhering to extreme diets, an incomplete cognitive grasp of the effect of present food intake on future health, and insufficient time to prepare or eat nutritious foods(1,2). The unfortunate consequence of this irony is reflected in a study finding that adolescents, ages 10 to 16, had the most unsatisfactory nutritional status of any other age group(3).

Nurses may be better prepared to help adolescents effectively meet their own nutritional needs if they are informed about the following issues: What are adolescents' basic nutrient requirements? What deficiencies exist in the present diets of young people and what influence do food fads and fast foods have on these deficiencies? What effects do pregnancy and participation in sports have on an adolescent's nutritional needs? What are some of the common nutritional problems which occur during adolescence?

*Copyright © 1977, The American Journal of Nursing Company. Reproduced, with permission, from MCN, The American Journal of Maternal Child Nursing, March/April, vol. 2, no. 2.
□Ms. Torre, R.N., M.A., is an instructor at Rutgers College of Nursing in the School Nurse Practitioner Program and also serves as a pediatric nurse practitioner in ambulatory care at Willets Health Center, Douglass College, Rutgers University.

BASIC NUTRITIONAL NEEDS OF ADOLESCENTS

While nutritional needs during adolescence vary individually and according to sex, they closely parallel velocity of growth in all individuals. That is, the period of greatest nutritional needs coincides with the peak rate of growth during the adolescent growth spurt(4).

A 1974 report on an analysis of the growth of approximately 7000 youths from 12 to 17 years old concludes that the growth spurt is occurring at an earlier age than past studies revealed. On the average the height spurt in girls begins at about age 10¼ and lasts for 2¼ years. In boys this period starts at about 11¾ years—nearly 18 months later than in girls—and lasts 2¾ years. The weight spurt in both boys and girls begins about 6 months after the onset of the height spurt and continues for 2¾ to 3 years. During this overall period of maximal growth girls attain about 9% of final adult height and 23% of adult weight; boys attain 11% of adult height and 23% of adult weight.

One can therefore roughly define the period of greatest nutritional need in adolescence as between approximately 10¼ and 13½ years for girls and approximately 11¾ and 14½ years for boys(5). But Young, among others, emphasizes the limitations of defining an individual's nutritional needs in terms of chronological age alone because the time of onset of puberty varies so widely(2). Since the growth spurt and the sequence of sexual development are related, it is useful to consider an adolescent's maturational status to assess accurately his nutritional needs.

Tanner found that in females the beginning of the growth spurt may precede the appearance of the breast bud, generally the first sign of puberty. The point of maximum growth in height usually occurs about 1 year prior to menarche(6). In males the beginning of the growth spurt coincides with an increase in the size of

Recommended dietary allowances for adolescents*

	Male			Female				
	11 to 14 years	15 to 18 years	19 to 22 years	11 to 14 years	15 to 18 years	19 to 22 years	Pregnant	Lactating
Weight (kg)	44	61	67	44	54	58		
Height (cm)	158	172	172	155	162	162		
Energy (kcal)	2800	3000	3000	2400	2100	2100	+300	+500
Protein (g)	44	54	54	44	48	46	+30	+20
Vitamin A activity (IU)	5000	5000	5000	4000	4000	4000	5000	6000
Vitamin D (IU)	400	400	400	400	400	400	400	400
Vitamin E activity (IU)	12	15	15	12	12	12	15	15
Ascorbic acid (mg)	45	45	45	45	45	45	60	80
Folacin (μg)	400	400	400	400	400	400	800	600
Niacin (mg)	18	20	20	16	14	14	+2	+4
Riboflavin (mg)	1.5	1.8	1.8	1.3	1.4	1.4	+.3	+.5
Thiamine (mg)	1.4	1.5	1.5	1.2	1.1	1.1	+.3	+.3
Vitamin B_6 (mg)	1.6	2.0	2.0	1.6	2.0	2.0	2.5	2.5
Vitamin B_{12} (μg)	3.0	3.0	3.0	3.0	3.0	3.0	4.0	4.0
Calcium (mg)	1200	1200	800	1200	1200	800	1200	1200
Phosphorus (mg)	1200	1200	800	1200	1200	800	1200	1200
Iodine (μg)	130	150	140	115	115	100	125	150
Iron (mg)	18	18	10	18	18	18	18+	18
Magnesium (mg)	350	400	350	300	300	300	450	450
Zinc (mg)	15	15	15	15	15	15	20	25

*Adapted from 1974 Recommended Dietary Allowances, Eighth revised edition, Food and Nutrition Board, National Research Council. National Academy of Sciences, Washington, D.C. and "Adolescents and Their Nutrition," by C. Young, in *Medical Care of the Adolescent,* Third Edition, edited by J. Gallagher *et al.* (New York, Appleton-Century-Crofts, 1976). Pregnant and lactating females are included as some nurses work with these individuals.

the penis, about 1 year after the onset of scrotal and testicular enlargement; peak velocity in height gains does not occur until the genitalia are already well developed(7).

On the basis of these maturational indices one can conclude that the period of greatest nutritional need in girls is early in puberty, *prior* to menarche. In boys, needs are greatest in mid to late puberty, *after* the genitalia are well developed. This is reflected in the Recommended Dietary Allowances (RDAs) most recently published by the Food and Nutrition Board, National Research Council(8). (See Recommended Dietary Allowances for Adolescents).

Because few studies have been done on adolescent nutritional requirements, however, the RDAs for this group have been extrapolated from findings on the needs of children and adults. Thus their accuracy is open to question. In an attempt to account for individual variations, the Food and Nutrition Board calculated the RDAs to contain a margin of safety for each of the nutrients listed. They hope to have been overgenerous rather than undergenerous in this regard(9).

Mueller stresses that RDAs are guidelines designed for groups of people and that they should not be used to assess the status of any one individual. Rather, he encourages that they be used as "guides to healthy eating patterns"(9).

Whether or not a given adolescent's nutritional needs are being met is probably best determined by assessing the adequacy of his growth rate. Patterns of height and weight are easily visualized by plotting values on a growth chart such as that devised for adolescents by Jaworski and Jaworski(10). Does the adolescent fall within the normal limits for height and weight for his particular chronological age? If not, nutritional deficiencies might be considered.

DEFICIENCIES RELATED TO EATING PATTERNS

The dietary patterns of adolescents, like those of Americans of other ages, have changed dramatically over the past three decades. A report on food consumption published by the United States Department of Agriculture in 1968 described a decline in the nutritive value of diets between 1955 and 1965 which continues to hold true today.

Parrish correlates this decline with changing sociological circumstances in the United States since World War II, including improved income levels, increased urbanization, and greater mobility. All of these factors have contributed to a decrease in the variety of foods eaten—notably to a decrease in the intake of fresh fruits and vegetables—and to increased consumption of "fast foods" which lack some vitamins(11).

Nutritional studies indicate no evidence of extensive calorie or protein deficiency among American adolescents today; they do, however, reflect deficiencies in both vitamins and minerals. The nutrients most often lacking in adolescents' diets are iron, vitamin A, calcium, and—to a lesser extent—vitamin C, riboflavin, and thiamine(3,12-16).

One of the changes in dietary patterns which has apparently contributed to nutritional deficiencies during adolescence is a tendency to skip breakfast. Steele and his colleagues reported that adolescents who consistently eat breakfast more nearly meet the recommended levels of all nutrients for their age group than those who miss breakfast once a week or more(17).

Breakfast foods tend to provide the major source of vitamin C; consequently skipping breakfast—a phenomenon especially common among adolescent girls—results particularly in less than adequate vitamin C intake(14). Among the reasons adolescents have mentioned for missing breakfast are that their parents did not prepare the meal, that they were not hungry in the morning, and that they arose too late on school days to take time to eat breakfast(11).

Since nutritional adequacy is positively correlated with increasing variety in the diet, it is difficult to achieve during adolescence. Many young people voluntarily restrict themselves to eating a relatively small number of favorite and familiar foods. The effects of this restriction are reinforced by the limited number of nutrients offered in the fast foods which contribute substantially to adolescent diets. Nutrients which have been cited as lacking in these foods are vitamins A, D, C, and folic acid.

Furthermore, in the quantity in which fast foods are typically eaten, they contain more calories than the average adolescent probably needs and may increase the risk of obesity(11,18). Finberg contends, however, that one fast-food meal a day does not constitute a "national disaster for adolescents" and notes that deficiencies in such diets could be amended by including two glasses of milk; a serving of green, leafy vegetables; and a glass of fruit juice daily(18).

For a variety of social and religious reasons an increasing number of young people are becoming vegetarians, another pattern which can affect their nutritional status. Parents particularly have expressed concern about the effects of this generally unfamiliar diet on nutrition. While it is true that extreme forms of vegetarianism—one level of the Zen Macrobiotic diet which consists solely of brown rice and tea, for example—may induce malnutrition, vegetarianism is certainly not now responsible for the deficient nutritional status of American youth. Indeed, it may provide long-term benefits in the form of reduced rates of cancer of the colon and of atherosclerosis to those who practice it consistently and well(19).

Strict vegetarians—those who eat no meat, fish, dairy products or eggs—are more susceptible to nutritional deficiencies in amino acids, calcium, iron, zinc, and vitamin B_{12} than others. But it is generally agreed that their diets will be adequate if they contain a variety of fruits, vegetables, unrefined cereals, legumes, seeds, and nuts and if they are also supplemented with vitamin B_{12}(19, 20).

Snacking has long had an apparently undeserved reputation for contributing to nutritional deficiencies in adolescents. What nurse cannot recall hearing parents protest to their ravenous adolescent, "But it (snacking) will spoil your appetite?" Evidence strongly indicates that adolescents obtain an important part of essential nutrients through snacks and that those who eat more than three times a day have better diets than those who eat less frequently(12,21).

Although young people undeniably consume their share of potato chips, soft drinks, and candy, the foods most often mentioned in one study as favorite snacking items of this age group were dairy products—milk, ice cream, and cheese(14). Considering that these are excellent sources of calcium, which is one of the nutrients most in need of being increased in adolescent diets, snacking on at least milk and cheese should be encouraged. Ice cream is less satisfactory as a snack because of its high calorie content as well as its cariogenic potential.

Another examination of adolescent food preferences revealed that adolescents did like foods which are good sources of nutrients commonly deficient in their diets, except for some which are richest in vitamin A—squash, spinach, and liver(15). It does not, therefore, seem to be impossible to provide young people with foods they like and which also fulfill their nutrient requirements.

Adolescents tend to eat whatever is closest at hand, so foods containing needed nutrients should be readily accessible to them for snacking (See Food Sources of Nutrients Commonly Deficient in Adolescent Diets). Parents and dietary personnel at school need to be encouraged to purchase items which are simultaneously low in calories and cariogenic potential.

In addition, through judicious dietary counseling which stresses the immediate and tangible effects of a good diet such as improved appearance and increased physical endurance, adolescents can be helped to recognize nutritious foods independently(2). Whether or not they then eat these foods is a decision which only they themselves can make.

ADOLESCENTS WITH SPECIAL NUTRITIONAL NEEDS

Conditions which alter normal nutritional needs often arise during adolescence. Nurses must understand the effects of these factors such as pregnancy, family planning, and athletic performance to provide effective dietary counseling.

Pregnancy during adolescence, as at other ages, increases the Recommended Dietary Allowances for protein, calories, iron, calcium, vitamins C and A, and the B vitamins (See Recommended Dietary Allowances for Adolescents, p. 531). It has been well documented that a large number of adolescents from low-income families suffer from dietary deficiencies. For example, Brewer describes toxemia as an "unofficial deficiency disease of late pregnancy" directly related to inadequate protein consumption(22). The highest rates of pregnancy at an early age are also found among the poor(2). When a girl becomes pregnant before she has

Food sources of nutrients commonly deficient in adolescent diets*

Common nutrient deficiencies	Foods high in these nutrients
Vitamin A	*Direct sources:* liver, fish liver oils, butter, cheese, eggs and milk *Sources of carotene:* yellow vegetables, green leafy vegetables, tomatoes, yellow fruits
Vitamin C	Citrus fruits, strawberries, broccoli, bell peppers, tomato juice, rose hips
Calcium	Milk, cheese, yogurt, ice cream, soybeans, mustard, and turnip greens
Iron	Red meats, especially liver, wheat germ, brewer's yeast, egg yolks, dark green leafy vegetables, apricots, whole grain cereals, fish
Riboflavin	Milk, liver, brewer's yeast, whole grains, green leafy vegetables, fish and eggs
Thiamine	Brewer's yeast, wheat germ, rice polish, pork, milk, nuts, whole grains, liver, peas, lentils

*Adapted from the *Dictionary of Nutrition* by Richard Ashley and H. Duggal, St. Martin's Press, 1975.

completed the growth spurt, the condition carries a special health risk for both mother and fetus, who will be competing for nutrients which may be in insufficient supply. Fortunately, however:

Growth appears to compete with pregnancy only in those rare instances when fertilization takes place before or soon after menarche. There is no evidence that the age group in which pregnancy is most likely to occur—15 and upwards—has special nutritional needs apart from those that may be created by the socioeconomic and cultural environment.(23)

The two most common complications of adolescent pregnancy, higher incidences of low birth weight babies and toxemia in the mother, are both associated with nutritional inadequacies(24). Birch writes that fetal malnutrition may also have more subtle consequences, including decreased brain myelinization, deficient brain cells, and impaired neurological development which may eventually be manifested in the form of epilepsy, mental retardation, cerebral palsy, or minimal brain dysfunction(25).

The nutrients most often cited as lacking in the diets of pregnant adolescents are, not surprisingly, iron, calcium, and vitamin A. In addition, pregnant young girls, particularly those from low-income areas, may consume insufficient protein, calories, and folic acid. Most nutritionists reportedly agree that the diets of pregnant women should be supplemented with iron and folic acid, but adolescents often fail to take supplements as directed(26). Nurses may improve the pregnant adolescent's compliance by spending time in providing an adequate explanation of the medication's purpose.

Many pregnant adolescents are simply not aware of the constituents of a good diet and can also profit from individual or group discussion of foods which supply essential nutrients, especially those they are likely to ingest in less than adequate quantity. Finally, the weight-conscious pregnant young girl needs to be made aware that a weight gain is vital to her own health and that of her child and will not impair her future figure.

The adolescent who takes precautions to prevent pregnancy may develop deficiencies in certain nutrients just as the pregnant young girl may. Both pregnancy and oral contraceptives alter tryptophan metabolism and increase the need for pyridoxine (vitamin B_6). Dosages of up to fifteen times the recommended level of 2 mg have been suggested as necessary to provide optimum pyridoxine under these circumstances (27).

Other nutrients probably needed at higher levels by women on "the pill" are vitamin C and folic acid, but the exact dosages required by these women have not yet been specified(28).

Serum iron levels are actually increased by oral contraceptives because they both stimulate iron absorption and reduce blood lost during menses(29). Contrarily, use of the intrauterine device tends to deplete iron levels by increasing menstrual flow and may warrant iron supplementation. All these factors should be taken into careful consideration by nurses who provide birth control counseling to adolescents.

Another group of young people whose nutritional requirements are altered to some extent by self-imposed circumstances are those involved in athletic activities. Their diets, like those of their more sedentary peers, should contain water, fats, proteins, carbohydrates, minerals, and vitamins in proportions appropriate for their ages. Some modifications in the quantity of nutrients are necessary, however, because of the demands produced by exercise.

For example, adolescent athletes require increased calories due to greater energy expenditures. Williams writes that 2300 calories per day should be regarded as a minimum level for individuals actively participating in sports and adds that a caloric intake of up to 5000 calories may be necessary for those involved in especially strenuous exercise(30).

An athlete's appetite will heighten with increased exercise and is probably the best gauge for determining how much he should eat. Excessive calories leading to significant weight gain are obviously not recommended since fat not only reduces one's capacity for exercise but also places added strain on the heart.

The optimum diet for athletes is probably attained when calories are derived in a proportion of 25% to 35% from fat, 10% to 15% from protein, and the remainder from carbohydrates (31). Contrary to popular opinion, a high-protein diet is not physiologically necessary for the athlete since even heavy exercise is not accompanied by significant protein catabolism. In fact, protein is an expensive and rather inefficient source of energy. On the other hand, high carbohydrate diets (70% of total calories) are reported to increase work capacity, particularly during strenuous exercise by (1) providing greater energy per liter of oxygen consumed than either fat or protein and (2) by contributing to glycogen reserves (32).

It has been suggested that athletes require increased levels of vitamins C and B complex (30). Whether or not this need can be met without supplementation is a debatable issue; certainly those involved in sports can be encouraged to eat foods high in these nutrients.

Another requirement increased by such activity is for salt. Quantities of up to 2 gms of salt per liter of water lost in sweat per day are warranted. This need can be met adequately by salting foods at meals. Water lost in perspiration also needs to be replaced daily. Small frequent sips of water during performance are preferable to larger, occasional drinks of water. There is no proof that commercial electrolyte solutions such as Gatorade® and Spartade® are superior to plain water, saline, or glucose solutions as fluid sources during strenuous activity(32).

Athletes are encouraged to eat at least three meals a day, delaying participation in strenuous games for 3 to 4 hours after a given meal. Liquid foods are preferred before games because they seem to be easier to digest than solid food and apparently relieve some of the common symptoms of nervous tension suffered by athletes such as nausea, vomiting, and abdominal cramps(32).

School nurses in particular have expressed concern about the drastic weight loss regimens frequently undertaken by wrestlers prior to a match in order to qualify for the lowest possible weight class. These regimens often include starvation and extreme water deprivation. Starvation depletes protein, glycogen, vitamin, mineral, and enzyme stores which are essential to optimum athletic performance and the adolescent's growth(32). Dehydration involving a loss of 5% of total body water decreases oxygen intake by cells and significantly reduces muscle capacity for sustained work(33).

Adolescents should be helped to recognize that their weight loss efforts may jeopardize their chances of performing well. A reasonable weight loss for wrestlers, according to Cooper, involves no more than 2 to 5 pounds per week (33).

COPING WITH ADOLESCENT NUTRITION PROBLEMS

Aside from the special nutritional considerations which accompany pregnancy, family planning, and athletic activity during adolescence, the nurse is likely to encounter problems which have arisen from young people's improper eating habits. Three of the most frequently mentioned problems are iron deficiency anemia, dental caries, and obesity.

Iron deficiency anemia

This problem has been found in 5% of low-income and affluent male adolescents, in 20% of low-income female adolescents, and in 12% of affluent adolescent girls(36). That adolescent girls are affected more often than boys is related primarily to their poorer iron nutriture but also to their lack of testosterone to stimulate erythropoiesis and to their blood loss during the normal process of menstruation.

Symptoms of the disease may include fatigue, irritability, inability to concentrate, headache, and, paradoxically, increased menstrual flow in females. Although the long-range effects are unknown, the disease can certainly impair an adolescent's school performance and limit his physical activity level.

Iron deficiency anemia may be suspected in an adolescent because of a dietary history reflecting inadequate iron intake; the presence of symptoms suggestive of the disorder; or a low hemoglobin or hematocrit level. In females, a hemoglobin under 11.5 and hematocrit under 35 are low. In males, values vary with age and changes in testosterone secretion. Cutoff values for males are as follows: 10 to 12 years old, same as for females; 13 to 16, hemoglobin below 13, hematocrit below 39; and 17 and older, hemoglobin 14 and hematocrit 42(37). These values may change according to the population group.

Serum iron levels, red blood cell indices, and iron binding capacity should be checked to confirm the suspicion. When the condition is present, red cell indices indicate hypochromia and microcytosis (MCH [mean corpuscular hemoglobin] $< 26.5 \mu\mu g$ and MCV [mean corpuscular volume] $< 79c\mu$), iron binding capacity is increased ($> 350 \mu g\%$), and fasting serum iron is reduced ($< 65 \mu g\%$)(37).

Because iron deficiency anemia is rather easily corrected using ferrous sulfate, efforts to change dietary habits through counseling, a time-consuming process, may be neglected, in which case the problem is likely to recur at a later date. Younger adolescents particularly are influenced by their mothers' attitudes toward nutrition, and efforts should be directed toward supporting mothers' attempts to purchase and serve foods that are high in iron(36). The successful prevention of the disease in adolescents may ultimately require iron supplementation of foods they commonly eat such as bread and milk(21).

Dental caries

An increase in incidence of tooth decay among adolescents in the past decade has directly paralleled the rising consumption of baked goods and sugary confections between meals(34). Foods that remain for longer periods in the mouth—hard candies, carmels, and pastry—are more cariogenic than those which have a low sugar content, are less sticky, or are quickly swallowed such as soda and peanuts. Adolescents who snack frequently on small amounts of cariogenic foods are at a greater dental risk than those who eat large quantities of such food once during the day(35).

While snacks can contribute substantially to the nutrient quality of adolescent diets and should not be eliminated, snack foods should be carefully selected. If a young person eats a sugary snack, it might contribute less to the formation of caries if immediately afterward he at least rinsed his mouth with water.

Adolescents may also need to be reminded about the importance of brushing their teeth after meals and especially before bedtime, and flossing should be introduced as a valuable adjunct to brushing. Disclosing tablets may stimulate an adolescent to improve dental hygiene practices. Similarly, body-conscious adolescents may be motivated to improve their dental health practices if they are fully informed about the effects of poor dental hygiene on their appearance(35).

Obesity

The prevalence of obesity in adolescence is estimated to be fairly high. It varies inversely with economic status. Adolescents whose parents are obese are at considerably greater risk for developing obesity themselves. Most obesity does not first occur during adolescence; rather, it is a condition which typically originates in infancy and childhood. Often, however, it is recognized as a problem only when the individual's body becomes sufficiently unattractive and unwieldy to impose social restrictions on him.

During adolescence a normal acceleration in the deposition of body fat may be misinterpreted by youth and health care provider alike as the onset of obesity. Normal fat deposition usually occurs in girls between 11 and 13 years and in boys between 12½ and 14½(38). By late adolescence the combined effects of differences in hormonal secretion and physical activity result in males being composed of 7.9% fat and females 22.8%(39).

The current cultural emphasis on being slim leads many young girls to attempt weight loss in the face of difficult natural odds; the result is often impaired nutritional status. *Anorexia nervosa,* an extreme form of obsession with weight loss, is presently on the increase in the United States. Although many physiological and psychological factors have been implicated in its development, there is no doubt that anorexics have a distorted impression of what constitutes normal body weight(40). Both parents and children should receive anticipatory guidance in preparation for the onset of puberty so that when body fat begins to increase, the process is expected and recognized as normal.

An adolescent may be classified as overweight if his weight falls farther than two stan-

Obesity standards for adolescents*

| Ages | Minimum triceps skin-fold thickness† indicating obesity (millimeters) | |
	Males	Females
10	16	20
11	17	21
12	18	22
13	18	23
14	17	23
15	16	24
16	15	25
17	14	26
18	15	27
19	15	27
20	16	28
21	17	28
22	18	28

*Reprinted from "A Simple Criterion of Obesity," by C. Seltzer and J. Mayer, *Postgraduate Medicine,* Vol. 38, August, 1965, p. A-105 with the permission of Harry L. Brown, publisher. The standards presented were developed for caucasian American adolescents.
†Thickness of the pinched skin at a point midway between the olecranon process of the ulna and the acromion process of the scapula.

dard deviations from the mean on available growth charts. Whether or not the adolescent is actually obese depends on what proportion of his excess weight is fat. This is an important distinction to make since weight due to muscle mass and skeletal size is not reduceable in the same sense as that due to fat.

An accurate method of indirectly assessing obesity which will probably be used with increasing frequency by nurses in the future is measuring the thickness of the triceps skin fold using a skin-fold caliper and the obesity standards developed by Seltzer and Mayer. (See Obesity Standards for Adolescents.) Directions for use of the skin-fold caliper are well described in the literature(39).

While obesity in childhood is undoubtedly the result of increases in both the number of fat cells and their size due to overeating, in adolescence it is probably maintained and exaggerated because energy expenditure is insufficient to use all the calories consumed. A study in California found that obese adolescents ate less total food and fewer meals daily, missing breakfast and lunch more often, and had more nutritionally inadequate diets than others. But obese adolescents exercised markedly less than those young people who were nonobese(41).

Guide to nutritional assessment of adolescents

History
Family
- Obesity, diabetes mellitus, or heart disease in close family members? Preventive diet may be indicated.

Dietary
- Appetite, total daily food intake, special diet, frequency of meals, snacking habits, food preferences and allergies, vitamin supplements.

Medications
- On oral contraceptive? May need increase vitamin C, pyridoxine, and folic acid.

Exercise
- Daily exercise pattern, if any.
- Participation in sports. Which sports? How often? May need increased calories, vitamins C and B complex, water and salt.

Past health problems
- History of significant weight gain or loss? History of obesity, anemia, thyroid imbalance, or diabetes?

Special considerations
- Pregnant? Consider needs for increased calories, protein, calcium, iron, B vitamins, and vitamins C and A.
- Intrauterine device in place? May need increased iron to replace losses during menstrual flow.

Review of systems
If the following symptoms are present, consider corresponding mineral and vitamin deficiencies.
- Dryness and cracking of skin or lips, itching of genital area—Riboflavin
- Nervousness, irritability, insomnia, muscle cramps—calcium
- Indigestion, constipation, nervousness, irritability, fatigue, mental depression—thiamine
- Night blindness, roughness of skin, dryness of hair—vitamin A
- Bleeding of gums, slow wound healing, easy bruising—vitamin C
- Fatigue, irritability, anorexia, headache, increased menstrual flow—iron

Physical assessment
Height and weight
- Far below mean on growth chart for age? Consider protein and calorie deprivation.
- Far above mean? Consider obesity, overweight.

Clinical signs
- Lethargy; general depression; dry skin or hair; lesions on lips, skin, or genitalia; dental caries; swollen or bleeding gums; tachycardia; and enlarged thyroid may indicate nutritional inadequacies.

Laboratory data
- Consider iron deficiency anemia if hemoglobin and hematocrit levels are low.

The physiological mechanisms underlying the preference of overweight subjects for inactivity are not clearly understood. It has been speculated that a higher rate of iron deficiency anemia among the obese may contribute to this preference or that they may simply give up physical activity since they must work harder to exercise their heavier bodies(39). Heald also reported that glucose is transferred less efficiently into muscle tissue as the size of the fat pad increases. It therefore seems logical to conclude, although he does not do so, that obese adolescents consequently have less energy available to perform physically(42). All of this evidence indicates that obese adolescents are caught in a frustrating cycle: the heavier they become, the less they exercise, and the less they exercise, the heavier they become.

Such adolescents may suffer both future physical ill effects in the form of increased rates of atherosclerosis, diabetes mellitus, and renal disease as well as immediate psychological disadvantages such as defective body image, low self-esteem, depression, and social isolation. The presently available evidence strongly suggests that obesity in adolescence is extremely difficult to reverse(43).

Experts agree that preventive efforts are essential and that they must begin in infancy when the problem begins. Accordingly, parents should be encouraged to breast-feed infants, to delay introduction of solid foods, and to avoid using food to reinforce good behavior(43).

The paramount goal in working with obese adolescents is to help these individuals to like and accept themselves. Significant weight loss may not be a realistic objective. In fact, the degree of caloric restriction necessary to achieve such a loss is best avoided since growing adolescents may respond by going into negative nitrogen balance(39). Further weight *gain*, however, can be prevented by eliminating high carbohydrate foods from the adolescent's diet.

To improve the quality of their diets, obese adolescents can also be encouraged to eat small portions of nutritious and personally acceptable food frequently (more than three times a day) and to eat high-protein breakfasts. Such breakfasts not only improve performance but are also associated with a lowered carbohydrate intake throughout the rest of the day(44).

Exercise is an integral part of any obesity treatment plan and should be modified to suit each individual's needs. Studies indicate that while obese adolescents are generally well informed about the elements of a nutritious diet and are motivated to and have attempted to lose weight, they are surprisingly ignorant about the value of exercise in achieving weight loss(45). Because obesity tends to be a family pattern, dietary counseling may be a wasted effort unless the entire family, particularly his mother, is willing to cooperate in reducing the carbohydrate content of the family diet.

The old axiom, "You are what you eat," is no less true for adolescents than for those of other ages. Overall attempts to promote adolescent health through improved nutritional habits should be based on the following considerations:

- Helping adolescents change their dietary habits requires a thorough evaluation of their present nutritional status. (See Guide to Nutritional Assessment of Adolescents.) Evidence of poor nutrition or potential nutritional imbalance is far more likely to be determined from the history than from the physical assessment process. Dietary counseling must be tailored to meet the individual needs and circumstances of the young person involved.
- To improve their nutritional intakes, adolescents themselves and not solely the nurses working with them must be motivated to change. Authoritarian approaches and judgmental attitudes by parents and nurses alike may serve only to turn adolescents off or to encourage them to assert their independence by pursuing extreme diets more actively.

Establishing sound nutritional habits begins long before adolescence. Information about nutritious foods and their effects on health need to be provided to expectant parents so that a proper eating pattern can be started from the baby's birth. Once a child reaches adolescence it may be possible to influence his dietary intake in a healthy direction by consistently reinforcing his attempts at selecting nutritious food and ignoring his "mistakes." Perhaps the most nurses can hope for is that given ample, accurate nutrition information, adolescents will voluntarily make the appropriate, sound choices in their daily diets.

REFERENCES

1. Caghan, S. B. The adolescent process and the problem of nutrition. *Am. J. Nurs.* 75:1728-1730, Oct. 1975.
2. Young, C. Adolescents and their nutrition. In *Medical Care of the Adolescent.* 3d edition, edited by J. Gallagher and others. New York, Appleton-Century-Crofts, 1976, pp. 15-24.
3. U. S. Center for Disease Control. *Ten State Nutrition Survey 1968-1970.* (DHEW Publication No. (HSM) 72-8134;72-8133) Washington, D. C., U. S. Government Printing Office, 1972. Vol. 1, pp. 1-12; Vol. 5, pp. v81-v85.
4. Heald, F. P. Adolescent nutrition. *Med. Clin. North Am.* 59:1329-1336, Nov. 1975.
5. PHS publications. *Am. J. Clin. Nutr.* 26:1031-1033, Sept. 1973.
6. Tanner, J. M. *Growth at Adolescence.* Philadelphia, J. B. Lippincott Co., 1962, pp. 37-38.
7. Marshall, W. A., and Tanner, J. M. Variations in the pattern of pubertal changes in boys. *Arch. Dis. Child.* 45:13-23, Feb. 1970.
8. National Academy of Sciences, National Research Council, Food and Nutrition Board. *Recommended Dietary Allowances.* rev. ed. Washington, D. C., The Academy, 1974.
9. Mueller, J. Current recommended dietary allowances in adolescents. In *Nutrient Requirements in Adolescence.* ed. by J. I. McKigney and H. N. Munro. Cambridge, Mass., M.I.T. Press, 1975, p. 137, 138-144.
10. Jaworski, A. A., and Jaworski, R. A. New teen-age boy and girl growth charts for pediatric office use. *Clin. Pediatr.* 10:410-413, July 1971.
11. Parrish, J. Implications of changing food habits for nutrition educators. *J. Nutr. Educ.* 2:140-146, Spring 1971.
12. Hampton, M., and others. Caloric and nutrient intakes of teenagers. *J. Am. Diet. Assoc.* 50:385-395, May 1967.
13. Wharton, M. A. Nutritive intake of adolescents. *J. Am. Diet. Assoc.* 42:306-310, Apr. 1963.
14. Hodges, R. E., and Krehl, W. A. Nutritional status of teenagers in Iowa. *Am. J. Clin. Nutr.* 17:200-210, Oct. 1965.
15. Schoor, B. C., and others. Teenage food habits: a multidimensional analysis. *J. Am. Diet. Assoc.* 61:415-420, Oct. 1972.
16. U. S. Public Health Service. *First Health and Nutrition Examination Survey, U. S. 1971-72.* (DHEW Publication No. (HRA) 74-1219-1) Rockville, Md., The Service, 1974.
17. Steele, B., and others. Role of breakfast and between-meal foods. *J. Am. Diet. Assoc.* 28:1054-1057, Nov. 1952.
18. Finberg, Laurence. Fast foods for adolescents. *Am. J. Dis. Child.* (Marginal comments department) 130:362-363, Apr. 1976.
19. Williams, E. R. Making vegetarian diets nutritious. *Am. J. Nurs.* 75:2168-2173, Dec. 1975.
20. Erhard, D. Nutrition education for the new generation. *J. Nutr. Educ.* 2:135-139, Spring 1971.
21. Thomas, J., and Call, D. Eating between meals—a nutrition problem among teenagers? *Nutr. Rev.* 31:137-139, May 1973.
22. Brewer, T. *Nutrition in Pregnancy.* Paper presented at a meeting of the New Jersey State Nurses Association, Division of Maternal Child Health, held June 2, 1975.
23. Thomson, A. Pregnancy in adolescence. In *Nutrient Requirements in Adolescence,* ed. by J. I. McKigney and H. N. Munro. Cambridge, Mass., M.I.T. Press, 1976, p. 250.
24. Grant, J. A., and Heald, F. P. Complications of adolescent pregnancy. *Clin. Pediatr.* 11:569, Oct. 1972.
25. Birch, H. Functional effects of fetal malnutrition. *Hosp. Pract.* 6:134-148, Mar. 1971.
26. Weigley, E. S. The pregnant adolescent. *J. Am. Diet. Assoc.* 66:588-592, June 1975.
27. György, P. Developments leading to the metabolic role

of B$_6$, *Am. J. Clin. Nutr.* 24:1250-1256, Oct. 1971.

28. Hodges, R. E. Vitamin and nutrient requirements in adolescence. In *Nutrient Requirements in Adolescence,* ed. by J. I. McKigney and H. N. Munro. Cambridge, Mass. M.I.T. Press. 1973, pp. 127-133.

29. Nutrition and the pill. *J. Am. Diet. Assoc.* 59:212-217, Sept. 1971.

30. Williams, J. Nutrition and sport. *Practitioner* 201:324-329, Aug. 1968.

31. De Wijn, J. Nutritional health in the adolescent period. *Nutritio et Dieta* 9:1-20, Jan. 1967.

32. Nutrition and athletic performance. *Dairy Council Digest* 46:7-10, Mar.-Apr. 1975.

33. Cooper, D. L. Wrestling and weight fluctuations. *J. Am. Coll. Health Assoc.* 21:451-454, June 1973.

34. Bibby, B. G. The carogenicity of snack foods and confections. *J. Am. Diet. Assoc.* 90:121-132, Jan. 1975.

35. Slattery, Jill. Dental health in children. *Am. J. Nurs.* 76:1159-1161, July 1976.

36. Faigel, H. C. Hematocrits in suburban adolescents: a search for anemia. *Clin. Pediatr.* 12:494-496, Aug. 1973.

37. Gilman, P. The reticuloendothelial system. In *Medical Care of the Adolescent.* 3rd edition, edited by J. Gallagher and others. New York, Appleton-Century-Crofts, 1975, pp. 645-650.

38. Faigel, H. C. A developmental approach to adolescence. *Pediatr. Clin. North Am.* 21:353-359, May 1974.

39. Heald, F., and Khan, M. Disorders of adipose tissue. In *Medical Care of the Adolescent.* 3d edition, edited by J. Gallagher and others. New York, Appleton-Century-Crofts, 1976, pp. 125-138.

40. Bruch, H. Management of anorexia nervosa. *Resident and Staff Physician* 22:61-67, Aug. 1976.

41. Huenemann, R. L. Food habits of obese and nonobese adolescents. *Postgrad. Med.* 51:99-105, May 1972.

42. Heald, F. P. ed. *Adolescent Nutrition and Growth.* New York, Appleton-Century-Crofts, 1969, pp. 37-41.

43. Hammar, S. L., and others. An interdisciplinary study of adolescent obesity. *J. Pediatr.* 80:373-383, Mar. 1972.

44. National Dairy Council. *A Source Book of Food Practices with an Emphasis on Children and Adolescents.* Chicago, The Council, 1975, pp. 1-19.

45. Kaufmann, N. A., and others. Eating habits and opinions of teenagers on nutrition and obesity. *J. Am. Diet. Assoc.* 66:264-268, Mar. 1975.

The special needs of the adolescent with chronic illness*

LOIS J. JELNECK

Teenagers who are chronically ill are often torn in two directions. They know they must adhere to restrictions on their activities imposed by their conditions. But society's expectation that they grow and develop into adults urges them to strike out on their own.

One of the long overlooked aspects of adolescent care has been that of chronic illness. Many times the psychosocial problems of teens with such illnesses can lead to social disability which is far more serious than the direct effects of their physical ailments. To prevent such disability, a concentrated, conscientious effort must be made by all those who provide care to the adolescent and her family.

In order fully to understand the complexity of the effects of chronic illness on the adolescent, one must also keep in mind the problems of the healthy adolescent. These alone can be overwhelming for both teen and parents. Add chronic illness to the picture and the challenge becomes significantly greater.

Behavioral scientists are far from unanimous regarding the principal sources of difficulties for adolescents. The biologically-oriented view these problems as primarily a reflection of the process of maturation. They attribute adolescent behavior either directly to the physiological changes of puberty such as increases in sex hormones and changes in body structure and function or to the psychological adjustments these changes require.

Others view adolescent adjustment problems as principally cultural in origin. They emphasize the many highly concentrated demands made upon teens by our society. In cultures in which these demands are neither as complex nor as restricted to one age group, they assert, adolescence is not viewed as a particularly difficult period. Among the tasks that face adolescents in our culture are achieving independence, making peer and heterosexual adjustments, choosing a course of education and vocation, and developing a workable set of personal and social values.

Aside from achieving these cultural goals, every adolescent must attain developmental goals for this phase of life. The first of these objectives, accepting the physical self, is hard to reach, for the adolescent's body is changing very rapidly. As a result, she sometimes has difficulty adjusting to these alterations. She may take moderately good care of the physical body by maintaining a proper diet, exercising, and practicing good hygiene. On the other hand, she may try to destroy her new self-image as well as her physical self by abuse, disuse, and neglect. If the teen truly accepts her physical self, she makes the most of her good points without dwelling on her imperfections. She also learns to accept the physical changes of growing up.

To achieve emotional control, the second goal, the teenager must strike a balance between childish expression of emotions without inhibition and complete suppression of all feelings. In addition, each adolescent faces the task of learning to expect and accept the inevitable frustration of failure without degrading herself

*Copyright © 1977, The American Journal of Nursing Company. Reproduced, with permission, from MCN, The American Journal of Maternal Child Nursing, January/February, vol. 2, no. 1.
□**Ms. Jelneck, R.N.,** is currently working as a private pediatric nurse practitioner in association with a physician in Ann Arbor, Mich. She has extensive experience in caring for adolescents.

or disintegrating into uncontrolled rage or immobilizing fear of future failures.

Aside from these two deeply internal goals, the teen must develop social maturity, which centers around the ability to establish good interpersonal relationships. Without friends and family to reflect one's wishes, attitudes, and feelings, a teen will remain a stranger to herself. The individual who is completely self-centered, striving only for her own welfare, is eventually cast out of society. But the person who places "belonging" above all else, sacrificing her individuality and thereby losing her identity, is no better accepted. The adolescent's task is to master the conflict by acquiring a unique identity and still functioning within the limits set by society. She must also learn to function independently of the family.

The final goal of adolescence is to develop intellectual sophistication and sensitivity. Intellectual sophistication demands that the teen attain a balance between gullibility at one extreme and a complete skepticism at the other. Neither position alone can ensure effective intellectual functioning. Sensitivity of intellect involves acquiring the ability to face reality. A major demonstration of such sensitivity is being able to come to grips with failure by gaining knowledge from an unsuccessful experience and going on from there.

ADDITIONAL PROBLEMS OF CHRONIC ILLNESS

The added difficulties that the teenager with chronic illness may face in achieving these four goals are apparent in many cases. The physical imperfection involved in such illness often dominates the teenager's life. Her special needs may inhibit her moving toward independence, and facing the reality of her condition may be extremely difficult because of the limitations and dangers of the disease. Furthermore, the chronically ill teen may employ a variety of involuntary defense maneuvers which are contrary to these developmental goals in an attempt to handle the anxiety, the threat to bodily integrity, and the changes in life-style that the illness may pose.

The defense mechanisms the teen uses are important not only for their effect on the teen herself but also because they compound the difficulties the rest of the family has to face. Parents are also struggling to cope. Understandably, the discovery of chronic disease in their child provokes a storm of emotions in them.

They are overwhelmed by feelings of helplessness, disappointment, disbelief, anger, confusion, and guilt. In short, right from its diagnosis, chronic illness produces family crisis, and how the family resolves this crisis will greatly determine how it will later function (1-8).

Among the defense mechanisms the teen uses that affect the way the family functions are the following:

In *regression* the adolescent reacts to the threat of illness by adopting earlier modes of behavior which she found comforting and useful. For instance, she may resort to whining and baby talk or seek assistance with tasks which she is perfectly capable of performing.

Denial protects the patient from conflict by preventing her emotional and intellectual recognition of the fact that the disease exists. This can be helpful in minimizing anxiety but can become destructive if as a result the patient does not seek medical care when she needs it or does not follow a treatment regimen.

Intellectualization for the adult patient consists of a feeling that the more she knows about the disease, the less likely it is to exist. When the adolescent is involved, however, more often the reverse is true. She may pretend to know all there is to know about her disease and will not ask questions. The teen, in her immature way of thinking, assumes that somehow the less she knows about the disease, the less likely it is to exist. As a result classes to acquaint patients with what to expect after corrective surgery for scoliosis are often not attended by those who need them most.

In *projection* the patient blames others, usually her parents or ancestors, or her environment for her illness. Consequently she accepts none of the responsibility for her own care. This mechanism is especially prominent in the case of hereditary diseases such as diabetes or hemophilia.

Displacement refers to the patient's expressing her anxiety over her illness by centering it upon a less threatening symptom than that which actually and severely afflicts her. For instance, the patient with congenital heart disease may become excessively concerned with her bowels and constipation rather than the shortness of breath and fatigue that characterize the problem.

Through *introjection* the patient turns all her feelings onto herself, blames herself for her illness, and feels strongly that she should be punished for what has happened to her. This occurs especially when the causes and the nature of the disease have not been adequately explained to the patient.

In addition to these defense mechanisms, there are three common psychological responses the adolescent may manifest. These are depression, overdependency, and nonadherence to the treatment regimen. The depressed individual feels hopeless and sad and has a bleak outlook on life as a reaction to her loss of bodily function, freedom, and independence. These deprivations are especially difficult for the adolescent, who is at a stage in life when she is trying to assert herself.

On the other hand, the adolescent may become too comfortable with the added attention that she receives as a result of her disease and may lapse into overdependence. In such a case the teen uses her illness as an excuse for not maturing and thus fails to accept the responsibility that goes with adulthood.

Finally, nonadherence to the prescribed course of treatment can take various forms— from the diabetic who refuses to take insulin to the patient on dialysis who rejects the treatment. For some people this response is a manifestation of denial. For other individuals it is an expression of independence. In either case the effects of nonadherence can be ravaging.

SPECIFIC CONDITIONS AND RELATED STRESSES

All of the above stresses and responses are common to all teenagers who are chronically ill. But each disease process poses problems which are specific to it alone and are just as important to consider. Thus, I have tried to explore the special needs of adolescent patients with some of the most common chronic conditions.

Diabetes mellitus

Eating well-balanced meals at regular times does not fit in with a teenager's way of life, and testing urine is embarrassing, especially when it must be done at school. Thus, as might be expected, fluctuations in the control of juvenile diabetes frequently seem related to emotional factors.

Often the discomfort of insulin injections does not bother the teen as much as having to get up each morning by a certain hour to administer it to herself. If she denies the disease altogether, ketoacidosis will result and the patient may have to be hospitalized, eliciting further antagonism toward the disease.

Both sexes worry about the effect their disease will have on their social and sexual acceptability(1,4,9). The effects of diabetes on pregnancy are important to include in any sex education for the teenage girl.

Fibrocystic disease

While the child with this disease can now expect to live through adolescence into adulthood, she is faced with constant medication, diet regulations, postural drainage, and perhaps even the cumbersome environment of pumps and steam tents. She suffers from poor exercise tolerance, frequent and sometimes prolonged periods of illness, and a troublesome cough.

The male teenager needs to be aware that he will probably be sterile due to hypospermia but that his sexual adequacy will not be affected. The possibilities of adopting children and artificial insemination are important to discuss at this time(1,4,10,11).

Asthma

Respiratory disease, including asthma, is responsible for 45% of chronic illness in children. The asthmatic teenager is constantly faced with the frightening prospect of an attack. These attacks frequently require medical intervention with injections of adrenalin and sometimes hospitalization(1,4,12). Since they can be brought on by exertion, infections, temperature changes, stress, or environmental factors such as smoke and dust, the teen's anxiety level may be great and warrants close attention.

Cardiac problems

The adolescent with congenital heart disease may be severely incapacitated. Exercise tolerance may be limited. Cyanosis or clubbing of fingers and toes increases her anxiety over body image. Simple procedures such as dental work take on awesome proportions with the ever-present possibility of subacute bacterial endocarditis. The thought of possible cardiac surgery and of a limited life expectancy further aggravate the adolescent's anxieties.

Ulcerative colitis, regional ileitis

This is probably one of the most embarrassing and uncomfortable of all chronic illnesses for the adolescent. First of all, no teenager enjoys the restricted diet which is required. Secondly, cramps, tenesmus, abdominal pain, bowel bleeding, and cortisone enemas assault the teenager's sensitivities. It is especially difficult for adolescent boys to have nurses or their mothers giving them enemas. If at all possible a male should perform this procedure when it's necessary.

The adolescent's normal anxiety over body image is heightened by her undernutrition leading to thinness and a sickly pallor. Moreover, the possibility of major surgery and perhaps an enterostomy is extremely frightening and repulsive to her. Should this become a reality, her membership in an ostomy club would be invaluable in providing support and encouragement from those who have successfully managed the problems involved and live full lives(1,13,14).

Kidney disease

Teens with such conditions live with the realization that their lives depend on a machine and the eventual finding of a suitable donor for a kidney transplant. Dialysis interferes with school attendance, choice of life-style, extracurricular activities, and diet. Adolescents are often very shy and particularly protective of their privacy. The medical and surgical treatment of kidney disease—with the frequent exposure, constant inspection and palpation of the body surface, and regular exploration of various body orifices—contributes to destroying the individual's sense of privacy, even when an attempt is made to be as sensitive as possible in approaching the patient.

Furthermore, sexual development in affected teens often does not proceed normally. Menarche may not occur or may be delayed, and the initial high-dosage steroid therapy after transplantation may again interfere with the normal menstrual cycle. Also, the typical moon face and buffalo hump this treatment causes can be devastating to one's self-image(1,4,15).

Orthopedic problems

These include such conditions as *osteogenesis imperfecta,* dislocation of the hip, clubfoot, scoliosis, various forms of paralysis, and gait disturbances. Confinement to a wheelchair can be devastating to the teenager. Even splints and other orthopedic appliances do not foster a healthy self-image. Also, stature and body contours may be greatly deviated from normal, and the adolescent has a great adjustment to make in relating to her peers. Teenagers can be very cruel to anyone who looks even the slightest bit different(1,4).

Chronic bleeding disorders

Disorders such as hemophilia often cause the adolescent to be concerned with fatal bleeding, resulting from physical trauma and medical procedures such as venous puncture. Emotional distress may increase the likelihood of bleeding with minor physical trauma or may even lead to spontaneous bleeding episodes without apparent injury. Joint hemorrhages frequently occur with even the slightest trauma, resulting in severe disfigurement and loss of mobility. These episodes severely limit the teen's activity and give her more time to brood about her disability(1,4).

NURSING CARE FOR TEEN AND FAMILY

Healthy personality development of the chronically ill adolescent depends to a great extent upon the parents' acceptance of the child's disability and their understanding of its possible impact on other members of the family. The parents must therefore be educated concerning the disease and normal patient and family responses to it in order to reduce their anxiety level, overattention, and overprotection. They need to be assured that their feelings, negative as well as positive, are a normal reaction to their situation and encouraged to talk freely about them. They also need encouragement to develop in their child increasing responsibility for her own care.

Constant assurance that they are doing a good job in handling the situation, even if only a spark of improvement has appeared since the previous visit with the family, is essential. During each visit the family as well as the patient should be given at least one goal to concentrate on in the interval before the next visit.

Since healthy siblings can easily suffer from neglect in such families, the nurse's role is to make sure they are receiving adequate parental love and attention. As with parents, siblings' feelings of anxiety, resentment, and guilt regarding their handicapped brother or sister should be discussed and explained.

In managing the chronically ill adolescent

herself, improvement in medical condition, if possible, is of primary importance. The adolescent needs to be allowed to make some of the decisions regarding her care and to be made aware of the exact nature of her illness, the limitations of present knowledge, and recent advances that might affect her future.

It is important that she be consulted regarding appointments for health care visits to give her a sense that her time is important, too. The nurse can also ensure that at least part of the teen's visit to the doctor is conducted without the parents in the room. Also, encouraging the teenager's participation in the scheduling of her home care and treatments is an important intervention.

In short, adolescents should be treated as adults as much as possible and helped to increase their responsibility for their own care. In this way their dependency on family and others will automatically decrease.

LEADING A FULL LIFE

The chronically ill teenager's overall lifestyle also warrants close attention from the nurse. Total dependence on television as an escape should be avoided at all cost. Instead she might be encouraged or perhaps required to read on a wide range of topics, with special emphasis on her own favorite subject, as part of her daily schedule. Indeed, a reward system for reading may be a good idea, especially in getting the teen to begin this worthwhile habit.

When the adolescent does watch television, the nurse, parents, or other health care providers might provide valuable help for her in learning to choose substantive television programs such as documentaries. Family sharing of knowledge and interests is important to encourage in this regard. On the other hand, occasional flights from reality through lighter television shows can also be beneficial to the incapacitated adolescent.

Skills and interests to compensate for limitations in other activities are vital to encourage in both boys and girls. Hobbies such as stamp collecting, model building, celebrity card collecting, sewing, knitting, and painting can be substituted for athletic achievements and will help fill many otherwise empty hours and lead to a much fuller life.

Like any other adolescent, the teen with a disability needs to be encouraged to join groups or clubs. Organizations which center on similar interests such as model trains, photography, chess, debating, and poetry reading rather than on similar disabilities are a better choice. It is important that at least some of the teen's experiences be with normal healthy adolescents rather than the handicapped and ill. However, sometimes membership in a club of people with similar problems can be beneficial. An ostomy club, for instance, offers information and skills in personal care and hygiene, which are so important to the teenager. If an adolescent belongs to such a group, she should also have other social outlets.

Most importantly, chronically ill teens must learn to live openly with their handicap and to answer graciously questions that their peers may have regarding their condition. This helps to allay fears that their friends may have regarding the relationship between them and so will encourage friendships.

Similarly, these youngsters are often better off in regular schools with modified activities suited to their specific needs. Their teachers, however, must also be dealt with honestly and forthrightly. Before the teen ever enters the classroom the teacher needs to be aware of the teen's special situation. Occasional contacts between parents and teacher may also be beneficial in clarifying the adolescent's particular educational and vocational needs and discovering any misunderstandings that may arise.

SPECIAL BUT CAPABLE

To develop their fullest potential and be equipped for adult life, teens with chronic illness must have their special educational and vocational needs met. One of these needs is for sex education geared to the limitations and lack of physical and emotional development which they may experience. Relationships with groups of boys and girls rather than one-to-one relationships with someone of the opposite sex are advisable. Such interaction allows them to make an easier transition to a more meaningful relationship with one person.

Opportunities for living away from home for short periods of time might also be encouraged in order to prepare these patients for possible admission to college. Many camps are set up to handle the handicapped and afford the adolescent a sense of independence.

Incidences of overindulgence, lack of discipline, or neglect which can endanger the teen's emotional growth must be tactfully called to the parents' attention. It may be necessary to suggest a psychiatric consultation in situations which seem stalemated both on the part of the parents and the child. This is especially true in instances of children showing defiant, risk-taking behavior; unduly fearful, passive dependence; or hostile, embittered attitudes toward their environment and life situation(1,4).

Finally, we must recognize our own feelings of frustration and helplessness in the dealing with children who never truly get well. Unrealistic optimism can be devastating not only to ourselves but to the patient, her parents, and her family. With knowledge, warmth, humanity, common sense, and realism, however, we can find the right approach to each adolescent's care.

REFERENCES

1. Mattsson, Ake. Long-term physical illness in childhood: a challenge to psychosocial adaption. *Pediatrics* 50:801-811, Nov. 1972.
2. Abram, H. S. Psychology of chronic illness. *J. Chronic Dis.* 25:659-664, Dec. 1972.
3. Poznanski, E. O. Emotional issues in raising handicapped children. *Rehabil. Lit.* 34:322-326, Nov. 1973.
4. Wolfish, M. G., and McLean, J. A. Chronic illness in adolescents. *Pediatr. Clin. North Am.* 21:1043-1049, Nov. 1974.
5. Steinhauer, P. D., and others. Psychological aspects of chronic illness. *Pediatr. Clin. North Am.* 21:825-839, Nov. 1974.
6. Pless, I. B. The challenge of chronic illness. *Am. J. Dis. Child.* 126:741-742, Dec. 1973.
7. Reif, Laura. Managing a life with chronic disease. *Am. J. Nurs.* 73:261-264, Feb. 1973.
8. Holaday, B. J. Achievement behavior in chronically ill children. *Nurs. Res.* 23:25-30, Jan.-Feb. 1974.
9. Guthrie, D. W., and Guthrie, R. A. Juvenile diabetes mellitus. *Nurs. Clin. North Am.* 8:587-603, Dec. 1973.
10. Crozier, D. N. Cystic fibrosis: a not-so-fatal disease. *Pediatr. Clin. North Am.* 21:935-950, Nov. 1974.
11. Gayton, W. F., and Friedman, S. B. Psychosocial aspects of cystic fibrosis. *Am. J. Dis. Child.* 126:856-859, Dec. 1975.
12. Greer, T. L., and Yoches, Carol. Modification of an inappropriate behavioral pattern in asthmatic children. *J. Chron. Dis.* 24:507-513, Sept. 1971.
13. Jackson, Betti. Ulcerative colitis from an etiological perspective. *Am. J. Nurs.* 73:258-261, Feb. 1973.
14. Krizinofski, M. T. Human sexuality and nursing practice. *Nurs. Clin. North Am.* 8:673-681, Dec. 1973.
15. Grushkin, C. M., and others. The outlook for adolescents with chronic renal failure. *Pediatr. Clin. North Am.* 20:953-963, Nov. 1973.

The neglect and abuse of children and youth: the scope of the problem and the school's role*

ROBERT W. ten BENSEL, M.D., M.P.H.,
JANE BERDIE, M.S.W.

INTRODUCTION

Although abuse and neglect of children and youth are not new phenomena, they have only recently received national attention. Professionals and the general public are becoming increasingly aware of the incidence, forms and ramifications of the physical and emotional maltreatment in childhood and adolescence. Just as abuse and neglect reach into all sectors of society, solutions require the concern and cooperation of communities and professions such as education, health, law and social work, all of which have the primary responsibility for reporting, assessing and making decisions in this complex area regarding children and their families.

This article will focus primarily on the school's role and responsibilities in this area and will cover the historical development of the phenomena, terminology of maltreatment, statistical data on the dimensions of the problem, characteristics of an abusive situation, physiological symptoms of abuse and neglect, and the relationship between past and current abuse and neglect and delinquency.

Suggested guidelines for schools will cover the need for comprehensive policy and training on a district-wide basis, ways to work with fam-

ilies and other agencies, and the special role of schools, i.e., (1) recognizing, identifying, and reporting abuse or neglect; and (2) providing a physically and emotionally secure environment for pupils. Since about half of all reported incidents of abuse involve school-age children,[1] the school plays an integral role in protection of its pupils.

HISTORICAL ASPECTS

In order to understand the neglect and abuse of children it is beneficial to have a historical perspective on the development of the issue. Violent abuse and physical neglect have been present in society and have been noted since early writings. Radbill suggests that children are exposed to less violence from their parents today than in the past and, in fact, many of the instances of maltreatment to children in the past would be defined as abuse and would be the object of intervention by social or legal authorities.[2]

Infanticide has been documented in almost every culture, both civilized and uncivilized, so much so that it can almost be considered a universal phenomenon.[3] Solomon states that infanticide has "been responsible for more child deaths than any other single cause in history, other than possibly bubonic plague."[4] Infanticide usually refers to the willful killing of a newborn with the consent of parents, family or community. It may also occur as part of the accepted life in a family. DeMause relates the story in sixteenth century France of a brother of King Henry IV who, while being tossed from one window to another, was dropped and killed. Tossing infants was a common form of amusement.[5]

*From ten Bensel, R. W., and Berdie, J.: 1976. J. School Health 46(8):453-461, Oct. Copyright © 1976, American School Health Association, Kent, Ohio 44240.

□**Robert W. ten Bensel, M.D., M.P.H.,** is Professor and Director, Maternal and Child Health, School of Public Health, Department of Pediatrics, University of Minnesota, Minneapolis, Minnesota. **Jane Berdie, M.S.W.,** is a doctoral student in Family Social Science and a Research Assistant for the Center for Youth Development and Research, Department of Home Economics, University of Minnesota, St. Paul, Minnesota.

Infanticide has been justified on several bases. Bakan[3] feels that infanticide has been practiced in many cultures both primitive and civilized for the purpose of controlling population or eliminating weak or deformed infants. Other rationales for this practice have been ascribed to religious appeasement or reactions to prophecies of doom. From a psychosociological point of view the individual responsibility for the killing of an infant under these guises is transferred to a higher authority, thus leaving the individual's psyche undamaged in the process.

Ritualistic killing, maiming and severe punishing of children in attempts to educate them, exploit them or to sometimes rid them of evil spirits have also been part of history since early biblical times. Forms of mutilation of children have been recorded over the centuries as part of religious and ethnic traditions.[6] This has been referred to as ritual surgery and has included castration to produce eunuchs or singers, footbinding of female children in China, wrapping the neck with wiring, splinting the lips and nose by certain cultures in Africa, tattooing and cranial binding as seen in North American Indians. In Roman times children were used as professional beggars after they were hamstrung, deformed, had eyes gouged, or been otherwise blinded.

With the advent of urbanization and the resulting technological changes, more economic value was placed upon the child by society; the phenomenon became defined as one of "maltreatment of children." Charles Dickens wrote about the problems of children growing up in an industrialized society.[4] Receiving "the Dickens" remains a euphemism for the beating of children.

Whipping children and youths has been the prerogative of teachers from the days of the early Greeks. Five thousand years ago there was a "man in charge of the whip" to punish boys upon the slightest pretext. In England and America teachers were pictured armed with the birch. The severity of punishment by schoolmasters led to Roger Ascham's writing of *The Schoolmaster* in the 16th century, in which he advocated love instead of fear in teaching children.[2] One nineteenth century schoolmaster who kept score of his disciplinary practices reported administering 911,527 strokes with a stick; 124,000 lashes with a whip; 136,715 slaps with his hand, and 1,115,800 boxes on the ear.[5]

Even today, most of the states have laws condoning the use of "reasonable" force against children, including pupils. "Reasonable" is limited, at least by law, only by the nature and extent of enforcement of state statutes regarding abuse and neglect of minors.

The first reported case of physical maltreatment of children in the United States was the Mary Ellen case in 1874.[7] Mary Ellen had been beaten by her foster parents and in an attempt to get help for the child, the social worker finally took Mary Ellen to the Society for the Prevention of Cruelty to Animals. It was out of this experience that the Society for the Prevention of Cruelty to Children was organized in New York in 1875.

In medical literature child maltreatment was not appreciated even in 1946 when Dr. Caffey[8] reported six infants having multiple fractures in the long bones and suffering from chronic subdural hematomas (bleeding between the brain and the skull). Dr. Caffey concluded that the "fractures appear to be of traumatic episodes and the causal mechanisms remain obscure."[8] Dr. Silverman in 1953[9] reached conclusions similar to those of Caffey and noted the "excellent prognosis of traumatic lesions compared with that of other diseases considered in the differential diagnosis." In 1955 Drs. Woolley and Evans[10] wrote an article suggesting the possibility that parents were indeed responsible for the fractures and subdural hematomas and concluded that "it is difficult to avoid the overall conclusion that skeletal lesions having the appearance of fractures, regardless of history or injury or the presence or absence of intracranial bleeding, are due to the undesirable vectors of force."

It was Dr. C. Henry Kempe's monumental work published in 1962[11] in the *Journal of the American Medical Association* which brought the full impact of physical maltreatment to the medical community and subsequently to the attention of the general public. His article was entitled "The Battered Child Syndrome." The introduction of this term was very helpful in attracting attention to this still neglected medical and social problem. However, it is important to realize that the "Battered Child Syndrome" is only one small but severe portion of the spectrum of physical maltreatment of children.[12] The impact of Dr. Kempe's publication led to the subsequent passage of laws (1963 to 1968) in all states mandating reporting of suspected abuse by health professionals to welfare departments and/or police departments. DeFrancis's summary of state laws in 1974[13] records thirty-two states as requiring reporting by school teachers and/or school personnel. This has been a legal impetus for the development of awareness, knowledge, policy, and procedures in school systems.

TERMINOLOGY OF MALTREATMENT

The terminology currently used to describe the spectrum of maltreatment includes both physical and emotional abuse and neglect (Table 1). *Physical neglect* refers to the failure by parents to provide the basic physiological needs for the child. This includes failure to provide for adequate nutrition and clothing for the child and also encompasses proper medical care (the child's right to medical diagnosis and treatment) and provision for a safe environment in which the child can live. Neglect is often manifested by poor skin hygiene, lack of adequate nutrition, and a poor physical environment. Moreover, there is a close correlation between children with "failure to thrive" (e.g., not gaining in weight or height), emotional neglect and concomitant physical retardation.[14]

Emotional neglect and abuse refer to the failure of the parents or other caretakers to provide an emotionally stable environment in which the child may "develop sound character." Emotional abuse is often expressed vituperously. Pemberton and Benady quote parents speaking of their rejected children: "She smells," "He's destructive," "A champion liar," "Not our child," "Not worth bothering about," "I don't care where he goes."[15] Emotional abuse and emotional neglect go hand-in-hand; the abuse is a way of rejecting the child and thus denies the child his right to an adequate and safe environment in which to live.

Emotional neglect and abuse can be as destructive to the healthy development of children as physical abuse. However, to define emotional abuse and neglect and, in juxtaposition, moral and emotional well-being, is difficult except in terms of behavioral or other observable manifestations.[16] Possible indicators include unusual or deviant behaviors such as excessive aggression, negative attitudes, stealing, lying, or inability to control bowel movements. Such behavior does not necessarily indicate mistreatment, but it serves as a signal that the child is experiencing difficulty and is in need of some form of help.

Because of the difficulty of identifying emotional neglect and abuse, it is important to confer with a psychologist, psychiatrist and/or social worker. Whatever the cause of the child's behavior, a multidisciplinary approach to assessing and treating the problem provides the most comprehensive and effective way of helping the child and his family.

Physical abuse is active abuse causing injury to the child by another person irrespective of age of the abuser. Physical abuse is often subdivided into mild, moderate or severe abuse, depending on the judgement of the physician, nurse, social worker or police. Physical abuse usually refers to either a single episode of abuse or repeated milder forms of abuse as seen in inappropriate disciplinary actions. Death can occur from a single episode of physical abuse in an infant or young child, but is extremely rare in school age children because they are physically stronger and have the capacity to run or fight back.

Most of the physical abuse to school age children results in soft tissue swelling, e.g., bruises, welts, abrasions, lacerations, and burns (cigarette or hot water). However, injuries sometimes are more severe. A recent article in the *Minneapolis Star* (March 1975) describes a 12-year-old boy who was severely and repeatedly beaten with a baseball bat by his father.

The Battered Child Syndrome applies to the infant or child who has had repetitive, severe injuries which usually involve the fractures of bones, internal injuries, severe repeated skin injuries (scarring and burning) with or without fractures, or central nervous system damage. As with physical abuse, the hallmark of this type of maltreatment is that the circumstances of the injuries as described by the parents or other caretakers often do not adequately explain the types of injuries sustained. The legal interpretation of abuse implies that the injuries were of a "nonaccidental" nature.

Table 1. Maltreatment of children

Neglect	Abuse
Emotional	Emotional
Physical	Physical
Medical	Mild
Nutritional —→ Death	Moderate
	Severe
	Battered child syndrome

Sexual abuse of children and adolescents runs a wide spectrum including incest, sodomy and rape. For instance, Minnesota law defines sexual abuse as "when a child's parents, guardian or person responsible for the child's care subjects a child under 16 years of age to the sex acts of rape, sodomy, intercourse, indecent liberties" and/or sexual contact or sexual penetration.[17]

The extent of sexual abuse is unknown. While there are data on reported cases,[18] they reflect only a fraction of the actual number. Sexual abuse against children often carries severe legal and social penalties. If the victim knows the offender, the victim is often afraid to report the incident. Symptoms are not usually as evident as with other physical abuse. Small children often do not know how to easily describe what has happened. A report of incest by an adolescent girl is sometimes interpreted by social workers, police, teacher, or counselors as "manipulation" or "revenge." Underlying all of this is general resistance to recognizing the existence of sexual abuse. As Sgori says, "It seems to be 'too dirty', 'too Freudian' or perhaps 'too close to home.' Recognition of sexual molestation in a child is entirely dependent on the individual's inherent willingness to entertain the possibility that the condition may exist."[19]

THE DIMENSIONS OF THE PROBLEM OF MALTREATMENT

Some hard statistics are available, but due to the lack of uniformity in definitions and hesitancy in reporting, there are inaccuracies in existing data. Reported statistics often include both cases of abuse (physical and sexual) and neglect. There appears to be an increasing rate of maltreatment of children.[11] This is due not only to better identification and reporting, but also to a probable absolute increase in the number of children who are maltreated, perhaps as a result of a combination of factors which Bronfenbrenner has identified as correlative with the increase of problems such as suicide and juvenile delinquency.[20] Bronfenbrenner compared families today with those of 25 years ago and found more mothers working full-time (and thus leaving the care of their children to others), a decrease of extended families living together or in close proximity, an increase in divorce, in desertion and an increase in unwed pregnancy (thus decreasing the emotional support and help in child-caring tasks of many parents) and a low median income level (creating more crises).

In New York City in 1968 there were 956 cases of abuse reported; in 1969, 1600; in 1970, 3000; and in 1972, 5200 cases. Data from California and Colorado when extrapolated yield a conservative estimate of 200,000 to 250,000 children in the United States who are maltreated annually.[4] The incidence (occurrence of new cases in a year) is given at approximately 350 per 100,000 preschool children and 40 to 120 per 100,000 school age children.[22] The Mershon Center Study estimates about 600,000 reports of child abuse and neglect are made each year.[23]

Some workers state that for every child reported a hundred children go unreported.[21] Abuse of adolescents is often not included in abuse data either because it is called or explained as something else (e.g., parent-adolescent conflict, discipline, adolescent-provocation, arrest, or training for sports) or the recording system (e.g., of a welfare department) may classify all adolescents in a separate category. Recent Congressional testimony stated that an estimated 6000 children die annually as the result of child abuse.[24] This represents about 10% of children who are reported as suffering from maltreatment.[24]

THE ABUSING PERSON(S)

It is now well known that not only parents but also other adults and even children may maltreat children. Dr. Adelson[25] has described the "battering child" where preschool children can experience homicidal rage and kill other children.

In order for abuse to take place, the potential for abuse needs to be present. As the type and degree of physical attack varies greatly, so does the psychology of the individuals involved. At the one extreme are those cases where only mild physical abuse may have occurred. In these latter cases (which represent the majority of abuse cases) the abusers may not differ greatly psychologically from a "normal" sample of people.

From the studies published there seem to be at least four categories relating to the parents' potential for physical abuse. These categories are taken from Dr. Helfer's article:[26]

1. *How the parents themselves were reared.* Thirty to sixty percent of abusing parents say they were abused as children themselves.[4] Some research-practitioners believe the problem of poor parent-

ing is "universal" for abusers.[26] This life style imprinting has an effect not only on the increased chance of abusive behavior when they become parents, but also is an etiological factor in juvenile delinquency and adult homicide.[28,29,30] Many individuals who were abused or neglected as children grow into an "isolated, trapped, hopeless pattern of living."[27]

2. *The inability of families and of the abusing parent in particular to use people to help them when they are "uptight" with their children.* Parents who abuse children have not developed sufficient skills or abilities to call upon other people to help them when they are in a crisis with their children. They are often isolated from their families, have low trust levels, and often have very low self-images.

3. *Unstable marital relationship.* There is a high proportion of premarital conception, youthful marriage, unwanted pregnancies, forced marriages, and emotional or financial difficulties in the lives of abusing individuals.

4. *How parents see the child.* The parents who have the potential for abuse often expect the child to do things for them at a very early period of life. They often have an inappropriate expectation of the child's level of functioning and the child's capacity to respond at any given developmental age.

Statistics from the 1960s indicated more mothers abusing and neglecting children because they were the principal caretakers. In 1974 in Hennepin County, Minnesota, there was an increase in males involved in physical abuse. Particularly striking is the rise in stepfathers (14%), mother's boyfriend and male babysitters (13%). Natural parents are involved in only 49% of the cases.[31] As suggested by Brofenbrenner and others, recent trends in divorce and remarriage patterns, change in adoption patterns, and change in sex work roles in part explain these shifts.

Reference has been made to the abusing parent or caretaker. However, abuse and neglect of children, particularly those of school age, occur in other environments and institutions. It is not only the individuals in the community such as police and teachers, who may perpetrate neglect and abuse, but also the very nature of the institutions, through their philosophy and organization, which creates an environment in which neglect and abuse may occur. Brenton quoting Kaplan's work (1959) on teacher maladjustment states that 25% of teachers "consider themselves unhappy, worried or dissatisfied." Seventeen percent were "unusually nervous" and 9% are "seriously maladjusted" by psychological testing.[32] This represents a consider-

able potential for abuse or neglect in the classroom. The potential for abuse and neglect may be heightened by the "alarming and dramatic trend" in violence and vandalism in the schools as reported by a recent congressional committee.[33]

It is, however, important to look for similar characteristics in whoever is abusing. It is equally important to look for abuse-provoking characteristics in the child and in the situation itself.

THE ABUSED AND/OR NEGLECTED CHILD

From national studies we see the typical abused child as an infant or young child under age 3,[4] more frequently a male than a female, and a child who is somewhat "different." Hyperactive children, mentally defective children or children with other physical handicaps have a higher frequency of being abused. The child who has had prolonged separation from the family, such as occurs in prematurity and neonatal diseases, has an increased risk of abuse.[35] Children may be unwanted from the financial or psychological perspective of the parents. Some abused children have characteristics which evoke negative associational responses in the abusing parent. The child may remind the parent by his looks, time of birth, or mannerisms of a time of crisis, a poor relationship, or a personal shortcoming in the parent's own life.

Abuse of adolescents and youth is being reported more frequently in some communities.[31] They may provoke adults into assaulting them ("conflict of values") or the abuse may represent an extension of the phenomenon of the abuse of infants and small children.[5]

THE CRISIS

It is generally conceded that many, but not all cases of physical abuse or repetitive abuse of children arise out of a single or multiple series of crises within a family. Sometimes the crises are seemingly minor, but to the parent who is experiencing loneliness and other emotional difficulties, any additional stress may be perceived as overwhelming and therefore a crisis.

Although abuse has been reported in all socioeconomic and educational groups, most abuse reported comes from the lower socioeconomic groups. Being poor does create extra stresses or crisis situations within families. Also, the poor are more vulnerable to reporting public institutions. Crisis situations are not basic etiological factors but rather precipitating ones.[26]

Neglected children have been subjected to acts of omission rather than commission.[34] Legal and operational definitions are therefore less specific and there is no widely accepted typology of the dynamics. Much of the literature on neglect deals with lower income families and concentrates on physical neglect to the exclusion of the important but elusive aspect of emotional neglect.

The patterns of neglect described by Polansky[34] emphasize economic stress, situational stress (e.g., one-parent family, marital problems, isolation), the "cycle of neglect," breakdown of the nuclear family, parental pathology (e.g., depression), and alcohol and drug use. The neglected child is often described as immature, behaving at a younger age level, being overly dependent and unable to carry out age-specific responsibilities, lacking inner controls and having poor or distorted judgement. As in situations of abuse, the parent's needs take priority over the child's.

THE PHYSICAL FINDINGS OF ABUSE AND NEGLECT

In the general physical examination of the abused or neglected child, the physician may discover a wide range of findings. There may be general signs of neglect manifested by poor skin hygiene or malnutrition ("failure to thrive"). The child may show aggressive or withdrawal tendencies, irritability, or repression of personality. Bruises, burns, abrasions, or old healed lesions may be present on examination of the skin. Old fractures or dislocations are suspected if the extremities are malformed. Intentional administration of drugs to children is a subtle form of abuse which is often very difficult to detect unless one has taken a thorough history and examination for drugs.[36]

School personnel cannot undress and examine the child in the same fashion as the physician, thus the suspicion of neglect and abuse must be based upon the observation by the teacher and other personnel regarding the child's behavior and external appearance. On occasion the child may volunteer information regarding abuse or neglect and if the observation of the child tends to substantiate the information given, this should meet the criteria of "suspected" abuse.

Physical observations important to school personnel include:

Skin. General signs of poor skin hygiene, other than cleanliness, include recurrent infections of the skin and bruises. Sussman[37] has characterized the skin lesions in child abuse so that one may distinguish them from other skin conditions. The ecchymosis or hematomas (bruises) are more often concentrated in clusters on the trunk and buttocks and to a lesser extent on the head and upper portions of the extremities. The lesions are morphologically similar to the implements used to inflict trauma, e.g., the hand, belt buckle, strap, coat hanger, etc. The bleeding into the skin is purpuric (bruises) and almost never petechial (pinpoint), which may represent systemic disease. The presence of old and new bruises at the same time suggests repeated injury. Hamlin has described a case of subgaleal hemorrhage (bleeding under the scalp) from hair-pulling as well as widespread and localized alopecia (absence of hair).[38]

Burns are fairly common and include cigarette burns to the skin used in physical discipline and immersing a child's extremities or buttocks into boiling or extremely hot water. Bruises to the face, mouth, and dental injury are common in some articles about abuse.[39,40]

Neurological manifestations. Early studies relating to child abuse showed that one-third of the children who survived child battering would be left with mental retardation. The major cause of death in all cases reported is due to brain injury. It is apparent from the nature of the forces applied to children's heads that they can be left with a variety of residual neurological signs.[41] The complex of forceful vomiting, irritability, excessive drowsiness and bruises about the head are serious signs and need immediate referral.

Children in school with neurological symptoms such as mental retardation and coordination problems may have had their problems begin in early infancy. Recent studies indicate these relationships.[42,43] Dr. Caffey has made a good case that shaking may be a common and often disregarded form of violence in child abuse.[42,43] X-ray changes seem to support traumatic factors in many cases of child abuse and due to rough handling of the infant's arms and legs such as by grabbing, wringing, and jerking motions. This also predisposes the child to whiplash-shaking injuries of the head. It is important to realize that all of these injuries can occur in the absence of visible bruises of the arms and legs.

The school's role is to help in the identification of children with neurological deficits and refer them for more complete evaluation. Abuse is obviously only one dimension of neurological problems and thus labeling or statements regarding abuse should be assiduously avoided.

Gastrointestinal manifestations. Children may be kicked or hit in the abdomen causing crushing or rupture of bowels against the vertebral bodies. A blow or kick may also rupture the liver or spleen. The cases are rare in the school age child, but a 6-year-old child did die of a ruptured liver after attending school that same day as the result of abuse.

The school nurse is an important resource to consult with on "suspected cases." The availability of a physician to discuss cases with would also be desirable. The evaluation of x-rays, blood studies and other studies to determine the nature of injuries in many cases needs to be made by the physician. X-rays in particular may be the only tool to ascertain the extent and seriousness of abuse.[44]

CONSEQUENCES OF ABUSE AND NEGLECT

Data is beginning to emerge which suggests an extremely high correlation between delinquency and prior neglect and abuse. In a 1972 study of youth in a county detention facility in Colorado by Hopkins and Steele, 80% of 100 youths interviewed said they had been abused as youngsters. This was corroborated by at least one parent of each child.[45]

Preliminary results of study by the State Assembly Select Committee on Child Abuse in New York indicate correlation between childhood abuse and later delinquency.[46] Of 5000 children who were reported as abused and/or neglected in 1952 to 1953, 35% to 40% were subsequently involved in family court as being delinquent or ungovernable. Family Court in New York is a legal resort for only "severe" cases. A related study analyzed data concerning 2000 youth who were reported as delinquent or ungovernable in 1971. In both studies it was found that approximately 60% of the families of these youth had at least one child adjudicated delinquent or ungovernable in juvenile court.

SUGGESTED GUIDELINES IN HELPING TO PROTECT ABUSED AND NEGLECTED CHILDREN AND YOUTH

Of all service-providing agencies and organizations, schools are in the best position to take the initial steps to protect abused and neglected children and youth. It is school personnel who see children and young people, observe their appearance and behavior, and interact with them daily. It is they who are able to identify the signs of neglect or "suspected" abuse and initiate the intervention of protective and therapeutic services.[27] Working in cooperation with other agencies, school personnel can sometimes provide support and understanding to the parents as well as to the children.

The guidelines which follow are intended to increase the capacity of school personnel to help protect abused and neglected children and youth. The guidelines are presented in two areas:
1. Gaining more understanding of the phenomena of abuse and neglect, of the importance of reporting, and of treatment; and
2. Developing a school policy including procedures for reporting abuse and neglect of school age children and youth to appropriate agencies and working with these agencies in a team approach to treatment and prevention.

Understanding abuse and neglect

The best method to increase the capacity of school personnel to understand and cope with abuse and neglect is to make training available at least once a year in the first month of school to all personnel. Training should cover identification, reporting, dynamics, medical evidence, implications for physical, mental and psychological development, treatment and follow-up, legal issues (including rights of children and youth), and the role of the schools. Experts including local service delivery personnel should be utilized.

It is also important to deal with the reluctance most people feel about reporting suspected abuse or neglect. Frequent reasons include:

1. The fear of having to deal with irate or hostile parents.[47,48] This is a realistic fear in some cases and the procedure of reporting should consider protection for the reporting party. This may be handled by the option of anonymity.
2. The uncertainty about whether the situation involves abuse or neglect, and, concurrently, the hope that, if ignored, the situation won't arise again.[48]
3. Not understanding or misunderstanding what will happen after the report is made. For instance, being unfamiliar with the difference between civil and criminal jurisdictions in abuse and neglect and unaware of treatment modalities.
4. Poor relationship and/or experience with the county welfare agency (protective services), the police, and/or the court.[48]
5. No assurance of support within the school system.
6. Fear of legal involvement, e.g., having to spend time in court and being subject to cross-examination. Being unaware of immunity from liability.[47]
7. Seeing the child or young person as unruly and in need of the punishment he has received. (Per-

haps similar treatment is practiced in the school itself.).[47,50,51,52]

Understanding the dynamics of abuse and neglect, medical, legal and therapeutic interventions, and developing a school policy of support and method for reporting should help to alleviate the hesitancy to report suspected abuse and neglect.[53]

If cases of neglect or abuse go to court, it is usually to civil court (family court). Cases go to criminal court usually only in instances where death or disability has occurred.

Most state laws also provide for immunity from liability for the person who reports a suspected case of child abuse and neglect as long as he or she is acting "in good faith."

Developing school policy and procedure

The school board of each district should have a policy and program regarding child abuse and neglect. Policy should include responsibilities and legal immunity of school personnel, specific guarantees to employees in case of harassment or abuse from parents,[48] and, as part of the overall purpose to protect as well as educate pupils, the commitment to provide a physically and emotionally secure environment.

The program should include training for all personnel in procedures for reporting and follow-up. As an example, the Montgomery County School Board (Maryland) has implemented a comprehensive policy and training program called PROJECT PROTECT.[54] Training reaches every level of school personnel, School public service staff, i.e., psychologists, social workers, public personnel workers and counselors, attend a 2-day workshop which prepares them to conduct training in individual schools. In this way, the people who interact daily with pupils receive training.

Many county welfare and police departments have developed standard reporting procedures and forms. If this has not happened, a reporting procedure should be worked out between the school district and the county welfare agency which will evaluate the case and provide or arrange for therapeutic and medical treatment. In cases of *physical abuse* state law often requires a report to be made orally and immediately to the county welfare agency and/or police and followed "as soon as possible thereafter" by a written report. It is important to be sure what is required in the report. The law probably requires identifying information, a description of

the nature and extent of the injury, the time and place you became aware of it, and what, it anything, the reporting party knows about the cause of the injury and when it occurred. "Nature and extent" is essentially an issue of medical evidence; however, a lay description can be crucial, especially if a medical examination or assessment has not been made prior to the report. The reporting party may not be required to identify the alleged perpetrator of the suspected abuse.

Reporting is best kept simple. It should include the child's name and address, his parent or guardian's name(s) and address(es), his date of birth, teacher and grade level, the date of the report, the name, title and telephone number of the person making the report, a description of the injury and/or condition of the child, and the basis for the belief that the injury or condition was nonaccidental or the result of negligence.[49]

A policy regarding the parents or guardians should be made and should involve them *prior* to the report being made to the county welfare agency. Although this often leads to confrontation with an angry parent, it is helpful to resolving the problem of abuse or neglect in the long run. It lets the parents know that the school is actively interested in the child's well-being and that the school is not acting without the parents' knowledge (due process).

The school's policy should also include a commitment to remain involved in whatever ways are determined in cooperation with the county welfare agency and other agencies to be in the best interest of the child or youth. The school can provide important follow-up by reporting long absences or subsequent suspected abuse or neglect. If abuse or neglect is confirmed and the family is receiving treatment, the child's teacher(s) and counselor can help to structure his school experience to complement the therapeutic intervention process. The school can be a source of support and a secure environment for children and adolescents who have been abused or neglected. The school can offer continuity of concern and involvement to parents as well.

The policy should also designate a coordinator within the school who will make reports to the county welfare agency. However, it should be clear that any personnel may make a report if abuse or neglect is suspected and if the administrator or coordinator refuses to file a report.[27,43]

The process of identification and reporting is

an important part of the intervention. The following is a suggested model:

1. Talk to the child or youth. Whoever has the best rapport with the child or young person (a teacher, coach, counselor) should talk to her/him. Most children and many youth are afraid of further abuse. Younger children in particular often believe the abuse or neglect was warranted by their misbehavior. Many want to protect their parents. Do not base your judgment solely on what the child says.[27] Look for nonverbal cues as well as other behavior and appearance. If you still suspect abuse or neglect after talking to him, explain what will happen; that is, his parents will be contacted, he will be examined by a physician, a report will be made to the county welfare agency, and a caseworker will talk to him and to his parents. Explain the reasons. Emphasize the fact that you do not wish to accuse or punish anyone, but to help insure that if it has occurred, the abuse or neglect does not continue. Talk to the child or young person about his ambivalence in discussing his situation and his fears of recurrence, encourage him to express his thoughts and feelings, and support him.
2. Report the situation to whomever has been designated as coordinator in the school system.
3. The coordinator should then call the parents and tell them of the school's concern regarding the situation. Tell the parents you will call the county welfare agency as required by law. Explain the procedure to them (i.e., a caseworker from the county welfare agency will call them).
4. Call the county welfare agency, having as much of the information on the form as possible. Let the county welfare agency know the reaction of the child's parents, and that you would like to know the results of their findings and the school's readiness to be involved in *follow-up* if necessary.
5. Obtain medical attention for the child or youth if needed. The method will depend on your school's policy regarding parental consent in obtaining medical examination and treatment. In addition, you will want to work out a policy with the county welfare agency regarding the place and time of medical intervention, taking into account the severity of the injury.

SUMMARY

We have attempted to define the spectrum of maltreatment of children seen in our current society. The potential for abuse in the child's caretaker, a child who is somewhat *different,* and a stressful situation are ingredients which often interact to produce maltreatment. The maltreatment rendered to the child includes many mechanisms ranging from direct blows from a variety of objects, to violently shaking the child, to neglect. The spectrum of the pathological findings is as varied as the means to inflict the trauma or neglect and involves every organ system. The predominate pathology of abuse is located in the central nervous system, bones and cutaneous tissues.

The school's role primarily involves awareness of the problem of maltreatment, a method of approach to identify and report "suspected" cases, and the documentation of the injuries or neglect which have been observed. The school plays an important role in the follow-up of individual cases in providing a supporting environment for the child and coordinating with other agencies dealing with the family.

The school personnel and all professionals must work together if adequate services are to be provided to protect children and rehabilitate families.

REFERENCES

1. Gil D: Statement before The Senate Subcommittee on Children and Youth, Hearings for the Child Abuse Prevention Act, 1973. US Gov't Printing Office, 1973, pp 13-21.
2. Radbill SX: A history of child abuse and infanticide, in Steinmetz S, Strauss M(eds): *Violence in the Family.* New York, Dodd, Mead & Co. 1973.
3. Bakan D.: *Slaughter of the Innocents: A Study of the Battered Child Phenomenon.* Boston, Beacon Press, 1972.
4. Solomon T: History and demography of child abuse. *Pediatr* 51(pt 2):773-776, 1973.
5. DeMause L: Our forebears made childhood a nightmare. *Psychol Today* 85-88, 1975.
6. Radbill SX: A history of child abuse and infanticide, in Helfer RE, Kempe CH(eds): *The Battered Child.* Chicago, The University of Chicago Press, 1968.
7. Fontana VJ: *The Maltreated Child: The Maltreatment Syndrome in Children,* ed 2, Springfield, Thomas, 1971.
8. Caffey J: Multiple fractures in the long bones of infants suffering from chronic subdural hematoma. *Am J Roentgenol Radium Ther Nucl Med* 56:163-167, 1946.
9. Silverman FN: The roentgen manifestations of unrecognized skeletal trauma in infants. *Am J Roentgenol Radium Ther Nucl Med* 69:413-427, 1953.
10. Woolley PV Jr, Evans WA Jr: Significance of skeletal lesions in infants resembling those of traumatic origin. *JAMA* 158:539-543, 1955.
11. Kempe CH: The battered child syndrome. *JAMA* 181: 105-112, 1962.
12. Fontana VJ: The diagnosis of the maltreatment syndrome in children. *Pediatr* (Supplement): Symposium on Child Abuse 51(pt 2):781-792, 1973.
13. DeFrancis V, Lucht C: *Child Abuse Legislation in the 1970's.* rev ed. Denver. The American Humane Association Children's Division, 1974.
14. Koel BS: Failure to thrive and fatal injury as a continuum. *Am J Dis Child.* 118:565-567, 1969.
15. Pemberton DA, Benady DR: Consciously rejected children. *J Psychiat* 123:575-578, 1973.

16. *Guidelines for Schools*. Denver, The American Humane Association Children's Division, 1971.
17. Minnesota Statutes, Chapter 374. *Minnesota Criminal Sexual Conduct Law,* 1975.
18. DeFrancis V: *Protecting the Child Victim of Sex Crimes Committed by Adults*. Denver. The American Humane Association Children's Division, 1969.
19. Sgori S: Sexual molestation of children: The last frontier in child abuse. *Child Today* 19-20, 1975.
20. Bronfenbrenner U: A look at the disintegrating world of childhood. *Psychol Today* 9:32, 1975.
21. Gil DG: *Violence Against Children*. Cambridge, Harvard University Press, 1970.
22. Drews K: The child and his school. *Helping the Battered Child and His Family*. Philadelphia, Lippincott, 1972, chap 8.
23. Nagi S: Child abuse and neglect programs: A national overview. *Child Today* May-June 1975.
24. Congressional Record-Proceedings and Debates of the 93rd Congress. First Session (Senate), USA 119(39): S4444, pp 1-9, Washington (Tuesday, March 13, 1973).
25. Adelson L: The battering child. *JAMA* 222:159-161, 1972.
26. Helfer R: The etiology of child abuse. *Pediatr* (Supplement): Symposium on Child Abuse 51(pt 2):777-779, 1973.
27. Kempe CH, Helfer RE: *Helping the Battered Child and His Family*. Philadelphia, Lippincott, 1972.
28. Duncan GM, et al: Etiological factors in first-degree murder. *JAMA* 168:1755-1758, 1958.
29. Steele BF: Violence in our society. *The Pharos* 42-48, 1970.
30. Silver LB, et al: Does violence breed violence? *Am J Psychiat* 126:152-155, 1969.
31. Child Abuse Report for 1974, Hennepin County, Minnesota.
32. Brenton M: Troubled teachers whose behavior disturbs our kids. *Today's Health* 17, 1971.
33. *Our Nation's Schools—A Report Card—"A" in School Violence and Vandalism*. Preliminary Report of the Subcommittee to Investigate Juvenile Delinquency, Senator Birch Bayh, Chairman, April 1975.
34. Polansky N, et al: *Profiles of Neglect: A Survey of the State of Knowledge of Child Neglect*. US Dept of Health, Education, and Welfare, 1975.
35. Klein E, Skin L: Low birth weight and the battered child syndrome. *Am J Dis Child* 122:15-18, 1971.
36. Dine MS: Tranquilizer poisoning: An example of child abuse. *Pediatr* 36:782-785, 1965.
37. Sussman SJ: Skin manifestations of the battered-child syndrome. *J Pediatr* 72:99-101, 1968.
38. Hamlin H: Subgaleal hematoma caused by hair-pull. *JAMA* 204:339, 1968.
39. Tate RJ: Facial injuries associated with the battered child syndrome. *Br J Oral Surg* 9:41-45, 1971.
40. Cameron JM, Johnson HR, Camps FE: The battered child syndrome. *Med Sci Law* 6:2-21, 1966.
41. Baron MA: Neurological manifestation of the battered child syndrome. *Pediatr* 45:1003-1007, 1970.
42. Caffey J: On the theory and practice of shaking infants. *Am J Dis Child* 124:161-169, 1972.
43. Caffey J: The whiplash shaken infant syndrome. *Pediatr* 54:396, 1974.
44. Caffey, J: *Pediatric X-ray Diagnosis,* ed 6. Chicago, Year Book Medical Publishers Inc, 1972, pp 1132-1147.
45. Hopkins, J (personal communication).
46. Alfaro, J, Project Director, NY Select Assembly on Child Abuse (personal communication).
47. Martin DL: The growing horror of child abuse and the undeniable role of the schools in putting an end to it. *Am School Bd J* 160:11.
48. Elseroad H: reACTION. *Hearings on Child Abuse,* US Senate, pp 558-575, 1973.
49. Amiel S: Child abuse in schools. *Northwest Med,* Nov 1972.
50. Gil DG: A holistic perspective on child abuse and its prevention. *J Soc and Soc Welfare* 2:110-125, 1974.
51. Gil DG: What schools can do about child abuse. *Am Educ,* April 1969.
52. Brenton M: Troubled teachers whose behavior disturbs our kids. *Today's Health,* Nov 1971.
53. Murdock G: The abused child and the school system. *AJPH* 60:105-109, 1970.
54. Broadhurst DD: Project protect: A school program to detect and prevent child abuse and neglect. *Child Today,* May-June 1975.

Index

□ *t* indicates table.